THE ENCYCLOPEDIA *of* MEDICAL BREAKTHROUGHS & FORBIDDEN TREATMENTS

Health Secrets & Little-Known Therapies for Specific Health Conditions from A-to-Z

Revised and Expanded

MEDICAL RESEARCH ASSOCIATES, LLC
P.O. BOX 55725, SEATTLE, WA 98155, USA

THE BOOK THAT NEVER GROWS OLD

With your purchase of *The Encyclopedia of Medical Breakthroughs & Forbidden Treatments*, you receive unlimited access to the Member's Area of our website, year after year. This password-protected area contains links to information that has become available since the last printing of *The Encyclopedia*. In this way we're able to keep our readers up to date on recent medical breakthroughs and other important medical information. *The Encyclopedia*, therefore, exists as a complete work in two locations: 1) in the physical world as a soft cover book (or online as an ebook), and 2) online in the Member's Area of our website. Without consulting the information contained within both venues, you will not have accessed the complete work.

"If it's not in the book, on our website you should look."

Please Visit Our Website Regularly for Important Updates at
www.medical-breakthroughs.com. **Enter Username and Password.**

Important Member's Area access: When you purchased *The Encyclopedia*, you were asked to create your unique access to the Member's Area. In addition, following your purchase you were emailed information on how to access the Member's Area had you not done so during the purchasing process. If at any time you need to acquire or recover your Username or Password, please visit medical-breakthroughs.com/support to submit a "Support Ticket" requesting additional information/directions.

To locate a holistic/integrative medical practitioner in your area, contact the American College for Advancement in Medicine at (800)532-3688, (949)309-3520, www.acam.org, or the International College of Integrative Medicine at (866)464-5226, (419)358-0273, www.icimed.com.

To order additional copies of *The Encyclopedia of Medical Breakthroughs & Forbidden Treatments*, visit www.RealMedicalHelp.com

TABLE OF CONTENTS

A Challenge to the Reader

Dear Health Enthusiast,

Congratulations. By owning this book, you've taken the first step toward better health. With this material in hand, you now have access to a new view of health and medicine provided by the hard-to-find, little-known information about treatments, products, and services contained within these pages. This information will open a new world of health options, allowing you to prevent and treat many ailments and diseases you previously may have considered beyond your reach. In a very real way, this book holds the key to your future good health.

Although you've taken the first step, there's another step yet to take. Even though you hold the key in your hands, you must use it in order to do any good. You must insert the key and open yourself to this new information now in your possession—both for your own benefit as well as that of your friends and relatives. Who among us doesn't have personal health challenges? Who doesn't have friends or relatives with health issues that need to be resolved—be it arthritis, asthma, cancer, heart disease, heartburn, osteoporosis, or the rest of the long list of health challenges that follow modern man throughout life's long journey?

If you accept the challenge of accessing the material contained within these pages, you will command more knowledge of new ways of resolving your health issues than is known by many in the healing professions. By reading and understanding this information, you will open the possibility of being no less than a hero amongst your family members and your circle of friends. Such is the power of information. But you must take the time and make the effort to read and understand the contents of this book. Whether you use it as a reference or read the book from cover to cover, you must make the effort in order to gain the benefits.

How would you answer if someone asked you the following question: "What's the most important thing in your life?" Would you say... money, fame & fortune, relationships such as a spouse, family or friends? Whatever your answer, there's one thing that's high on most peoples' list: good health and longevity—a long, healthy life. It's really your continued good health that forms the foundation for all of the other good things that may come your way in life—friends, family, a good job, money, notoriety, and so forth. In fact, you've probably heard it said many times that without your good health, all the money in the world would be useless! Good health is indeed priceless, and all other things in life pale in comparison without its robust presence. It is indeed your most important asset.

As we age, good health is progressively more difficult to maintain. But this understanding isn't new to modern man. For as long as there has been a recorded history, man has searched for ways of living a longer, more healthful life. This perpetual quest for long-lived youth has been referred to variously as the "elixir of life," the "universal panacea," the "philosopher's stone," and the "fountain of youth." From historical times to present, this never-ending search has been of the highest importance to people—even as today's fast-paced Western society pushes it to the background, making the trivial seem important while often obscuring the most important thing—our long-lived good health.

So then, will you accept the challenge? Will you take the next step? Are you prepared to learn valuable new information about your most important asset and put it to good use? You hold the key. Though a long journey begins with one small, first step, the destination is gained only through effort and perseverance. In this case, the destination is your good health and longevity. The life you influence for the better will be your own, or that of a loved one.

USING AND PURCHASING DIETARY SUPPLEMENTS

During the last 100 years or so—and especially in the last 50—the American (Western) diet has changed so radically that virtually no one younger than an octogenarian can remember what the human diet consisted of prior to the advent of modern foods of convenience. The process of eating has remained unchanged. The substances still enter through the orifice directly below the nose; it is chewed; then swallowed. The nature of the food stuffs, however, has changed radically. So much has it changed that those substances presently masquerading as foods no longer maintain human life at an optimal level—not even at an advantageous level; not even at an acceptable level; not even at a level sufficient to maintain the body in a state free from illness and disease. This is a remarkable circumstance given the fact that we depend upon these vital substances for our very existence.

The radical changes in our society over the span of the last 100 years have not come without other significant, detrimental consequences. If it weren't for these consequences, the endless variety of our modern, high-tech wonders would be a joy, as most currently believe them to be. Little do we realize the toxicity associated with most of our high-tech accoutrements is killing us—and making us crazy—even if slowly. For many in the Western world, the connection between our toxic environment and disease, both physical and mental, is not readily apparent. Even those who understand this insidious connection cannot escape our polluted fish bowl Earth.

Over the last 50 years or so, many health conditions of relatively non-obvious origins have skyrocketed, including allergies; asthma; attention deficit and hyperactivity disorder (ADD & ADHD); autism; birth defects (3-5% of U.S. babies are born with birth defects); chronic fatigue syndrome; fibromyalgia; infertility (5-10% of American couples are infertile); insomnia; migraines; neuropathies; miscarriage; and more.

Even more disconcerting is the rise in the more serious conditions of heart disease and cancer, America's number one and number two killers of humans, respectively. In 1900, heart disease accounted for 8% of all deaths in the U.S., and cancer about 3.5%. Since 1900, the number of cases of heart disease has increased some 400%, and the number of cases of cancer by over 700%. Mathematically speaking, for a person living in the United States there is a 75% probability for men and more than a 50% probability for women of being afflicted either with heart disease,

cancer or both. These are unacceptable odds, even for a confirmed gambler.

Part of the solution to these types of health challenges of our modern world is the use of dietary (nutritional) supplements. These are a vast array of various compounds and substances—vitamins, minerals, amino acids, enzymes, essential fatty acids, herbs, plant extracts, etc.—typically purchased in health food stores. An example of the importance of these substances is the recent discoveries of the many benefits of supplementing with vitamin D, including the prevention of at least 17 different types of cancers.

Throughout the book you'll be presented with descriptions of a wide range of supplements that have been shown effective in treating a host of illnesses and diseases. The proof of their effectiveness is documented in the scientific research literature which is noted in the product descriptions—even though by law, this information can't be disclosed by the companies marketing these products. In the United States, only pharmaceutical companies are allowed to make claims relating to the treatment and cure of diseases by their (patented) prescription medications.

Our discussion of dietary supplements generally focuses on individual ingredients, e.g., vitamin C, vitamin D, ginkgo, lipoic acid, green tea extract, etc. At the end of the discussion, dosages are suggested. Keep in mind that combination formulations are sometimes available, i.e., products containing multiple ingredients. When combination formulations are available, they're less expensive than purchasing multiple single ingredients. The only caution is that combination formulas often do not contain optimal amounts of the individual ingredients. You can be guided by our dosage recommendations for individual ingredients.

Also important in protecting our good health in these challenging times are what can rightly be termed "superfoods," such as stabilized rice bran, salba (chia), and various algae including spirulina and chlorella. (See the Index). "Super extracts" such as resveratrol and Seanol® have recently become available, each providing a multitude of health benefits.

In Appendix A, you will find a listing of several online companies that market dietary supplements at a significant discount—usually 30-50% or more below retail. Whenever we discuss a particular supplement, even though we may give the contact information of the manufacturer, please keep in mind that product can be ordered online from one or more of the companies listed in Appendix A, as well as a host of additional online companies not mentioned.

THE BOOK THAT NEVER GROWS OLD

With your purchase of *The Encyclopedia of Medical Breakthroughs & Forbidden Treatments*, you receive unlimited access to the Member's Area of our website, year after year. This password-protected area contains links to information that has become available since the last printing of *The Encyclopedia*. In this way we're able to keep our readers up to date on recent medical breakthroughs and other important medical information. *The Encyclopedia*, therefore, exists as a complete work in two locations: 1) in the physical world as a soft cover book (or online as an ebook), and 2) online in the Member's Area of our website. Without consulting the information contained within both venues, you will not have accessed the complete work.

"If it's not in the book, on our website you should look."

Please Visit Our Website Regularly for Important Updates at www.medical-breakthroughs.com. Enter Username and Password.

Important Member's Area access: When you purchased *The Encyclopedia*, you were asked to create your unique access to the Member's Area. In addition, following your purchase you were emailed information on how to access the Member's Area had you not done so during the purchasing process. If at any time you need to acquire or recover your Username or Password, please visit medical-breakthroughs.com/support to submit a "Support Ticket" requesting additional information/directions.

To locate a holistic/integrative medical practitioner in your area, contact the American College for Advancement in Medicine at (800)532-3688, (949)309-3520, www.acam.org, or the International College of Integrative Medicine at (866)464-5226, (419)358-0273, www.icimed.com.

To order additional copies of *The Encyclopedia of Medical Breakthroughs & Forbidden Treatments*, visit www.RealMedicalHelp.com

Part One:
The Background

Preface

*T*he *Encyclopedia of Medical Breakthroughs and Forbidden Treatments* contains a wealth of information on a wide diversity of topics—much of which will be new to many readers. By bringing this new information to your attention, we point the way so that you will be able to continue your exploration and experimentation on your own, or with the assistance of your physician or other medical professional(s). Due to length limitations, however, the subjects covered in this book by no means exhaust the full knowledge and understanding of the topics discussed, nor is it suggested they are fully inclusive of all medical information that may be relevant.

To a considerable extent, but not exclusively, our approach to healing and the medical arts involves holistic/alternative/integrative, more natural approaches rather than the application of traditional Western medicine (allopathy) which relies heavily on surgical procedures and the use of pharmaceutical drugs. This more natural field of medicine is referred to as the field of Complementary & Alternative Medicine (CAM).

In many other cultures, the core understandings of medicine and healing center around the use of treatment techniques that are less invasive and accompanied by far fewer adverse reactions (side-effects) in comparison to many of the Western methods. The same or better results are usually achieved with CAM, but without the consequences that may accompany the practice of often unnecessary surgery and the use of side-effect-producing pharmaceutical drugs. We believe this approach represents the medicine of the future, as it was to a considerable extent in the past—before big money and big business became involved in the healing arts.

For example, traditional Chinese medicine (TCM) is an art dating back thousands of years into antiquity. TCM relies heavily on the use of herbs and herbal formulations, diet, exercise, and massage. It also incorporates the use of acupuncture, a medical technique relatively recently introduced to Western medicine—and scoffed at for years by traditional Western physicians. Ayurveda, another complementary treatment modality, is the ancient Hindu system of healing dating to the first century A.D., and centers around the use of herbs, oils, purgatives, and other natural forms of healing. Scores of additional non-invasive, side-effect-free "alternative" treatment modalities are also readily available.

Even in the U.S. prior to 1900, the American physicians' mainstay treatment was homeopathy—practiced by America's best and brightest physicians—a very effective form of medicine against which massive publicity was directed in order to discredit its effectiveness. These campaigns to discredit were launched just prior to the formation of the American Medical Association, which functioned then and still functions to this day in support of large financial conglomerates with the specific intention of promoting pharmaceutical drugs and expensive medical procedures including surgery. Most Americans are unfamiliar with the origins of contemporary Western medicine and the facts behind the formation of organizations such as the English Society of Apothecaries, the British Medical Association and the American Medical Association. Nevertheless, for those who care to explore these matters at greater length, these organizations have a well-documented, deep and sordid history including clandestine and less-than-admirable intentions, as you shall see.

It is neither our desire nor intention to belabor the issues surrounding the questionable policies and practices of the current Western medical establishment—some of the results of which bring much suffering and hardship into the lives of many. On the other hand, in addition to informing our readers of tried-and-true "complementary" techniques of healing—the main focus of this writing—we feel obligated at least to touch upon some of the main highlights of what, in our opinion, are questionable medical treatment modalities which are currently offered to the public, the harmful effects of which have been thoroughly documented for all who care to spend the time and energy in pursuit of the details. Without informing you about what you or your loved ones currently might be doing that is medically detrimental to your health—or what you unknowingly might do in the future as the result of your lack of knowledge and understanding concerning the various medical choices available to you—we would be obscuring a significant part of the story as well as denying our responsibility to you by not waiving a red flag of caution.

At the same time we must be careful not to paint the story with such a broad brush as to indict all of Western medicine, and the thousands upon thousands of innocent, well-meaning people employed within the health and medical community. Many to most of those so employed are largely unaware of the width and breadth of the entire story, and the harm that is brought to the population at large as the result of the misguided policies and practices of a few. It is the Directors and those who guide the course and set the policies of both the companies that provide medical care and related products and services, as well as the institutions that continue to allow them to function unimpeded, who deserve the blame.

Also sharing the responsibility are all those who may have come to a personal understanding of the reality of these unfortunate situations and circumstances and have done nothing to correct them, be they employees in the medical profession, physicians, news reporters, researchers such as the

writers of the present document, or the like. Many pressures come to bear which may subtly and not-so-subtly prevent people from speaking out and acting in line with their consciences. Fear is a strong motivating factor which helps maintain the silence. Fear of losing one's job is so strong it can be overcome only by the most courageous. For most, going with the flow is the most comfortable path of least resistance. We go along to get along. "In a time of universal deceit," spoke George Orwell, "telling the truth is a revolutionary act."

The story is simple if not alarming. In search of gigantic profits the large pharmaceutical companies have lost their hearts in favor of financial profit margins. If they ever were, they are no longer in touch with the real needs of real people. These companies, in cooperation with government bureaucracies, allow many prescription pharmaceutical drugs to remain on the market even though both the manufacturers of the drugs and the government agencies know very well that some of these drugs are the direct cause of thousands of deaths annually.

In 2008, U.S. physicians wrote 3.84 billion prescriptions for pharmaceutical drugs.[1] This is prescription writing at the rate of one each month for every person residing in the United States. With Americans spending over $290 billion per year on prescription pharmaceutical drugs, we can see there's a very powerful impetus on the part of the pharmaceutical companies to maintain this foothold in the bleeding pocketbooks of Americans, as well as the rest of the world.

Unfortunately, it's not only our pocketbooks that are bleeding. In the May 2002 issue of the *Journal of the American Medical Association*, Dr. Karen Lasser and colleagues from Harvard Medical School reported their analysis of 548 drugs approved from 1975 through 1999. Fifty-six of these drugs—slightly more than 10%—were later given serious side-effects warnings, or removed altogether from the market for safety reasons. When the researchers focused on the drugs that were approved toward the end of the study, the number grew to 20%.[2]

Dr. Lasser and her fellow researchers concluded that most of the troublesome new drugs don't represent any advance in treatment capability and are at best no better than the older, safer drugs already on the market.[3] If this is indeed the case, what would motivate the pharmaceutical companies to develop these new, potentially unsafe and life-threatening drugs when they already had developed better, safer products? The answer, we believe, is as crystal clear as the "ka-ching" coming from the cash register. Prescription drugs have a 20-year patent lifetime. After that, other companies are permitted to sell these previously patent-protected drugs. In order to maintain a monopoly in the marketplace, new patentable drugs must be created. An example of this is the recent switch from the USD $6 billion per year purple progenitor Prilosec®—whose patent had run its course—to its newly-patented purple replacement, Nexium.® Prilosec is now doing double duty in its second incarnation as an over-the-counter product.

The general idea behind most pharmaceutical drugs has been the discovery of *un*patentable, natural plant substances which are effective in treating specific ailments, and then to slightly alter the molecular structure of these substances so that patent protection can be obtained. By so doing, invariably the new, "molecularly-modified/me too" substances are fraught with side-effects ranging from bothersome to life threatening to lethal. In our opinion, this simply is not an acceptable approach to pharmacy and medicine. There are exceptions, of course, the opiate pain medications and properly-administered antibiotics being two specific areas that generally benefit humanity. Even with the potentially life-saving antibiotics, however, we have witnessed the creation of antibiotic-resistant superbugs that have come back to haunt us. Only the future will reveal the ultimate result of this pharmaceutical approach to infectious diseases.

As reported in the July 2000 issue of the *Journal of the American Medical Association*,[4] Dr. Barbara Starfield of the Johns Hopkins School of Hygiene and Public Health confirmed that every year in the United States more than 100,000 hospital deaths occur as the result of adverse reactions to prescription pharmaceutical drugs that are prescribed by physicians in accordance with the directions given by the pharmaceutical companies who manufacture them. These deaths are called Drug Adverse Events. (If hospitals were war zones, they would be termed "collateral damage.") They do not include data from other medical settings such as doctors' offices or outpatient deaths. Additionally, these numbers are only for deaths and do not reflect negative effects associated with non-lethal adverse reactions but are nevertheless associated with disability and/or pain and discomfort.

In addition to the 100,000 annual hospital deaths caused by correctly-prescribed pharmaceutical drugs, an additional 125,000 deaths occur in the U.S. each year as the result of incorrectly-prescribed prescription drugs. To put this into perspective, these numbers are equivalent to a World Trade Center disaster every week for a year-and-a-half.

In Europe, Drug Adverse Events are kept secret by the national governments. In October 2008, however, a team of Danish and Dutch journalists used freedom of information legislation in Denmark and Holland to obtain secret pharmaceutical company documents revealing that pharmaceutical drugs are the fifth most common cause of death in European hospitals.[5]

It has been recognized that the majority of injuries and deaths caused by prescription drugs go unreported or under reported. When drug-related statistics are published, it is often stated that the numbers quoted are gross underestimates compared to what is likely to be the true incidence.

The following example gives an indication of how blatant and deep-seated the pharmaceutical problem is. In 1999 in a Federal Court in Dallas, Texas, Attorney General Janet Reno of the U.S. Department of Justice prosecuted the world's two largest vitamin (pharmaceutical) manufacturers for conspiring to fix the world-wide prices of vitamins. Every year for a decade, top executives of the world's largest pharmaceutical companies would meet clandestinely in various posh settings to establish production quotas, prices and distribution channels for vitamin ingredients used in a diversity of ways—from ingredients used to enrich foods (bread, butter, cereals, meats, milk, orange juice, etc.) to vitamin pills. The global markets of various vitamins such as A, B_2, B_5, C, E and beta carotene would be divided among the companies to the level of one half of one percent.[6]

Hoffman-LaRoche Ltd., a Swiss company having a 40% world-wide share of the vitamin market, pleaded guilty to violating the Sherman Antitrust Act and agreed to pay a penalty of USD $500 million. The company stated they expected substantial further fines in Europe and Canada. A second company, the German firm BASF A.G., which commands 20% of the international vitamin market, agreed to pay a fine of USD $225 million for their participation in the "conspiracy." (Reno's word, not ours.) Dozens of lesser companies were also investigated.

The third largest company in the cartel, the French conglomerate Rhône-Poulenc, agreed to testify against Roche and BASF in order to receive amnesty from prosecution. Good-hearted as this may seem, it was not a pang of conscience that convinced Rhône-Poulenc to drop a dime on their co-conspirators. Rhône had a pending $22 billion merger with Hoechst A.G. which could not be completed without the approval of antitrust officials in both the U.S. and Europe.[7] (BASF and Hoechst were part of the I.G. Farben breakup following the Nurenberg Trials of WWII. For those who would like to know more about the astonishing I.G. conglomerate, do an online search for "ig farben.")

Following the antitrust trial in Dallas, Hoffman-LaRoche's CEO Franz B. Humer stated, "I'm personally, absolutely shocked at what has happened." But then, so were we as kids when we got caught with our fingers in the cookie jar.

All of this is particularly puzzling, especially in light of the recent admission of Dr. Allen Roses, worldwide Vice President of Genetics at Glaxo-SmithKline, the fourth largest pharmaceutical company in the world, and Britain's largest pharmaceutical firm. Dr. Roses made a most astounding admission—one that has been an open secret within the pharmaceutical industry but never before publicly voiced by such a senior drug boss. Speaking at a scientific meeting in late 2003, Dr. Roses admitted most pharmaceutical drugs are ineffective for most of the people who take them. He stated that "The vast majority of drugs—more than 90%—only work in 30-50% of the people. I wouldn't say that most drugs don't work. I would say that most drugs work in 30-50% of people."[8] Some industry analysts commented that Dr. Roses' statements were reminiscent of a 1991 gaffe by Gerald Ratner, a British jewelry store magnate who famously said that his high street shops are successful because they sell "total crap."

Having a formidable reputation in the field of pharmacogenetics, Dr. Roses explained that most drugs are effective in fewer than one in two patients primarily because persons taking the drugs carry a genetic makeup that in some way interferes with the drugs' effectiveness. He cited statistics on the effectiveness of different classes of drugs, as follows: Alzheimer's: 30% effective; Asthma: 60%; Cancer: 25%; Depression: 62%; Diabetes: 57%; Hepatitis C: 47%; Incontinence: 40%; Migraine: 52%; Rheumatoid arthritis: 50%; Schizophrenia: 60%.[9] The French philosopher Voltaire summed up the issue over two hundred years ago when he stated, "Doctors give drugs of which they know little, into bodies of which they know less, for diseases of which they know nothing at all."

In addition to the foregoing, the following statistics offer undeniable evidence that conventional Western medicine has failed to fulfill the medical needs of the American public: The number of unnecessary medical and surgical procedures performed annually in the U.S. is 7.5 million.[10] The number of people exposed to unnecessary hospitalization annually is 8.9 million.[11] These two figures combined indicate that every day 45,000 Americans are being unnecessarily hospitalized or subjected to unnecessary surgery. Additionally, the total number of U.S. deaths caused by medical errors of all types ranges from 800,000 to one million every year.[12] This figure represents at least six jumbo-jet crashes every day for an entire year. Further, the cumulative 10 year estimate of deaths from all types of medical errors is more than eight million Americans, which is almost three times more human lives than all the deaths from all the wars that America has fought in its entire history.[13]

Medical bills are the leading cause of bankruptcy in the U.S. despite the fact that more than 75% of those declaring bankruptcy had health insurance at the start of their illness.[14] Currently, 16¢ out of every U.S. dollar is spent on healthcare.[15] Even though healthcare spending is 350% higher than America's 2009 Department of Defense budget,[16] at least 44,000 adults die each year due to lack of health insurance.[17] The uninsured have a 40% higher risk of death than those with private insurance.[18]

Of the roughly 200 countries assessed, the U.S. ranks #1 in healthcare spending,[19] #50 in life expectancy,[20] and #37 in the overall healthcare system performance.[21] The odds of being killed in the

U.S. by conventional medicine are almost 20 times (2,000%) greater than being killed in an automobile accident[22] and almost 30 times (3,000%) greater than being killed by a gun.[23] The conclusion is that the American medical system is the leading cause of death and injury in the United States.[24]

On a more positive note, there are alternatives to conventional medicine which have an excellent track record in treating a multiplicity of illnesses and diseases. In the information which follows, we tend to focus on treatment methods rather than methods of prevention. That's because we assume many readers already have medical problems for which solutions are presently being sought. Nevertheless we realize—as you should as well—that whatever medical ailments may presently plague you, they have originated for some reason—probably having to do with poor dietary habits (e.g., eating too many processed foods which contain unhealthy oils, chemical additives, etc.) and unhealthy lifestyles (e.g., little or no exercise, lack of sleep, etc.). Therefore, in order to maintain any progress you may achieve from the information contained within this work, dietary and lifestyle changes must be made. Otherwise, the underlying problem(s)—the disease-causing mechanism(s)—may still be in operation. For general prevention strategies, see **Nutrition: Detoxification and Deficiencies** under **General Treatment Methods.** Furthermore, many/most treatment methods are also effective preventives.

This book contains many potential solutions covering a diversity of ailments. We suggest that most of the time your medical disorder can be fixed or at least significantly improved. However, it should be pointed out that, generally speaking, no single remedy works for everyone, and that you may have to experiment with several prospective treatment methods before finding one or a particular combination that is personally effective. You must have the fortitude, both financial and emotional, to follow up on this. You must be consistent, persistent and patient.

One last item. We would like to explain what is meant by the term "forbidden" as used in the title of this book. Simply put, many medical researchers have noticed over the years that, for one reason or another, a larger-than-expected number of important medical discoveries/treatments do not

find their way into everyday use by the general public. It's as if these technologies have fallen silently into a medical black hole, never to be seen by the needy public. Or, more subtlty, even though some of these modalities may be made available to some extent, they have not been in the past and are not currently publicized and allowed to prosper in the open marketplace. They are either subtly or not-so-subtly ignored and/or criticized when compared to the more popular treatments currently available. Consequently, they are known only to a relatively small number of people. There are a number of reasons why this happens.

On the one hand, there are certain medical procedures/treatments/medications that are banned for use within specific countries,—i.e., they are illegal. In the U.S., for example, many drugs popular in Europe are prevented from being sold, even when they have been shown to be safe and effective by reputable monitoring agencies. Memantine (Namenda®) is one example of a drug used successfully in Germany for over 10 years in the treatment of Alzheimer's disease. It was made available to the American consumer only in 2004, after much lobbying by consumer groups who knew of the drug's benefits.

If memantine accidently slipped through the cracks and was inadvertently ignored by the medical establishment, strophanthin has suffered the same fate—but more egregiously. Brought to England in 1862, strophanthin was quickly recognized as a miraculous heart tonic. Today, its widespread use could save hundreds of thousands of lives globally each year. There is currently no other pharmaceutical preparation that fully replicates strophanthin's benefits. Nearly a century-and-a-half after its discovery, why is strophanthin readily available only to people living in Germany?

In addition to drugs, many life-saving treatment methods/technologies find their way into perpetual obscurity. It is not that these methods are replaced by superior technology as time progresses. On the contrary, many of the forgotten treatment methods are arguably some of the most effective technologies ever discovered by man. One would think such discoveries would be difficult to forget—particularly when they save lives and especially considering that no more effective technologies have replaced them.

Photoluminescence, for example, discussed under **General Treatment Methods**, is a technique developed by American physicians during the early 1900s. It uses simple light rays of a certain wavelength to treat the blood of the ailing patient. Although Photoluminescence is effective against a multiplicity of problems, one of its specialties is infection. Considering that infectious diseases are an ever-growing problem in today's world, why have the tremendous benefits of this technology been virtually ignored by the medical authorities in so many countries throughout the world including the U.S.? Although there are American physicians who practice Photoluminescence, they are under the constant eye of their local Medical Boards and often feel intimidated. If this technology were more widely known, the grip infectious diseases have over man would be significantly lessened.

Insulin potentiation therapy (IPT) is another important life-saving technique that has been virtually passed over by traditional medicine. IPT was developed by a family of three generations of Mexican physicians. It is one of the most effective, simple, and least expensive therapies for treating a host of ailments. Why are there barely more than 100 practitioners worldwide more than sixty years after the discovery of the technique? The answer will become painfully clear when you read about IPT under **General Treatment Methods**.

Before becoming a veritable poster child for alternative cancer treatment, not only was Dr. Stanislaw Burzynski's discovery of cancer-defeating *antineoplastins* forbidden, the American medical authorities tried for years to jail the doctor. Only public outcry saved the career of this courageous physician. Antineoplastins have saved countless lives and Burzynski's discovery is now available to the public, but only after many trials and tribulations for him and his loyal and respectful colleagues and patients.

Whether there is a "formal" legal ban as in the case of some pharmaceuticals, or more subtle forms of "banning" certain medical practices by not allowing them to prosper (for example, as the result of negative or even no publicity, etc.), many proven, life-saving modalities never reach the surface of public awareness. And the physicians who practice these methods often feel uneasy about offering a "non-standard" medical treatment to their patients, and in certain countries may be fearful of legal and professional recrimination for using an "unapproved" or even an "unknown" technique.

The list of "forbidden" medical treatments goes on and on, and you will discover many more as you continue to explore these pages. We believe it will become increasingly apparent that many important medical discoveries remain unknown or little known to large segments of people, even those who are interested in so-called alternative and complementary medicine.

The principal thread running through the "disappearance" of many of the little-known therapies discussed in this book is an active interest by competitors to see that their competition (or even the potential competition) does not survive. Most readers recognize this as a free-market economy in action. Under these circumstances, however, where literally millions of human lives are at risk, more conscious behavior on the part of those involved would spare much suffering and death to those in need. The fact that humans would knowingly trade lives to increase the profit margin of a company is a sad commentary on the present state of human consciousness, and a wakeup call for change.

For additional information about treatment methods discussed in this book, or to locate a medical practitioner in your area skilled in a particular treatment method, contact the American College for Advancement in Medicine at (800)532-3688, (949)309-3520, www.acam.org, or the International College of Integrative Medicine at (866)464-5226, (419)358-0273, www.icimed.com

Wishing you the best of luck in your search for a harmonious and healthful life,

—The Staff of Medical Research Associates

INTRODUCTION

The human being is an intricate organism composed of several aspects—mind, body, spirit. Some would argue only two aspects exist—mind and body. Nevertheless, when the aspects are functioning properly, all is well with the world, life is a happy event, and there is no experience of illness or perception of pain, either mental or physical. However, with age, injury, and stress, illness and pain become serious factors in our lives.

The primary object of this writing is to focus on remedies which treat the underlying causes of illness and disease. If we are able to rid ourselves of these maladies, life can be extended and lived to the fullest. Otherwise, life is shortened and accompanied by illnesses' byproduct—the experience of pain. It is because pain causes such turmoil and upheaval in peoples' lives that it is so necessary to focus on the pain-reduction aspect of illness and disease. Clearly, more attention must be given to reducing pain, and that means new treatment methods must be found that are capable of effectively resolving its underlying causes.

The incidence of illness and disease, and the accompanying pain that it causes, is significant. In a 2003 study called Pain in Europe,[1] one in five Europeans, or about 75 million people, were found to be living with pain—often agonizing, long term pain. According to the report, this has led as many as 15 million Europeans to contemplate suicide. One in five chronic pain sufferers reported they had lost their job as a result of their condition. Thirty-four percent reported their sex lives had been affected, and 73% said their pain interfered with normal sleep. Similar unfortunate statistics are found in other industrialized populations.

The human being—the pinnacle of evolution, called the Crown of Creation—must also be Earth's most sensitive sensing being. Eagles and other birds of prey can see much farther, dogs have a keener sense of smell, and most animals have a more highly-developed sense of hearing—but the human must surely be the being with the most highly-developed sense of pain perception.

No doubt a series of environmental factors plays a role in how we experience pain—i.e., to some extent we learn to hurt. There is no better example of this than Napoleon's soldiers who, during the Russian campaign of 1812, would soon return to battle on horseback after having a limb amputated.[2] This type of experience is difficult for most contemporary Westerners to comprehend. Nevertheless, for whatever reason(s), modern-day humans are the creatures that seem to experience pain more acutely in comparison to other living beings—or at least this is how most people would judge the perception of our pain in comparison to that of other animals.

This is particularly true of mental pain. Even though our highly-developed mental faculties are able to solve problems our pets can't dream of formulating, this same mental sophistication can turn on us with a ferocity not experienced by either domesticated pets or animals in the wild. For example, when is the last time you noticed your love-torn, jilted dog or cat losing sleep over a relationship gone bad? Have you noticed your canary being upset about her feathers being the "wrong" color, or panic stricken when her plumage changes color with age?

True, this is a simplistic way of looking at animals' emotions (feelings). We know, for example, that elephants mourn their dead, that our old cat doesn't want to deal with a new, fuzzy house guest, and that dolphins have sex seemingly only for fun; nonetheless, the basic point is valid—namely, that human beings are mentally developed in quite different ways from other animals, and it's this sophistication that makes us the leader in the pain perception department.

THE BODY-MIND-BODY LOOP

In humans, physical pain most often becomes mental pain as well, and vice versa. For us, the pain simply can't be separated—the two are inexorably intertwined. We all have noticed that we're not at our mental (emotional) best when experiencing the throbbing of a painful tooth, or even a stubbed toe. The physical sensation of pain seeps into our psyches like melting butter on a hot piece of corn-on-the-cob. Physical pain disrupts sleep, produces anxiety and can lead to depression and myriad other physical involvements. On the other hand, researchers at the Johns Hopkins University have found that relieving or preventing pain tends to strengthen the body's immune response.[1] No pain, big gain.

Just as the body can exert powerful influences on the mind, it is well established that the converse is also true—the human mind can exert powerful effects on the body. It is known that negative psychological states such as depression and anxiety can lower the body's immune function, opening the door to various types of illness and disease. For example, depression has been linked to dramatic reductions in immune function, including the reduction of white blood cell activity and lowered antibody responses.[2] In one dramatic study, a team of researchers at the University of Bergen in Norway monitored a group of more than 60,000 Norwegians from 1995 to 1997. Those participants who had the highest levels of self-reported anxiety in 1995 were 25% more likely to develop premalignancies[3]—abnormal cells that can turn cancerous. Witnessing studies such as this, immune system researchers have commented that it is almost as though the immune system itself is expressing grief.

One of the most dramatic pieces of evidence of mind influencing matter (body) was a study performed by the Cleveland Clinic Foundation in 1992. Subjects trained for 15 minutes a day, five days a week, for a period of 12 weeks to *imagine* (via intense concentration) they were flexing muscles in either the little finger or the elbow. At the end of the three month period it was found that muscle strength in the finger increased by 35%, and elbow flexor strength was enhanced by 13.4%. Physiological monitoring of the supplementary motor area of the brain showed cortical signal increases with increased mental practice. Magnetic resonance imaging (MRI) studies indicated the prefrontal lobes were involved, as well as the primary sensory motor cortex. It was also found that the strength gained during the training was maintained even after the training ended, especially in the group that exercised the abductor muscle of the finger. The study director reported that "all you have to do is sit in a quiet place where you can concentrate. You don't need any equipment. You don't need to spend a cent."[4]

We all have experienced the acute pain of bumping an elbow, dropping something on our foot, a sore throat, or the like. The best thing about these types of pain is that even though it hurts, we know the acute pain will be short lived. Just this knowledge alone somehow makes the pain more bearable. In a few minutes, hours, or days at the most, the pain will dissipate and life will resume its normal pace. Chronic pain, on the other hand, is an ongoing burden with no end in sight. Pain is labeled as chronic when it goes unrelieved for at least three months. Nearly 50% of adult Americans experience this type of pain.[5] According to a recent *Wall Street Journal* article, the economic price tag for medical costs, lost income, lost productivity, compensation payments and legal costs related to pain exceeds $50 billion annually.[6]

DIFFERENCES IN PAIN PERCEPTION

Despite conventional wisdom—probably related to the function of childbearing—it has been shown that men generally have a higher pain threshold than do women, i.e., men tolerate pain better than women. In a recent study published in the *Proceedings of the National Academy of Sciences*,[1] researchers discovered a protein called GIRK2, which is part of the physiological system by which a drug or the body's neurotransmitters dampen the pain signal within a nerve. This protein seems to be more active in males than females. By removing GIRK2, the sexes become more equal in their ability to withstand pain.

Another fascinating study shows that when it comes to pain perception in general, a tiny variation in a single gene separates the men from the boys...and the women from the girls, so to say. Researchers at the University of Michigan and the National Institute of Alcohol and Alcoholism have discovered a gene that differentiates how men and women withstand both physical pain and emotional stress. The gene produces an enzyme called COMT (catechol-O-methyl transferase), which is critical in mopping up the dopamine neurotransmitter (secreted in the brain) linked to the experience of sensing pain.[2]

Macho men (and women), believed to be about 25% of the population, carry a more robust form of the gene than do the "wimps"—those who experience pain more easily, accounting for an additional 25% of the population. Those individuals with both forms of the gene—the more robust from one parent and the weaker form from the other parent—experience intermediate pain. This group accounts for the remaining 50% of the population. Those with the most active genotype from each parent produce the COMT enzyme which is three to four times more active in uptaking the dopamine chemical.[3] These are generally considered to be the more stoic people, as opposed to those much more sensitive to physical pain and emotional stress.

PAIN RELIEF THROUGHOUT HISTORY

Over the centuries, different cultures have held various ideas concerning the subject of pain. Some have felt pain to be a "necessary evil." Others have felt, "No pain, no gain"—for both physical and mental pain. "These are experiences which strengthen the character of an individual," so it is said. Still others have believed God wants us to experience pain—for example, the pain of childbirth is the so-called "duty" of the mother. Any medication given to the expectant mother would be an act against God, according to this view. Some have thought the Earth to be flat.

Throughout the ages humans have used many different forms of pain relief—some quite enlightened, and others patently ludicrous. On the ludicrous side, the ancients practiced a form of pain relief called blood-letting, wherein blood would be drained from various parts of the body. To stop the bleeding, a branding-iron-type device would be used. This practice persisted even into the late 1700s. Another form of pain relief practiced by the ancients is called *trepanning*, or *trephination*. This practice involved chiseling a hole into the skull in order to let out whatever evil was suspected to lurk therein. The procedure is still practiced today, although rarely, because it obviously goes against modern medical ethical practices. Other forms of pain treatment have ranged the gamut, from contact with electified fish to being subjected to bee stings. Pharmacological agents, i.e., drugs, have evolved alongside these other methods.

The Opiates. There is an historical record of man's use of the opiates for pain relief dating back as long ago as 4,000 years. Derived from the opium plant (poppy), the opiate drugs include heroin, morphine, and codeine. Heroin—about five times the strength of morphine—was first synthesized in 1874. Known chemically as *diacetylmorphine*, heroin was sold world wide during the early 1900s by the Bayer

Company, the German company founded by Dr. Bayer which later become part of the infamous (German) I.G. Farben conglomerate (cartel). In 1906, the American Medical Association (AMA) approved the use of heroin as a replacement for morphine for general public consumption, and painful conditions in particular. By 1924, heroin was outlawed in the U.S. because of its addictive properties. In 1659, Sir Christopher Wren administered the first successful intravenous anesthetic in the form of an opiate. Nevertheless, it would be another 200 years before intravenous anesthesia gained general medical acceptance.

Cocaine. Cocaine, a derivative of the leaves of the coca plant, has been used by indigenous peoples throughout history where the plant grows naturally. The leaves are still chewed today by many South American natives as a matter of routine daily practice, providing an energy-enhancing and general palliative effect. Partially due to the efforts of the famous psychiatrist Sigmund Freud, cocaine became very popular during the late 1800s. Coca Cola derives its name from the plant, as early formulations (but not the "classic" Coke...) contained ingredients from the coca plant. During the early 1900s in the U.S., many drugs were banned from use, including cocaine. Even today in the U.S., the clinical use of cocaine is all but non-existent, as most physicians fear legal repercussions from the Drug Enforcement Agency and their local Medical Boards. Many other countries continue using the drug for appropriate clinical applications.

Up in Smoke. For better or for worse, man's use of marijuana is also documented in the historical record. Used both medicinally for pain and other benefits, and recreationally for over 5,000 years, the *Bible* makes reference to reefer in at least three instances, calling it kaneh, kannabus, and aromatic or sweet cane. History tells us the Father of America, George Washington, may have had a particular affinity for the plant. During the mid-to-late 1800s in the U.S., there were many favorable articles published in reputable medical journals recommending its use for a wide variety of physical and mental disorders. In 1937, cannibus fell out of political favor and was outlawed in the U.S. Recently, several states have approved medical marijuana ballot initiatives, much to the chagrin of many politicians and religious conservatives. Even still, the federal government won't honor what citizens support at the local level, and continue to spend billions of dollars annually to stop purveyors of smoke. Canada, on the other hand, has recently all but legalized the personal use of pot, making small quantities a minor offense. Belgium has recently legalized the substance. For decades Holland has led the way in the decriminalization of marijuana. In August 2003, the Dutch government made marijuana available as a prescription drug offered in two strengths, in addition to its continued "legal" street use.

Got Gas? Nitrous oxide (N_2O), also known as laughing gas, was identified in 1772. N_2O was the first gas recognized to have analgesic properties—initially observed by scientist Sir Humphry Davy—and it is still in use today by many dentists as an anesthetic. In 1846, Boston dentist W.T.G. Morton successfully and routinely used the gas ether in his dental practice. This marked the acceptance of anesthesia in general medical practice, with the exception of childbirth, in which case pain was viewed by the religious community as a "requirement" of childbearing. Also around the mid-1850s, chloroform gas started to become widely used as an anesthetic in general medical practice.

Modern Pain Pills. Concerning the opiates, these drugs represent modern medicine's principal armamentarium against the war on serious pain. Opiate derivatives are widely prescribed throughout the Western world, generally with effective results and minimal side-effects. The caveat to this is that in the U.S., this classification of drug is often withheld from patients most in need of their use—even terminal patients in severe pain—resulting from the current political climate. In cases such as this, the War on Drugs becomes a War on Patients.

Other pain relievers of lesser ability also are prominent in Western medicine. Acetylsalicylic acid (aspirin) came into use in about 1830 and has been sold world wide as a pain reliever since the early 1900s. In 1955, acetaminophen was introduced into the U.S., and in the 1970s ibuprofen was introduced as a prescription drug, followed by over-the-counter (OTC) approval in 1984.

Today throughout the Western world, there are many new anti-inflammatory drugs—including Non-Steroidal Anti-inflammatory Drugs, or NSAIDs—which are available both by prescription and over-the-counter. Many physicians understand that NSAIDs are of limited use in reducing pain, and may cause bleeding of the stomach lining (GI tract) and/or kidney and liver difficulties. Typical NSAIDs include naproxen (Aleve,® Naprosyn,® and Anaprox®), indomethacin (Indocin®), and ibuprofen (Midol IB,® Advil,® and Motrin®). Aspirin and acetaminophen (Paracetamol® and Tylenol®) are also considered non-steroidal drugs.

According to a 1998 article in the *American Journal of Medicine*,[1] more than 16,000 arthritis patients die each year in the U.S. from the use of Non-Steroidal Anti-inflammatory Drugs, and over 100,000 people are hospitalized due to NSAID use, generally due to gastrointestinal bleeding or perforation. Although these numbers are alarming, they are little known to the unsuspecting public. What should be a big clue is the October 2004 removal from the market of Vioxx, Merck pharmaceutical's sales blockbuster—which was shown to significantly increase the risks of heart attack and stroke. Modern pills? Yes. A better form of treatment? Probably not. You can read more about NSAIDs in the section on *Arthritis*, and more about how Merck literally "made a killing" on Vioxx in Appendix B.

The remainder of this book will focus on Specific Ailments as well as Treatment Methods which have been found effective in treating a wide variety of maladies. It should be noted that *wherever applicable*, the recommended treatment methods focus on the cause of the ailment rather than simply ameliorating pain and other symptoms. The exception to this is the group of treatments for pain relief, which generally offer pain amelioration without particular regard to the underlining cause of the problem, with certain exceptions. Nevertheless, pain amelioration by itself can be a godsend. Please note that many of the topics discussed in the **Pain Relievers** and **General Treatment Methods** sections are applicable to many ailments discussed in the **Specific Ailments** section.

Part Two:
Specific Ailments

In addition to the treatment methods discussed in this section, also review **PART III: Pain Relievers** *and* **PART IV: General Treatment Methods,** *which offer additional strategies for many of the specific ailments discussed below.*

ACNE. See *Iodine* and *Sodium Chlorite* under **General Treatment Methods**. See also the **Index**.

ACQUIRED IMMUNE DEFICIENCY SYNDROME (AIDS/HIV).

From its contested origin...to its questioned ability to cause AIDS singlehandedly, if at all...to its potential of annihilating a significant portion of the human species, the subject of the HIV virus is fraught with controversy. Some "experts" believe the virus is a *zoonosis*, a disease which initially infects animals before crossing species to infect humans. In the present case, some researchers believe monkeys and chimpanzees have been infected with the virus known as Simian Immunodeficiency Virus prior to "jumping species" to man.

In his book *Emerging Viruses: AIDS and Ebola*, Dr. Len Horowitz argues that HIV is the product of a biowarfare laboratory, having originally been developed in the U.S. by the National Cancer Institute in conjunction with U.S. military biowarfare researchers. The joint project was known as the Special Virus Cancer Program (SVCP) and was in operation from 1962-1977.

> This research program was responsible for the development, the seeding, and the deployment of various animal viruses, which were capable of producing cancer and immune system damage when transferred between animal species and into human cells and tissue...The SVCP

marshaled many of the nation's finest virologists, biochemists, immunologists, molecular biologists, and epidemiologists, at the most prestigious institutions in a coordinated attempt to assess the role of viruses in causing human cancer. Many of the top AIDS scientists, including Dr. Robert Gallo (the co-discoverer of HIV), Myron (Max) Essex (of "cat AIDS" fame), and Peter Duesberg...were connected with the Program.

The scope of the program was international and included scientists from Japan, Sweden, Italy, the Netherlands, Israel, and even Uganda, Africa. A main mission of the SVCP was to collect various human and animal cancers from around the world and to grow large amounts of cancer-causing viruses. In the process, many animal viruses were adapted to human cells. These cultured viruses would then be shipped to researchers throughout the world...Special attention was given to primate viruses (the alleged African source of HIV) and 'the successful propagation of significant amounts of human candidate viruses...' Candidate viruses were animal or human viruses that might be capable of initiating human cancers. And primate cancer-causing viruses were adapted to 'normal' human cells.[1]

Despite the fact that animal viruses such as Simian Immunodeficiency Virus *may* have jumped species into humans as the result of natural evolutionary processes, the Special Virus Cancer Program accomplished in 15 years what may have taken Mother Nature millenia—not discounting the fact that cross-species transmission may never have occurred by evolutionary forces alone. In addition to the SVCP, research to develop/engineer pathogens that degrade the human immune system was openly called for during the congressional testimony of Dr. Donald MacArthur, Deputy Director of Defense Research and Engineering, on July 1, 1969, before the House Committee on Appropriations, Subcommittee on Department of Defense Appropriations. Congress subsequently approved the appropriation. A copy of this revealing congressional testimony can be viewed at http://panindigan.tripod.com/aidsdodhear.html.

Following its "development," HIV was "introduced" into two populations which were administered the hepatitis B vaccine developed from chimpanzees infected with the SVCP's immune-suppressing viruses, according to Horowitz and others. The two populations were: 1) various Central African countries in the 1970s via the World Health Organization's Hepatitis B Vaccination Program, and 2) the gay populations of New York, Los Angeles and San Francisco in 1978-1981 via the Centers for Disease Controls' gay hepatitis B vaccine experiments.

Entire books have been written on this subject, including Dr. Horowitz' aforementioned book, as well as Dr. Alan Cantwell's 1988 classic *AIDS and the Doctors of Death: An Inquiry into the Origin of the AIDS Epidemic*. Before a naive reader declares these possibilities patently absurd, these books and copious additional compelling information on the subject should be carefully reviewed. Truth is often stranger than fiction, and this may be one such case. For more information on these topics, see www.whale.to/v/hepb1.html and www.originofaids.com/articles/early.htm.

AIDS is a set of symptoms including various infections resulting from damage to and suppression of the immune system. Because the immune system is weakened, these opportunistic "secondary infections" are often lethal. Some researchers believe the HIV virus doesn't cause AIDS at all. Others believe it is the sole cause, while yet others believe HIV doesn't cause AIDS without the involvement of additional co-factors such as other pathogens or nutrient deficiencies.

Many compelling anomalies suggest the presence of co-factors is necessary for HIV to produce AIDS. One such anomaly is that among HIV-infected nursing mothers, mortality is three times higher in the breastfeeding group than in the group of mothers whose babies receive infant formula. In fact, studies show the risk of mater-

nal death due to breast feeding is almost 70%.[2] If HIV is the sole cause of AIDS, why does breast feeding increase the death rate of the breast feeding mothers? Some have suggested certain nutrients, including selenium, are being depleted, further weakening immunity. This seems particularly relevant since blood serum selenium levels are a more accurate predictor of death from AIDS than the much-discussed CD4 T-cell count.[3]

Several additional anomalies also implicate selenium deficiency as a major co-factor necessary for an HIV-infected person to acquire AIDS. For example, despite widespread unprotected promiscuous sexual activity in Senegal, Africa, HIV is spreading very slowly, if at all.[4] In Africa, differences in soil selenium levels seem to greatly influence the prevalence of HIV/AIDS. A similar relationship has been documented[5] in the U.S., especially in the African American population where there is an inverse relationship between AIDS mortality and adequate soil selenium.

AIDS victims are characteristically deficient in selenium. In fact, AIDS as well as Hepatitis B and C viruses and the Coxsackie B virus encode the seleno-enzyme *glutathione peroxidase*,[6] the enzyme that stops viral replication. According to Harold Foster, Ph. D., Professor of Geography at the University of Victoria in British Columbia, Canada, author of the book *What Really Causes AIDS*, and member of the boards of the *Journal of Orthomolecular Medicine* and the Canadian Schizophrenia Foundation, "as these viruses replicate, because their genetic codes include a gene that is virtually identical to that of the human enzyme glutathione peroxidase, they rob their hosts of selenium."[7] Moreover, HIV "depletes its host not only of selenium but also of the other three components of this enzyme: namely, cysteine, glutamine, and tryptophan."[8]

■ *Selenium, Cysteine, Glutamine, and Tryptophan*. Accordingly, Foster maintains significant benefits can be gained in both prevention and treatment by supplementing with selenium as well as cysteine, glutamine, and tryptophan. Early clinical reports from South Africa, Uganda, and Zambia support this contention. Some patients have had a complete remission of symptoms. Unless HIV-positive individuals supplement with each of these nutrients, these deficiencies will likely culminate in AIDS, according to Foster.

Oral dosages of selenium ranging from 200-400 micrograms (mcg) are suggested by Foster and other researchers. Cysteine is easily obtained by supplementing with N-acetyl cysteine, a more stable form of the sulfur amino acid L-cysteine. A daily amount of 1,500-2,500 mg in divided doses with or without food is recommended. A dosage of 1,000 mg (1 gram) three times daily of the amino acid L-glutamine is recommended, preferably between meals. The amino acid L-tryptophan is readily available and should be taken separately from food or supplements containing protein or other amino acids at the level of 1,500 mg daily in divided doses, preferably with 6-8 ounces of water or a small amount of fruit juice.

■ *Glutathione*. Reduced glutathione (GSH) is the precursor of glutathione peroxidase. Some research indicates that orally administered glutathione is degraded in the harsh environment of the stomach. Therefore, it is best taken either sublingually, or from products having a liposomal delivery system. Either Source Naturals' Reduced Glutathione Sublingual Complex, or the two liposomal products Lipoceutical™ (www.autism coach.com) or ReadiSorb™ Liposomal Glutathione (www.readisorb.com) are recommended.

■ See **Olive Leaf Extract, Photoluminescence**, and **Sodium Chlorite** under **General Treatment Methods**, and Blood Electrification and Magnetic Pulsing under **Herpes**. These treatment modalities have shown the potential of curing HIV/AIDS.

Some people have benefitted from *colloidal silver*, itself a controversial topic. For more information, visit www.silver-colloids.com and www.purecolloid.com/mesosilver.htm. A free copy of Dr. Foster's e-book *What Really Causes AIDS* is available at www.hdfoster.com. See also the **Index**, and the Member's Area of *The Encyclopedia's* website.

ADDICTION. See **Stress**.

ALLERGIES

An allergic reaction is a hypersensitive, exaggerated or pathological reaction of the immune system to substances or situations that usually cause no reaction in the average individual. These reactions are typically triggered by something in the environment such as cat or dog dander, chemicals, foods, insect stings, molds, odors—any stimulus that may cause a person's immune system to overreact. The physical symptoms can manifest as itching, sneezing, respiratory distress, skin rashes, and the like. Allergic reactions range in severity from merely being bothersome to life threatening, and in some situations can actually cause death.

The immune system produces *antibodies* which attack the foreign *allergens*, substances which produce the allergic reactions. The antibody *immunoglobulin* E (IgE) binds to the allergen at one end and to mast cells lining the respiratory tract at the other end. The antibody attacks the mast cells, causing them to rupture and release histamine and other inflammatory chemicals. Allergic reactions result largely from the release of these chemicals and not from the allergen itself.

Genetics plays a significant role in allergies. If one parent has allergies, there is one chance in three of the offspring having an allergy. If both parents have an allergy, the likelihood is 70%.

■ *NAET*. Another effective treatment for allergies is referred to as *Nambudripad's Allergy Elimination Techniques*, or NAET. The brainchild of Devi Nambudripad, D.C., L.Ac., Ph.D., NAET is a non-invasive, drug-free approach to eliminating allergies of all types and intensities using a combination of techniques from several disciplines of medicine including acupuncture, acupressure, allopathy, chiropractic, kinesiology and nutrition—but focusing on acupuncture. According to Dr. Nambudripad, it is often possible to desensitize the person to a specific allergen in one treatment.

NAET is able to eliminate adverse, allergic reactions to a host of allergens, including animal dander, aspirin (and other medications), chemicals, cigarette smoke, cold, flowers, foods, grass, heat, latex, makeup, pathogens, ragweed, and many other environmental triggers.

Over 5,000 medical practitioners around the world have been trained in the NAET techniques. To learn more, read Dr. Nambudripad's book *Say Goodbye to Illness*, or visit www.naet.com for a directory of certified NAET practitioners.

■ *Methyl-Sulfonyl-Methane* (MSM). Sulfur is found in every cell of all animals and plants on Earth. MSM is an easily-absorbable, odorless, organic form of sulfur which is a derivative of DMSO. If the body is deficient in sulfur, there is a stiffening and hardening of cell walls which acts to trap allergy-producing foreign substances within the cells. MSM combats both environmental and food allergy symptoms by increasing the permeability of cell membranes, enabling allergenic foreign particles including free radicals to be more easily excreted from the cells. MSM has been shown to be as effective in the treatment of allergies as traditional antihistaminic drugs such as Chlor-Trimeton,® Benedryl,® and Allegra.® MSM is discussed in detail in the section on *Arthritis*.

■ *AllerPhase*.® Only recently available in the West, AllerPhase is a natural formulation consisting of 10 traditional Chinese herbs. It not only quickly and safely relieves allergic symptoms, but also attacks the root problem by exerting an immune-normalizing (balancing) effect. Many who have used AllerPhase report that after using only one bottle, their symptoms did not return even after discontinuing the product. To order AllerPhase, contact Tango Advanced Nutrition, (866) 778-2646, or visit www.puretango.com.

■ The flavonoid *quercitin* in combination with the pineapple enzyme *bromelain* is very effective in treating allergies. Two additional products are Xlear® (pronounced "clear") and vitamin C. Each of these remedies is discussed in detail in the section on *Asthma*. See also **Del Immune V** and **Seanol** under **General Treatment Methods**, the **Index**, and the Member's Area of *The Encyclopedia's* website.

ALZHEIMER'S DISEASE

In 1906, the German neuropathologist Alois Alzheimer microscopically identified the two specific markers characterizing the disease that now bears his name: sticky, abnormal clumps that form within the empty spaces between brain cells, and tangled bundles of fibers that erupt from within the clumps. The clumps are referred to as *amyloid plaques* (also called *senile plaques*) and the fibrous bundles are known as *tau neurofibrillary*

tangles. A loss of nerve cells in the areas responsible for memory and other higher mental abilities is also characteristic of the disease.

Alzheimer's disease (AD) is a progressive, neurodegenerative disease that affects the areas of the brain responsible for thought, memory, and language. Symptoms typically begin slowly, and progress over a period of 5-20 years with the average life span of the affected person averaging from 8-10 years following the initial diagnosis.[1] In the beginning, one may experience absentmindedness such as trouble remembering formerly familiar things and events such as people's names, dates, times of activities, and the like. As the disease progresses into its later stages, thought processes become increasingly less clear. There may be increased difficulty in speaking, reading, writing, and comprehension of everyday activities. Anxious or aggressive behavior also may occur, as well as mood swings, disorientation and depression. Specific symptoms and the progression of the disease may vary from person to person.

Alzheimer's disease is the most prevalent type of dementia, accounting for up to 60% of all dementia cases. AD affects from four to five million Americans generally over the age of 60, although younger people less commonly contract the disease. Over the age of 65, the incidence of AD doubles every five years, with about 3-10% of both males and females between 65-74 and roughly 50% of all those over 85 having some form of dementia, many of these being Alzheimer's victims.[2]

Diagnosis. Until recently, a definitive diagnosis for Alzheimer's was provided either by a biopsy or an autopsy. In 2001, Dr. Jorge Barrio of UCLA announced that a positron emission tomography (PET) brain scan in conjunction with an intravenously injected radioactive tracer chemical (called [18F]FDDNP) can identify those with Alzheimer's. The tracer chemical is retained longer in the areas of the brain where the amyloid plaque is present and can be viewed via PET. Barrio suggests that PET is able to differentiate between the various forms of dementia, and enables physicians to diagnose AD at an early stage with almost total certainty.[3] Previously, doctors struggled to differentiate AD from other types of senile dementia using medical tests (blood, urine, and spinal fluid), neuropsychological tests, and by collecting a complete medical history. Hypothyroidism, drug reactions, neurovascular disease, brain tumors, and Mad Cow Disease are among the other ailments that can be mistaken for AD. Some researchers believe a significant percentage of Alzheimer's diagnoses are actually misidentified cases of Mad Cow. This issue is discussed in more depth in the section on **Mad Cow Disease**.

Causes. The specific cause of AD is not fully understood, and it's likely that multiple causes exist. Although there is a rare genetic (inherited) form of AD that affects people between 30-60 years of age, most cases are not related to family history. Other than age which is the greatest risk factor, another factor is the presence of a specific form of the compound *apolipoprotein E* (apoE; specifically e4), believed to be caused by a genetic variant which may predispose a person to the disease. About 20% of all Americans have this genetic variant, although many remain unaffected by any symptoms of the disease.

In a 2002 study reported in the *Archives of Neurology*,[4] the eating habits of 980 dementia-free elderly participants were followed for a four year period. Those with the apolipoprotein-producing gene (e4) in the highest 25% of fat consumption had double the risk of developing Alzheimer's as those eating the lowest amount of fat. The presence of the e4 gene can be determined by a simple blood test. If present, the predisposition often can be modified by dietary factors (discussed below) so that the disease is less likely to manifest.

In 1998, researchers at the Philadelphia College of Osteopathic Medicine's Center for the Study of Chronic Diseases of Aging reported that 17 of 19 people who had died of AD had traces of the bacterium *Chlamydia pneumoniae* in their brains. This contrasted with only one of 18 autopsied brains of people known not to have AD showing signs of the microbe.[5] Although other respected researchers doubt the possibility of an infectious agent such as *C. pneumoniae* being responsible for the disease, pathogenic infection nevertheless remains a possible causative factor.

Hugh Fudenberg, M.D. is perhaps the world's leading immunogeneticist, with nearly 850 papers published in peer-reviewed scientific journals. From 1970-1980 Dr. Fudenberg studied the connection between flu vaccinations and the incidence of Alzheimer's. According to Dr. Fudenberg, those who received five consecutive flu vaccinations during the 10 year span he investigated have a 10-fold increased risk of developing AD than those who received no shots, one shot or two shots.[6] Fudenberg attributed this finding to the presence of both mercury and aluminum contained in influenza (and some other childhood) vaccinations.

One of the premier researchers in the field of mercury toxicity is Dr. Boyd Haley, Professor and Chair of the Department of Chemistry at the University of Kentucky, Lexington. Haley's research has established a likely link between AD and mercury toxicity. In a 2001 article published in *NeuroReport*, he states that "seven of the characteristic markers that we look for to distinguish Alzheimer's disease can be produced in normal brain tissue, or cultures of neurons, by the addition of extremely low levels of mercury."[7]

The levels of mercury exposure used by Haley and his co-researchers was considerably lower than those found in many people with mercury/silver amalgam dental fillings.[8] In the study which was conducted at the University of Calgary, it was further discovered that exposure to mercury caused one of the two hallmark signs of AD—neurofibrillar tangles.[9] Other research has shown that exposure to mercury can cause the formation of amyloid plaques, the second marker of Alzheimer's.[10] In the researchers' experience, no other metal has produced even remotely similar results.[11] To view a video demonstrating the toxic effects of mercury on nerve cells, visit http://commons.ucalgary.ca/mercury.

Aluminum, long recognized as a neurotoxin, is another serious culprit related to the development of AD. Seven studies have linked concentrations of aluminum in drinking water to an increased incidence of Alzheimer's.[12] In a study that analyzed lifetime exposure to aluminum contained in antiperspirants and antacids, the more these two modern-day conveniences were used, the greater the risk of developing AD. In frequent users, the risk was as high as 300%.[13]

Another modern chemical highly implicated in the development of Alzheimer's is fluoride, which is present in drinking water in many countries including the U.S., and in most toothpastes [1,000-1,500 parts per million (ppm), and mouth washes 200-900 ppm]. Chinese scientists have shown that fluoride at levels of only 3-11 ppm can directly affect the nervous system, and that the attention span of humans is reduced by consuming fluoride at 100 ppm. Furthermore, aluminum and fluoride have an affinity for one another, and fluoride may promote the absorption of aluminum.

In a 1998 study reported in the *Journal of Brain Research*,[14] researchers compared the effects on laboratory rats of amounts of elemental fluoride in the drinking water equal to the amounts of fluoride found in human fluoridated drinking water. The study authors concluded that changes in brain tissue caused by fluoride administration were similar to pathological changes present in human AD sufferers. Contained in the authors' summary were the following comments:

> One of the most remarkable findings was that animals administered the lowest dose of aluminum-fluoride (0.5 ppm) exhibited a greater susceptibility to illness and a higher incidence of mortality than animals administered the higher levels (5 ppm, 50 ppm) of aluminum without the fluoride...Chronic administration of aluminum-fluoride and sodium-fluoride in the drinking water of rats resulted in distinct morphological alterations of the brain, including the effects on neurons and cerebrovasculature.[15]

Speaking of rats, it is a little-known fact that sodium fluoride, the main source of fluoridation of the U.S. water supply, was for years the active ingredient in many varieties of rat poison. This has led veteran medical investigator Eustace Mullins to quip, "Whether the adding of this compound to our drinking water is also part of a rat control program has never been publically discussed."[16]

A further disquieting fact, reported by many researchers including Lono A'o in his book *Don't Drink the Water*, is that,

> ...sodium fluoride is a byproduct of aluminum manufacture, and...the transformation of sodium fluoride from dangerous chemical to benign cavity fighter came as the result of promotion from the Mellon Institute, the chief research facility of ALCOA Aluminum Company, North America's largest fluoride producer.[17]

The February 5, 1990 edition of *Newsweek* magazine reported that information obtained through the Freedom of Information Act (FOIA) showed that research pointing to the health risks associated with fluoridated water was deliberately withheld from the public for many years by the U.S. Public Health Service.[18]

Treatment. Several pharmaceuticals, including tacrine (Cognex;® first introduced in the U.S. in 1993), rivastigmine (Exelon®) and donepezil (Aricept;® first introduced in the U.S. in 1997) may offer some help in the short term. It is well known these drugs are more effective during the early stages of the disease. As with most pharmaceuticals, they have significant potential side-effects including liver and kidney toxicity.

■ *NSAIDS.* In a 2001 study published in the *New England Journal of Medicine*,[19] it was reported that Non-steroidal Anti-inflammatory Drugs (NSAIDS) are useful in preventing AD. Researchers reviewed pharmacy records of 7,000 people 55 years of age and older. It was found there was an 80% reduced rate of developing AD in those who used NSAIDS (aspirin, ibuprofen, and naproxen—but not acetaminophen) for at least two years, as compared to persons who took the drug for less than two years or not at all. This is not surprising, as AD has been associated with elevated levels of C-reactive protein (CRP; discussed in more detail under *Cardiovascular Disease*), a sensitive indicator of systemic inflammation. Also not surprising is the fact that drug companies are in constant search of opening new markets for their already-existing, already "tested" drugs. While this makes good financial sense, the approach may not be altogether medically sound, as NSAIDS have been shown to have significant side-effects including life-threatening gastrointestinal bleeding that results in thousands of deaths each year. (See *Arthritis* for a discussion about the dangers of NSAIDS). There are safer means of reducing inflammation than by using drugs known to have significant side-effects.

(In addition to C-reactive protein, AD has been associated with elevated levels of the amino acid homocysteine. Homocysteine levels increase substantially with age, and high levels are associated with many common diseases including vascular occlusion, kidney failure, and dementia including AD. What's unclear is whether elevated levels of homocysteine are a cause or a consequence of Alzheimer's. For additional information on homocysteine, see **Cardiovascular Disease**.)

■ *Curcumin*. The *Journal of Neuroscience*[20] reported in 2001 that curcumin, an extract of the spice turmeric, reduces inflammation and amyloid plaque deposits in animals. The study authors reported that although long-term use of ibuprofen suppressed inflammation and amyloid plaque-related pathology in an Alzheimer's transgenic mouse model, excessive use of NSAIDS can cause gastrointestinal, liver, and kidney toxicity. With low-dose but not high-dose curcumin, insoluble beta-amyloid (Abeta), soluble Abeta, and plaque burden were significantly reduced by 43-50%.

Other natural, side-effect free anti-inflammatories include fish oil, serrapeptase, ginger, flax oil, and Lyprinol.® Seanol,® an extract of brown algae, is also a powerful anti-inflammatory. For a discussion of its many medicinal uses, see **Seanol** under **General Treatment Methods**. (As anti-inflammatories, these substances also are useful in treating arthritis and many other conditions where inflammation is a component.)

■ *Statin Drugs*. At the annual meeting of the American Academy of Neurology in April 2002,[21] researchers announced the results of a study upon which they base the recommendation that the statin class of drugs should be used to prevent Alzheimer's disease. In a six year study of nearly 2,600 participants from over 800 families, a 79% reduction in the incidence of AD was noted. (There was no reduction in people with a higher genetic risk of developing AD.) Although these results are significant, the difficulty associated with statin use is similar to the problems associated with NSAID use—too many significant side-effects.

Although statin drugs such as Lipitor,® Zetia,® Vytorin,® Crestor,® Zocor,® Pravachol,® Lescol,® and Mevacor® are well tolerated by many, liver and kidney toxicity, impotence, muscle soreness, and serious breakdown of muscle cells (rhabdomyolysis) are potential side-effects.[22]

It is well known that statin drugs inhibit the production of coenzyme Q10. CoQ10 deficiencies are associated with many disease states including cardiovascular disease,[23] and should be a matter of serious concern to those using statins. (See **Cardiovascular Disease** for a discussion of the critical vitamin-like nutrient CoQ10). In addition to these drawbacks, statin drugs are quite expensive in comparison to more natural cholesterol-reducing substances such as policosanol—a sugar cane extract. Red yeast rice, another natural cholesterol-lowering product, has natural compounds that statin drugs attempt to mimic and is as effective as the pharmaceuticals. See **Cardiovascular Disease** for more information on these two substances.

■ *Memantine*. Also known by its trade name Namenda,® memantine is one pharmaceutical drug that may be of significant benefit to AD sufferers. The drug only became available in the U.S. in 2004, although previously it had been used in Germany for over 10 years. While the majority of other AD drugs such as Cognex, Exelon, and Aricept work by inhibiting the enzyme *acetylcholinesterase* in order to prevent the characteristic reduction of the neurochemical *acetylcholine*—which drops by 90% in advanced AD patients— memantine blocks the process of *excitotoxicity*, where nerve cells in the brain become overexcited and die.

For the majority of users, memantine slows the course of mental deterioration, allowing AD patients to perform certain daily functions that otherwise wouldn't be possible. Numerous research studies have demonstrated its safety and efficacy in treating all degrees of severity of Alzheimer's, vascular, and other dementias. Additional studies indicate it also may be effective in treating Parkinson's disease,[24] alcohol cravings,[25] and diabetic and other neuropathies. One study administering 40 mg/day showed significant alleviation of nighttime pain in neuropathic patients.[26]

In a 1999 Swedish study reported in the *International Journal of Geriatric Psychiatry*, memantine demonstrated its effectiveness in treating late-stage AD patients. The study authors concluded, "The results of the trial support that Memantine treatment leads to functional improvement and reduces care dependence in severely demented patients."[27] A study of 252 patients over a 28-week period, reported in the *New England Journal of Medicine* in 2003, found that memantine reduced clinical deterioration in moderate to severe AD patients. Lead researcher Hans Joerg Moebius stated that, "These promising results represent a breakthrough in terms of significant patient and caregiver benefit...compared to other anti-dementia drugs, Memantine showed an excellent safety and tolerability profile."[28]

■ *__Galantamine__.* An extract from the snowdrop flower, daffodil, spider lily, and other plants, galantamine has shown an ability to halt the progression of AD, and in some cases improve and rejuvenate cognitive function. It is marketed under the trade name Reminyl,® and has been used in more than a dozen European countries since 2000. The U.S. FDA approved Reminyl for use with AD patients in 2001.

Similar to Cognex, Exelon, and Aricept, galantamine works by blocking the acetylcholine-reducing enzyme acetylcholinesterase, thereby increasing the levels of acetylcholine and promoting brain function. It also has been shown to increase the production of new acetylcholine in addition to merely preventing its destruction.[29] As reported in *Clinical Geriatrics*[30] in 2000, New Zealand researchers administered galantamine at 24 mg/day for three months to one year to hundreds of AD patients. Significant improvements in cognitive function and daily activities were noted. The development of behavioral disturbances and psychiatric symptoms were delayed. After one year, galantamine-treated patients maintained their cognitive and functional abilities. In comparison to the other cholinesterase inhibitors, the positive effects of galantamine seem to be long lasting. Also, those implicated with a genetic predisposition obtained similar, positive benefits.[31] Many other studies have confirmed these results.

Galanta-Mind,® marketed by Life Enhancement Products, is a non-prescription version of the pharmaceutical Reminyl. It contains 24 mg of galantamine (the optimal dosage determined by clinical trials), vitamin B_5 and choline. Galanta-Mind can be ordered from Life Enhancement Products by calling (800)543-3873.

■ *__Ginkgo Biloba__.* The Ginkgo tree is one of the oldest trees known to man, having grown on Earth for over 50 million years. Of the various species, only the *Ginkgo biloba* tree survives to this day. *Ginkgo biloba* leaf extract is the most widely sold phyto- (plant) medicine in Europe, and one of the best-selling herbal medicines in the U.S. The European designation of the standardized product used in clinical trials is EGb761, while in the U.S. the herb is sold as a dietary supplement. Standardized preparations of Ginkgo contain 24% ginkgo flavonoid glycosides, 6% terpene lactones, and less than 5 ppm ginkgolic acids. Ginkgold,® Ginkoba,® and Ginkai® are standardized products that have been used in clinical trials.

Ginkgo biloba has been the subject of more than 100 clinical studies, mostly European. In several studies of AD patients using a placebo-controlled design, the positive overall effects were comparable to the benefits of donepezil (Aricept).[32] A review of clinical studies lasting six months or more also found Ginkgo to be as effective in treating mild to moderate AD dementia as cholinesterase inhibitors such as Aricept.[33]

Although some studies have produced conflicting/inconsistent results, most studies show improvement in cognitive function among patients taking 120-180 mg daily in divided doses. Over the past 20 years, upward of two billion individual doses of Ginkgo have been sold with only minor side-effects noted, the most significant being the potential problem of blood thinning. As such, *Ginkgo biloba* should not be used in conjunction with other blood thinning agents such as aspirin, warfarin (Coumadin®), and blood-thinning herbs such as dong quai, feverfew, garlic, ginseng, and red clover. To prevent the possibility of post-operative bleeding, its use should be discontinued at least one week before surgery. Standardized Ginkgo preparations are available in health food stores in the U.S., and on the internet.

■ *__Alpha Lipoic Acid__* (ALA). A sulfur-containing fatty acid and universal antioxidant capable of fighting free radicals in both aqueous (watery) and lipid (fatty) environments, alpha lipoic acid has been used as a treatment for multiple ailments including nerve damage caused by diabetes. In addition to being a master antioxidant, ALA is a blood glucose regulator and is significantly involved in the energy production of cells. Researchers are now beginning to notice its positive effects in neurodegenerative diseases. In a 2001 study reported in the *Archives of Gerontology & Geriatrics*,[34] participants were given 300 mg of ALA twice daily for one year. During the course of the study, their condition stabilized with no additional loss of cognitive function. While test scores of untreated AD sufferers would be expected to drop 8-11 points during a one year period, the fact that the patients' scores remained unchanged was noted by the study authors as being quite significant. R-lipoic acid, a potent new form of lipoic acid having 50% more biological activity, is likely to substantially increase the benefits of this substance. To learn more, visit www.r-lipoic.com.

■ *Huperzine A*. For hundreds of years traditional Chinese healers have used a healing tea brewed from the club moss plant (Shen Jin Cao; *Huperzia serrata*) to treat a variety of mental disorders. Contemporary Chinese researchers from the Chinese Academy of Sciences in Shanghai have now isolated the active components, known as *huperzine A*. As with tacrine and donepezil, huperzine A functions as a cholinesterase inhibitor, preventing the destruction of the neurotransmitter acetylcholine, thereby facilitating memory and learning. Huperizine A appears to be at least as effective[35] and is less toxic than the pharmaceutical cholinesterase inhibitors even when administered at levels 50-100 times the therapeutic dose. Also, its effects last at least 10 times longer than tacrine, according to researchers at Georgetown University's Institute of Cognitive and Computational Sciences. Researchers at the Chinese Academy of Sciences conducted a randomized, placebo-controlled study of 100 participants with mild to moderate AD. Participants were given 400 mcg (micrograms) of huperizine A for 12 weeks. The study authors concluded that huperizine A is a safe and effective medicine which "remarkably improves the cognition, behavior, activity of daily life, and mood of AD patients."[36]

■ *Vitamin E*. A 1997 article published in the *New England Journal of Medicine*[37] reported that a daily dosage of 1000 IU of vitamin E was effective in slowing the progression of AD in the participants studied.

■ *Chelation Therapy*. As mentioned, ingestion of aluminum is implicated in the causation of AD. Two agents helpful in chelating aluminum from the body are malic acid and silicon. Malic acid is an ingredient in the oral chelation formula Essential Daily Defense,® formulated by chelation specialist Dr. Gary Gordon. Silicon is available from some foods but preferably as a supplement such as BioSil® from Jarrow Formulas. Some evidence indicates those receiving an aluminum chelating agent deteriorate more slowly compared to those not receiving the agent.[38] Mercury is also implicated in the development of AD. The compound DMSA is a powerful oral mercury chelator, available in Dr. Gordon's product Heavy Detox.® Both Essential Daily Defense and Heavy Detox can be ordered by calling (800)976-2783. TD-DMPS, a transdermal DMPS lotion, is a powerful chelator of mercury and lead. Details regarding TD-DMPS and its availability are discussed in the section on *Autism*.

■ *Infrared Helmet*. In January 2008, news services were abuzz about a new British invention. Among others, the British newspaper *Daily Mail*[39] printed a story about an unusual Alzheimer's treatment device being developed by researchers at the University of Sunderland in cooperation with the British medical research firm Virulite. The device is a helmet containing an array of about 700 LED lights which focus infrared light on the brain. The low level light penetrates the skull and is thought to encourage brain cell repair by stimulating the growth of all cell types. Dr. Gordon Dougal, medical director of Virulite and co-researcher Dr. Abdel Ennaceur of the University of Sunderland, believe the apparatus has the potential of not only halting the progression of the disease, but at least partially reversing the symptoms of dementia such as memory loss and anxiety when worn for 10 minutes a day for a period of only four weeks.

The technology is based on a study conducted at the University of Sunderland that exposed middle-aged mice to infrared light for six minutes a day for ten days. The treatment significantly increased the performance of the mice in a three-dimensional maze. In related research, it has been discovered that about 90% of humans with dementia show improvement when treated with infrared lasers. Human trials on roughly 100 patients with Alzheimer's and other degenerative brain diseases are due to begin during the summer of 2008. The trials will use levels of infrared light that occur naturally in sunlight in the near infrared range of 1,072 nanometers. Stated Dr. Dougal, "...what if there was a technology that told the cells to repair themselves and that technology was something as simple as a specific wavelength of light...The implications of this research at Sunderland are enormous."[40] To view a photo of the experimental helmet, visit www.dailymail.co.uk. Enter "infrared helmet" in the search box.

■ *Etanercept* (Enbrel®). In January 2008, an article bringing hope for Alzheimer's patients and families was published in the *Journal of Neuroinflammation*.[41] The article reported the results of a study performed by Dr. Edward Tobinick of the Institute for Neurological Research and Dr. Hyman Gross of the University of California. According to the article, the perispinal administration of the pharmaceutical drug etanercept, tradenamed Enbrel,® to an 81 year old Alzheimer's patient demonstrated marked and long-lasting cognitive improvement within ten minutes of injection of the drug into the neck of the patient.

The doctors stated the patient was calmer, less frustrated, and more attentive. Over the next several hours, he showed additional improvement in a formal cognitive examination that began two hours following the injection. He demonstrated significantly better performance on tests requiring him to identify pictures, list words, and name animals. The patient also showed similar improvements on some but not all of the additionally-administered cognitive and memory test. The patient received one injection per week for five weeks. Prior to treatment, his score on the Montreal Cognitive Assessment test (MOCA) was 7 out of 30, indicating moderate to severe dementia. Two hours after the initial injection, his score had more than doubled to 15. Two weeks following the fifth and final injection, his score was 14.

This study of one Alzheimer's patient is a follow-up to an open-label study published by Dr. Tobinick in 2006 in which 15 patients received perispinal etanercept injections. The patients in the previous study showed improvements in cog-

nitive function which lasted the entire six month term of the study. Although Dr. Tobinick believes perispinal administration is necessary to enable the large molecule of etanercept to cross the blood-brain barrier, it has been pointed out that etanercept's use on psoriasis patients found the drug has anti-depressant effects, suggesting its availability in the brain even after ordinary systemic dosing.

In this study, etanercept was administered as an "off-label" use of the drug. (See the discussion of off-label drug use in Appendix B). The drug is currently FDA approved for treating rheumatoid arthritis and similar conditions. It is postulated the improvement following etanercept is related to the amelioration of the negative effects of excess *tumor necrosis factor alpha* (TNF-alpha) on the synaptic mechanisms in Alzheimer's patients. Researchers believe this is a promising area for further research, and a controlled trial of perispinal etanercept has been funded and is being designed in collaboration with an academic institution.

Sue Griffin, Ph.D., Director of Research at the Donald W. Reynolds Institute on Aging at the University of Arkansas for Medical Sciences (UAMS) and an editor-in-chief of the *Journal of Neuroinflammation*, visited Dr. Tobinick's clinic to witness the treatment first-hand. She stated,

> I noticed clinical improvement in each of the three patients within minutes following treatment. My first impression was that there was a clear, easily discernable, difference in each. They were more cheerful, more at ease, and more attentive.[42]

She further stated in a lengthy journal commentary,

> It is unprecedented that we can see cognitive and behavioral improvement in a patient with established dementia within minutes of therapeutic intervention...Even though this report discusses a single patient, it is of significant interest because of the potential insight it may give into the processes involved in the brain dysfunction of Alzheimer's.[43]

■ *NADH*. Nicotinamide Adenine Dinucleotide (Hydrogen)—abbreviated NADH, one of the most important coenzymes in the human brain and body—is the coenzyme (reduced, active) form of vitamin B_3. Dr. Georg Birkmayer, head of the Division of Neurochemistry at the Department of Medical Chemistry, University of Graz, Austria, has studied the effects of NADH on Alzheimer's patients. In a study of 17 mildly to severely demented Alzheimer's patients, Birkmayer found that treatment with NADH not only halted the progression of the disease, but significantly reversed the cognitive and behavioral symptoms—even in the most severe patients. In some cases, patients who were "virtual vegetables" were restored to a semblance of normalcy. To learn more about NADH and Alzheimer's disease, visit www.enadh.com/case_show.html. See also NADH under *Parkinson's Disease.*

■ A device that's shown effectiveness in treating Alzheimer's is the Magnetic Molecular Energizer (MME). The MME offers hope for many difficult-to-treat medical conditions, including AD. To learn more, see *Magnetic Molecular Energizer* under **General Treatment Methods**.

■ Other substances that may be helpful in the treatment of AD include acetyl-L-carnitine, CoQ10, creatine, inositol, omega-3 fatty acids, sage, and vinpocetine, all of which are available both in health food stores and on the internet.

■ See *Seanol* in **General Treatment Methods**.

■ See *Lyme Disease*. Some researchers believe Lyme is implicated in many AD cases. See also *Stem Cells*, and Alzheimer's Disease in the Member's Area of *The Encyclopedia's* website.

Prevention. Especially with such a devastating disease as AD, an ounce of prevention may be worth many grams of brain cells. First of all, a healthy diet rich in fruits, vegetables, whole grains, seeds and nuts (preferably organic) will go a long way in helping to maintain normal brain function. In addition, there are several other actions one can take that offer general protection from AD.

❑ Ingestion of aluminum, implicated as a probable cause of AD, should be avoided. This would include avoiding antiperspirants (nearly all of which contain aluminum salts); aluminum-containing antacids (such as Mylanta,® Maalox,® and many others); aluminum cans (even those with protective liners can degrade); and aluminum cookware (that can leach aluminum ions).

❑ A 2004 article[44] documented the protective capability of supplementing with vitamins C and E. Researchers at The Johns Hopkins Bloomberg School of Public Health tracked 4,700 people over the age of 65. They found those taking 500-1,000 mg of vitamin C and up to 1,000 IU of vitamin E had a 78% reduced risk of developing AD. Lower doses did not confer protection.

❑ In a 2001 study of elderly nuns, The Nun Study,[45] those who had the lowest blood levels of the B vitamin folic acid were significantly more likely to develop AD. A good B-complex vitamin having several times the recommended daily allowance of the ingredients folic acid, B_6, and B_{12} is recommended—all of which have been shown to lower homocysteine levels.

❑ The ingestion of pesticides and other toxic chemicals, either by inhalation, through skin absorption, or oral ingestion, should be avoided.

AMYOTROPHIC LATERAL SCLEROSIS (ALS)

Also known as Lou Gehrig's disease, ALS is a progressive, usually fatal neurodegenerative disease caused by deterioration of nerve cells in the central nervous system that control voluntary muscle movement. Rilutek® (riluzole) is the only FDA-approved drug for the treatment of ALS. A study reported in 2008 in the *Proceedings of the National Academy of Sciences*[1] compared a group of ALS patients taking Rilutek to a group taking Rilutek along with 150 mg of prescription lithium carbonate twice daily. The addition of lithium significantly extended the lifespan and slowed or halted the progression of the disease. See *Hyperbaric Oxygen Therapy*, *Stem Cells*, and Robson Splint under *Sleep Apnea*. See also the Member's Area of *The Encylopedia's* website.

ANDROPAUSE. See Testosterone under *Diabetes*.

ANGINA. See *Cardiovascular Disease*.

ANXIETY. See *Stress*.

APPENDICITIS[1]

The appendix is a small, worm-like appendage attached to the colon, and is usually located in the lower right quadrant of the abdomen, although for various anatomical reasons its position can vary somewhat. Appendicitis occurs when bacteria invade and infect the wall of the appendix. The symptoms include abdominal pain, often accompanied by nausea and vomiting.

Abdominal pain can be caused by a number of physical problems including diverticulitis, ulcers, and pelvic inflammatory disease. Also, the pain may be originating from the kidney or gallbladder. For this reason, pain in this area of the abdomen is often difficult to diagnose.

Various techniques are used in an attempt to accurately diagnose appendicitis, including:

♦ White blood cell count—may be elevated if infection has set in.

♦ X-ray—may detect (pea sized) fecal blockage causing pain.

♦ Ultrasound—appendix can be seen in only 50% of patients.

♦ CT Scan—useful in diagnosing appendicitis and excluding other diseases. The helical CT scan is about 98% accurate in diagnosing appendicitis.

Subsequent to performing a helical CT which will define the state of the appendix with high accuracy in most all cases, the most definitive technique in diagnosing appendicitis is *laparoscopy*, which is a surgical procedure wherein a small fiberoptic tube with an attached, miniaturized camera is inserted into the abdomen through a small puncture made in the abdominal wall. Laparoscopy allows the appendix as well as other abdominal and pelvic organs to be viewed directly. If appendicitis is found (and is not treatable), the inflamed appendix can be removed at the same time. Laparoscopy is performed under general anesthesia.

Surgery of any type is a serious procedure, and should be considered only as a final option. Particularly in the case of appendectomy (removal of the appendix), there is an additional factor to consider. The wall of the appendix contains lymphatic tissue which is part of the immune system, the body's front-line defense against illness and disease. Before consenting to (possibly unnecessary) surgery, it would be prudent to first employ helical CT imaging and, if indicated, laparoscopy to finalize the diagnosis and ensure its accuracy. Also, if appendicitis is caught in the early stages

of infection, a large dose of antibiotics will sometimes resolve the problem, according to British researchers. A word to the wise: never rush into surgery before less invasive options are explored. Hopefully, that's sufficient.

ARTHRITIS

The word "arthritis" is derived from its two components, "arth" and "itis." The prefix "arth" means joint, and the suffix "itis" means inflammation. Therefore, arthritis is roughly defined as inflammation of the joints which, depending on the type, can cause pain, swelling, stiffness and sometimes deformation or destruction of the joint(s) and consequent loss of function. The three primary types of arthritis are 1) osteoarthritis, 2) rheumatoid arthritis, and 3) gout, or gouty arthritis. It is not uncommon for a person to have varying degrees of combinations of the different types. Symptoms can range from aggravating to crippling.

Osteoarthritis—also called degenerative arthritis or degenerative joint disease—primarily affects the large, weight-bearing joints of the hips and knees. It is sometimes called the "wear and tear" disease because the bone and cartilage of one or more joints become worn down by the friction of the opposing joint surfaces. To some degree, osteoarthritis affects more than 50% of the Western world by the age of 55. This disease has been known throughout all of recorded history. It is also thought to be strongly influenced by dietary habits and may involve allergic reactions.

Rheumatoid arthritis, on the other hand, is a disease characterized by symptoms of pain, inflammation, stiffness, and swelling of the joints and sometimes the surrounding muscles and fibrous tissues. Approximately one percent of all adults in Western societies have this disease. Concerning its origin, several hypotheses have been offered. Some believe the disease is an autoimmune disease, where the body's own immune system attacks the joints. Other researchers believe there is no such thing as autoimmune diseases, and that rheumatoid arthritis is an infectious disease, i.e., it is caused by some type of microbial infection. As with osteoarthritis, the course or even the cause of the disease may be influenced by dietary habits—in particular, the consumption of sugar, and may involve allergic reactions.[1]

Gout, or gouty arthritis, is a metabolic disease characterized by painful inflammation of the joints, usually the feet (toes), but the ailment also can affect other joints, especially the hands, ankles, knees, elbows, wrists, and sometimes the tissues of the ears. It is caused by a systemic buildup of uric acid within the blood and tissues which crystallizes to form deposits of urates in and around the joints—especially the joints at the base of the big toes. The condition is thought to be significantly influenced by dietary habits, particularly excessive consumption of animal meats, fermented beverages including wines, coffee, soft drinks, ice cream, sugar, fats, white flour, and whole grains. Poor digestion and assimilation, food allergies, chemotherapy, hypothyroidism, lead poisoning, antibiotic and diuretic use, dehydration, joint injury, and surgery can also play a role. It is estimated about two million Americans have gout, 75-90% of whom are middle-aged males. It can be inherited, and about 25% of gout sufferers have family members with the condition.[2]

Western medicine's primary treatment for arthritis focuses on pain control through the use of analgesics such as the Non-Steroidal Anti-inflammatory classification of drugs (NSAIDs) which include naproxen (Aleve,® Anaprox,® and Naprosyn®), ibuprofen (Advil,® Midol,® Motrin,® Nuprin,® and Pamprin®), diclofenac (Cataflam® and Voltaren®), and indomethacin (Indochron E-R® and Indocin®). Aspirin and acetaminophen are also considered NSAIDs.

As mentioned above in the section on **Modern Pills**, according to a 1998 article in the *American Journal of Medicine*,[3] more than 16,000 arthritis patients die each year in the U.S. from the use of Non-Steroidal Anti-inflammatory Drugs, and over 100,000 people are hospitalized due to NSAID use, generally as the result of gastrointestinal bleeding or GI tract perforation. This would mean that every day in the U.S. an average of 44 people dies from the direct effects of taking these drugs. These figures are not generally known to the innocent victims—a.k.a. the loyal customers of the pharmaceutical companies—and are certainly not highly publicized by either the pharmaceutical firms or the popular mainstream media.

Reading from the manufacturer's (G.D. Searle, LLC, a subsidiary of Pharmacia Corp., former-ly Monsanto) product insert for Celebrex,® one of the "new, improved" NSAIDs, we find the following warning:

> Serious gastrointestinal toxicity such as bleeding, ulceration, and perforation of the stomach, small intestine or large intestine, can occur at any time, with or without warning symptoms, in patients treated with non-steroidal anti-inflammatory drugs...Therefore, physicians and patients should remain alert for ulceration and bleeding, even in the absence of previous GI tract symptoms...upper GI ulcers, gross bleeding or perforation, caused by NSAIDs, appear to occur in approximately 1% of patients treated for 3-6 months, and approximately 2-4% of patients treated for one year...However, even short-term therapy is not without risk...Borderline elevations of one or more liver tests may occur in up to 15% of patients taking NSAIDs...Long-term administration of NSAIDs has resulted in renal [kidney] papillary necrosis [death of living tissue] and other renal injury.[4]

Does this sound like a drug you'd want to take, or have a loved one take? Does this sound like a drug that should have been approved for marketing to humans? For analgesic medications such as this, Americans spend over $6 billion annually. Over 100 million prescription are written each year in the U.S. for NSAIDs. The unknowing public is being asked to "bend over" for this (mis)treatment. Could this be why these medications are called *anal*gesics?

If you think this is too strong a statement about the NSAID class of drugs, this is the mere beginning of the story. In a May 2003 article that could have been titled "More Pain for NSAIDs" (but was actually titled "Camera Pill Reveals 'Inside' Story on Pain Relievers"), Baylor College of Medicine reported on the work of Dr. David Graham, Professor of Medicine and Molecular Virology at Baylor University and Chief of the gastroenterology section of the Veterans Administration Medical Center in Houston, Texas. Dr. Graham used a miniature disposable video camera contained within a capsule that was swallowed by 40 patients to investigate the condition of the small bowel (intestine) following the use of NSAIDs such as ibuprofen, indomethacin and naproxen. The tiny camera is able to traverse the entire digestive tract while relaying color images to the doctors monitoring the study. The high-tech capsule is able to go where no other diagnostic tool, including an endoscope, has gone before.

In the study, 20 patients took NSAIDs daily for at least three months and 20 patients, the control group, took either acetaminophen or nothing at all. Seventy-one percent of the NSAID users had at least some injury to the small intestine and 23% had "severe damage." Those in the control group had only a five percent incidence of minor lesions and none had major damage as did the NSAID group.[5]

Capsule endoscopy, as the technique is called, became FDA approved in 2001. As it continues on its fantastic voyage throughout the intestinal tract, the encapsulated camera snaps two color photos per second, about 50,000 in total, which it transmits to a hard drive worn on the patient's belt. The images are able to be replayed at a later date as a movie sequence. The cost of the procedure, which is covered by some insurance companies, is about USD $1,700—$500 for the camera and $1,000-$1,200 for the accompanying diagnostic analysis.

Aspirin and other traditional NSAIDs target cyclooxygenase (COX-1 & -2) enzymes which serve as biochemical pathways of pain signals. Celebrex (and formerly Vioxx® and Bextra®) targets COX 2 enzymes. These new, highly-touted COX-2 inhibitors are probably only slightly less corrosive to the GI tract than their predecessors, and may bring with them additional adverse side-effects which are unique to these new NSAIDs. Since the introduction of the COX-2 inhibitors such as Celebrex, there has been a significant amount of published research on their effects upon the gastrointestinal tract, although the research results have been somewhat convoluted—including being both defended and contested.

In 1995, a writer for the publication *Rachel's Environment and Health Weekly* coined the term "cigarette science" to describe the corporate manipulation of scientific evidence linking cigarette smoking to human disease. The research and marketing tactics regarding NSAIDs may be yet another example of cigarette science. In the case of cigarettes, the tobacco companies continue to sell a product which kills 10% of all those who use it as directed. Trade organizations such as the To-bacco Institute make statements such as, "Smoking may cause illness; it may not. We don't know and we don't think anybody knows."[6] Statements such as this serve to muddy the waters of the issue in service of the companies which produce the questionable product.

In the case of NSAIDs, the scientific literature contains much back-and-forth bantering about whether the new COX-2 inhibitors constitute a better product than their predecessors, the traditional NSAIDs such as ibuprofen, naproxen and indomethacin. What seems clear to a discerning reader is that whereas the COX-2 inhibitors may (or may not) be less corrosive to the GI tract—a side-effect that kills thousands of people annually—overall they are judged inferior to traditional NSAIDs (and that's quite an accomplishment...) because of the additional side-effects that accompany their use. Namely, COX-2 inhibitors bring with them an increased risk of other serious adverse events, specifically an increase of serious cardiovascular problems including an increased risk of myocardial infarction (heart attack).[7]

But wait, there's more...heartbreaking news about NSAIDs. According to a 2000 article published in the *Archives of Internal Medicine*,[8] researchers at the University of Newcastle in Australia have discovered that NSAID use is a significant contributor to congestive heart failure (CHF). CHF is failure of the heart muscle including its inability to maintain adequate blood circulation throughout the body or to pump out the venous blood as it returns to the heart.

The Newcastle doctors found the odds of a first admission to a hospital for CHF was positively correlated to the dosage of NSAIDs consumed during the previous week. In a study of 365 CHF patients, NSAIDs, they reported, were responsible for approximately 19% of first-time hospital admissions for CHF. Other than low-dose aspirin, the use of NSAIDs during the previous week doubled the risk of hospital admission with CHF, and increased it by ten-fold in persons with a history of heart disease. The researchers concluded that "the burden of illness from NSAID-related CHF may exceed that resulting from gastrointestinal tract damage." In this study, traditional NSAIDs were not differentiated from COX-2 inhibitors.

When considering the extremely high incidence of heart disease in developed countries, coupled with the fact that NSAIDs are among the most widely used drugs throughout the developed world, this information is nothing short of alarming. It's also not widely recognized that in addition to these drugs being available both as prescription and over-the-counter medications as painkillers and anti-inflammatories, they are also ingredients in everyday products such as cold, flu and other preparations commonly assumed safe.

There's yet a further condemnation of NSAIDs. As reported in the August 2003 edition of the *British Medical Journal*,[9] researchers have discovered the use of NSAIDs significantly increases the incidence of miscarriage. Over 1,000 women were recruited for a study and interviewed immediately after testing positive for being pregnant. Fifty-three women reported using NSAIDs around the time of conception or during pregnancy. It was found that prenatal NSAID use increased the risk of miscarriage by 80%. There was a stronger relationship if the initial NSAID use was around the time of conception or if there was more than one week's usage. Aspirin usage, but not paracetamol, was also associated with increased risk of miscarriage.

The ultimate revelation came in October 2004, when pharmaceutical giant Merck removed the $2.5 billion per year COX-2 blockbuster Vioxx from the market. Company executives admitted 18 months of Vioxx use nearly doubled the risk of heart attack and stroke.

If we remember, the target of the COX-2 NSAIDs such as Celebrex is arthritis pain. Aside from the significant side-effects discussed, are the COX-2 NSAIDs effective in treating arthritis? On the contrary, the COX-2 inhibitors perpetuate the basic, underlying degenerative arthritic process even though the disease's superficial symptoms may be lessened.

In technical parlance, COX-2 inhibitors increase the production of the proinflammatory cytokine signaling molecules *tumor necrosis factor alpha* (TNF-alpha) and *interleukin-1 beta* (IL-1b). As reported in 2000 in the *Journal of Immunology*, the study authors comment that,

the short-term effects of COX-2 inhibitors on the pain and swelling of inflammation and ar-

thritis may be achieved at the cost of an increased propensity to long-term tissue damage with which these cytokines have been associated.[10]

It will probably come as a surprise for most readers to learn it is a well-established fact that traditional NSAIDs are plagued by the same drawback—accelerated cartilage destruction and inhibition of cartilage formation. Many studies have confirmed this, and it has been known for decades. In 1979, physicians in Norway made X-ray evaluations of the hips of 58 patients taking Indicin® (indomethacin). Patients taking the NSAID experienced significantly more rapid destruction of the hip than the control group taking no NSAIDs. Studies with aspirin and other NSAIDs have repeated these results.[11]

Western medicine's primary treatment for gout focuses not only on NSAIDS, but a small group of pharmaceutical drugs that target uric acid reduction. These drugs include allopurinol [including Aloprim,® Zyloprim® (U.S.), Apo-Allopurinol,® Purinol,® and Zyloprim® (Canada)] and febuxostat (Adenuric®). Colchicine is an anti-inflammatory pharmaceutical used to treat acute flare-ups of gout.

Although allopurinol is effective for some, it comes with a group of potentially serious side-effects, the most frequent of which is skin rash. Further, the drug should be discontinued immediately at the first appearance of rash, painful urination, blood in the urine, eye irritation, or swelling of the mouth or lips, as these can be signs of impending severe allergic reaction, which can be fatal. Rarely, allopurinol can cause nerve, kidney, and bone marrow damage.

Febuxostat is a new addition for the pharmaceutical treatment of gout. It was approved for use by the European Medicines Agency in April 2008—but its approval in the U.S. is still pending as of that date. In a 2005 study published in the *New England Journal of Medicine*[12] comparing allopurinal to febuxostat, the treatment goal of a serum urate concentration of less than 6 mg/dL following 50 weeks of treatment was achieved by 21% of participants taking allopurinol daily, 53% of those taking 80 mg of febuxostat, and 62% of those taking 120 mg of febuxostat daily. A major difference between allopurinol and febuxostat is that allopurinol is metabolized by the kidneys while febuxostat is metabolized by the liver.

Colchicine, an alkaloid derived from the dried seeds of the plant *Colchicum autumnale* (also known as autumn crocus and meadow saffron) is the preferred pharmaceutical treatment for acute gouty flair-ups. The alkaloid's use for treating gout dates to the early 1800s, and its medicinal value was noted as far back as the 1ˢᵗ Century AD. Colchicine was approved for use by the FDA in 1939. Although it's considered highly effective for treating acute gouty arthritis, its use comes with a long list of potentially serious side-effects including abdominal pain, abnormal bleeding/bruising, bone marrow depression, hair loss, nausea, peripheral neuritis (numbness in the hands and feet), purpura (purple-colored spots on skin, organs, and mucus membranes such as the lining of the mouth), sperm reduction, vomiting, and weakness.

There are many alternatives to side-effect-producing drugs for osteoarthritis, rheumatoid arthritis, and gout. The following is a discussion of some of the most powerful treatments that are not only effective, but generally side-effect free.

■ ***Univestin.*** Another pain pathway not treated by NSAIDs is the enzyme *lipoxygenase*, also called 5-LO (not to be confused with J-LO). 5-LO produces *leukotrienes*, another group of chemicals which promotes inflammation. Several new pain-reducing products target both COX 2 and 5-LO. They typically contain standardized extracts of two herbs: *Scultellaria baicalensis* (Chinese skullcap) and *Acacia catechu*. A compound called Univestin® (60% Free-B-Ring flavonoids and 10% flavans) contains a mixture of these two herbs. To locate a product containing Univestin, contact the manufacturer of the compound, Unigen, at (360)486-8200 or visit www.unigenusa.com.

■ ***Glucosamine and Chondroitin.*** Complementary medicine offers many effective treatments for arthritic conditions, some of which are quite familiar even to the general public. Glucosamine sulfate (GS) and chondroitin sulfate (CS) are two substances that have been highly advertised in recent years. (The sulfates are the specific forms of the substances evaluated in the research.) Over a period of time, generally at least one month, these substances *do* stimulate the growth of cartilage cells and rebuild cartilage damage caused by osteoarthritis[13]—but for some the process is seen as too long-term and not the immediate solution they may wish. Therefore, those taking these substances should understand the long-term nature of this therapy. On the other hand, restoration of cartilage may offer a permanent solution to pain.

Research has shown that GS and CS work synergistically, and therefore should be taken together.[14] It also has been shown that low molecular weight CS is preferred, as it is absorbed much more readily than the higher molecular weight form. This allows it to more easily enter the bloodstream which is the highway to the synovial fluid of the joints.[15] When shopping for a GS/CS product, look for the low molecular weight form of CS. One such product is CosaminDS, manufactured by Nutramax Laboratories, Inc., (800)925-5187. Enzymatic Therapy also markets a GS/CS product using a low molecular weight condroitin sulfate.

■ ***Methyl Sulfonyl Methane*** (MSM). The yellow, non-metallic mineral sulfur is the 16ᵗʰ most abundant mineral element in the soil and the 4ᵗʰ most prominent mineral found in the human body, following calcium, phosphorus and potassium. The fact that sulfur is found in every cell of all animals and plants on Earth underscores its essential role in all living things.

MSM, also known as *dimethylsulfone*, should not be confused with sulfa drugs, sulfite (a food preservative), or sulfate (a salt of sulfuric acid), which are inorganic forms of the mineral. The use of MSM does not typically affect those who are allergic or otherwise sensitive to these inorganic forms of the mineral.

MSM is a derivative of DMSO, discussed in the section on **Pain Relievers**. Although MSM and DMSO are chemically similar, each substance has its own unique set of properties. Of the two, MSM is considered the "nutritional" sulfur. Sulfur maintains the permeability within cell membranes, making certain that nutrients reach critical cell components, and that cellular waste byproducts are efficiently excreted. It is this specific attribute of MSM that is the basis of many of its health-enhancing benefits.

Roughly 50% of the body's total sulfur content is found in the muscles, skin and bones. Sulfur is a constituent of *keratin*, the tough fibrous protein substance that forms the principal matter of nails, hair and skin, as well as the horns of animals. It is a required ingredient in the production of collagen, which is the principal ingredient of cartilage as well as the body's connective tissues.

Supplementing with MSM in the range of 2,000-10,000 mg daily in divided doses with meals often provides effective and prolonged relief to arthritis sufferers, particularly when taken over a period of several months. It is an analgesic, anti-inflammatory, and blood vessel dialator. Additionally, it reduces muscle spasms, and has a normalizing effect on the immune system.[16]

MSM is a powerful healing agent and its use should not be overlooked. Although many "arthritis formulas" include MSM in their list of ingredients, because the best effectiveness is obtained at relatively high dosages, it should be considered being taken by itself at the quantities mentioned, up to 15 gm daily. MSM is available as crystals, in capsules or as a gel. For more information, visit www.jacoblab.com, or search online for "methylsulfonylmethane."

■ *Cetyl Myristoleate* (CMO, also CM). Known chemically as *cis*-9 cetyl myristoleate (mir-is-TOE-lee-ate), CMO was discovered (isolated) in 1964 by Harry W. Diehl, a researcher for U.S. the National Institutes of Health (NIH) for over 40 years, although his discovery was made privately. Diehl was issued three patents on his discoveries: U.S. No. 4,049,824, Cetyl Myristoleate, 1977; U.S. No. 4,113,881, Method of Treating Rheumatoid Arthritis, 1978; and U.S. No. 5,569,676, Method for the Treatment of Osteoarthritis, 1996. The results of Diehl's research were published in 1994 in the *Journal of Pharmaceutical Sciences*.[17]

CMO is believed to work in three ways: 1) It is a surfactant that not only lubricates joints, but also other parts of the body. It allows muscles to function more smoothly; 2) It functions as an immune system modulator, which may make it effective against auto-immune diseases, such as some believe rheumatoid arthritis to be; and 3) It functions as a fatty acid in the mediation of histamine and leukotrine responses.[18]

Several forms of CMO are currently marketed. Diehl's version of the product is derived from a bovine source, while others are derived from a vegetable source. A modification of Diehl's original formulation was made by the late Dr. Len Sands of the San Diego International Immunological Center. Sands' version, also from a bovine source, is known as "cerasomal-*cis*-9-cetyl myristoleate." According to the Sands contingent, the cerasomal version is better assimilated, and is therefore more effective. On the other hand, both the Diehl and Sands' formulations are effective.

Several well-known companies are currently marketing a vegetable-sourced version of CMO, including Source Naturals, Now Foods and Longevity Science. Because of the current, potential problem related to bovine-sourced products—specifically, Mad Cow Disease, or Bovine Spongiform Encephalopathy (discussed in detail under **Mad Cow Disease**)—the vegetable-sourced version of CMO may be the wiser choice. Further, after speaking with various experts about the different formulations, the Longevity Science product CM Plus comes highly recommended.

CMO may or may not be available in your local health food store, but is readily available on the internet. Visit www.authenticcmo.com to order animal-sourced CMO. An example of animal-sourced cerasomal-*cis*-9-cetyl myrastoleate is True CMO™ by Jarrow Formulas. Celadrin® is the trade name of an animal-sourced proprietary blend of cetylated, esterified fatty acids, including cetyl myristoleate. Various vegetable-sourced CMO products are available at www.iherb.com. To purchase CM Plus,® search online for "cm plus longevity science." As to which form of CMO is most effective, we're uncertain. Nevertheless, this substance is so important to arthritis sufferers that we recommend you try one form of the product. If one version is ineffective, try another.

■ *Lyprinol*.® The Maori are the indigenous peoples of New Zealand. Traditionally, Maori believe that eating a specific type of mussel—the green-lipped mussel (*Perna canaliculus*)—brings them good health and a long life. Among the Maori living in the costal areas where there is ready access to the mussel, both osteo- and rheumatoid arthritis are virtually unknown.

Research into the anti-arthritic qualities of the green-lipped mussel began in 1973. Over decades of painstaking research, the active ingredients were identified, stabilized, and subsequently marketed under the trade name Lyprinol. The active ingredients of Lyprinol are a specific type of polyunsaturated fatty acids known as *eicosatetraenoic acids*, which are related to omega-3 fatty acids found in fish, flax seed, and other oils known for their significant anti-inflammatory effects.

Direct comparison tests have been made between Lyprinol and other oils known for their anti-inflammatory and anti-arthritic qualities including flax, evening primrose, Norwegian salmon, and the high-potency fish oil MaxEPA.® Lyprinol proved to be the most effective by reducing swelling 79%. MaxEPA reduced swelling by 50%, but at a far higher dosage. The anti-inflammatory constituents in Lyprinol are some 200 times more potent than high-potency fish oil and 350 times more potent than evening primrose oil.

Comparing the effectiveness of Lyprinol to the mainstream pharmaceutical indomethacin, at 5 milligrams per kilogram (mg/kg) for both treatments, Lyprinol reduced swelling in 97% of the cases versus 83% for the indomethacin group. Lyprinol was found non-toxic and side-effect free.

Lyprinol is typically taken orally, but can also be administered topically by opening the capsule and rubbing the liquid into the affected areas. To determine its availability worldwide, visit www.lyprinol.com/home.htm. In the U.S., it's available as Lyprinol from Enzymatic Therapy.

■ ***Hyaluronic Acid***. Also called *hyaluronan* and *hyaluronate*, hyaluronic acid (HA) occurs naturally in many tissues of the body including connective, neural, and epithelial tissues. It is also present in the skin, cartilage, vitreous humour of the eye, and is a major component of *synovial fluid*—a thick, stringy fluid that reduces joint friction. When osteoarthritis is present, the synovial fluid decreases in viscosity (thickness) and concentration. For many years, HA has been used to treat joint pain via a course of injections directly into the affected joints, where it has a lubricating and cushioning effect. It is now understood that in addition to providing an analgesic effect by improving lubrication and thus reducing joint fric-

tion, the administration of HA also stimulates the body's production of additional HA.[19]

The vast majority of research studies on HA—which have demonstrated its efficacy in the treatment of osteoarthritis—have been on the injectable method of administration using one specific form of HA: high molecular weight (700,000+ daltons) derived from either animal or vegetarian-compatible sources such as bacterial synthesis. Oral use of HA came into public awareness in November 2002 when ABC News aired a segment on the possible anti-aging effects of dietary HA. Subsequently, various forms of HA have been offered in dietary supplements.

The three principal forms of HA currently offered in dietary supplements are derived from various sources and have different physical properties : 1) hydrolyzed chicken sternal cartilage—a natural source of HA such as the branded (trademarked) ingredient BioCell Collagen II™ which is offered as an ingredient in various dietary supplements; very low molecular weight of 50-10,000 daltons 2) dried rooster combs—a natural source of HA such as the branded ingredient Injuv™ which is offered as an ingredient in various dietary supplements; low molecular weight of 50,000-200,000 daltons, and 3) sodium hyaluronate from animal (rooster combs) or vegetarian-compatible material (microbial fermentation) with a high molecular weight of 700,000-1,000,000+ daltons.

Perhaps not surprisingly, each of the manufacturers of the branded ingredients used in a multiplicity of currently available dietary supplements claim their product is superior to the others. While considerable research has demonstrated the efficacy of injectable HA, there is much less scientific evidence supporting the claims of HA's oral use—although there is some. One example is a recent double-blind, placebo-controlled study[20] of 20 participants with osteoarthritis of the knee who received either a placebo or 80 mg orally of the Bioiberica branded ingredient Hyal-Joint™ daily for two months. The group taking HA experienced a 33% improvement in pain scores compared to 6% for the placebo group. According to Bioiberica, Hyal-Joint stimulates HA within two to four weeks of beginning the supplement.

A selection of HA-containing supplements can be found online or in healthfood stores. To view some of these, visit www.iherb.com. Enter "hyaluronic acid" as the search term.

■ *Avocado/Soy Unsaponifiables* (ASU). Sapon is the latin word for soap. Various vegetable oils are used in the making of soap. The portion of the oil appropriate for soap-making is called saponifiable, while the discarded portion is referred to as unsaponifiable. Avocado and soy unsaponifiables, as the name implies, are derived from avocado and soybean oils and are rich in anti-inflammatory plant sterols including beta-sitosterol, campesterol, and stigmasterol. Studies have shown ASU relieves osteoarthritis pain, reduces inflammation, and stimulates cartilage repair. Unlike glucosamine and chondroitin, ASU seems to work best in persons who have more severe cartilage loss. It aids in the production of four types of collagen in the exact proportions found in normal, healthy joints. Use of ASU increases production of *aggrecan*, an important component that helps keep cartilage hydrated, and decreases levels of interleukin-1-beta, a compound that destroys cartilage-producing cells.[21]

In a double-blind clinical study[22] of 260 persons with arthritis of the knee, three months of using ASU at either 300 mg or 600 mg daily resulted in significant improvement of symptoms including greater mobility, less pain, and a reduction of use of other remedies. No significant difference was found between the two dosages examined. The ASU-containing products Piascledine 300™ and Avocado 300™ can be purchased online. Advanced Joint Support™ from Healthy Resolve is available by calling (800)728-2288.

■ *ArthriPhase*.™ A combination of 12 Chinese herbs comprise the ArthriPhase formulation, which has been shown to be effective in treating both rheumatoid and osteoarthritis. The ingredients function synergistically to help soothe inflammation, reduce swelling, and increase circulation—thus assisting in the formation of new cartilage. The ingredients are specifically formulated to calm overly-excited nerves and to act on nerve receptors that are directly related to chronic pain.

ArthriPhase has been tested on both animals and humans. In a Chinese human study, 310 participants received ArthriPhase for 30 days. By the 10th day, 70% of the participants reported a significant reduction in joint pain. At the end of the study, blood evaluations showed that 50% of the participants had a normal ESR (*erythrocyte sedimentation rate*—a marker of inflammation). In the group that had rheumatoid arthritis, 63% registered negative for RF (*rheumatoid factor*—a marker of rheumatoid arthritis). To purchase ArthriPhase, visit www.puretango.com.

■ *Water*. It is well known that arthritis sufferers should drink plenty of pure (not tap) water. In his books *Your Body's Many Cries For Water* and *Water Cures: Drugs Kill*, Dr. F. Batmanghelidj argues convincingly that arthritis, as well as many other diseases, is caused principally by the body being in a state of chronic, unintentional dehydration. According to Dr. Batman, as he is affectionately referred to, there is a common factor to most all bodily pain: regional shortages of water, including within the cells of the pain-sensing nerves. The nerve endings sense an increase of toxic buildup within cells as the result of insufficient water to remove the waste products of cellular metabolism. These nerves then broadcast pain to force the individual from continuing to make actions which add to the toxic cellular buildup. At this point, the area is shut down, and there is loss of function in the painful area.

Rheumatoid arthritis, for example, is a signal of inadequate water in the painful joint. Low back pain and arthritis of the spine, according to Dr. Batman, are signs of a water shortage in the spinal column and discs, water being necessary to cushion and support the weight of the body. Drink two to three quarts per day of pure water—and take a little sea salt—and KaPow!, according to Dr. B., your symptoms will vanish faster than a speeding Batmobile. To learn more about the water cure for arthritis, visit www.watercure.com.

■ *Exercise*. Although it may be painful at first, exercise is helpful in preventing and treating arthritis. Low-impact exercises are best, such as walking, swimming and cycling. Exercise helps the body circulate synovial fluid into and out of the cartilage, keeping it moist and healthy. Begin slowly and build your ability to exercise more vigorously. A healthy exercise regimen also helps reduce weight, the goal of which is to attain a reasonable height/weight proportion. Proper height/weight proportion reduces the load on the major weight-bearing joints—the hips, knees and ankles. Motion also helps to circulate lymph fluid, which bolsters the immune system. Exercise also helps promote restful sleep, optimal bone density, as well as strengthening the cardiovascular system and optimizing lung function.

For those who are limited in their ability to take on a rigorous exercise program, a unique new exercise product may be just what you need. Designed by an internationally recognized rheumatologist and Clinical Professor of Medicine at UCLA, Dr. Robert Swezey—an expert in back pain, arthritis and osteoporosis—the OsteoBall is an inflatable, canvas-covered ball with attached straps that allow the user to perform a series of 10 isometric resistance exercises which target key muscle groups at the sites where they attach to the bone. This results in the strengthening of both muscles and bones.

Each exercise takes only five seconds, and can be accomplished even by most people with physical limitations. The total time for the complete workout is just 10 minutes, including warm up and cool down. The exercises can be done even while watching TV. The OsteoBall is portable, as it deflates for easy travel. It comes complete with a user's manual and detailed instructional video. To learn more about the OsteoBall or to place an order, visit www.bonefitness.com or do a key word search for "osteoball."

While on the subject of exercise, there's an amazing exercise technology that's relatively new to the U.S., but has been available in Europe for about 10 years. Originally developed in the Soviet Union and used by both their Olympic athletes and their cosmonauts, the technology is called Whole-body Vibration Therapy.

If you are old enough to remember the U.S. cartoon series *The Jetsons*, vibration therapy is the closest you'll ever come to the exercise techniques used by George Jetson. In the cartoon, as each episode began, George Jetson would get his quota of "exercise" by turning on the T.V. and watching someone else exercising. After only a few seconds he would be exhausted, having gotten his own vicarious daily workout just from watching

someone else make the effort. Vibration therapy is probably the closest thing you'll ever encounter that approaches this level of effort, or non-effort.

To receive your workout—not more than three times per week for a maximum of 10 minutes each session—a person simply stands on a small platform attached to the apparatus...period. The plate produces a vibration which transfers energy to the body. The plate itself vibrates at adjustable frequencies that cause the body's postural muscles to contract very vigorously from 30-60 times per second. As the body moves back and forth slightly, the muscles contract and relax. A full workout is accomplished in only 8-10 minutes. More time than this provides no additional benefits. In addition to just standing, a series of other exercises can be done on the plate which strengthens other muscle groups. For example, one can do pushups to strengthen the arm muscles.

In this short 8-10 minute time period, the body receives tremendous benefits in several ways. The muscles receive a thorough workout, and increase in strength 20-30% more than in conventional strength training with an 85% reduction in training time. Tendon, fasciar and connective tissue loosen, and joints become more flexible yet stronger. There is a strong increase in blood and lymph flow throughout the body.[23] Levels of testosterone, serotonin, neurotrophine, and IGF-1 increase; and levels of growth hormone (HGH) increase as much as 360%.[24] Bone strength and density are significantly increased, making the technology useful for the prevention and treatment of osteoporosis.[25] All of this is accomplished with less strain on the body, and with no risk of training injury.

Whole-body vibration is also very effective in reducing both acute and chronic pain. In one study of over 700 patients who had not been helped by other pain-relieving therapies and medications, over 80% experienced at least some level of relief using vibrational therapy.

Many professional sports teams have adopted vibrational therapy. Some of the teams using the technology include the Chicago Cubs, Dallas Mavericks, Dallas Stars, Germany's National Bobsled Team, Kansas City Chiefs, Los Angeles Dodgers, Miami Dolphins, New York Giants, New York Mets, Oakland Raiders, Pittsburgh Pirates, San

Diego Chargers, San Diego Padres, St. Louis Cardinals, Tampa Bay Buccaneers, Tennessee Titans, Toronto Blue Jays, and Toronto Maple Leafs.

Although the technology was originally developed in Russia, several companies currently manufacture the equipment. Prices range from about USD $2,000 to $15,000. There are presently units available for use at gyms and training facilities in many locations in Europe, but they are less available in the U.S. To learn more about whole-body vibration and to compare various models, visit www.powerplate.com and www. turbosonicusa.com.

■ *Antibiotics*. Many research studies have shown the prescription antibiotic *minocycline* (my-no-CY-kleen; trade named Minocin®) to be an effective treatment for rheumatoid arthritis, especially if the condition is of recent origin. The studies have shown that from 50-60% of the participants have at least 50% improvement in physical symptoms as well as physiological indicators such as IgM rheumatoid factor, erythrocyte sedimentation rate, and platelet count. The beneficial effects have been maintained for long periods as has been observed in monitoring for up to three years.

The typical dosage is 100-200 mg twice daily for several months to two years, depending on the patient's progress. Minocycline is usually well tolerated, but some side-effects can occur such as dizziness, headaches, rash and stomach upset. Dozens of studies evaluating minocycline's effectiveness in treating rheumatoid arthritis have been published over the past two decades in such journals as *Arthritis and Rheumatism, Drug Safety, Rheumatology International, Annals of Pharmacotherapy, Journal of Rheumatology* and *Annals of Internal Medicine*.[26] Henry Scammel, author of the 1998 book *The New Arthritis Breakthrough*, describes the treatment of RA with minocycline. Scammel discusses the positive results of the Harvard clinical trial (the MIRA trial) of rheumatoid arthritis' treatment with the antibiotic.

It has long been suggested that rheumatoid arthritis is caused by microbial infection. It is hypothesized that organisms such as bacteria (e.g., proteus and klebsiella) and viruses, but especially difficult-to-detect organisms such as L-form bacteria and mycoplasma, stealthily attack joints and surrounding tissue. (To learn more about these hidden pathogens and how they may be affecting your health, read Dr. Lida Mattman's book *Cell Wall Deficient Forms: Stealth Pathogens*.) If pathogens are indeed the cause, or one of the principal causes of rheumatoid arthritis, this would explain why minocycline is an effective treatment. Some researchers, however, offer alternative explanations such as minocycline's beneficial immune system and anti-inflammatory effects.

If you would like to be tested for infection by mycoplasma, contact Medical Diagnostic Laboratories at (877)269-0090, (609)570-1000, or visit www.mdlab.com.

The corticosteroid Prednisone® is often used to treat rheumatoid arthritis. For a discussion of this drug's serious side-effects, see *Asthma*.

■ *Biodegradable Scaffold*. Dr. Pertti Törmälä and a group of surgeons at the Tampere University of Technology in Finland have pioneered a unique treatment for damaged joints caused by rheumatoid arthritis.[27] The surgeons have successfully regrown new finger and toe joints in over 100 patients with damaged joints using this technique. Törmälä and colleagues have designed a mold or scaffold-type device which is fitted in the gap between the bones of the fingers or toes. Tissue grows through the tiny holes which perforate the scaffolding, filling the empty space between the bones, thereby creating a new joint. Constructed of a biodegradable "yarn" 10 mm in diameter and 3 mm thick, the structure disappears in about 18 months.

According to the Finnish surgeons, patients can begin to move their previously-afflicted joints almost immediately after the operation. The procedure effectively reverses the damaged condition, restoring movement and eliminating pain so that the joint functions normally. The new procedure was tested in Finland, Germany, Italy, Sweden and Turkey, and should be widely available.

What Törmälä and his colleagues are doing is one small segment of a larger body of research in the emerging field known as *tissue engineering*—the development of biological structures to restore, maintain, or improve tissue function. Although still in its infancy, doctors of tomorrow will be able to repair or replace damaged or aging body parts, including skin, bone, and organs. Scientists are targeting virtually every tissue and body part for engineering, including blood vessels, bone, cartilage, eyes, liver, muscle, nervous tissue, and pancreas. To learn more, Google "biodegradable scaffold."

Dr. Tom Minas of the Brigham and Women's hospital in Boston is another leading-edge tissue engineering researcher specializing in cartilage transplantation, especially in the knees. The technique is simple and straightforward. Weeks prior to knee surgery to repair damaged cartilage, a tiny piece of cartilage is removed from the patient's knee during arthroscopic surgery. The tissue is then grown in a laboratory to the volume of cells needed, after which they are reinjected into the damaged knee.[28] Such procedures offer hope to millions of suffering people.

■ *Salt & Vinegar*. Bet you thought we were going to recommend eating a lot of salt and vinegar potato chips, eh? Not quite. This age old remedy is an effective treatment for gout, according to Dr. Goodenough's book *Home Cures and Herbal Remedies*, as reported in the book *Practical Guide to Home Remedies*. Place all the salt that will dissolve into a small quantity of hot vinegar. For the first four days, rub the treatment into the affected body parts for 15 minutes, four times per day. Repeat the treatment for the next four days, but applied only twice daily; then once a day for four additional days. Thereafter, apply as needed. Sometimes remedies such as this are a lifesaver.

■ *Suma*. According to the book *Amazing Medicines the Drug Companies Don't Want You to Discover*, an incredibly informative book published in 1993 by University Medical Research Publishers of Tempe, AZ, USA—this book is a classic—the dietary supplement "Suma" is an effective pain reliever for gout. Brazilians call the tonic "para toda," meaning "for everything" and "Brazilian ginseng," as it's recognized as a popular adaptogen. Known botanically as *Pfaffia paniculata* (and by other names), the shrubby ground vine has a deep root system, and it is this part of the plant that has been used traditionally for a wide range of medicinal purposes. Suma has also been called "the Russian Secret," as it's been used for many years by Russian Olympic athletes for muscle building

and endurance. For more information and to order Suma, visit www.rain-tree.com/suma.htm.

■ *Cherries & Cherry Juice*. In recent historical times, Texas physician Dr. Ludwig Blau discovered cherries' beneficial effects on gout. After personally benefitting, Dr. Blau studied 12 additional gout sufferers who had a similar result. His findings were reported in 1950 in the journal *Texas Reports on Biology and Medicine*.[29] Several follow-up studies in reputable scientific journals have supported Blau's findings. Either fresh or dried cherries, or cherry juice/juice concentrate lower uric acid levels by as much as 15%. It's believed the plant phytonutrient *anthocyanins* contained in cherries is responsible for the reduction of inflammation and uric acid levels. Black, sweet, and tart cherries contain similar amounts of anthocyanins, so each should perform equally well. Although there are differences between people, a starting point for consuming cherries is one to two servings of fresh or dried cherries, two tablespoons of tart cherry juice concentrate daily, or 32 ounces of cherry juice at the initial sign of an attack.

■ *Additional Gout Remedies*. 1) It's been reported that drinking the juice of one fresh lemon in a glass of room-temperature water will prevent gout attacks by stimulating the production of calcium carbonate which neutralizes uric acid. 2) 500 mg of celery seed extract taken two times daily is effective. 3) One thousand milligrams of the flavonoid quercetin along with 1-1.5 gm of the enzyme bromelain two to three times daily between meals is a useful remedy. 4) B complex vitamins along with 500 mg of pantothenic acid in divided doses daily help reduce uric acid levels. 5) Eating a cup of strawberries with each meal is also an effective prevention/treatment. 6) For the prevention of recurring attacks, take 10-15 mg of lithium orotate twice daily together with two grams of the ascorbic acid form of vitamin C twice daily. Vitamin C reduces uric acid levels while lithium helps dissolve uric acid crystals.

■ *Dog-Gone Pain*. If your pooch has an arthritis problem, there's a very effective product you'll want to try. Called DGP—for Dog-Gone Pain—this product was pioneered by Dr. C.D. McKellar of Melbourne, Australia, one of the most respected Australian veterinarians. DGP consists of 12 herbs, many of which are native to Australia, and organically-processed shark cartilage. DGP has been used on racing greyhounds, working dogs and house pets alike, with remarkable results. From hip dysplasia to spondylosis (fusing of the spinal vertebra) to inflamed joints, DGP seems to do it all. It is also effective in the treatment of acute injuries and severe trauma. Results often occur relatively quickly, sometimes within a week or two. Because of the digestive differences between humans and animals, DGP is recommended only for animals, and especially dogs, although it has been shown to be effective on other small animals including pigs. DGP can be ordered on the internet by searching for "dog gone pain."

■ Many additional orally-administered substances have been shown effective in treating arthritis. Among these are herbs, oils, vitamins and enzymes. Some of the most effective include aniseed myrtle, borage oil, *Boswellia serrata*, capsaicin, curcumin (turmeric), devil's claw, DHA, EPA, fever few, flax oil, ginger root, lemon myrtle, mountain pepper, Nexrutine® (derived from the bark of the phellodendron tree), olive oil (extra virgin only), perilla oil, proteolytic enzymes (especially serrapeptase), vitamins C, D & E, white willow bark, wild rosella, yucca and zinc.

■ ***Cortisone.*** The administration of low-dose cortisone therapy, as discussed under ***Chronic Fatigue & Fibromyalgia***, can be a most effective solution for arthritic conditions.

■ ***NAET.*** If allergies are involved NAET therapy, as discussed under ***Allergies***, may be useful.

■ See **Pain Relievers** for additional arthritis treatments. See also ***Prolotherapy*** and ***Seanol*** under **General Treatment Methods**, and the Member's Area of *The Encyclopedia's* website.

■ See also ***Stem Cells***.

ASTHMA

The word "asthma" is derived from the Greek word "panos," which means "to pant." Ancient Chinese healers called it *xiao-chiran*, or wheezy breath, and believed asthma to be caused by an imbalance of the life force they call *chi* (Chee), also called *Qi* (Key). They re-balanced the life force by means of acupuncture, diet, exercise, herbs and massage. These techniques continue to be used in the Chinese tradition to treat asthma. Ancient Hindus used meditative techniques to control the breath and help manage the disease. Practicing medicine in the court of the sultan of Egypt, 12th Century rabbi and physician Maimonides recommended less food, drink and sex as a treatment, along with eating chicken soup. By the 1800s, asthma treatment had "progressed" to blood-letting and tobacco smoking. Live and learn.

Asthma is so prominent in Western societies it hardly needs a definition. Almost 15 million Americans and 150 million people worldwide suffer with the ailment. Nine million American children suffer with the illness.[1] It is estimated that the health care costs in the U.S. for treating asthma exceed USD $6 billion annually, with over 500,000 annual asthma-related hospitalizations and more than 5,000 annual deaths.[2]

Asthma differs from emphysema in that asthma is seen as only a temporary obstruction or blockage of the bronchial airways—caused by inflammation, swelling and constriction of the bronchial tube linings, and an increase in mucus production which blocks the passage of air. Modern medicine considers from 70-90% of asthma cases to be an allergic reaction to environmental stimuli such as cat dander, dust mites, foods, molds, etc. The remaining cases can be caused by varying factors including exercise, viral and bacterial infections, and genetic predisposition.[3]

Pharmaceutical drugs and inhalers are modern medicine's approach to asthma symptom control. Prednisone® is a commonly-prescribed corticosteroid drug (different from anabolic steroids) used to treat asthma, as well as rheumatoid arthritis. Dr. John Wong of Tufts-New England Medical Center in Boston tracked the use of Prednisone for 15 years in 4,993 patients with rheumatoid arthritis. He recently reported that even low doses of the drug can cause serious side-effects. Patients taking a daily dosage of only 5-10 mg of oral Prednisone were 200% more likely to develop hip fractures and 250% more likely to develop cataracts than those who took no Prednisone.

Even though asthmatics usually inhale the drug, studies have shown both methods of administration lead to similar absorption characteristics.[4]

The hormone *epinephrine*, also called *adrenaline*, is an additional drug used in over-the-counter (OTC) inhalers—and is yet another drug that can cause serious side-effects. In a study reported in the journal *Chest*,[5] researchers found 13 deaths linked to the use of epinephrine inhalers.

■ ***Neural Therapy.*** Dr. Harry Philibert of New Orleans, LA is the originator of an asthma-treatment technique which is a form of Neural Therapy, discussed under **General Treatment Methods**. Dr. Philibert discovered that following an injection of a local anesthetic such as procaine into a "trigger point" over each shoulder blade (scapula), asthma symptoms disappeared or were significantly reduced for most patients. As reported in the *Journal of Family Practice*,[6] Dr. Philibert achieved an 84% total remission rate in over 4,000 of his asthmatic patients.

There's more science to this than may first meet the eye. Trigger points such as the two over the scapulas are connected to the autonomic nervous system which controls involuntary actions such as constriction and relaxation of the bronchial airways. It is in this way the technique gains its effectiveness. To contact Dr. Philibert, call his office at (504)837-2727. To learn more or to locate a practitioner, contact The Institute of Neurobiology at (425)637-9339. See also **Neural Therapy** under **General Treatment Methods**.

■ ***The Buteyko Method.*** During the late 1940s, a Russian medical student named Konstantin Buteyko noticed that patients in the acute respiratory ward became more ill when their breathing rate increased (hyperventilation), and that those who reduced their breathing rate began to recover. Although this phenomenon had been noticed previously, Buteyko went beyond the observation to develop a set of breathing techniques which effectively treat the symptoms of asthma. (This is somewhat reminiscent of the Indian meditative techniques of using breath control to reduce the symptoms of asthma.)

Dr. Buteyko noticed that asthmatics breathe two to three times the rate of normal, non-asthmatics. His research over more than a 30-year period defined the effects of hyperventilation on the human body. Based on his observations, Buteyko developed techniques to normalize breathing patterns, reverse symptoms, and decrease the need for medication. In a research study published in the *Medical Journal of Australia*,[7] after 12 weeks of practicing the techniques, patients were able to reduce their bronchodialator medication by 96%, and their anti-inflammatory medication by 49%. To learn more about Buteyko Asthma Education, visit www.buteyko-usa.com.

■ ***Xylitol.*** Xylitol (ZY-li-tol) is a five carbon sugar alcohol with a sweetening power similar to sucrose, the common sugar obtained from sugarcane and sugar beets. It was first isolated by French and German chemists during the 1890s. The word is derived from the Greek word "xylan," meaning wood (e.g., the wooden bars of the xylophone), one of the sources from which it is commercially derived.

Xylitol functions by occupying the receptor sites that bacteria would ordinarily use to attach themselves to other cells. Also, bacteria are unable to ferment xylitol in their metabolism, and are reduced up to 90%. It combats three species of bacteria that live exclusively in the nasal passages and are responsible for most respiratory infections: *Streptococcus pneumoniae*, *Haemophilus influenza* and *Moraxella catarrhalis*.

In addition to a number of asthma symptoms which are caused by bacterial infections, it has been found that by spraying a solution containing xylitol directly into the nasal passages, the allergens and irritants that are the primary cause of asthma are effectively washed away. Developed by Dr. Lon Jones, a Texas physician and researcher, Xlear® (pronounced "clear") is a nasal wash containing xylitol, saline, purified water and grapefruit seed extract as a preservative. It is used to aid in the relief of irritation caused by allergens, pollutants and nasal infections. Xlear has been found to be particularly effective in treating asthma and allergy-induced respiratory symptoms, as well as sinus and middle-ear infection.

To learn more about Xlear or to place an order, visit www.xlear.com or call (877)599-5327 (within the U.S.) or (877)332-1001 (outside the

U.S.). See the **Index** for additional information on xylitol.

■ ***Vitamin C.*** Considerable research has shown that vitamin C is a very effective asthma treatment as well as an effective treatment for other allergies. It not only works as a preventive, but is effective in altering the course of an attack in progress. Physicians have observed that a teaspoon of powdered (crystalline) vitamin C (about 4,000 mg) is able to immediately halt an asthma or allergy attack. As a preventive, two to four grams (2,000-4,000 mg) per day is recommended.

According to the *Tufts University Diet & Nutrition Letter*,[8] as vitamin C intake increases, the risk of asthma and other allergic attacks decreases. In a recent 14-week double-blind study of asthmatic patients, the vitamin C group who took one gram (1,000 mg) per day experienced more than a 75% decrease in asthma attacks compared to the placebo group, and the attacks were less severe. All thirteen of the 22 patients in the vitamin C group who had no attacks during the 14-week testing period had at least one attack in the two month period following treatment.

Had the daily dosage been higher—in the 2,000-4,000 mg range—the results likely would have been even better. Lending credence to this is a recent study reported in the *American Journal of the Dietetic Association*[9] in which it was found that participants given 2,000 mg of vitamin C per day for two weeks experienced a 40% reduction in blood histamine levels, whereas a dosage of 500 mg had an insignificant effect.

Persons taking the *ascorbic acid* form of vitamin C need to develop a "bowel tolerance" to the substance by taking it in gradually larger doses. Diarrhea results when bowel tolerance is surpassed. Bowel tolerance is not an issue when taking the buffered form of the vitamin, as Ester C does not cause diarrhea. However, many believe ascorbic acid to be significantly more effective.

■ ***Lyprinol.***® A powerful anti-inflammatory oil extract from the New Zealand green-lipped mussel is marketed under the name Lyprinol. Its use for asthma became known when elite European marathon runners and cyclists began using the product to combat exercise-induced bronchial

constriction caused by inflammation and swelling. Many studies have shown Lyprinol to reduce the need for inhalers by as much as 50%, increase lung capacity, and reduce the frequency and severity of asthma attacks without adverse side-effects. For ordering information and to learn more, see Lyprinol under **Arthritis**.

■ ***Water.*** As discussed above, Dr. F. Batmanghelidj believes that chronic dehydration of the body accounts for many of the body's ills, including asthma. It is drought management, according to Dr. Batman, that constricts the free passage of air so that the body retains the water vapor normally expelled in the breath. The solution—drink two to three quarts of pure (not tap) water daily.

■ See *Allergies* and *Emphysema*. See also *Seanol* under **General Treatment Methods**, and the Member's Area of *The Encyclopedia's* website.

AUTISM

Autism—sometimes called classical autism—is the most common condition in a group of neurobehavoral/developmental disorders referred to as *autism spectrum disorders* (ASDs). Autism is a complex disorder which has been linked to early childhood abnormalities of brain development, and varies widely in both its severity and manifestation of symptoms. Although there are differences in the anatomy and function of the central nervous system in those with autism, the definitive cause of the disorder is yet unknown—although a genetic link may play a role. This, at any rate, is the opinion of "mainstream medicine." Other researchers provide persuasive evidence of certain environmental factors being intimately linked to the cause of the disorder.

A group of ASD symptoms characteristically manifests as one or a combination of the following, which can range in severity from mild impairments which are hardly detectable to totally disabling: impaired social interaction (unresponsiveness to people or a fixation on one item for long periods of time); difficulty with verbal and nonverbal communication (typically including delayed speech, regressed language skills, or attention deficit disorder); and unusual, repetitive, or limited or obsessive activities and interests (movements such as rocking and twirling or self-abusive behavior such as biting or head-banging).

Other sub-categories of ASD include Asperger syndrome (a high-functioning form of autism characterized by poor social skills but with no delay in language or cognitive development); Rett syndrome (a sex-linked genetic disorder characterized by social withdrawal, regressed language skills, and hand wringing); childhood disintegrative disorder; and pervasive developmental disorder not otherwise specified (typically referred to as PDD-NOS). Autism was once an uncommon disorder in the U.S., but has progressively grown to epidemic proportions. According to the Centers of Disease Control's recent estimate, one in 166 American children are autistic to some degree. Other legitimate researchers estimate autism is even more prevalent, with as many as one in 100, or possibly one in 50 U.S. children being affected with some level of severity of the disorder.

In recent years, vaccinations have come under scrutiny as a possible causative factor of autism, a subject which is a controversial topic in modern American medicine. American's receive 30 childhood vaccines, the majority of which are given before 18 months of age. There are additional vaccines given in subsequent years. Because they have been used so widely, it would be difficult for governmental agencies whose task it is to protect citizens from harmful medicines—as well as manufacturers who reap billions of dollars from vaccine sales—to admit there are health difficulties associated with vaccines even if it were a proven fact, which many maintain it is. Admitting a causative connection would open the flood gates of parents' demands for just compensation.

Virtually every "official" agency maintains there is no connection between autism and vaccines, including the Centers for Disease Control, the American Academy of Pediatrics, and the Food and Drug Administration. The Institute of Medicine Report on Vaccines and Autism has concluded that "the hypothesis regarding a link between autism and MMR vaccine and thimerosal [ethyl mercury, a substance added to many vaccines as a preservative] -containing vaccines lacks supporting evidence and are only theoretical."[1] Although studies have been performed which supposedly show no connection to autism, critics of these studies point to their sources of funding—which are often the very manufacturers of the vaccines, who have a vested interest in declaring them safe.

Nevertheless, given the meteoric rise of autism in recent decades, vaccinations are a plausible explanation for the disorder and many credentialed researchers believe there is a causal link. Prior to the government-established nationwide vaccine initiatives of the 1970s and 80s, the incidence of autism in the U.S. was one in 10,000. The mandatory immunizations program was instituted in 1998. With today's 97% vaccination compliance in public schools, the statistics have steadily crept to roughly one in 100. Some have naively explained this increase as merely the result of improvements in diagnostic capability.

The neurological damage characteristic of autism is remarkably similar to the well-established side-effects of several toxic substances contained in vaccines including aluminum, mercury, and formaldehyde. Further, multiple vaccines are often administered on the same day, providing a brew of potentially-toxic substances. It's difficult to believe that no damage is caused to the immature immune systems of children by such a pervasive and extreme series of toxic insults.

Although autism is running rampant in mainstream America, one small segment of American society has all but escaped the disorder—the Amish, a religious sect living mostly in rural Pennsylvania and the mid-west. The Amish live a simple life of self-imposed isolation from modern society—no cars, no power-line electricity, and... no vaccinations. In mid-2005 Dan Olmsted, an investigative reporter for United Press International, published a series of articles entitled *Age of Autism: A Glimpse of the Amish*. Olmsted reported that, according to the national statistic of one autistic child in 166, there should be as many as 130 among the Pennsylvania Amish. Instead, he discovered only three—two who had been vaccinated and the third having an unknown status.

Olmsted also visited an Amish community in Middlefield, Ohio where he found the prevalence of autism to be about one in 15,000. He also located a group of about 35,000 children in metropolitan Chicago who were cared for by Homefirst Health Services. This group had two things in common with the Amish: they had never been vaccinated and they didn't have autism. According to Dr. Mayer Eisenstein, Homefirst's medical director who founded the practice in 1973, "We have about 30,000 or 35,000 children that we've taken care of over the years, and I don't think we have a single case of autism in children delivered by us who never received vaccines."[2] No matter how you slice it—and it's been tried—it's difficult to argue with Olmsted's findings.

Another factor that's unrecognized by most people, including physicians, is that the efficacy of vaccines is questionable. The question is, are vaccines able to confer immunity to humans against the diseases they are designed to combat? The answer is controversial, but many medical researchers believe that vaccines are in fact ineffective—i.e., they do not work as proposed (and advertised). In spite of the fact that vaccines are heavily promoted by trade organizations such as the American Medical Association, and government agencies such as the National Institutes of Health, the Centers for Disease Control, the Food and Drug Administration, and the World Health Organization, there are many reasons to believe they are ineffective, if not harmful.

Most people view vaccines as a modern wonder medicine that has rescued humanity from the ravages of many once-highly-feared diseases—including diphtheria, influenza, measles, pertussis (whooping cough), smallpox, and tetanus. A more thorough investigation paints a different picture altogether. If one examines the annual incidence from 1900 to present of the many diseases for which vaccines are available, a most revealing pattern becomes apparent. All of the diseases, without exception, show a steady decline from 1900 directly through the points at which these vaccines were introduced. By the time vaccines were introduced in the mid-1940s to the mid-1960s, the diseases they were designed to fight were almost nonexistent—already having declined by some 95%. Improved nutrition and sanitary conditions are generally believed to be the reasons for this gradual but steady decline in the incidence of most diseases against which we continue to vaccinate. With such questionable efficacy and such a strong link to autism, it gives pause for thought why so many vaccines are administered to so many people—including the most vulnerable, children.

There's a veritable vaccination frenzy currently occurring in the U.S. Some states continue their push to enforce mandatory school vaccinations. Gardasil,® Merck's new human papillomavirus (HPV) vaccine which claims to protect females from cervical cancer and genital warts, is being given to non-sexually active, underage girls. In addition to questioning the logic of this, the safety of the Gardasil vaccine is indeed questionable, as there have been many adverse reactions including seizures, rashes, paralysis, and even deaths.[3] (Even school-age boys are now being advised to be vaccinated with Gardasil, according to mainstream media reports. This recommendation is based on the notion that a boy could contract throat cancer if he has oral sex with an HPV-infected girl.) Several vaccines don't appear to be medically necessary, including the hepatitis B, human papillomavirus, Gardasil, and chicken pox vaccines. Flu vaccines are not medically necessary, of questionable efficacy (see a discussion of flu vaccines in the **Colds and Flu** section), and as of early 2009 still contain mercury (thimerasol)—yet they are recommended and may become mandatory for school children in some states.

Mainstream medicine offers no cures for autism, but palliative measures such as educational and behavioral interventions focusing on the development of social and language skills, and a range of medications including antidepressants, anticonvulsants, and stimulants—e.g., ADD medications.

The term detoxification refers to the elimination of bodily toxins (poisons). Throughout the ages the body has evolved complex systems which enable the excretion of a wide range of toxins never previously encountered—such as ingredients in vaccinations. Even though the body has a powerful capability to detoxify, the extent of the pollution present in today's world often exceeds the body's ability to do so, especially when multiple vaccines are administered on the same day.

Researchers recognize that every individual has a specific detoxification profile characterized by his/her own unique detoxification capacity. One's capacity to detoxify is a function of both individual environmental and genetic factors. This explains why, when presented with the same toxic stimuli, some persons become ill while others do not. This is particularly relevant in the present case, as children having a genetic predisposition to autism may be those most adversely affected by toxins such as those present in vaccines.

This is, in fact, the thesis of Amy Yasko, N.D., Ph.D., co-author of the 2006 book *The Puzzle of Autism: Putting It All Together*.[4] Dr. Yasko has found that 100% of autistic children have a defect in *methylation*—a complex biochemical process that, among other functions, protects cells from toxins. Although about 20% of the population has such a defect, no ill effects occur unless the body is unable to overcome its toxic overload. In such cases, brain diseases such as Alzheimer's, Parkinson's, and autism can result. The predominant cause of autism, according to Dr. Yasko, is the defect in methylation which compromises the ability to detoxify, combined with a toxic overload resulting from the heavy schedule of vaccines.

[A short side note about Alzheimer's and vaccines. Hugh Fudenberg, M.D., a leading immunogeneticist, studied the connection between flu vaccinations and the incidence of Alzheimer's between the years 1970 and 1980. According to Dr. Fudenberg, those who received five consecutive flu vaccinations during the 10 year span he investigated have a 10-fold increased risk of developing Alzheimer's than those who received no shots, one shot or two shots.[5] Fudenberg attributed this finding to both mercury and aluminum that are contained in flu (and some other) vaccinations].

An additional factor that may be contributing to the high incidence of autism is our increasingly polluted, toxic environment. It's now known that the bodies of adult Americans are burdened with at least 500 xenobiotic (foreign; industrial/household) chemicals, and about half of these toxic chemicals are passed to newborn babies from their toxic mothers. To read an expanded discussion of this issue, see Toxic Consequences on p. 274.

■ *Vitamin D*. Respected psychiatrist John Cannell, executive director of the Vitamin D Council, believes an undeniable link exists between low levels of plasma vitamin D and autism. Following extensive research on the subject, Cannell has put forth the "vitamin D deficiency theory" of autism—pointing to a likely causal relationship.

Although vitamin D is popularly recognized as assisting in bone mineralization, it is less well known as an important neurosteroid hormone which is intimately related to brain development and behavior. *Calcitriol*, the active form of vitamin D in the blood, controls brain cell growth and acts on brain cell receptor molecules beginning with embryo formation.[6] It acts as a molecular switch targeting at least 1,000 genes which influence brain development. Recent research has shown that vitamin D provides "neuroprotection, anti-epileptic effects, immunomodulation...[and] regulation of behaviors."[7] A disruption of 36 important brain proteins during fetal development has shown to result from a vitamin D deficit.

Dr. Cannell believes it is a change in our *behavior* over the last 20 years that accounts for the rapid rise of autism. Specifically, he believes it is our lack of obtaining sufficient sunshine needed to generate adequate levels of vitamin D that has caused the epidemic, as sunshine's UV rays interacting with the skin is the only means of obtaining the vitamin short of pill-form supplementation. Information about the dangers of sun exposure expounded over many years by governmental agencies and groups such as the American Medical Association has created a sun-phobic populace, leading to severe deficits in vitamin D which in turn have brought about the current epidemic of autism, according to Cannell.

Considerable evidence supports the vitamin D theory. Low levels of calcitriol are related to lower levels of glutathione, the body's most powerful heavy metal detoxifier. Estrogen seems to enhance the beneficial effects of vitamin D, helping to explain the prevalence of male autistic children versus female. High- and low-latitude populations receiving less sunlight (UV energy) have a higher incidence of autism. Rural areas have a lower incidence than urban areas, which may be accounted for by the assumed lesser amount of sunshine received by city dwellers. Geographic areas having the highest rates of precipitation—as well as the lowest amounts of sunshine—have the highest rates of autism. Darker-skinned individuals, whose skin pigment blocks the production of vitamin D, have a higher incidence of autism.

While the evidence linking vitamin D deficiency and autism does not demonstrate a conclusive causal link, it is sufficiently cogent to suggest erring on the side of caution. Pregnant women, infants, and young children should maintain vitamin D levels equal to those living in mid-latitude, sun-rich environments—50-80 ng/mL (nanograms per milliliter) of 25-hydroxyvitamin D—by supplementing with vitamin D$_3$, also known as *cholecalciferol*. A beginning point for daily supplementation with cholecalciferol is 2,000 IU for pregnant women; 800 IU for breast-feeding infants; 400 IU for formula-feeding infants; and 1,000-2,000 IU for toddlers and young children not receiving regular sun exposure. Current Food and Nutrition Board guidelines state daily doses of up to 2,000 IU are safe for children over one year of age. See Vitamin D under **Colds and Flu**.

■ *Glutathione*. One of the most important protective substances synthesized by the body is *glutathione* (GSH)—which has a major presence in the liver and kidneys, the body's two principal detoxifying organs. Glutathione is a master antioxidant, fighting damaging *free radicals* and specifically reducing free radical damage caused by exposure to toxins. It also plays a major role in eliminating toxins from the body, including heavy metals such as mercury and aluminum, present in many vaccines. Researchers have found that many autistic children are deficient in glutathione (and folic acid, vitamins B$_6$, and B$_{12}$). A new, oral form is *liposomal* glutathione, which is glutathione encapsulated in tiny bubbles formed of the same material as cell membranes—making it highly bioavailable. Two liposomal glutathione products are Lipoceutical™ Glutathione, available at www. autismcoach.com, and ReadiSorb™ Liposomal Glutathione, available at www.readisorb.com.

■ *DMPS*. Another substance effective in eliminating toxins is DMPS (dimercaptopropane sulfonate), which assists in removing mercury and lead. Physician Rashid Buttar, who is also a Visiting Scientist at North Carolina State University, has developed a DMPS skin lotion (TD-DMPS). Dr. Buttar not only cured his son, but also has helped countless other children reverse autism. His autism treatment protocol can be viewed at www.defeatautismyesterday.com/ddmpspro.pdf, and important links relating to his work are found at www.defeatautismyesterday.com/buttar.htm. A list of physicians who practice Dr. Buttar's au-

tism protocol is available at www.centerforadvancedmedicine.com/listcenters.php.

■ *L-Carnosine*. L-carnosine is a di-peptide, a combination of the two amino acids beta-alanine and histadine. A 2002 study published in the *Journal of Child Neurology*[6] evaluated the use of the L-carnosine in 31 austic children. Administering 800 mg of L-carnosine daily for eight weeks had significant beneficial effects in behavior, socialization, communications, and other markers.

A complete list of dozens of researcher Dan Olmsted's articles on autism can be viewed at www.vaccinationnews.com/age_of_autism.htm. A list of vaccine ingredients can be viewed at www.cdc.gov/vaccines/pubs/pinkbook/downloads/appendices/B/excipient-table-2.pdf. If you choose not to have your child vaccinated, information on this link will be helpful: www.mercola.com/article/vaccines/legally_avoid_shots.htm. Dr. Amy Yasko's website is www.dramyyasko.com. Her book *The Puzzle of Autism* is available on her site as well as other online sites. *Vaccine Nation*, Dr. Gary Null's must-see video on the dangers of vaccines, can be viewed at http://curezone.com/forums/fm.asp?i=1240062#i. See also www.autismcoach.com, "detoxification" in the **Index**, and the Member's Area of *The Encyclopedia's* website.

BACK

Within the industrialized Western nations, back pain is the most common form of chronic pain—affecting about 15% of the entire population. It is the single largest cause of missed work days.[1] According to Dr. Thomas A. Zdeblick, Director of Orthopedic Surgery at the University of Wisconsin, most people are able to treat back problems, even disc degeneration, without surgery.[2] Chiropractic manipulation and physical therapy are often very effective. An exercise program including sit-ups and crunches is able to strengthen the back muscles, often reducing pain.[3]

Sometimes a brace or weightlifting belt is effective. Acupuncture also has been found effective in treating chronic back pain. In a 1985 study,[4] following chiropractic treatment 74% of the 204 participants experienced significant relief that lasted over three months.

According to the Cleveland Clinic, roughly 85% of Americans will experience significant back pain at some time during their life. About 5% of these people will develop persistent, chronic pain lasting four to six months or longer.[5] The cause of chronic back pain is often difficult to diagnose.

■ *Epiduroscopy*. Several years ago a new method was pioneered which often aids in locating the source of back pain. The technique, known as *epiduroscopy*, uses a small fiberoptic scope to evaluate the *epidural space*, which is the area on the exterior of the sheath surrounding the spinal cord. This space contains a network of nerve fibers which travels from the spinal cord to various parts of the body. Under local anesthesia, the fiberoptic scope is used to evaluate the presence of scar tissue on or near the nerves which could be the source of the originating pain. This technique also allows the physician to remove scar tissue from the irritated nerve root. In some patients, epiduroscopy assists in providing pain relief.[6]

Research from Australia, New Zealand and the United Kingdom has shown that in a group of over 9,500 patients undergoing major surgery, the pre-surgical administration of an anesthetic such as lidocaine into the epidural space reduces the surgical death rate by about 30%.[7] Further results were as follows:[8] vein clotting was reduced by 44%; pulmonary embolisms by 55%; pneumonia by 39%; and respiratory depression by 59%.

These beneficial results are explained as resulting from altered coagulation; improved ability to breathe free of pain; increased blood flow; and reduction in surgical stress responses.

■ *Chiropractic*. In May of 2000, *Consumer Reports*[9] magazine published a survey of 46,000 back pain sufferers. Much to the surprise of many mainstream physicians, chiropractic was rated as the most effective treatment for back pain. This was a surprise to many, as Americans spend more than $6 billion per year for prescription and over-the-counter analgesics. In the same *Consumer Reports* survey, deep tissue massage ranked number two behind chiropractic for relief of back pain.

■ *Prolotherapy*. One of the most potent techniques for treating the underlying cause of back pain is the method Prolotherapy. Prolozone® therapy, a variation of Prolotherapy, is also very effective. To learn more about both techniques, see *Prolotherapy* under **General Treatment Methods**.

■ See also *Spinal Cord Injury* and *Sciatica*.

BALDNESS. See *Hair Loss*.

BIOWARFARE AGENTS. See Biowarfare Agents and Infection in the **Index**.

BOILS AND MINOR SKIN INFECTIONS

Perhaps the simplest and most effective technique for treating boils and superficial skin infections is a technique practiced by many old-timers. It's simply the application of hot compresses to the afflicted area. Apply a hot compress for 20-30 minutes every two to three hours until improvement is noticed. Thereafter, apply the compresses several times daily until the condition is resolved. Needless to say, if this doesn't resolve the problem, consult a medical professional.

BURNS

■ *Honey*. The medicinal properties of honey have been recognized for thousands of years. Ancient Ayurvedic (Indian) medical practitioners used honey as dressing aids to purify sores and promote wound healing.[1] The Egyptian Edwin Smith Papyrus dating to 1500 B.C. recommended the use of honey in the treatment of burns. During WWI, Chinese and Russian soldiers used honey as a wound-healing agent.[2] According to an article recently published in the *American Journal of Clinical Dermatology*,[3] honey provides a moist healing environment, deodorizes, rapidly clears infection, and reduces inflammation, edema and exudation (oozing). Healing is also stimulated by the processes of *angiogenesis* (formation of blood vessels), *epithelialization* (growth of membranous cellular tissue), and *granulation* (growth of specialized tissue), thereby preventing the need for skin grafts. Excellent cosmetic effects are also noted.

Many clinical studies have demonstrated honey's effectiveness in treating burns. An article in the *British Journal of Surgery*[4] compared the topical use of honey with silver sulfadiazine (SSD)—one of the most widely-used, common treatments for burns—in 104 cases of superficial burn injuries. In the honey-treated group of 52 patients, 91% of the burns were infection free within 7 days, compared to only 7% of the 52 patients in the SSD group. Healthy granulation tissue averaged 7.4 days versus 13.4 days, and 87% of the burns healed within 15 days in the honey-treated group compared to only 10% in the SSD group. Additionally, pain relief and lower incidence of scarring and skin contracture were observed. Another recent study comparing honey to SSD in the treatment of burns showed better control of infection and inflammation, and better wound healing in the honey-treated group.[5] In fact, clinical studies have shown honey kills the seven species of bacteria that most commonly produce wound infections—even when the honey is diluted up to 10 times its original strength.

In the above-referenced studies, raw unprocessed honey was used. These honeys maintain their enzymes and other active ingredients. Two therapeutic honeys—MediHoney, an Australian product, and Manuka Honey, a New Zealand product—are specifically-formulated medicinal honeys. Both are derived from bees which forage the flowers of the manuka shrub, *Leptospermum scoparium*, also known as tea trees. These products are available in some health food stores and can be ordered on the internet. While any raw honey may provide acceptable results, the best wound-healing honeys are rated UMF (unique manuka factor) 10 or greater. In addition to burns, raw honey has been used effectively in the treatment of abrasions, acne, amputations, bacterial infections (including MRSA, Methicillin Resistant Staphylococcus Aureus), eczema, gunshot wounds, leg ulcers, puncture wounds, psoriasis, septic wounds, and surgical wounds. For abscesses or deep wounds that have been cleaned, honey is used to fill the cavity, after which an adhesive dressing is applied.

The Trenton, New Jersey firm Derma Sciences, Inc. markets Medihoney,™ a wound dressing saturated with manuka honey. One version is sold to hospitals, clinics and doctors in the U.S., while another is available in many U.S. drug stores. The dressing's germ-fighting and fluid-absorbing qualities last up to a week. Comvita, which controls about 75% of the world's manuka honey supply, markets similar products worldwide.

Ordinary granulated table sugar can be used for all wounds treatable by honey. When packed on or inside a wound, it dissolves in the fluid exedate forming a medium in which bacteria cannot survive and proliferate. Sugar draws fluid out of the wound; reduces swelling; encourages the removal of dead tissue; promotes granulation and the growth of new skin; and significantly reduces pain. Do not use sugar on a bleeding wound, as its use promotes bleeding. Further, sugar is ineffective in treating abscesses or pustules covered with skin. To view the exact treatment protocol for treating wounds with sugar, visit www.naturalnews.com/z026812_sugar_antibiotic_honey.html.

■ ***Proteolytic Enzymes.*** Taken orally, proteolytic enzymes such as *papain*, *bromelain* and *serrapeptase* (see the **Index**) are natural compounds that support the body's healing processes. These enzymes have demonstrated success in speeding the wound healing of burns, flesh wounds, surgical trauma and sports injuries, as well as reducing pain and postoperative swelling.[6]

■ ***Myskin® Bandages***.[7] Professors Sheila MacNeill and Robert Short of the University of Sheffield, England, have developed a "living bandage" made from the patient's own skin cells. The product comprises a flexible polymer coated with a special polymer nutrient film that supports the growth of skin cells. Upon this substrate are placed new skin cells which are grown from the patient's own skin—usually taken as a small skin biopsy from the patient's thigh. The Myskin bandage is placed directly in contact with the wound site, after which the bandage releases the cultured skin cells into the wound, prompting new layers of skin growth in the damaged area. According to Cell-Tran, the British manufacturer of the device, the cells delivered to the wound site have a high proliferative capacity, and accelerate healing significantly. After the cells have migrated into the wound site, the bandage is removed.

Myskin can be used in place of *cultured epithelial autografts* (CEAs), another technique of growing skin cells initially derived from the patients own skin. Myskin also accelerates healing of the donor sites from which the patient's skin is initially taken. With large wounds, contiguous applications of the dressing are used. To learn more about Myskin, visit www.celltran.co.uk, or call CellTran at +44(0)114 2220980.

■ *Ice.* One further tip for minor burns. If you ice the burn (moist washcloth with ice), run cold (ice) water on it, or immerse the burn in ice water *within 15 seconds of the burn*, the wound will be less extensive and deep. After 15 seconds there's not only no benefit, but a risk of frostbite damage.[8]

■ Chelation Therapy (see *Cardiovascular Disease*), *Photoluminescence*, and *Hyperbaric Oxygenation* (under **General Treatment Methods**) are also effective systemic treatments. Also see **Pain Relievers** where applicable, especially *Light* and *Magnets,* Stem Cells in the **Index**, and the Member's Area of *The Encyclopedia's* website.

CANCER

Cancer afflicts 50% of American men and 30% of American women with some form of the disease during their lifetimes. Other Western countries have similar statistics. Cancer accounts for roughly 25% of all deaths in the United States and is currently the number two killer of Americans.

The treatment aspect of the disease occupies much of the present attention in both the traditional and alternative medical communities. The truth is that early detection can be critical to the success of any treatment modality. Step one, obviously, is detecting the potential problem.

Presently, we rely on procedures such as the mammogram for early detection of breast cancer, the PSA (Prostate Specific Antigen) along with a DRE (Digital Rectal Exam) for detecting prostate malignancy, as well as other tests which seek to measure the presence of certain "markers" that indicate tumor growth. Most of the early-detection methodologies currently in use are fraught with difficulties ranging from mere inaccuracy to possibly causing bodily harm.

In the October 2001 issue of the British medical journal the *Lancet*, Danish researchers Peter Gotzsche, M.D. and Ole Olsen, M.Sc., analyzed the seven major studies that have been the foundation upon which the cancer establishment rests its proclamation that mammograms save lives. The Danish study concluded that the case for screening mammography (evaluating women of certain age groups with no known presence of breast disease) remains unproven at best. "At present, there is no reliable evidence from large randomized trials to support screening mammography programs,"[1] the study concluded. The test is largely ineffective as a screening tool for detecting cancer in sufficient time to influence survivability.

Because mammography is such a large revenue earner, any studies challenging its safety or effectiveness are themselves challenged. Is one witnessing honest disagreement within the medical community regarding discrepant analyses of the same data, or unscrupulous sales tactics masquerading as scientific inquiry?

University of Toronto's Cornelia Baines, M.D., Deputy Director of the Canadian National Breast Screening Study, has pointed to an almost willful silence concerning both the dangers and ineffectiveness of screening mammography. Regarding the dangers, she states an unacknowledged harm of mammography is that,

> ...for up to 11 years after the initiation of breast cancer screening in women aged 40-49 years, screened women face a higher death rate from breast cancer than unscreened control women, although that is contrary to what one would expect...three years after screening starts, their chance of death from breast cancer is more than double...[2]

Although these findings are counter intuitive, Baines further points out that in clinical trials conducted on two continents spanning 30 years, excess deaths in screened women 40-49 have been observed for up to 10 years after mammography is begun. Even those who disagree with Dr. Baines' disturbing conclusions regarding the increased mortality rates in this age group generally agree that the benefits of mammography are smaller in women younger than 50 years of age compared to those over 50. Many researchers now admit that any reduction in mortality in the 40-49 age group that may result from screening mammography is modest at best; and, when these modest benefits have been reported in the research literature, they have been statistically insignificant when compared to those not receiving mammography.

If the increase in the incidence of breast cancer in mammogram-screened pre-menopausal women ages 40-49 continues to be demonstrated in future studies, as Dr. Baines maintains it will be, it may ultimately be explained by a combination of factors, including: 1) Early detection of a tumor leads to surgical intervention. Removal of a primary tumor can induce the growth and proliferation of dormant micrometastases which already exist at distant sites, 2) In response to surgery, the body produces growth factors to accelerate healing. This, in turn, accelerates tumor growth, 3) The trauma of surgery is known to suppress the immune system, and 4) The exposure of breast tissue to ionizing radiation produces damaging free radicals. (Digital mammography, a more recent technology, uses a slightly lower dose of radiation.)

Mammography is one of the pillars of America's War on Cancer. Many doctors, government-related institutions, and industry lobbying groups recommend an annual screening mammogram for all women beginning at 40 years of age. Yet, the scientific literature shows screening mammography provides little if any survival benefit in premenopausal women, and it may increase the risk of dying compared to women who do not receive mammograms. In April 2008, an influential physician's group publicly declared their opposition to the general practice of giving annual screening mammograms to women 40-49, stating that women within this age group aren't at a uniform risk of cancer and that mammograms themselves could expose them to harm from needless treatment because of false positive evaluations. In women 50 and older, the benefit of increased survivability becomes more pronounced.

Diagnostic mammograms, as opposed to screening mammograms, are administered when cancer is suspected and when any possible tumor(s) would be presumed to be larger and more easy to detect. From 1996 through 2003, a three-state study[3] led by Group Health Cooperative of Seattle, Washington demonstrated that even the most skilled radiologists fail to detect 20% of breast cancer cases evaluated by diagnostic mammograms. The researchers examined 35,895 mammograms which had been evaluated by 123 radiologists. Accuracy of the evaluation varied greatly, with the worst radiologists missing nearly 40% of the existing tumors and misidentifying 8.3% of the patients as having non-existent

tumors (false positives). The top evaluators tended to be physicians at academic medical centers and/or practitioners specializing in breast imaging with at least 20% of their time dedicated to breast evaluation. Even these radiologists failed to detect 20% of the existing tumors while having a 2.6% false positive rate.

One additional fact women should know is that in 2000, researchers published the results of a review of the medical records of 2,227 women between the ages of 40-69. They concluded that after an average of nine mammograms, the risk of a false positive test was more than 43%.[4] A (false) positive mammogram may lead to unnecessary procedures such as lymph node removal or mastectomy—"just to be safe."

The PSA is another of modern medicine's means of diagnosis that is fraught with difficulties. Many in the medical community now realize the test is highly inaccurate and non-predictive. An expanded discussion of the PSA is included in the section on **Prostate**. Prostate biopsy—a procedure which evaluates whether or not there is malignancy (cancer)—involves multiple puncturings of the prostate gland. This may contribute to increased symptoms, and may also increase the possibility of spreading cancerous cells.

Modern medicine also relies heavily on detection/diagnostic techniques using electromagnetic radiation such as X-rays, CT and fluoroscopy. These techniques use energy from the most energetic portion of the electromagnetic spectrum, and are damaging to cellular structures, including DNA. This is the thesis, among others, of Dr. John Gofman, M.D., Ph. D., Professor Emeritus of Molecular and Cell Biology, U.C. Berkeley.

An atomic pioneer who worked on the famous Manhattan (A-bomb) Project during the WWII era, Dr. Gofman is author of the 1999 book *Radiation from Medical Procedures in the Pathogenesis of Cancer and Ischemic Heart Disease: Dose-Response Studies with Physicians per 100,000 Population.* Gofman believes a significant percentage of both cancer and ischemic heart disease is the direct result of exposure to medical radiation. In fact, he believes medical radiation is the primary cause of these two diseases.

For several years, full-body scans have been used as an aid in the early detection of disease, including cancer and heart disease. Some of this technology uses a series of CT scans (ionizing radiation), although it is promoted as a non-invasive means of diagnosis. Unfortunately, what recipients of this technology don't realize is that one full-body scan is approximately equalivalent to a person standing within two kilometers of the atomic blasts at Nagasaki or Hiroshima. Also, the deliterious effects of multiple full-body scans are cumulative, increasing the recipient's odds of developing diseases such as cancer and heart disease.

Early Detection. There are several tests that provide effective yet harmless and non-invasive detection of cancer at its earliest and often most treatable stages. The following is a summary of the most effective of these tests.

■ *Digital Infrared Thermography.* In the 1950s, the military began to develop infrared systems as a surveillance technique to monitor nighttime troop movement. Most people are familiar with night vision technology, where a person's body heat generates a visible image on a monitoring screen. Similar technology is used to detect tissue abnormality within the body. In 1982, the U.S. FDA approved thermography as an adjunct (additional, but secondary) screening procedure.

Thermography is recommended *in addition to* a mammogram even though thermography is clearly superior to the mammogram in many respects. While both procedures together are better than either one separately, if only one or the other were to be given, it's likely that most physicians who have knowledge of both tests (which they don't...) would recommend thermography to their wives and other family members. Mammography evaluates the *structure* of the tissues via X-rays, while thermography observes the *function* in terms of the metabolic activity of the tissues.

Breast cancer is the most common cancer in women, afflicting about 13% of women during their lifetimes and killing 40,000 American women annually. It is the leading killer of women aged 35-54. Seventy percent of breast cancers occur in women who have no family history of the disease, and 90% are diagnosed by palpation (physical examination involving touch).[5] By the time an abnormality (lump) can be felt, it is likely the tumor

has been growing for years, as most breast cancers take 8-10 years to grow to the size of one centimeter [10 millimeters, or about 3/8 of an inch (0.375 inches)].[6] After reaching this size, it typically takes only 1.5 additional years to grow to the size of 3.5 cm (about 1.375 inches).[7] About 25% of women with breast cancer die within five years and 40% die within 10 years of diagnosis.[8]

Mammography detects disease in roughly 60-80% of women who have tumors. In women who have been taking hormone replacement therapy, the percentage can be lower due to the increased density of breast tissue caused by estrogen intake. Also, breast implants obscure the breast tissue, making mammograms less than adequate.

As mentioned, by the time a mammogram is able to detect an abnormality, the tumor is likely to have been growing for years. Thermography, on the other hand, is able to detect tissue abnormality *in advance of the formation of a tumor*. Even before tissue becomes cancerous, i.e., while it is still in a precancerous state, the metabolic activity increases in the potentially-problemed area in comparison to the surrounding tissue. As cells begin to multiply abnormally, new blood vessel growth is necessary to deliver nutrients to the site and dispose of cellular wastes. This increase in blood circulation produces an increase in regional surface heat which can be detected by the sensitive thermographic equipment.[9] Therefore, even before the actual tumor develops, pre-cancerous tissue can be detected and a medical plan of action can be taken to treat the affected area, and enhance the overall immunity of the patient. Even after a tumor begins to develop, cure rates can be increased if treated in the earliest stages.[10]

While mammography has a high rate of false positives (an incorrect positive indication), and detects only 60-80% of cancers—most of which have been growing for years—thermography is able to detect 90% of the malignancies with only 10% false positives. It also detects pre-cancerous tissue having increased metabolic activity, which registers as a relative increase in skin surface heat.

A 1986 study reported in the journal *Thermology*[11] evaluated both thermography and mammography in their ability to detect breast cancer. The study included 4,716 women with confirmed cancer, 3,305 women with confirmed benign breast disease, and 8,757 women who were non-cancerous. Physical examination detected 75% of all tumors (which is higher than normally observed), but only 50% under two centimeters in size. Mammography detected 80% of the tumors two centimeters or smaller, but 27% of the detections were false positives. Thermography detected 88% including 85% under one centimeter, with only a 15% rate of false positives.

The following are important additional facts about thermography:[12]

❖ More than 800 peer-reviewed studies on breast thermography appear in the medical literature.

❖ Strict, standardized interpretation protocols have existed for at least the past 20 years.

❖ Thermography has an average 90% detection accuracy, with only a 10-15% false positive rate.

❖ While a first order of family history of breast cancer is a significant future risk indicator, an abnormal thermogram is 10 times more significant.

❖ An abnormal thermogram is associated with a higher risk of breast cancer by a factor of 22.

❖ An abnormal breast thermogram is the single most significant marker of high risk for the development of breast cancer.

❖ Infrared thermography can detect the first signs of pre-cancerous development up to 10 years in advance of any other diagnostic procedure.

❖ Clinical studies that span at least 40 years have shown that breast thermography contributes to the long-term survival rates by as much as 61%.

❖ When thermography is used in conjunction with a clinical examination and mammography, 95% of early-stage cancers can be detected.

To locate a certified practitioner of thermography, visit www.breastthermography.com or www.iact-org.org, the International Academy of Clinical Thermography. Also see www.thermology online.org/breast_thermography_clinics.htm.

■ ***Magnetic Resonance Spectroscopy***. Following the detection of a breast abnormality by a various means including a mammogram or MRI, a needle biopsy is typically performed—which has been the gold standard method of differentiating malignant from non-malignant tumors. However, about 80%

of breast tumors are benign, which means most biopsies are unnecessary—a determination that's made after the fact. A new diagnostic technique accurately differentiates malignant from non-malignant breast tumors by providing biochemical information about the tissues being examined. Called Proton Magnetic Resonance Spectroscopy (^{1}H MRS; also called the 3.0 Tesla MRI), the test is able to detect elevated levels of choline compounds which are present in cancerous tumors. Although MRIs are able to detect breast abnormalities proficiently, they have a high rate of false positives. When MRS is added to the MRI, the evaluation reduces the number of false positives by over 50% while being extremely accurate in diagnosing malignancy. As of spring 2009, the MRS is not widely available in the U.S.

■ ***Ultrasound***. A diagnostic technique on the horizon may also be able to replace biopsies as the means of differentiating between cancerous and non-cancerous breast tumors, as does Magnetic Resonance Spectroscopy. Scientists at Duke University have been working on a system that uses ultrasound waves to differentiate between malignant and benign tumors. Tissues have different mechanical properties in terms of their elasticity and recovery time when acted upon by sound waves such as those produced by ultrasound. Sophisticated analyses determine whether the tissue is cancerous or benign. If this technique proves viable, it would be another replacement of invasive biopsies as a means of evaluating tumors.

Aside from being painful and stress producing, many enlightened physicians believe needle biopsies provide a path for cancer cells to traverse, whereas without the biopsy the cancer would have been contained. This is true for tumor biopsies in other locations of the body. If an evaluation could be made with soundwaves, this would be a significant medical step forward and a boon to everyone—except the laboratories that perform the biopsies. Whether or not this test ever comes to fruition, there already exists a non-invasive blood test that easily and accurately determines the presence of cancer within the body—the AMAS test.

■ ***The AMAS Test***. For years, husband and wife team Samuel Bogoch (BO-Gosh), M.D., Ph.D. and

Eleanor Bogoch, M.D., both of the Boston University School of Medicine, were in search of a less harmful, less invasive technique for the early detection of cancer. In 1974, the Bogoch's isolated *a new antigen located on most (if not all) malignant cancer cells*. They called this antigen "malignin." (An antigen is a substance the body recognizes as foreign, in this case a protein. Thereafter, the body mounts a response to the antigen by producing *antibodies* which attack the invaders.)

Dr. Samuel Bogoch, a Harvard-trained neurochemist, discovered that the outer coating of cancer cells contains sugar molecules covering an inner layer of glycoprotein. As cancer cells bump into each other, this outer layer is worn off, exposing the inner protein layer as well as the *malignin* antigen. The body perceives the malignin as foreign, and mounts a defense against the antigen, producing *anti-malignin antibodies* (AMAs). The Bogoch's devised a test to measure these anti-malignin antibodies, which they call the Anti-Malignin Antibody in Serum, or AMAS. Their Boston-based company is Oncolab, Inc.

The Drs. Bogoch worked for seven years before demonstrating that malignin is related to *most all cancer cell types and locations*, not just various select types and locations of infection. Therefore, the AMAS test detects both common and uncommon varieties of cancers throughout the body, including cancers of the anus, brain, breast, cervix, colon, esophagus, kidney, lung, ovary, prostate, skin, stomach, testes, thyroid, urethra, and uterus.[13] Classifications of malignancies detected include fibrosarcoma, hemangioblastoma, leimyosarcoma , leukemia, liposarcoma, lymphoma, melanoma, mesothelioma, and osteogenic sarcoma.

AMAS measures a well-defined antibody whose serum levels rise early in the course of the disease, as opposed to other standard tests such as CEA which measures a less well-defined antigen whose blood serum levels tend to be inconsistent and rise primarily in the latter disease stages. In cases where sera is evaluated *twice within a 24-hour period*, the false positive (test inaccurately indicates positive) and false negative (test inaccurately indicates negative) rates are less than 1%.

This means the AMAS test is 99% accurate when sera is evaluated in this manner. When only one AMAS is evaluated, the accuracy rate drops to 95% or greater—a result which has been demonstrated on more than 6,000 patients. When sera is stored (frozen) for more than 24-hours, false positives are 5% and false negatives 7%.[14] More than 95% of patients with malignancies have AMAS levels higher than 135 micrograms per milliliter (mcg/ml). If the AMAS is below 135 mcg/ml, either the patient has no malignancy, or the disease is in remission.

In some cases, detection of malignancies is as early as 1-19 months in advance of any other clinical signs of disease. Dr. William Friend of the Friend Foundation of Seattle, Washington believes AMAS "can detect cancer cells so early that your doctor may not be able to find it."[15] On the other hand, because the production of the anti-malignin antibody often fails during the latter stages of the disease, AMAS is an accurate diagnostic aid *only during the early course of the disease* when plentiful antibodies are being produced.

It follows that AMAS will test negative when: 1) there is no malignancy detected, 2) the disease is in the latter stages of malignancy, no AMA is being produced and is therefore undetectable, and 3) the malignancy has been treated successfully with no remaining evidence of disease. In 96% of patients, AMAS normalizes upon remission.[16]

In 1990 a study was published in the *Proceedings of the American Association for Cancer Research*[17] which is indicative of the typical results produced by the AMAS test. A group of patients with suspicious mammograms was evaluated with the AMAS test, as well as four other tumor markers: CEA, CA 15-3, CA 19-9 and CA 125. The control group consisted of 154 healthy women whose average AMAS was 77 mcg/ml. Three of the control patients had a positive AMAS of >135 mcg/ml. Subsequently, one of these patients was diagnosed with *in situ* cancer of the cervix, another had basal cell (skin) cancer, and the third had ulcerative colitis with no malignancy. The experimental group consisted of 20 patients with biopsy-positive breast cancer whose average AMAS was 220 mcg/ml. The study detected 95% of the malignancies in this group, compared to zero percent for the CEA marker, 11% for CA 15-3, 5% for CA 19-9 and 16% for CA 125.

Another representative study found that of 118 patients who were evaluated with AMAS, 21 patients showed elevated levels >135 mcg/ml—all of whom were documented to have cancer. AMAS was negative in the remaining 97 patients. In 56 patients who were undergoing treatment for cancer, 94.1% showed a response to treatment as indicated by AMAS levels returning to normal.[18]

Screening. With a 95-99% accuracy rate, AMAS is a front runner in the early detection of malignancy. Because it's inexpensive, accurate and easy to perform, at times such tests as the CT and X-ray might be required only following a positive indication on the AMAS.

Monitoring. After a course of treatment, patients can be monitored effectively using the AMAS. Following surgery, for example, it can be determined whether or not all of the cancerous cells have been removed. If malignant cells were missed, the AMAS will remain positive following surgery. Also, at any time following surgery, a patient's status can be assessed effectively.

Differential Diagnosis. A common clinical situation involves a questionable or inconclusive diagnosis obtained by an X-ray, CT or other diagnostic tool. For example, if an X-ray shows a shadow or a CT shows a spot on the lung, liver or kidney that may or may not be malignant, or if a PSA is significantly elevated, how does modern medicine determine an invasive biopsy, AMAS est is a relatively definitive measure of malignancy.

AMAS data were presented at a Proceedings of the Association for Cancer Research showing that, in general, the anti-malignin antibody level rises with age, as the body apparently attempts to offer more protection as risk factors increase. Also, higher-risk populations have increased levels of AMA. In both cases, the AMA rise is significantly lower than in cases of malignancy.

Supporters of the AMAS test believe it should be used routinely as an annual cancer screening tool for all adults, beginning as early as age 35, particularly if there is a family history of cancer. Also, Dr. Samuel Bogoch believes it will be possible to develop a vaccine either by active immunization with a malignin derivative, or passively with the anti-malignin antibody.

There are two separate expenses related to the AMAS test. Oncolab provides free of charge an *AMAS Cancer Test Kit* which can be shipped directly to the customer. They charge USD $135

to evaluate the blood sample (for anti-malignin antibodies) which is returned to them by your local lab drawing the blood. There is also the additional charge of having the blood drawn (and prepared according to a specific protocol, described below) by your local lab.

Because the AMAS test is not a routine, off-the-shelf procedure such as the PSA, there are two ways to best locate a laboratory in your area that would be able to withdraw the blood sample and prepare it according to Oncolab's special protocol: 1) Call Oncolab at (800)922-8378 to inquire whether there is a lab in your area familiar with their procedure. If there are none, they will supply a protocol to a local lab in your area that can draw the blood and prepare it for shipment to Oncolab; or 2) Contact the American College for Advancement in Medicine (ACAM) for a list of alternative/complementary medical practitioners in your area who may use the test in their clinical practice. Call (800)532-3688 or visit www.acam.org.

In contrast to the preceding positive comments regarding the AMAS test, some physicians who have used the test in clinical practice have complained it suffers from a higher level of false positives and false negatives than has been reported in the literature. Could this be accounted for by improper administration of the test? Because this doubt has been cast upon the level of accuracy of the AMAS, if cost is not a factor and the likely area of cancerous involvement is defined, it is advisable to receive an evaluative scan using the highest technology apparatus available as of spring 2009—the 3.0 Tesla MRI Spectroscopy scanner, which is available at some large U.S. hospitals.

■ **_Breath Test_**. A new, high-tech twist on an ancient idea is making inroads in the diagnosis of diseases, including cancer. Medical practitioners have known since the time of the ancient Greek physician Hippocrates that the aroma of human breath can provide insights into the diagnosis of many disease states. Experienced practitioners have recognized such abnormal aromas as a sweet, fruity odor in patients with uncontrolled diabetes; the musty, fishy smell of advanced liver disease; the ammonia-like smell that's associated with kidney failure, and so forth.

The French nobleman Antoine Lavoisier, known as the father of modern chemistry, was the first to analyze breath in the eighteenth century. Chemists developed breath tests for alcohol and acetone in the nineteenth century. The brilliant scientist and two-time Nobel Prize winner Dr. Linus Pauling analyzed compounds contained within the breath by gas chromatography, and discovered that human breath contains many different volatile organic compounds (VOCs) in very low concentrations. Today it is known that the human breath contains more than 200 VOCs, mostly in infinitesimal quantities of about one part per trillion. It is now known that some of these breath VOCs are markers of disease states.

Researchers at Menssana Research of Newark, New Jersey, have developed a portable *breath collection apparatus* (BCA) which can collect breath samples at virtually any location. The person whose breath is being analyzed breathes into the BCA for two minutes while it captures breath VOCs onto a small sorbent trap which looks like a stainless steel cigarette. This trap is then sent to the laboratory for analysis by gas chromatography and mass spectroscopy. Each analysis usually identifies more than 200 different VOCs. The device also collects a sample of the room air which is subtracted from the breath VOCs.

The BCA has identified a new and comprehensive set of markers of oxidative stress known as the *breath methylated alkane contour* (BMAC). Changes in the BMAC reveal distinctive changes in a number of different diseases, each of which can be identified with its own unique "breath fingerprint." The goal of the test is to identify diseases in their earliest and most treatable stages.

Menssana Research's breath test is currently being evaluated in several clinical studies for its ability to diagnose lung and breast cancer as well as other medical conditions including heart transplant rejection, kidney disease, ischemic heart disease, and diabetes mellitus. Some day in the not-to-distant future this test may become as commonplace as a blood test or X-ray. To learn more about Menssana Research's BCA, visit www.menssanaresearch.com.

Stopping Metastasis. Most cancers in and of themselves are not lethal when restricted to a localized growth. They can expand in size by invading surrounding tissue, but this is not typically life-threatening unless a primary organ is affected and the progression of the disease can't be stopped. It is only when cancerous cells spread to other parts of the body, particularly the vital organs such as the brain, lungs or liver, that cancer becomes a killer. The process whereby cancer cells travel from the initial site of origin to invade other parts of the body is referred to as *metastasis*. (Meta = after; stasis = equilibrium; i.e., the cancer is no longer stable.) Almost two decades ago Dr. H.V. Honn, writing in the journal *Science*,[19] stated that metastasis is the principal cause of failure in curing human cancers.

The two main vehicles through which cancer cells spread to distant areas of the body are:

❋ The lymphatic system, wherein malignant cells can spread to both local and distant lymph nodes.
❋ The bloodstream, wherein cancerous cells can detach from the tumor site of origin, travel throughout the body and invade any organ—thus seeding a new growth. Cancerous cells bind to cells on the outer membrane (vascular endothelium) of healthy organs, and in time penetrate to the interior of the target organ.

Several known methods exist which have a significant capability of preventing the spread of most/all types of life-threatening cancer. For those diagnosed with cancer in any location throughout the body, it would be prudent and potentially lifesaving to employ the following strategies:

■ ***Strategy #1: Preventing Adhesion with Modified Citrus Pectin.*** Throughout the past several decades, researchers have studied various substances which have shown at least some degree of anti-metastatic capability. It has been discovered that malignant cells which shed from a primary tumor site *have a particular "stickiness" that allows them to adhere to the cell walls of distant organs.* This is related to the ability of the blood to clot (coagulate). Therefore, various anticoagulants have been studied in an attempt to reverse this process. Anticoagulants are substances which reduce the thickening/clotting ability of blood.

Some of the anticoagulants researchers have evaluated include: heparin,[20] warfarin,[21] prostacyclin,[22] qian-hu,[23] trigramin,[24] antistasin,[25] and mo-ehr.[26] While some of these substances hold promise for further research, another approach to preventing metastasis is gaining momentum. In this approach, the stickiness which leads to clumping of individual cancer cells is directly targeted.

The Sticky Culprit Identified. In order for cancers to spread, it has been suggested that clumps of cells are likely required rather than a single cell or several individual cells.[27] The ability of cancer cells to clump together is thought to be controlled largely by a specialized protein known as *galectin*, specifically *galectin-3*. Galectin molecules occupy receptor sites on the surfaces of many cancer cells types, including cancers of the breast, colon, prostate, as well as glialblastoma, laryngeal epidermoid carcinoma, lymphoma and melanoma.[28] It is this compound that is thought to be the sticky, glue-like substance which allows malignant cells to adhere to each other, as well as to normal cells of the blood vessels and vital organs distant from the primary site of origin.[29]

Human studies of colon, stomach and thyroid cancers have shown that as the cancers progress from the initial to the most advanced stages, the presence of galectin increases proportionally. Researchers believe that higher galectin levels permit increased adhesion and clumping of the cancer cells to each other and to potential sites of metastasis.[30] Also, it has been observed that metastasized cells have significantly more galectin-3 than tumor cells at the primary site of origin.[31]

Citrus Pectin & Modified Citrus Pectin. Citrus pectin is a (branched-chain) carbohydrate found in most plants, but especially in the peel and pulp of citrus fruits—and particularly in apples, grapefruit, lemons, oranges, plums, and tangerines. Pectin is used as a thickening agent in the pharmaceutical, cosmetic and food industries. It is citrus pectin that puts the gel in jellies. This form of pectin serves mostly as a bulking agent, and the stomach's digestive enzymes do little to break it down.

Modified citrus pectin (MCP), on the other hand, is citrus pectin that has been modified (by heating and modifying the pH) by breaking down the long branched chains into shorter non-branched segments, with a reduced molecular weight. These smaller, less complex molecules dissolve more readily in water, and are more completely absorbed by the micro-villi of the intestines allowing them to pass directly into the bloodstream, and then to the entire body.[32] For thousands of years Chinese medicine has used boiled tangerine peel (Qing Pi) as a cancer treatment. Even though the specific mechanisms of action were unknown at the time, the treatment apparently was effective, as it is used even to this day.[33]

How Modified Citrus Pectin Works.[34] Modified citrus pectin contains particularly large amounts of the sugar *galactose* (galactosides and galactosyl residues). The sticky galectin-3 molecules have a pronounced affinity (attraction) for galactose, and bind with it within the bloodstream and lymph. Researchers believe this binding process of galactose with galectin-3 blocks (inhibits) the cancerous cells from being able to adhere to each other and to other sites throughout the body. Because the malignant cells are isolated—without being able to clump together to form colonies—they eventually atrophy and are eliminated from the body. While MCP may not be able to stop cancerous cells from detaching from the original host site, it does inhibit the chemical footholds needed to colonize other organs.

Supporting Clinical Research (in chronological order):

❏ In a 1992 article published in the *Journal of the National Cancer Institute*,[35] researchers studied the effects of MCP on lung colonization of human B16-F1 melanoma cells in laboratory mice. Injection of MCP decreased metastases by over 90%. Those mice not receiving MCP had an increase in tumor colonies as much as 300%. The study concluded that MCP may lead to a reduced ability to form emboli (tumor particles circulating in the bloodstream) as well as metastasis.

❏ A 1995 study published in the *Journal of the National Cancer Institute*[36] marked the first evaluation of the effectiveness of orally-administered MCP in living systems. In this animal study, MCP was given in the drinking water to rats injected with one million prostate-tumor cells (MAT-LyLu). One group received no MCP; another 0.1% MCP (wt/vol); the third received 1.0% MCP. Ninety-four percent of the group receiving no MCP developed metastases, compared to only

50% of the MCP-treated group. Additionally, the 1% MCP group developed an average of only one tumor colony in the lungs compared to nine colonies in the non-MCP-treated group. The researchers concluded that the oral intake of MCP acts as a potent inhibitor of spontaneous prostate carcinoma metastasis in the animal model studied.

❏ It was reported in 1995 that human cancer cell lines including prostate adenocarcinoma cells, breast carcinoma cells, melanoma cells, and laryngeal epidermoid carcinoma cells showed significantly reduced adhesion to an endothelial base *in vitro* with the use of MCP.[37]

❏ In a study presented at the *International Conference of Diet and Prevention of Cancer*[38] in Tampere, Finland in 1999, researchers at the Prostate Cancer Research Institute in Los Angeles evaluated the ability of MCP to influence Prostate Specific Antigen (PSA) scores in men with prostate cancer. Seven patients participating in the study had either relapsed or failed previous treatment for prostate cancer. PSAs ranged between 0.63 and 7.5. All patients were orally administered MCP (PectaSol®, Econugenics, Inc., San Rafael, CA) at the dosage of 15 grams per day in three divided doses. In 57% of the patents there was a 30% lengthening of PSA doubling time (a standard measure of disease progression. Lengthening of the doubling time represents a slowing of the disease progression); one patient had a partial response; one patient's disease stabilized; and one patient did not respond. Researchers concluded that administration of MCP significantly slowed the PSA doubling time in prostate cancer patients having low levels of PSA. Additionally, it was compelling that all patients were still living three years after study completion.

Also presented at the Conference was an *in vitro* assessment of the cytotoxicity of MCP on PC-3 prostate cancer cell lines. At a 0.1% concentration, the cytotoxic effect was 76.9%; it was 80.7% at the 1.0% concentration; with a corresponding 3.8% cytotoxicity for the control group.[39]

❏ In 2000 a study examining the size and weight of tumor reduction in colon-25 tumors implanted in mice was published in *Alternative Medical Review*.[40] The animals were administered MCP either 0.8 mg/ml (low dose) or 1.6 mg/ml (high dose) on a daily basis beginning about a week after implantation. The low-dose group had a 38% reduction in tumor size, while the high-dose group had a 70% reduction. This was the first evidence that MCP reduces solid primary tumor growth.

❏ A 2001 study reported in the *Journal of Cancer Research and Clinical Oncology*[41] defined the gene expression pattern of all presently-known human galectins in tumor cell lines of various origin. The presence of human galectins-1, -2, -3, -4, -7, -8, and -9 was determined by RT-PCR analysis in a panel of 61 different human tumor cell lines originating from brain, breast, colon, kidney, lung, skin, urogenital and hematopoietic system. Galectin-8 expressed a presence in 59 of the panel of 61 cell lines. (Galectin-8 is thought to be associated with suppressor activity.) Galectin-1 and -3 were frequently expressed (with differences between individual cases) throughout the panel of cell lines with the exception of the tested lung tumors. The expression of galectin-2 and -4 was confined to a significant portion of colorectal and neural tumors. The presence of galectin-9 was restricted to colorectal carcinoma cell lines with the same incidence as that of galectin-4.[42]

❏ Wayne State researchers studied tumor growth, angiogenesis (formation and growth of blood vessels), and metastasis *in vivo* in mice fed MCP in their drinking water and injected with human breast carcinoma cells (MDA-MB-435). Also, galectin-3-mediated functions *in vitro* were studied by assessing the effect of MCP on capillary tube formation by human umbilical vein endothelial cells (HUVECs) in Matrigel. It was found that *in vitro*, MCP inhibited the growth of capillary tube formation in a dose-dependent manner (i.e., the higher the dose, the more pronounced the effect, and vice versa.) At concentrations of 0.1%, MCP inhibited the binding of galectin-3 to HUVECs by 72.1%; concentrations of 0.25% MCP inhibited the binding by 95.8%. *In vivo*, tumor growth, angiogenesis and metastasis were statistically significantly reduced in mice receiving oral MCP. These data suggest the importance of dietary carbohydrate compounds (MCP) as agents relevant to the treatment and prevention of cancer.[43]

❏ At the National Institute for Cellular Biotechnology of the Dublin City University, Ireland, researchers investigated the significance of galectin-3 in human (non-small cell) lung (DLKP) and nasal carcinoma cells. Galectin-3 over-expression resulted in three findings: 1) increased adhesion to extracellular matrix components, 2) cell motility, and 3) *in vitro* invasiveness in both lung and nasal tumor cells.[44]

❏ To evaluate the potential contribution of galectin-1 and -3 to colon malignancy, 67 colonic surgical resections were studied at the Laboratory of Gastroenterology, Erasmus Hospital, Brussels, Belgium. Ten normal resections, 10 mild dysplasias, 10 severe dysplasias and 37 cancers were evaluated. Galectin-1 and -3 were expressed in varying amounts in the epithelial cells and connective tissue of the normal colons. As the degree of dysplasia increased, there was found a corresponding significant increase in galectin-1 and -3 expression, suggesting that galectin-1 and -3 are related to malignant disease progression.[45]

❏ The data from a Phase II human clinical trial using MCP to prevent biological recurrence of prostate cancer was reported in 2003 in the journal *The Prostate*. Twelve patients were enrolled in the study after their PSA began to rise following treatment to eliminate the primary tumor. Patients were administered 15 grams of MCP (Pecta Sol,® EcoNugenics, Santa Rosa, CA) in three divided doses per day for a one year period. Nine of the 12 patients, 75%, had a statistically significant response, while another patient experienced a 78% lengthening of the progression. Six of the 12 patients more than doubled their PSA doubling times, with an increase in doubling times varying between 129-941%. Two additional patients experienced a decrease in their PSA values.

The decrease in PSA values for these two subjects was unexpected, and could not be accounted for by previously-outlined mechanisms of action of MCP—inhibiting metastasis and emboli formation. Only destruction or inhibition of the active tumor site could produce this result, it has been postulated. Also, reduction in PSA values occurred soon after administration of the MCP began, a further possible sign of MCP's direct action on the active tumor. Galectin-3 is believed to be involved in angiogenesis. It is possible that galectin-3 acts as an anti-angiogenesis agent.[46]

Two additional studies are relevant to this discussion:

♦ U.S. and Swedish researchers have modified galectin-3 by removing the key part of the molecule that allows cell-to-cell adhesion. The modified molecule also occupies sites on cell surfaces blocking normal galectin-3 from binding. The modified galectin protein decreased the number of mice developing metastatic tumors by over 50%. Only four of the mice injected with the modified protein had lymph node involvement, compared to 11 of the 20 control animals.[47] Could this research represent a new phase of the pharmaceutical industry's approach to anti-metastatic therapy?

♦ Researchers at the University of Michigan Medical School have shown the presence of a protein designated as RKIP (Raf kinase inhibitory protein) prevents the metastasis of prostate cancers. Lacking RKIP, tumor cells are more likely to enter the vascular system. RKIP was present at high levels in all ten samples of non-cancerous tissue evaluated, and at only slightly lower levels in all 12 of the non-metastatic tissue evaluated. The protein was completely absent in all 22 of the prostate metastatic tissue evaluated. Further, in a gene therapy approach designed to alter the amount of RKIP produced by cells, metastatic cancer cells that received additional RKIP showed a 48.5% decrease in their invasive ability. The invasive ability more than doubled in non-metastatic cells whose RKIP levels were artificially reduced. The researchers concluded that in prostate cancer cells, and possibly more generally, the presence of RKIP inhibits metastatic cells from invading nearby normal cells. Two new avenues of possibilities are, 1) RKIP or similarly-functioning molecules could be measured to determine the potential of a tumor to metastasize, and 2) gene therapy may one day replace RKIP, or its similarly-functioning counterparts, in RKIP-deficient cells so that metastasis to other, distant areas of the body can be prevented.[48]

Patents. Two patents have been issued relating to the use of modified citrus pectin in the treatment of cancer:

❖ Raz, A. and Pienta, K.J. *Method for Treatment of Cancer by Oral Administration of Modified Citrus Pectin.* United States Patent Number 5,895,784. Date of issuance: April 20, 1999.

❖ Eliaz, I. and McCulloch (EcoNugenics®). *Modified Citrus Pectin and Modified Alginates in the Control of Cancer Metastasis in Humans*. United States Patent Number 6,274,566. Date of issuance: August 14, 2001.

Method of Use. The evidence that modified citrus pectin is effective in inhibiting human cancer metastasis in many types of cancers is still in its infancy. Nevertheless, even the casual reader should be impressed with the weight of the present evidence. Especially because the substance is totally non-toxic at treatment levels, there seems only an upside to its use.

Many brands of modified citrus pectin are available in the marketplace. According to the research, the most effective form of this substance conforms to certain specifications. The molecular size must be small enough to be absorbed, but large enough to fulfill its binding function effectively. According to what is currently known, the most effective molecular weight ranges from about 10,000-20,000 kilodaltons (kD). Some marketed products have molecular weights in excess of 34,000 kD, or smaller than 8,000 kD. Also, the number of available binding sites is determined by the degree of methylation. The higher the degree of methylation, the fewer binding sites. Some marketed products have 50-70% methylation, while 10% is optimal. Near neutral pH is also considered optimal, while some products have pH values greater than 7 or less than 3.2.

PectaSol,® manufactured by EcoNugenics of Santa Rosa, CA, has a molecular weight ranging from 10,000-20,000 kD, is 10% methylated, and has a pH value of 6.3. This conforms to the research which has established the most effective treatment parameters. A refined version of PectaSol is PectaSol-C. An enzymatic process further lowers the molecular weight of pectin so that more reaches the bloodstream and is available to target more cancer cells. To order PectaSol or PectaSol-C, visit www.econugenics.com, or call (800)308-5518. Source Naturals and Now Foods also market PectaSol under license from EcoNugenics.

■ ***Strategy #2: Tissue Strengthening & Collagen-Dissolving Enzyme Blocking***. The body's cells can become damaged as the result of various influences. Some of these include the ingestion of toxic chemicals such as pesticides and food preservatives which are consumed in the diet. Pharmaceutical drugs also can damage cellular structures. In 1996, for example, the *Journal of the American Medical Association*[49] issued a warning that all cholesterol-lowering (statin) drugs being marketed at that time were carcinogenic, i.e., they could damage cells which in turn could become cancerous. Viral infection and exposure to radiation are other influences which also have the ability to damage cells, turning them malignant.

When cellular damage occurs, it often involves damage to the DNA, the cell's genetic software. If this occurs, it can trigger two processes that facilitate the inception of a cancerous growth:

1) *Uncontrolled cell multiplication*. The cell becomes reprogrammed to reproduce and multiply without restraint. This is the first step.[50]

2) *Mass production of collagen-dissolving enzymes*. The vastly increased number of cells begins to produce tissue-degrading enzymes which allow the malignant growth to spread. Without the production of these enzymes, the intact surrounding tissue would confine the cancer's growth.

The rate of spread of a primary cancerous growth, i.e., its aggressiveness, is a direct function of the amount of collagen-dissolving enzymes it produces.[51] Therefore, this mechanism plays a major role in the process of metastasis.

Tumors receive their nourishment from capillaries—the tiny blood vessels that surround the tumor mass. By means of collagen-dissolving enzymes, the cancer cells migrate their way into the capillaries which lead to the major blood vessels of the body. Once inside these vessels, the malignant cells can travel to remote locations where they can attach themselves, dissolve tissue, and gain access to other body parts or organs. As in the case of the primary tumor site, the more tissue-dissolving enzymes a specific cancerous cell line produces, the faster it is capable of spreading to other locations and forming secondary tumors.[52]

Stopping Cancer's Growth and Spread. In order to stop the progression of both the initial cancerous growth and the possibility of metastasis, two strategies have been put forward by the renowned German physician Dr. Matthias Rath : 1) strengthening the stability of normal, healthy tissues so that they provide a strong defense against the movement of cancerous cells, and 2) further preventing the offensive advance of cancer cells by preventing the collagen-dissolving enzymes from attaching to the anchor sites of the collagen.

Details of Dr. Rath's two protocols for blocking metastasis as well as the physiological processes by which cancer cells migrate through the cellular matrix of skin and other tissue are discussed in the section on **Herpes**. Although the discussion pertains to the herpes virus, it also applies to the method of migration used by cancer cells and other pathogens, as well as healthy cells. See especially *Cell Movement Within the Body; The Defense; Vitamin C, Lysine and Proline;* and *Crippling the Offense* in the **Herpes** section.

Therapeutic Success. Although only a limited number of studies have been performed using the collagen-blocking technique as a treatment against cancer, its results have been positive and dramatic. It is likely the technique will be successful on both hormone-independent and hormone-dependent types of malignancies, according to Dr. Rath.[53] Hormone-independent cancers include cancers of the colon, stomach, lung and skin, whereas hormone-dependent cancers include cancers of the breast, ovary and uterus.

As reported in *Acta Medica Scandinavica* in 1977, a Swedish research group from the University of Lund successfully treated a case of advanced, metastatic breast cancer using a lysine enzyme block. The medication used was tranexamic acid, a synthetic derivative of the natural amino acid lysine. Dr. Rath suggests that high doses of lysine will produce similar results as the synthetic, but with no side-effects. The journal article included the following:

> Secondary tumors were already developing in the brain of the patient with breast cancer. Radiation and chemotherapy were without results. While under the treatment with enzyme blocks the brain metastasis and other symptoms of the illness began to diminish. One year after the treatment the patient was free of complaints.[54]

Again in 1997, the same Swedish research group reported in the *Journal of the American Medical Association*[55] dramatic success in treating advanced, metastatic ovarian tumors using

lysine as an enzyme block. The tumors were encapsulated, and prevented from spreading.

In an obstetrics and gynecology journal in 1980, University of Tokyo researchers reported on the treatment of another case of ovarian cancer. The scientists concluded,

> The treatment was successful in a patient with advanced, inoperable ovarian cancer. The disease had already caused secondary tumors and fluid accumulation in the stomach. Even in this advanced stage the cancer was brought to a standstill with the help of enzyme block therapy...three years after the start of the treatment the patient had no more complaints.[56]

Why is it that so few studies have been performed using enzyme-block therapy, especially in light of the spectacularly-positive potential it offers to those suffering from cancer? The answer seems to be that, similar to the heart disease market, cancer and chemotherapeutic pharmaceutical drugs represent a huge profit potential for their manufacturers—in the neighborhood of USD $100 billion annually. Even if the patentable, synthetic analogs of lysine were to gain popularity, some in the know feel their use would likely bring about the end of the cancer industry.

Conclusion. For persons who have been diagnosed with cancer, whether it be of the hormone-dependent or hormone-independent variety—no matter what the stage of progress of the cancer—the use of both modified citrus pectin *and* enzyme blocking therapeutics should be seriously considered.

■ ***Tetracycline***. Prostate cancer is the most common type of cancer in men, and breast cancer is the most common type in women. Both of these cancer types have a tendency of spreading to bone, which is thereafter very difficult to treat. Traditionally, radiation therapy is used to treat bone cancer, which may help alleviate pain and slow tumor growth but also may destroy bone tissue.

In 1978, Dr. Gurmit Singh of the Hamilton Regional Cancer Centre in Ontario, Canada, discovered the common antibiotic *tetracycline* is effective both in preventing metastases from forming in bone, but also is able to kill bone tumor cells. In the mouse model, Dr. Singh's team found tetracycline reduced the spread of certain cancers to the bone by 70%, and in some ways improved and healed the bone.

The tetracycline family of broad-spectrum antibiotics includes tetracycline, *doxycycline*, and *minocycline*. For decades, tetracycline has been used to treat acne and periodontal disease. It is absorbed into both bone and teeth, where it inhibits *matrix metalloproteinase* (MMP), an enzyme which dissolves collagen and other proteins that bind cells together, allowing cancer to spread. Thus, by blocking the action of MMP, tetracycline helps prevent bone metastasis. The researchers also believe tetracycline slows the development and reduces the survival of bone-dissolving *osteoclast* cells.

■ ***Cimetadine***. Cimetadine, better known by its trade name Tagamet,® has been used for decades as an over-the-counter antacid to help manage heartburn/indigestion, now called gastroesophageal reflux disease (GERD). In the late 1980s, it was used as an anti-emetic to prevent and treat nausea and vomiting in cancer patients undergoing chemotherapy. Physicians noticed that patients taking cimetadine along with chemotherapy had significantly increased survival rates compared with those only receiving chemotherapy. Although several mechanisms of action responsible for this effect have been proposed, cimetadine has been shown to help prevent metastasis by blocking the adhesion of certain types of cancer cells. Therefore, in addition to the two general anti-metastasis strategies discussed above, the use of cimetadine deserves consideration, particularly in the case of certain types of cancers.

In a 1988 randomized, placebo-controlled study, 181 patients with gastric (stomach) cancer received either 400 mg of cimetadine twice daily or a placebo for two years. Patients taking cimetadine had a significantly increased survival rate compared to the placebo group.[57] In a 1994 study reported in the *Lancet*,[58] colorectal cancer patients taking 400 mg of cimetadine twice daily for five days preoperatively and intravenously for two days postoperatively experienced a decrease in the three-year mortality rate from 41% to 7%. The cimetadine group also showed an increase in immune response, as indicated by increased tumor infiltration of lymphocyte white blood cells.

In a 2002 study reported in the *British Journal of Cancer*,[59] the results of a colon cancer study conducted by 15 Japanese clinics were examined. All patients initially had surgical removal of their colorectal tumors followed by intravenous chemotherapy. Thereafter, the patients were divided into two groups, one receiving chemotherapy only (200 mg of fluorouracil daily for one year), while the other received the same chemotherapy treatment plus 800 mg of oral cimetadine daily for one year. Eighty-five percent of the cimetadine group survived for 10 years compared to only 50% of the control group not taking cimetadine.

In addition to helping prevent metastasis, cimetadine has been shown to boost immune function, inhibit angiogenesis (the formation of tumor blood vessels), and increase apoptosis (cell death) of cancer cells. Additional studies have confirmed the increased survivability conferred by cimetadine use in malignant glioma brain tumor patients, as well as other possible applications for breast, esophageal, skin, liver, and pancreatic cancers.

Treatment Methods. If the moment ever comes that you or a loved one is given the unpleasant news of being diagnosed with cancer, it's difficult just to think clearheadedly, not to mention embarking on a comprehensive research project to determine what method(s) of treatment might be best for a particular type/location of cancer. Because of this, coupled with the life-threatening nature of the disease, there is usually a heightened willingness on the part of the patient and family members to turn the treatment recommendations over to "the experts,"—their doctor(s)—and rely totally on *someone else's* decisions. Although this is perfectly understandable, it may not be the best course of action in achieving the desired goal of long-term healing and wellness for the afflicted person.

Western medicine has gained little ground in its battle against cancer. Although the "war" on cancer has been waged for decades, its ability to heal many/most types of cancers in the long term is *not* what we would hope for ourselves or those closest to us. Traditional, allopathic medicine offers a three-pronged approach to cancer treatment: surgery, radiation, and chemotherapy—and often various combinations of the three.

■ **_Surgery_**. The approach of surgery attempts to remove the cancerous growth from the body, with the hope that all of the malignancy can be identified and removed. Although surgery is the most invasive of the three traditional approaches, it's sometimes useful in removing a growth that is immediately life threatening, or possibly in preparation for a more effective, long-term treatment—as they say, to "buy some time." However, the overall, long-term success rate for surgery of a *primary* cancer—a cancer that has *not yet metastasized*—is about 10-15%.[60] Once cancer metastasizes, surgery's only hope is to provide some palliative, short-term benefit. Of the three traditional approaches however, surgery alone, without chemo and/or radiation, accounts for most of the long-term successes.[61]

The negative side-effects of cancer surgery include infection, immune suppression, and complications with anesthesia. However, the most significant problem with the surgical removal of cancer is that *the procedure itself—in about 20% of surgical patients—stimulates the growth of dormant micrometastatic lesions* which already exist in different locations.[62] Upon removal of a primary tumor, two substances secreted by the tumor itself that help control metastasis—*endostatin* and *angiostatin*—are significantly reduced. The reduction of these substances, along with the considerable immune suppression that typically accompanies surgery, helps explain why the surgical removal of cancer has been unable to meaningfully prolong the lives of most cancer patients.

The pre- and postoperative administration of endostatin and angiostatin is currently being evaluated in clinical trials. It's likely the success rate of surgery will increase if these drugs are approved for use. Anti-metastatic drugs currently in use are sometimes helpful in preventing the postoperative spread of malignant cells. As described above, the use of Modified Citrus Pectin and Tissue Strengthening and Collagen-Dissolving Enzyme Blocking could provide significant benefit if used in advance of metastisis and following the removal of a primary malignancy. Other substances which may be useful in this regard—to help prevent new blood vessel formation in secondary tumors—are curcumin, green tea extract, quercetin, resveratrol, selenium, and vitamin D_3.

■ **_Radiation Therapy_**. Approximately 60% of all cancer patients in the U.S. receive radiation (radio) therapy. The goal of radiotherapy is to trigger programmed cell death (apoptosis), and/or to prevent the malignant cells from replicating. This is accomplished by damaging the cancer cells' DNA by the powerful ionizing radiation which generates massive amounts of free radicals within the cells. Several techniques of radiation therapy are currently practiced, including 1) External Beam Therapy (EBT), 2) Intensity-Modulated Radiation Therapy (IMRT), 3) Gamma Knife, 4) CyberKnife (for the treatment of tumors anywhere in the body. Visit www.accuray.com), 5) Proton Beam, 6) Seeding techniques (implantation), and 7) Intravenous administration of "liquid radiation," such as the pharmaceutical drug Bexxar.®

Even though these protocols endeavor to use only the minimum amount of radiation necessary—some less than others—as discussed earlier in this section, ionizing radiation is believed by some researchers to be a/the major cause of cancer and ischemic heart disease. Also, radiation therapy can cause 1) significant damage to normal, healthy cells, causing debilitating physical symptoms such as the inability to swallow, with subsequent weight loss, 2) the development of secondary diseases such as pneumonitis and radiation fibrosis, 3) both acute and delayed disturbances in the patient's nutritional status, and 4) the development of secondary cancers.[63]

■ **_High-Intensity Focused Ultrasound_**. In the same manner a magnifying glass can focus the energy of sunlight into a single point of intense heat, High-Intensity Focused Ultrasound (HIFU) uses focused sound energy to kill cancerous tissues with heat. HIFU raises the temperature of cancer cells to 175-212 degrees Fahrenheit (80-100 degrees Celcius) in about one second without damaging tissue surrounding the targeted area. The sound energy of HIFU can not travel through gas or bone, and therefore requires a direct path to the tumor site through tissue or fluid.

Although the first use of HIFU on humans took place in 1992 at Indiana University School of Medicine, as of early 2009 the technique is still considered "experimental" in the U.S. and is used only in clinical trials for investigational purposes to treat prostate cancer. The procedure is approved for use in Asia, Canada, the Carribian, Central America, Europe, and Mexico. In Europe, HIFU is used to treat prostate and other soft tissue cancers such as liver and pancreatic cancers. In China, it has been used with great success to treat more than 3,000 patients with liver and pancreatic cancers. Cancerous tissues the size of a small orange can be ablated. HIFU offers an alternative for patients too ill to undergo conventional surgery. It does not use radiation; can be used for repeated treatments; can be used in conjunction with other therapies; and shortens hospital stays. For more information, visit http://panamhifu.com.

■ *Chemotherapy*. Chemotherapy is prescribed to approximately 80% of all cancer patients in the U.S. This approach utilizes one or more cytotoxic drugs—administered orally or intravenously (IV)—in an attempt to shrink a tumor at its primary site, slow tumor growth, and destroy malignant cells that may have metastasized. These drugs typically function by destroying (poisoning) cancer cells at specific stages in their growth cycle.

Unfortunately, as they circulate systemically throughout the body, conventionally-administered chemotherapeutic drugs—which are typically prescribed in high doses as opposed to low-dose chemotherapy discussed below—are also toxic to healthy cells. This typically causes debilitating symptoms which may include hair loss; loss of appetite with attendant weight loss; nausea and vomiting; sores in the mouth and throat; and immune system suppression. Not unlike radiation, chemotherapy can cause secondary cancers even several years after treatment, including cancer of the bone marrow and lymph nodes.

A revealing study on the ineffectiveness of chemotherapy drugs was published in the journal *Clinical Oncology*[64] in 2004. Australian researchers searched the medical literature in both Australia and the U.S. in an effort to assess the effectiveness of chemotherapy on adult malignancies. The results of the study showed that the overall curative contribution of chemotherapy to the 5-year survival rates of adults was 2.3% in Australia and 2.1% in the U.S. (These results are so low they may not have been statistically significant, i.e., outside of the statistical margin of error of

the study. The researchers did not specify this.) The researchers concluded that "to justify the continued funding and availability of drugs used in cytotoxic chemotherapy, a rigorous evaluation of the cost effectiveness and impact on quality of life is urgently required."[65] Stated another way, the benefits of using chemotherapeutic drugs are so small in comparison to the significant reduction in the quality of life experienced by chemo patients, their use should be seriously questioned if not abandoned. For an expanded discussion on chemotherapy and to learn about a more effective method of using chemotherapy without the typical side-effects, see *Insulin Potentiation Therapy* under **General Treatment Methods**.

With these weapons of mass cellular destruction and/or removal, the Western cancer establishment wages its War On Cancer. In the United States, the governmental agencies that comprise this establishment include the American Cancer Society (ACS), the American Medical Association (AMA), the National Cancer Institute (NCI), and the Food and Drug Administration (FDA). According to these agencies, mainstream medicine is curing 40-50% of cancer patients, and the prognosis is good when the malignancy is treated in its earliest stages, prior to metastasis.

Unfortunately, these statistics are often "massaged" in various ways, so that the traditional techniques of surgery, radiation, and chemotherapy are made to appear more effective than they truly are. Although this is *not* how we would like to view these agencies whose task it is to assist us in achieving a healthful and prolonged life, financial concerns play such a dominant role in the affairs of our modern world that the human side of the struggle often plays second fiddle to the more important concerns of bottom-line profitability of the very large industry that offers the bulk of cancer treatments, particularly in the United States.

According to several prominent cancer researchers,[66] the "books are cooked" on cancer statistics in various ways, including 1) misleading definitions of the word "cure." At its *best*, this word merely means survival beyond five years after treatment. Sometimes the term "response rate" is used interchangeably to misleadingly *imply* "cure rate," while its more accurate meaning is a 50% reduction in tumor size over a period of time, usually about one month. Tumor response rates are not synonymous with long-term survival. It doesn't take an oncologist to understand that whatever cancer remains will likely continue to grow between breaks in treatment, 2) by not including certain groups of people in the statistics, such as non-whites, 3) by deleting certain categories of cancers, such as lung cancer—the leading cause of cancer death in both American men and women, 4) by including non-lethal types of cancers such as non-malignant skin cancers, 5) by deleting patients from the statistics who die before study termination—and by various other deceptive means. Although this may be difficult for some to believe—as it challenges all that is right and decent about humanity—because the stakes are so high and the potential consequences so unforgiving, personal naiveté on the part of those who have this disease can be costly indeed.

In the U.S., 65-75% of all cancer patients are diagnosed *after the cancer has metastasized*.[67] Most honest physicians and medical researchers agree that the long-term survival rate of patients who have metastatic cancers treated by conventional methods is generally less than 1%,[68] with certain notable exceptions for specific cancers. For example, chemotherapy achieves its greatest successes in the treatment of Hodgkin's disease; acute lymphocytic leukemia; ovarian and testicular cancers; and some rare, mostly childhood cancers.[69] With these few exceptions, even in primary, non-metastatic cancers, the conventional methods of treatment—surgery, radiation, and chemotherapy—score very low in their ability to produce long-term survival. Although it's difficult to know with accuracy, the long-term survival rates are probably in the low single digits—only several percent.

Methods for the effective treatment of cancer are a controversial subject in some countries. In addition to surgery, chemotherapy, and radiation, governmental agencies may frown on the discussion and dissemination of what are labeled "unproven" treatment methods—particularly in the U.S. Of course, what *has* been proven is that the War On Cancer has been lost, and the "approved" treatments are largely ineffective for most cancers, with certain exceptions, as noted.

On the other hand, there is no lack of so-called "alternative" cancer treatments (i.e., treatments other than surgery, chemotherapy, and radiation) vying for recognition in the marketplace. Because of this, it's often difficult to identify the cream that's risen to the top—i.e., those treatments that are effective, and those that are *most* effective. Immediately following is a discussion of three most promising alternative treatments, all of which can be accomplished on an "in-home" basis, although preferably under the care of a medical professional. These treatments are: 1) Protocel Therapy, 2) Cesium High pH Therapy, and 3) Dr. Johanna Budwig's Flax Oil Therapy. Following the discussion of these three treatments is a further discussion of several "in-patient" techniques requiring more direct care and supervision either in a doctor's office or hospital.

It should be understood by the reader that the current discussion of cancer treatments by no means exhausts all of the information available either on these specific topics or the subject of cancer treatments in general. This, in fact, is part of the difficulty facing individuals with recently diagnosed cancer—an *information overload* which, to some, may seem insurmountable.

Nevertheless, unless we are prepared to surrender our decision-making capabilities to "the experts" and blindly accept their guidance in whatever direction it may lead—especially in light of the abysmal long-term success rate of the traditional approaches—one must be prepared to take personal responsibility for one's own state of health. This entails being an active partner in the decision-making process, which would include doing *at least* a minimum amount of independent investigation and study. If you are reading the words on this page, and understanding them, then you have the capability of spending several hours of your time investigating treatment options for yourself or a family member. After all, the life you save may be your own or that of a loved one.

Our goal in the several pages that follow is to point the reader in the direction of some of the most effective, promising "alternative" treatment methods, and to provide information on how to access additional details on both these as well as additional alternative therapies. It should be understood that each of the following therapies has detailed treatment protocols that *must be followed explicitly* in order to achieve the desired result.

Any variations or departures from the established protocol may render the method ineffective.

IMPORTANT: It should also be understood that in order to achieve the best possible outcome, it's often appropriate to use multiple treatment methods simultaneously—the coordination of which requires a considerable degree of medical expertise. Therefore, even if your plan of action includes "self-treatment" methods, any cancer treatment regimen is best planned with and carried out under the supervision of a competent holistic/integrative physician who is familiar with the treatments discussed in this section. To locate such a physician, contact the American College for Advancement in Medicine [(800)532-3688; www.acam.org] or the International College of Integrative Medicine (www.icimed). Even while under the care of a competent physician, however, it's always incumbent upon the patient to ask questions and make suggestions.

■ *Protocel® Therapy.* James Vincent Sheridan was born in a small Pennsylvania mining town in 1912. Even as a high school student, he prayed to be able to find a cure for cancer. While in high school, Sheridan began having a series of recurring dreams, the focus of which was a certain chemical formula. At the time, neither he nor anyone he knew was able to decipher the formula.

As a college student, Sheridan came face-to-face with the chemical formula that had been so prominent in his recurring dreams. It was listed in a large resource book relating to cancer and carcinogenic substances. This, apparently, was one piece of the puzzle. Then, in 1936, Sheridan had a profound dream that brought together several meaningful events of his life, including the formula. The dream "suggested the controlled altering of the pathway of energy flow and energy production"[70] within cells.

(An interesting aside is that many famous inventors throughout history have gleaned marvelous insights through dreams. One such man was Nikola Tesla—the true inventor of the radio and other ingenious devices—known as one of the most brilliant inventors ever to live. The infamous Albert Einstein was also an insightful dreamer.)

These prophetic events marked the beginning of Sheridan's lifelong study of the cause of cancer, and his search for a cancer cure, which ranged from the 1930s to the 1990s. Although he became a chemist and was employed by Dow Chemical Company, most of his research was done independently as time allowed. He eventually became a patent attorney and left Dow Chemical in 1946 to practice law. In the early 1950s he worked under a private grant at the Detroit Cancer Institute, where he further perfected his formula, known as Entelev® (and later, Cancell®), to consistently cure 80% of the cancerous mice he treated.

Sheridan understood that cancer cells thrive in a low oxygen, or *anaerobic*, environment, and obtain their energy from the fermentation of glucose—a process known as *glycolysis*. Some cells other than cancer cells are anaerobic, but all such cells are also abnormal and unhealthy. Normal, healthy cells, on the other hand, thrive in an *aerobic*, or oxygen-rich environment, and obtain their energy through the process of oxidation. In fact, the German biologist Dr. Otto Warburg was awarded the 1931 Nobel Prize in Physiology/Medicine for determining this very fact.

Because they obtain their energy primarily through glycolysis, cancerous cells are relatively more primitive in comparison to healthy cells, and possess a lower energy level than healthy cells in terms of the very small micro-voltages (electrical charge/potential) they carry. Sheridan came to realize that if the energy level of cancer cells could be decreased slightly, say, by 10-15%, they would degrade to an even more primitive level that would not support their life function. Hence, the cancerous cells would die, and thereafter be harmlessly eliminated from the body by normal excretory processes. At the same time, healthy cells would be unaffected by the slight lowering of their energy level—having energy to spare—and would continue to function normally.

Sheridan's product, currently called Protocel, accomplishes this slight lowering of cellular energy by interfering with the production of *adenosine triphosphate* (ATP),[71] the chemical manufactured in the cells' mitochondria that produces energy for the body's many metabolic reactions. Likewise, other anaerobic, unhealthy cells such as those present in other disease states such as arthritis, chronic fatigue, diabetes, high blood pressure, and viral infections, would likely be eliminated using this therapy.[72]

Throughout the years, Sheridan made many attempts to have Protocel investigated by the official medical establishment for efficacy as a cancer treatment. Needless to say, with his life's work and lifelong dream of a cancer cure on the line, he exerted maximum effort to bring his remedy to the world. Sadly, the story of Protocel is not unlike many other effective treatments of both the past and present that aren't given a fair chance in the marketplace. This suppression invariably takes many forms, both subtle and blatant. Although the details vary from instance to instance, the stories of such maligned products/treatments always bear an uncanny resemblance. The ultimate result is most often the same: the product is not allowed an opportunity to prosper in the open marketplace as a treatment for which it was designed and developed. Protocel is one such casualty.

Because it has not been (allowed to be) evaluated for efficacy by the FDA, Protocel is not marketed as a cancer treatment. It is currently sold over-the-counter as a cell cleanser. Persons interested in taking this product should review the detailed treatment protocol and other relevant information which can be found online at www.protocel.com; www.protocelglobal.com; www.cellremoval.com; and www.elonnamckibben.com. Also highly recommended is Tanya Harter Pierce's 80-page ebook on Protocel, or her softcover book *Outsmart Your Cancer*, either of which can be ordered at www.outsmartyourcancer.com. Both books discuss over a dozen case histories of patients using Protocel.

Protocel Therapy has been very effective against many forms of cancer, both primary and metastatic. It is simple to use, inexpensive, and easy to self-administer in the home setting. Protocel is a liquid preparation taken with water, juice, or other beverages. The Protocel formulation consists of the following ingredients: copper (4 mg); sodium (50 mg); potassium (20 mg); and a blend of tetrahydroxyquinone; rhodizonic acid; inositol; croconic acid; triquinoyl; pyro-catechol; leuconic acid (244 mg); and distilled water.

In the U.S., Protocel can be ordered online at www.protocel.com, or by calling Renewal and Wellness, LLC, at (888)581-4442. Orders outside the U.S. can be placed at www.protocelglobal.com, or by calling International Internet Services, Ltd. (in the Bahamas), at +41-1355-3777.

■ ***Cesium High pH Therapy***. Another approach to defeating both primary and metastatic cancers is the use of cesium, a soft, silver-gold, metallic chemical element. Cesium is the most electropositive of all the chemical elements, having the ability to give up more electrons than any other element. Although radioactive cesium 137 is used in the radiation treatment of cancer, the present therapy utilizes a *non-radioactive form* of cesium, either as a powder or a liquid preparation.

Non-radioactive cesium has been used in the treatment of cancer since the 1980s. Its use was pioneered by Aubrey Keith Brewer, Ph.D. (1893-1986), an American research physicist and pioneer cancer researcher. Dr. Brewer was a highly esteemed scientist who at one time held the position of Chief of the Mass Spectrometer and Isotope Division of the National Bureau of Standards (renamed the National Institute of Standards and Technology in 1988).

Dr. Brewer focused his studies on the physiology/physics of cell membranes. He noted that cancer cells function in an *acidic*—as opposed to an *alkaline*—environment. This is due to the cancer cells' fermentation of glucose, the principal means by which they produce energy. Lactic acid, the source of much of the pain associated with the disease, is produced as a byproduct of glucose fermentation and lowers the intracellular pH of the cancer cells, making them more acidic. (Cells maintain a delicate balance between acidity and alkalinity, referred to as the pH balance, which ranges from 0, the most acidic, to 14, the most alkaline.) Based on these facts, Brewer reasoned he could specifically destroy acidic cancer cells by increasing their alkalinity to the point they could no longer function, thereafter dying and being harmlessly excreted by the body. (He also found that cesium reduces the cellular uptake of glucose, the cancer cells' main source of nourishment.) Just how to target the acidic, malignant cells was Brewer's next insight.

Dr. Brewer demonstrated in his laboratory that cesium has an affinity for cancer cells, i.e., it is attracted to and readily absorbed through their cell walls. In fact, present-day chemotherapy uses a radioactive isotope of cesium as a cancer cell marker to indicate the degree of penetration of the chemotherapeutic agent into a tumor mass. Of the 118+ chemical elements presently known (which are listed in the Periodic Table of Elements), cesium is the most alkaline of them all. Therefore, cesium is able to perform a "search and destroy" mission on cancer cells. It first searches out the malignant cancer cells, and then destroys them by raising their pH level away from acidity toward alkalinity, to the point the (formerly) acidic cancer cells are no longer viable.

In the late 1970s, Brewer began a series of animal experiments at three American universities—initially using the second most alkalizing element, rubidium, and thereafter using cesium salts to destroy cancer cells. All of the trials showed that high pH therapy produced a rapid and effective destruction of malignant tumors in mice.[73] In 1981, he initiated a series of trials using cesium to treat terminal cancer patients who had exhausted all conventional forms of treatment and were given up for dead by their physicians. As reported in *Pharmacology Biochemistry and Behavior*[74] in 1984, all participants using this therapy "showed great success."

Dr. Brewer reported on one trial of 30 patients, stating that, "In each case the tumor masses disappeared. Also, all pains and effects associated with cancer disappeared within 12 to 36 hours,"[75] due to the cessation of lactic acid production. In another study of 50 terminal patients with metastatic cancer, pain in all 50 patients disappeared by the third day of treatment. Twenty five of the initial 50 participants survived beyond three years.[76] This is quite remarkable given the initial terminal prognosis of all the enrolled patients. Famed German physician and cancer researcher Dr. Hans Nieper also conducted clinical trials using cesium therapy on cancer patients. He reported great success using this type of therapy.[77]

This treatment method also has been shown particularly effective in quickly reducing the size of large tumor masses. Because it is able to rapidly relieve the pain associated with advanced states of malignancy, cesium therapy should be seriously considered as a treatment option in such cases.

Until recently, cesium was available only in the powdered form of cesium chloride which, due to potential toxic build up, was typically administered only under the supervision of a physician. It's currently available in liquid form as an ionic mineral solution of cesium chloride (which can be sprayed on and massaged into the skin in situations where the patient is unable to eat or retain food). The only precaution in taking cesium is that it is known to lower potassium levels. Because potassium is critically involved in many bodily processes, including healthy heart function, those taking cesium are advised to supplement with potassium, as well as having potassium blood levels monitored. Persons with cardiac problems are advised to take cesium only under the supervision of a physician. Cesium taken on an empty stomach may cause stomach upset or nausea.

A series of dramatic case histories can be read in *Outsmart Your Cancer*, mentioned above, available by calling (800)266-5564, or by accessing www.outsmartyourcancer.com. Additional, must-read information is available at www.newswithviews.com/howenstine/james14.htm; www.mwt.net/~drbrewerhighpH.htm; www.mwt.net~drbrewer/brew_art.htm (where you can order Dr. Brewer's books, *High pH Cancer Therapy with Cesium*, and *Cancer: Its Nature and a Proposed Treatment*); www.mwt.net/~drbrewer/intro.htm; or by reading Kathleen Deoul's 2001 book *Cancer Cover-Up*. Liquid ionic cesium can be purchased online at www.essense-of-life.com, or by calling (800)760-4947.

An additional approach to increasing the alkalinity of cancer cells is put forth by Italian oncologist Dr. Tullio Simoncini. Simoncini maintains that cancer is a fungus, and can be destroyed by increasing its pH by administering sodium bicarbonate (baking soda) directly into the artery that nourishes the cancerous mass, or sometimes into the mass itself. Simincini has reported significant success with many types of cancers. To learn more about this technique, visit www.cancerfungus.com or read his book *Cancer is a Fungus*.

■ *Dr. Johanna Budwig's Flax Oil & Sulphur-Based Protein Therapy*. German-born biochemist Johanna Budwig (1908-2003) was acknowledged as perhaps the world's leading expert on lipid biochemistry—the field of study dealing with fats (lipids that are solid at room temperature) and oils (lipids that are liquid at room temperature), and their activity within biological systems. She held a Ph.D. in Natural Science, with emphasis in chemistry and physics, and was also formally trained as a physician, botanist, and biologist. On seven different occasions she was nominated by her peers to receive a Nobel Prize.

Dr. Budwig was familiar with the work of 1931 Nobel laureate Otto Warburg who demonstrated that, unlike normal cells which receive their energy from oxygen gas, the energy that maintains cancer cells is derived principally from the fermentation of glucose. In Warburg's words,

> Cancer, above all other diseases, has countless secondary causes. But, even for cancer, there is only one prime cause. Summarized in a few words, the prime cause of cancer is the replacement of the respiration of oxygen in normal body cells by a fermentation of sugar [glucose] ...*all* cancer cells without exception must ferment, and no normal growing cell ought to exist that ferments in the body.[78]

Warburg's work never fully postulated the cause(s) of this reversion of cancer cells to the more primitive anaerobic state. He did, however, theorize that he could raise the oxygen levels in anaerobic cells through the consumption of saturated fats. Pursuing this reasoning, he unsuccessfully attempted to increase oxygen transfer into cancer cells using the saturated fat *butyric acid* (which Budwig later determined was not sufficiently energetic to effect oxygen transport). Building on Warburg's work, 1937 Nobel laureate Albert Szent-Györgyi demonstrated that essential fatty acids (EFAs), combined with sulphur-rich proteins, *are* able to increase cellular oxygenation.[79]

Budwig understood that cancer cells revert to the more primitive fermentation of glucose because they are deprived of oxygen to the extent they must find another source of energy in order to survive. One of her greatest contributions is the discovery of *the reason* this oxygen deprivation and subsequent reversion occurs. Simply stated, the anaerobic environment that spawns the proliferation of cancer is caused by the lack of sufficient omega-3 and omega-6 essential fatty acids in the diet, as well as the overconsumption of modern foods containing unhealthy forms of fats and oils, according to Budwig.

Essential fatty acids are so labeled because they are essential for life and cannot be manufactured by the body. Consequently, they must be supplied through the diet. If these health-providing fatty acids aren't consumed in sufficient amounts, physical processes within the cells degrade to the more primitive form of energy production—fermentation of glucose within a poorly oxygenated environment. Also, and equally important, is the fact that the modern-day overconsumption of unhealthy forms of fats and oils so prevalent in today's processed foods, competes with the uptake and use of healthy EFAs, further limiting their availability. Although this is a simplified explanation of the physical/chemical processes involved, a more detailed explanation can be found in the references listed below.

Based on her own extensive research over many decades, as well as probable knowledge of Szent-Györgyi's findings regarding the use of essential fatty acids combined with sulphur-rich proteins to raise cellular energy levels, Dr. Budwig pioneered a protocol for cancer prevention *and* treatment based on the use of small amounts of flaxseed (linseed) oil combined with a rich supply of sulphur-based proteins. She recommended the products Quark® (a German cottage cheese-like dairy product), and more commonly cottage cheese, as the best sources of sulphur-based protein. Flax oil is one of the richest sources of the EFAs omega-3s and -6s, and cottage cheese is perhaps the most convenient, richest source of sulphur-based protein.

Budwig found that *neither ingredient alone* is effective in either the prevention or treatment of disease. The flax oil must be "activated" by *thoroughly mixing it* with the cottage cheese in an electric blender at a ratio ranging from 1 tablespoon flaxseed oil per ¼ cup of (preferably organic) low-fat cottage cheese, to 3-4 tablespoons flax oil per ½ cup cottage cheese, depending on the severity of illness—taken on a daily basis. Other ingredients such as fruit and honey may be added to taste.

For those who are lactose intolerant or simply want to avoid animal-derived foods, alternatives to cottage cheese can be found in the references below. One possibility is the product Companion Nutrients® by Nature's Distributors (800-624-7114), an Arizona-based company that claims one capsule of the dried, sulphurated protein in Companion Nutrients can activate the EFAs in one tablespoon of flaxseed oil. Because the precise treatment of cancer is so critical, Companion Nutrients might best be used in addition to but not as a substitute for cottage cheese.

As amazing as it may sound to some—especially to oncologists who practice traditional forms of cancer therapy, not to mention the unsuspecting and naive public who have observed for decades the many twists and turns of the War On Cancer—the use of these two inexpensive (and unpatentable) food substances provides a powerful and effective means of treating even the most advanced cancers. According to Dr. Budwig,

> ...99% of the sick that come to see me...are cancer patients who have had operations and radiation sessions, and were diagnosed as being far too advanced for another operation to be of any help. Even in these cases health can be restored, usually within a few months, I would say in 90% of cases.[80]

Writing in the *Townsend Letter for Doctors and Patients* in 1990, cancer researcher and physician Dan C. Roehm, M.D., F.A.C.P., states that,

> What she [Dr. Budwig] has demonstrated to my initial disbelief but lately, to my complete satisfaction in my practice, is: CANCER IS EASILY CURABLE; the treatment is dietary/lifestyle, the response is immediate: the cancer cell is weak and vulnerable; the precise biochemical breakdown point was identified by her in 1951 and is specifically correctable...[81]

According to Robert E. Willner, M.D., Ph.D., writing in his book *The Cancer Solution*,

> Numerous independent clinical studies published in major medical journals worldwide confirm Dr. Budwig's findings...Over 40 years ago Dr. Budwig presented clear and convincing evidence, which has been confirmed by hundreds of other related scientific research papers since, that the essential fatty acids are at the core of the answer to the cancer problem...You will come to your own conclusions as to why this simple, effective prevention and therapy has not only been ignored—it has been suppressed![82]

Dr. Budwig recommended the Flaxseed Oil & Cottage Cheese treatment protocol be followed precisely, according to her explicit directions. The caveat to this is that many people have successfully used only the flax oil and cottage cheese, without adhering to the other detailed food recommendations her works suggest. Detailed descriptions of the protocol and other useful information including case histories can be found at http://curezone.com/books/best/book.asp?ID=476; www.budwigflax.com/Articles/Dr%20Budwig .htm. Useful books include Tanya Harter Pierce's *Outsmart Your Cancer*; Dr. William L. Fischer's *How to Fight Cancer and Win*; and Dr. Budwig's books, *Flax Oil as a True Aid Against Arthritis, Heart Infarction, Cancer, and Other Diseases*. At the least, the Budwig protocol could be used easily and safely along with other treatments.

■ ***The Moss Reports.*** If you want to explore *all possible avenues* for the treatment of a particular type of cancer—leaving virtually no stone unturned—a *Moss Report* is what you need. For the past 25 years, Ralph W. Moss, Ph.D., has been investigating, and then continually updating, the latest, most effective alternative and conventional cancer treatments from around the world for dozens of different cancer types (diagnoses). He is considered the best-of-the-best in his area of specialty—researching the efficacy of cancer treatments. Dr. Moss is an internationally-known medical writer, having written 11 books and produced three documentary films relating to cancer research and treatment, including *Cancer Therapy*; *Antioxidants Against Cancer*; *Questioning Chemotherapy*; and *The Cancer Industry*. One documentary is the award-winning PBS film *The Cancer War*. In 1994 he wrote a section on alternative medicine for *The Encyclopedia Britannica*.

Dr. Moss now provides reports to individuals and their families about treatment possibilities specific to their individual situations. Each *Moss Report* provides the client 400-450 pages of specialized discussion of one out of some 200 different types of cancers. It includes his top recommendations on the best alternative and complementary treatments from around the world, as well as conventional therapies which may be applicable. All material is continually updated, and for that reason individual reports are printed only after an order is received. Each person who orders a *Moss Report* has access to Dr. Moss' monthly telephone update as well as the Member's Area of his website. To order, call (800)980-1234 or (814)238-3367. For more information or to order online, visit www.cancerdecisions.com.

One last item relating to self treatment: nutrition—the dos and don'ts. The food we take into our bodies provides the source of energy that, in the physical realm, powers the grand symphony of life. In a very real way, we are what we eat. In the section ***Nutrition: Detoxification & Toxicity***, under **General Treatment Methods**, you will learn many of the basics of good nutrition, as well as the importance of detoxifying the body.

As for the don'ts, virtually all cancer doctors and researchers—with the possible exception of traditional oncologists—agree that cancer patients would be well served by significantly reducing, or preferably totally eliminating, the following three items from their diets: 1) red meat, 2) sugar, including processed foods containing any form of sugar such as fructose, dextrose, glucose, and high dextrose (and fructose) corn syrup. Honey, xylitol, the herb *stevia*, or extracts of the *Lo Han Kuo* fruit (such as Jarrow Formulas Lo Han Sweet®) can be substituted. Remember, cancer's favorite food is sugar (glucose), which is consumed up to 15 times more by cancer cells than by normal, healthy cells, and 3) refined carbohydrates such as pastas, bread, cereal, cakes (anything made with refined white flour), and white rice, to name a few. Refined carbohydrates are one small, chemical step away from sugar. If it's sweetness you're looking for, your continued, uninterrupted breath on planet Earth will undoubtedly suffice.

Treatment in Germany. If you find the self treatment, do-it-yourself approach less than appealing and are in search of top-of-the-line in-patient treatments, many specialized clinics in Germany are at the forefront of state-of-the-art cancer treatment technology. Simply put, German doctors have access to high-technology equipment and other modalities which are currently not available in the U.S. This is due, in large part, to the incessant focus of American cancer treatment on surgery, radiation, and chemotherapy—and their extensive financial underpinnings—rather than being open to new and effective cutting-edge therapies available in some other countries, especially Germany. It is not a matter of Americans' being unable to keep pace with the state-of-the-art medical developments of other countries. Rather, it is more a matter of unwillingness to do so, based upon financial rather than technological considerations. Although no known cancer treatment is a "silver bullet" yielding a miraculous cure in every case, certain treatments have demonstrated a high degree of effectiveness.

Many specialty cancer clinics in Germany offer *hyperthermia*, *magnetic-field therapy*, and other advanced cancer-treating techniques including *dendritic cell vaccines* and intravenous *laetrile* (amygdalin). See the Member's Area of *The Encyclopedia's* website for an expanded discussion of these therapies. Some clinics send blood/tissue samples to a specialized laboratory for testing to determine a patient's specific tumor sensitivity to a range of chemotherapeutic drugs. This relatively new technology—offered by a select group of oncologists in both Germany and Mexico—greatly increases the success rate of chemotherapy, and should not be overlooked by anyone who selects chemotherapy as part of their treatment regimen.

Onkokonsult Laboratory is Germany's premier facility for the molecular (genetic) analysis of blood and bone marrow. Such analyses, which include the Polymerase Chain Reaction (PCR) test, are able to determine with 80% accuracy specific cancer cells' sensitivity to specific chemotherapeutic drugs. Head of the laboratory is Michael Giesing, M.D., Professor of Biochemistry at the University of Bonn. Dr. Giesing and others believe that in addition to the primary tumor mass are latent micrometastases disseminated throughout the body which may have a different genetic makeup than the primary tumor. Genetic analysis of the blood is the only means of determining the effectiveness of a specific chemotherapy drug against these cancers, and the most advanced means of preventing a recurrence. Giesing and others have shown that administering chemotherapy "blind"—i.e., without the aid of genetic analysis—is 80% ineffective, and that about 50% of blind chemo is harmful and even facilitates metastatic formation.

Several years ago when Dr. Giesing met with officials of the U.S. National Cancer Institute (NCI), he was told his research discoveries would revolutionize cancer treatment. Unfortunately, upon his return to Germany, he was never again contacted by the NCI. To learn more about Dr. Giesing's work, visit www.onkokonsult.com/cms/index.php?id=2.

As mentioned, German doctors tend to combine several methodologies as opposed to using a single treatment. Radio wave hyperthermia, discussed below, combined with low-dose chemotherapy can be a particularly effective combination—especially when a specific chemotherapeutic drug has been identified which is effective against a specific tumor type.

Other treatment methods include colonic hydrotherapy, which is widely used as a means of detoxifying the body. Special diets are given to live-in patients, and massage therapy, art therapy, and psychological counseling are also common.

In-patient treatment typically lasts from two to four weeks, but can last longer depending upon the specific case. Prices for cancer therapy in Germany are reasonable in comparison to American hospitals. The atmosphere of German clinics is much different than in American hospitals. Patients wear their own clothes as opposed to the typical American hospital attire. The staff-to-patient ratio is much higher, providing a more personalized approach, and each patient is treated as an honored guest. Germany is a beautiful country and most clinics are located in picturesque environments that encourage health and healing.

One of the most highly esteemed German clinics is the Fachklinik in the town of Nidda, near Frankfurt. The clinic is directed by Dr. Alexander Herzog, who has performed 2,500 hyperthermia treatments and is one of the few physicians having the equipment and experience to perform extreme hyperthermia. Fachklinik has a staff of four doctors and 11 nurses (all of whom speak English), and accommodates 25 in-patients. To learn more about Fachklinik, visit their website at www.fachklinikdrherzog.de. The Veramedica Institute of Munich, Germany specializes in assisting patients wishing to travel to Germany for cancer treatment. Their staff will help you determine which of the many clinics is best suited for your specific needs. Contact information is available on their informative website http://veramedica.net.

■ *Radio Wave Hyperthermia*. One of the most advanced German treatments—which is applicable to most types of cancer—is radio wave (frequency) hyperthermia. Using very sophisticated equipment, the body' temperature is elevated several degrees for short periods of time. Because cancer cells are more sensitive to heat than healthy cells, they become damaged and are more susceptible to attack by the immune system as well as low dose chemotherapeutic drugs, as mentioned, and/or other therapeutic substances which are often used in conjunction with hyperthermia.

Hyperthermia can be applied to specific, selected areas of the body—called local hyperthermia (as discussed under *Prostate*)—or the entire body—called whole-body hyperthermia. There are three ranges of temperatures used in whole-body hyperthermia: *moderate hyperthermia* (101-103 degrees Fahrenheit for about two hours; treatment can be given daily) simulates a natural fever; *systemic hyperthermia* raises the body's core temperature to about 105 degrees Fahrenheit; *extreme hyperthermia*—which is administered no more than once weekly—raises the body's temperature up to 107 degrees, and is practiced by only the most accomplished and experienced physicians using precise, state-of-the-art equipment. Patients being administered hyperthermia are often under anesthesia, with vital signs carefully monitored. Both local and whole-body hyperthermia are mainstay treatments in virtually all German clinics specializing in cancer treatment. (Interestingly, intravenous mistletoe is also used to induce short-term temperature elevation called fever therapy.)

Treatment in Mexico. Needless to say, cancer treatment in Mexico is less expensive than in the U.S. For those in North America not wanting to travel to Europe, some Mexican cancer clinics offer treatment methods similar to those available in Europe, including hyperthermia. An example of one such facility is the Stella Maris (Star of the Sea) Clinic in Tijuana. Gilberto Alvarez, M.D., the clinic's director, uses a combination of treatments not available in the U.S., including intravenous laetrile and DMSO, as well as both local and whole-body hyperthermia. Dendritic cell vaccines and intravenous vitamin C are also used at Stella Maris, as well as other therapies not provided by U.S. physicians. For more information, visit www. stellamarisclinic.com. Another respected Mexican oncologist is Dr. Filiberto Muñoz of the San Diego Clinic in Tijuana, who uses Dr. Giesing's laboratory to determine the effectiveness of specific chemotherapeutic drugs. Visit Dr. Muñoz' website at www.cancercure.org/san_diego_clinic.htm.

Dr. Ralph Moss, discussed above, makes regular visits to Mexican cancer clinics. In one of his newsletter articles, he discussed some of his impressions of these clinics.

> Typically, the physicians who run these Tijuana clinics are graduates of the Autonomous University of Gudalajara or the Autonomous University of Baja California, both of which are licensed facilities. A few have also trained or practiced in the United States or Europe. For example, Francisco Contreras, MD, medical director of the Oasis of Hope Hospital [www.oasisofhope.com], states at his website that he specialized in surgical oncology at the University Hospital in Vienna. Dr. Rodrigo Rodriquez of International BioCare [www. ibchospital.com] trained at Maimonides Hospital in Brooklyn. Dr. Tony Jimenez [www. hope4cancer.com] grew up in New Jersey but attended medical school in Mexico. All of the doctors...speak good, colloquial English.

> ...Many of these clinics are staffed by doctors who are very knowledgeable about alternative treatments. They are bright and resourceful people who have lots of hands-on experience of what seems to work and what doesn't. In this respect, they could run circles around the average American oncologist. Some can and do hold their own with European Complementary & Alternative Medicine specialists.[83]

About 35 specialized cancer clinics are located in or around Tijuana, Mexico. Several companies offer guided tours of these clinics. For more information on clinics and tours, visit www.alternative-cancer.net/mexican_hospitals.htm. For a list of clinics world wide specializing in cancer treatment, visit http://cancercure.ws/clinics.htm.

■ ***Cancer Conquest DVD***. A must-see DVD by medical researcher Burton Goldberg is *Cancer Conquest*. This DVD brings to life the best of alternative and conventional medicine in both Ger-

many and Mexico. To view or purchase this DVD, visit www.burtongoldberg.com.

■ ***Curaderm BEC5® and Cansema.***® Most skin cancers can be easily resolved using topical creams. Renowned alternative medical practitioner Dr. Jonathan V. Wright heralds Curaderm BEC5 as "the skin cancer cure...yes cure...that works." For more information, visit www.curaderm.net. Although less documented, Cansema has been used successfully by many skin cancer sufferers. Visit www.altcancer.com/cansema.htm.

Short Stories of Two "Suppressed" Treatments: Paw Paw and Antineoplastons. Paw Paw, known botanically as *Asimina triloba*, is a tree indigenous to the eastern half of the United States. The fruit, called the Indiana Banana, was eaten as a food by Native Americans, and the bark was used both medicinally and for making fish nets.

Paw Paw is proving to be one of the most promising new anticancer, antiviral, antifungal, antiparasitic, antimalarial, and pesticidal natural products. Over a 28 year period—20 years of which were supported by the National Cancer Institute—Jerry L. McLaughlin, Ph. D., Professor Emeritus of Pharmacognosy at Purdue University, tested 3,500 species of plants in search of anticancer substances. Of the thousands of plants investigated, Paw Paw led the pack.

McLaughlin's research, published in over 100 scientific papers relating to its chemistry and biology, re-opened the door to Paw Paw, but this time as a new treatment modality for cancer. However, even though he holds eight patents protecting his research discoveries—and even though 20 years of his research were supported by funding by the National Cancer Institute—in the end, the major pharmaceutical firms weren't willing to adopt the product. This is because the industry giants seek to adopt single-compound rather than multi-compound substances, and substances whose molecular form can be slightly modified, thereby enabling patent protection. Because it was looked over—not overlooked—this ultimately resulted in the relegation of Paw Paw to a significantly lesser position in the marketplace, which is a form of the subtle suppression that occurs frequently to such products.

In March 2003, Paw Paw became commercially available as the botanical dietary supplement Paw Paw Cell-Reg,® the result of McLaughlin's research. Although there are other Paw Paw products, Cell-Reg is the only product he recommends. For more information and to order, visit http://alternativecancer.us/pawpaw.htm. A lecture by Dr. McLaughlin can be viewed at www.pawpaw.tv.

The second example of a "suppressed" treatment is that of antineoplastons, an alternative cancer therapy that fought its way to legal use. In the early 1960s, Polish medical researcher Stanislaw Burzynski discovered certain small protein fragments (peptides) produced in the liver—antineoplastons. Many years of research led him to understand these peptides turn off genetic signals that allow cancer cells to divide, while turning on (reactivating) genes that prevent cancer's growth (tumor suppressor genes). Some of these antineoplastons actually stop cancer's runaway cell growth and allow the cells to normalize their function.

Dr. Burzynski came to the U.S. in 1970 where he taught at Baylor College of Medicine before establishing a private practice. He has developed a method of synthesizing antineoplastons, which are then given both orally and intravenously.

Although brain cancers are Dr. Burzynski's specialty, he successfully treats additional types of cancers where other methods have failed. He believes that if every antineoplaston produced by the body could be isolated and synthesized, it may be possible to cure virtually any type of cancer.

Before becoming a veritable poster child for alternative cancer treatment, not only was Dr. Stanislaw Burzynski's discovery forbidden, the American medical authorities tried for years to jail the doctor. Only years of public outcry saved his career and brilliant discovery. Today, antineoplastins have saved countless lives, and Burzynski's discovery is available to the public. To learn more, read *The Burzynski Breakthrough*, visit his website at www.cancermed.com or call (713)335-5697.

Some of the most important additional therapies which have shown success include but are certainly not limited to: 1) Intravenous Vitamin C, 2) Intravenous Laetrile, 3) The Max Gerson (dietary) Protocol, 4) Dr. Kelley/Dr. Gonzales Enzyme Therapy, 5) BryoMixol (www.bryomed .net), 6) Herbs and plant extracts such as artemisenim, carnivora, graviola, fucoidan, AHCC, and paw paw, 7) Galvanotherapy, 8) Dendritic cell vaccines, 9) Poly-MVA. DNA repair prevents cancer formation. Poly-MVA is an over-the-counter nutritional supplement that helps repair malfunctioning bits of DNA. See www.polymva.com, and 10) Insulin Potentiation Therapy, discussed in detail under **General Treatment Methods**. See the Member's Area of *The Encyclopedia's* website for additional information on these and additional therapies. As mentioned, with the assistance of and supervised by a holistic physician, many of these treatments can be used simultaneously to produce a more optimal result.

You may be asking yourself, "Does my doctor know about these treatment methods and, if so, what are his/her opinions?" First, it's unlikely a traditionally-trained physician would be familiar with many of the therapies discussed in this writing. Although doctors are highly educated people, Western doctors are trained to treat cancer principally with the techniques of pharmaceutical drugs, surgery, radiation, and combinations thereof. In some U.S. states, in fact, it's against the law to treat cancer by any means other than these traditional methods.

With these newly-discovered tools added to your inventory of knowledge, realize there's good reason to be optimistic. So engage your brain, be sensitive to your intuition, raise your sails to the winds of hope, and set out to take personal responsibility for your circumstances. At the very least, be an active participant in your recovery.

Cancer Pain. In the United States, cancer pain is often grossly undertreated—even in terminal patients—having much to do with the current political climate relating to the "War on Drugs," whether prescription or otherwise. Many American physicians are fearful of being sanctioned by their local Medical Boards for over prescribing narcotics. Any paper trail that can be used to monitor doctors' prescribing habits is enough to instill the fear of God (spelled DEA) in many physicians.

■ ***Pain Medications**.* Cancer patients *do* have some effective alternatives. In addition to Cesium Therapy, morphine is very effective in stopping or significantly reducing the pain of cancer.

One effective narcotic analgesic is the pharmaceutical *fentanyl*, having 100 times the potency of morphine.[84] Fentanyl is available either as a transdermal patch (Duragesic®) or a lollipop-style "lozenge-on-a-stick" (Actiq®) that dissolves transmucosally in the mouth over a 10-15 minute period.

A recent study published in the *British Medical Journal*[85] indicated that cancer patients preferred the transdermal Fentanyl patch over the use of time-released oral morphine. They reported less constipation and daytime drowsiness, but more insomnia on the Fentanyl patch.

Instanyl,® an intra-nasal fentanyl spray, is recommended for managing breakthrough cancer pain in adults already receiving maintenance opioid therapy. Studies have concluded that Instanyl is significantly faster acting than Actiq, offering patients much more effective pain control.[86]

■ *Morphine Pump*. The implantable morphine pump can work wonders for chronic pain sufferers, and cancer patients in particular. Using such a pump, the patient is able to stay in front of the pain, thereby reducing the overall amount of narcotic needed. The SynchroMed® is one of the most effective of these types of devices, delivering the medication directly to the spinal cord, thus substantially reducing the amount of medication required in comparison to oral administration.[87] The SynchroMed pump allows patients to avoid the "systemic effect" of oral medications which flood the entire body with medication, sometimes causing drowsiness and confusion.

■ *Cannabis*. As of winter 2010, 13 U.S. states have enacted some form of medical marijuana provision granting those with a physician's prescription legal use of the substance for treating and ameliorating the pain of various medical conditions including cancer. It is alleged—but has been difficult to verify—that persons other than those residing in this select group of states also use the substance for medicinal and other purposes.

Research from many countries has shown that cannabis contains many compounds which are effective in various aspects of cancer treatment.[88] It's also well known that cannabis exerts a powerful analgesic effect on intractable pain caused by many diseases, including cancer. For additional information, visit www.lewrockwell.com/orig5/armentano-pl.html and http://norml.org.

■ For pain, see also *Electricity* and *Sphenopalatine Ganglion Block* under **Pain Relievers**.

■ *Laser Therapy*. Low-level laser therapy (LLLT) is used to heal certain types of skin cancer. For more information, visit www.lazrpulsr.com.

■ See *Insulin Potentiation Therapy* and *Sodium Chlorite* under **General Treatment Methods**, Blood Electrification & Magnetic Pulsing under **Herpes**, and the Member's Area of our website.

CANDIDA ALBICANS. See Candida Albicans and Infection in the **Index.**

CARDIOVASCULAR DISEASE

Cardiovascular disease is the occurrence of disease relating to the heart or blood vessels, including the blood vessels of the brain. Heart disease and stroke are the two principal components of cardiovascular disease, and are the first and third causes of death in the United States, respectively—together accounting for more than 40% of all deaths.[1] Heart disease accounts for about one third of all deaths in the Western world.[2]

Heart disease is a physiologically abnormal heart condition, typically caused by a blockage (occlusion), while *coronary heart disease* (CHD), also called *coronary artery disease* (CAD), is characterized by a blockage of one or more of the main arteries that supply blood—hence oxygen and nutrients—to the heart. CHD is the most common form of heart disease. A *stroke* is a sudden diminishing or loss of consciousness, sensation or voluntary motion caused by a rupture or obstruction (such as a clot) of an artery in the brain.

The term *heart attack*, technically referred to as *myocardial infarction*, refers to the necrosis (death) of a portion or portions of the heart muscle due to loss of blood supply, hence oxygen. According to the American Medical Association, one-third of all people who suffer a heart attack never experience any pain.

All known types of heart disease—including a heart attack and CHD in general—can lead to *sudden cardiac arrest* (SCA), where the heart stops beating either temporarily or permanently, stopping the blood flow to the rest of the body. The victim thereafter loses consciousness within a few seconds and often dies. SCA usually results from an electrical disturbance in the heart muscle, as opposed to a heart attack which results from a blockage of blood flow to the heart. Persons are at a particularly high risk for SCA in the month following a heart attack. Most occurrences of SCA are accompanied by an acute episode of *cardiac arrhythmia*, where the heart beats irregularly and suddenly stops beating. The irregular beating can be rapid (*ventricular tachycardia*), chaotic (*ventricular fibrillation*), or slow (*bradycardia*).[3] An SCA leading to death is termed a *sudden cardiac death*.

Brain death, hence permanent death, begins in just four to six minutes after the heart stops. The chances of survival of someone who suffers cardiac arrest decrease by 7-10% each minute that passes without being administered an electric shock, called *defibrillation*, in an attempt to "jump-start" the heart muscle. After 10 minutes with no heart function, few attempts at resuscitation are successful.[4] Cardiopulmonary resuscitation (CPR) can keep a person alive until defibrillation is attempted.

About 90% of SCA victims have CHD, where the major arteries of the heart are narrowed by fatty deposits. About 65% of those who suffer a sudden cardiac arrest have been found to have scarring from a previous heart attack, where loss of blood supply has caused part of the heart muscle to die.[5]

In 1900, heart disease accounted for about 8% of all deaths, and heart attacks were so rare that most physicians spent their entire careers never having witnessed a single episode. The first mention of the term "heart failure" appeared in the medical literature in 1912.[6] By the early 1920s, heart disease had attained epidemic proportions, and by the 1950s it had become the leading cause of death in the Western world. As the population ages in the U.S., the toll on the health care system grows proportionally. In 2008, the total cost of all cardiovascular diseases in the U.S. was over $450 billion.[7]

What Causes Cardiovascular Disease?

Many factors contribute to heart disease including diabetes, high low density lipoprotein (LDL; so-called "bad") blood cholesterol, high blood pressure, obesity, physical inactivity, poor dietary practices, smoking, and stress. Another culprit has been suggested as a contributing factor—infection by pathogenic microorganisms. In 1999, an article published in *Science*[8] reported chlamydia, cytomegelovirus (CMV) and herpes to be implicated in the occurrence of cardiovascular disease. Still other pathogens could be involved. That same year, the *New England Journal of Medicine*[9] reported that more than half of all heart attacks might be prevented with proper antibiotic treatment.

A May 2009 article in *PLoS Pathogens*[10] reported that a persistent CMV infection of the arterial vessels leads to an increase in inflammation, hence an increase in high blood pressure. When CMV is present while consuming a high-cholesterol diet, the infection was found to induce *atherosclerosis* (see below) in a mouse aorta.[11] CMV is a member of the herpes virus family and is present in 60-99% of adults globally by age 40.

The brilliant scientist Dr. Linus Pauling, discussed below under Linus Pauling Protocol, believed heart disease has at its root a physical weakness of the arterial walls resulting from insufficient dietary intake of vitamin C. Whatever its ultimate origin, various physiological processes are hallmarks of its development and progression.

Inflammation of the inner lining of the arteries plays a major role in the origin of cardiovascular disease. The *endothelial cells* that comprise the inner lining become inflamed—irritated or injured in some way—causing *endothelial dysfunction*. This compromise of the normal biological processes of the endothelium results in several damaging effects including increased platelet adhesion, coagulation of the blood, and an underproduction or increased destruction of *nitric oxide* (NO)—a key chemical involved in the dilation of blood vessels.[12] These processes of inflammation and endothelial dysfunction can begin early and reinjury can occur over a period of years, with many factors compounding the problem—diet, hypertension, metabolic syndrome, stress, infection, etc.

Endothelial dysfunction is a key determinate in atherosclerosis, the formation and accumulation of *plaque* along the inside of the artery walls—and the resultant narrowing of the blood vessels, *stenosis*. The progressive accumulation of plaque over time—sometimes decades—predisposes arterial vessels to the formation of *vulnerable plaque(s)* which are unstable and can break away, occlude a blood vessel, and cause a heart attack (*cardiac infarction*) or stroke (*cerebral infarction*).[13]

The metabolite *homocysteine* is also intimately involved. Homocysteine is a product of the normal metabolism of the essential amino acid methionine. Adequate levels of the vitamins B_6, B_{12} and folic acid co-function with enzymes to dispose of harmful levels of the metabolite. However, when these vitamins aren't present in sufficient quantities, or the enzyme cofactors aren't present for other reasons, cardiovascular problems develop. A Harvard study of 15,000 physicians, reported in the *Journal of the American Medical Association*[14] in 1992, revealed those participants with the highest 5% homocysteine levels had more than a 300% increased risk of heart attack compared to those with normal levels. It is known that homocysteine levels increase substantially with age, and that high levels have been linked to vascular occlusion, dementia and kidney failure. *Hyperhomocysteinemia*, having excessive blood levels of homocysteine, is associated with poor nutritional status.

Homocysteine is used by the body to build and sustain tissue. But without being properly disposed of, it causes the smooth muscle cells which lie just beneath the surface of the artery to multiply out of control, creating a bulge that forces other cells apart. Eventually, as a result of inflammation and this shredding of the artery from the inside out caused by excess homocysteine, these microfractures protrude into the artery itself causing the inner walls to become rough and uneven.[15] Other factors also contribute to the formation of abnormalities in the arterial walls, a complete discussion of which is extremely technical and beyond the scope of this writing. Inflammation, nevertheless, is intimately involved in the formation and development of these abnormalities, and usually plays a significant role in all stages of their progression.

It is this formation of rough surfaces on the inside of the arterial walls that causes fats and cholesterol to begin to adhere to the walls—in an effort to repair (cover) the damage. This is the process which eventually forms a plaque buildup comprising a variety of substances including calcium, cholesterol, and other fatty molecules—which narrows the inside of the artery, thereby reducing blood flow.[16]

Over a number of years, plaques may grow or decrease in size, depending upon a number of factors including the level of infection/inflammation in the body, and the degree to which a person practices a healthful lifestyle.[17]

Plaques are classified as either stable (calcified) or unstable (soft, vulnerable). Stable plaques are relatively dense and are those that are detectable by an *angiogram* (or *arteriogram*), which is an X-ray visualization of the blood vessels following the injection of a radiopaque substance. Arterial vessels may become significantly occluded, producing various symptoms including angina, high blood pressure, and intermittent claudication.

Contrary to a previous belief, even though stable plaques occlude the vessel, they are not usually life threatening. In fact, it is now known the body can often create its own bypass by growing new blood vessels around long-term, stable plaques in a process of revascularization—the body's growth of collateral blood vessels.[18] Only 15% of heart attacks, it is now believed, are caused by stable plaques. Therefore, when a significant occlusion on an angiogram/arteriogram is observed, more than likely this will not lead to a heart attack or stroke as the plaque is firmly calcified and unlikely to rupture.[19]

It is the soft, or unstable (vulnerable) plaques that pose a significant danger. Although these plaques are not observable by angiogram, they are detectable by other techniques discussed below. Soft plaques are particularly subject to tearing or rupturing, after which they are covered by a blood clot (fibrous cap) in an attempt to mend the rupture in the same manner in which the body attempts to close any wound. The clot may obstruct the vessel, diminishing the supply of blood. If the clot breaks away and occludes the vessel significantly, a heart attack or stroke may ensue. The body produces anti-clotting chemicals that can prevent a clot from forming; however, inflamed plaques secrete chemicals that impede this process.[20]

Do You Have Cardiovascular Disease?

If you have suffered a heart attack or stroke, there is no question that cardiovascular disease has been a part of your life—and likely still is. As mentioned, roughly two-thirds of adults who are victims of sudden cardiac arrest have scarring from a previous heart attack.[21] If you experience pain in the chest or calf muscle(s), this also can be a sign of cardiovascular problems. However, even if you have never had a heart attack, and even if you don't experience cardiovascular-associated pain, this by no means rules out the presence of cardiovascular disease. Also, even if you have had angiography and your doctor has given you a clean bill of health, you are still not in the clear—as angiography detects only stable (calcified) and not vulnerable plaque.

There are several means of helping to determine if you have cardiovascular disease.

❖ Homocysteine, a contributor to the formation of arterial plaques, is easily measured by a simple blood test. Where high homocysteine levels are present, cardiovascular disease is likely to be present, or an indication of a potential future problem. A score of 7 mmol/L (micromoles per liter) or under is preferred. Levels over this value may represent an ongoing problem. Older persons may find it difficult to keep homocysteine levels under 7-8. Some physicians continue to tell their patients that a score of 15-18 is "normal." However, it is now known from epidemiological studies that homocysteine levels above 6.3 cause a steep progressive risk of cardiac infarction.[22]

A 1996 article published in the *American Journal of Epidemiology*[23] reported that each 3-mmol/L increase in homocysteine levels corresponds to a 35% increased risk of heart attack. A 2003 article published in *Circulation Research*[24] revealed that homocysteine levels as low as 10 mmol/L can cause massive damage to arterial walls.

❖ C-reactive protein is a substance that has been implicated in the formation of arterial plaques. Its elevated presence within the blood is an indication of inflammation, and a strong indication of atherosclerosis. For both men and women, C-reactive protein is a far better predictor of cardiovascular problems than high LDL cholesterol. The *New England Journal of Medicine*[25] reported in 2002 that women with elevated C-reactive protein levels were twice as likely to suffer a heart attack or stroke compared to women with high LDL cholesterol levels. Levels of C-reactive protein can be measured with a simple blood test. Ideally, the level should be under 0.5. If elevated, there's inflammation within the body which likely includes inflammation in the major blood vessels.

❖ Cardiac Recovery Rate. A common technique of determining whether the heart receives adequate blood flow is the Cardiac Stress Test—the treadmill test. We all have heard stories of this test being too stressful, and the patient has a heart attack and possibly expires on the spot. While this test is an indicator of heart disease—death would be a good clue—there is another, less stressful predictive test that has recently gained recognition—the Exercise Recovery Test.

As reported in the *Journal of the American College of Cardiology*[26] in 2003, 3,000 patients near 60 years old received a treadmill stress test. Some also received a cardiac ultrasound. All were measured for a decrease in heart rate within the first minute following termination of the treadmill exercise. The patients were followed for six years, at which time 300 had died. It was found that those whose heartbeats didn't decrease by at least 12 beats per minute within the first minute after concluding the exercise were two-and-one-half times more likely to have died during this time. These findings held true whether or not the person was diagnosed as suffering from coronary artery disease. Therefore, slow heart-rate recovery was not seen as being predictive of CHD. Be that as it may, they definitely had a "heart problem" that was predictive of their future death. Therefore, if you notice your heart rate does not begin to slow significantly after exercising, e.g., a decrease of at least 12-18 beats per minute during the first minute after exercising, there's likely a problem.

Several techniques are useful in assessing various aspects of cardiovascular disease:

❖ Two non-invasive high-tech diagnostic techniques show a significant ability to diagnose plaques within the arterial vessels. 1) High-speed Magnetic Resonance Imaging (MRI), and 2) High-speed helical (spiral) contrast-enhanced 3-D cardiac Computer-aided Tomography (CT) scans [also referred to as multi-slice detector computed tomography (MDCT)].[27] The 64-slice CT is the most advanced as of early 2010.

[A slightly older technology, Electron Beam Computed Tomography (EBCT; also called the Ultrafast CT Scan) has been widely advertised but is somewhat controversial. The test is designed to measure calcium deposits within the arteries. However, some patients showing small amounts of calcium actually have significant blockages (false negatives), and almost half the patients showing significant calcium deposits do not have significant arterial blockages (false positives)].

❖ Three ultrasound techniques are capable of detecting early atherosclerotic plaque/endothelial dysfunction. A non-invasive, externally-applied ultrasound apparatus can accurately measure the pathological thickening of the carotid arteries of the neck. This is referred to as a measurement of the *intima-media thickness* (also called intimal medial thickness), or IMT—or CIMT, carotid intima-media thickness. Often, IMT readings are taken at more than one segment of the carotid. Although factors other than atherosclerosis contribute to intima-media thickening, highly abnormal values are predictive of atherosclerotic pathology, heart attack, and stroke. As of early 2010 much of the clinical carotid software does not reach this level of accuracy, and many ultrasound technicians remain unfamiliar with state of the art CIMT protocols.

❖ An invasive (interventional) technique known as *intravascular ultrasound* (IVUS) is an imaging technology capable of accurately quantifying arterial plaque as well as detecting vulnerable plaque with a high degree of accuracy. A miniaturized ultrasound probe is attached to a catheter which is guided from outside the body through angiography catheters into the blood vessel to be examined. Although arteries of the heart are the typical targets of IVUS, CIMT can also be measured. By visualizing from inside the blood vessels out through the vessels, IVUS is able to measure both the size of the lumen (opening) within the arteries as well as the level of plaque accumulation within the artery walls.

❖ Healthy endothelial function is at the basis of cardiovascular health. An advanced means of evaluating endothelial function is to measure the blood flow-induced dilation and contraction of the *brachial artery* which runs from the shoulder to the elbow. The *flow mediated dilation test* assesses blood flow in this artery by means of a highly sensitive ultrasound instrument. An abnormal reading is indicative of cardiovascular disease.

❖ It has been suggested that elevated cholesterol is one of the principal factors in the origin of heart disease—at least in the mainstream media where

pharmaceutical companies air their incessant advertising campaigns for their cholesterol-lowering drugs. Although most physicians agree that cholesterol does play a part in the causation of cardiovascular disease—especially elevated levels of LDL—it is also known that half of all heart attacks in men and 65% in women occur in persons with normal cholesterol levels and no previous symptoms.

The standard cholesterol blood test measures total cholesterol, LDL, high-density lipoprotein (HDL; the so-called "good" cholesterol), and triglycerides. Although physicians have relied upon these factors, they're very limited in assessing the status of heart disease and predicting heart attacks.

An advanced method of measuring cholesterol has been developed which is considerably more accurate in both the assessment of the presence of heart disease and in predicting the risk of cardiovascular events. Known as the *Vertical Auto Profile* (VAP), the test supplies the four standard measurements as well as additional, expanded cholesterol information including LDL pattern density, and lipoprotein subclasses which include HDL_2 and HDL_3, IDL (intermediate-density lipoproteins), $VLDL_1$, $VLDL_2$, $VLDL_3$ (very low-density lipoproteins), and Lp(a) [lipoprotein (a)].

These expanded data include inherited risk factors that can predispose a person to heart disease. Persons testing in the normal range on the standard cholesterol test often test at risk on the VAP. The VAP identifies about 90% of persons at risk for cardiovascular disease compared to the standard test which identifies about 40%.

■ *PLAC®Test*. The PLAC Test is a simple blood test that measures the enzyme *lipoprotein-associated phospholipase A2* (Lp-PLA2), which is specific to vascular inflammation implicated in the formation of rupture-prone (vulnerable) plaque. It is the only FDA-approved test that aids in assessing the risk of an atherosclerosis-induced stroke or heart attack/sudden cardiac arrest.

■ Elevated blood pressure and pulse pressure, both of which are discussed below, are also indicative of cardiovascular disease.

Surgery
Various manifestations of heart disease—including atherosclerosis and arteriosclerosis—are often

treated by one of Western medicine's mainstay approaches—surgery. Angioplasty (percutaneous transluminal coronary angioplasty, aka balloon angioplasty) is one such method, wherein a catheter with an attached balloon is inserted into the artery, advanced to the blockage, inflated to open the vessel (hopefully...), and then withdrawn. It has been reported in the medical literature that the average death rate for those receiving balloon angioplasty is 400% higher than the death rate caused by the disease.

Other treatments include laser angioplasty, wherein a laser-tipped catheter is advanced to the blockage; and atherectomy, wherein a rotating-shaver-tipped catheter is advanced to the blockage site to do the work of clearing the blockage. The most invasive of all the techniques—short of a heart transplant—is coronary artery bypass graft surgery, first performed in 1967, wherein a (spare?) blood vessel is taken, usually from the leg, and used as a detour around the blocked cardiac vessel(s). Although these procedures sound like a lot of fun—what with balloons, swirling cutters, and all—our best medical journals, including the *New England Journal of Medicine* and the *Lancet*, have reported that neither angioplasty nor coronary bypass surgery prevent heart attacks or increase survivability.[28] Nevertheless, over one million angioplasties and bypass surgeries are performed each year in the U.S.

More than 30 years ago, writing in the *New England Journal of Medicine*, Dr. Eugene Braunwald, Chief of Cardiology at Harvard Medical School, commented on bypass surgery in less than complimentary terms, as follows,

> ...an industry is being built around this operation...[it] is developing a momentum and constituency of its own, and as time passes it will be progressively more difficult and costly to curtail it...[29]

Aside from being ineffective in saving lives, bypass surgery is plagued by several serious side-effects, including brain damage. In 2001, the *New England Journal of Medicine*[30] reported that from 10-30% of all bypass patients undergo a period of postoperative delirium, sometimes experienced as extreme disorientation. The journal states that from 1.5 to 5.2% of all bypass patients suffer a stroke while on the operating table, which sometimes results in death, but more often causes either tempo-

rary or permanent brain damage. Fifty to 80% of patients experience short-term changes in cognitive function. Six months following the operation, 10-30% continue to experience impairment.

Reported in 2001 in the *New England Journal of Medicine*,[31] researchers at Duke University confirmed the previous evidence of long-term cognitive brain impairment following bypass surgery. The researchers administered tests measuring cognitive function to 261 patients before bypass surgery, after discharge, after six weeks, six months and five years. More than 50% of the patients scored significantly worse immediately following surgery. At six weeks, one-third exhibited cognitive deficits. At six months, 25% still had deficits. Alarmingly, at the five year retest, 42% showed signs of impairment.

In 2000, Harvard Medical School professor Dr. Peter Libby stated,

> We have also come to realize that none of our high-technology therapies...including surgery and angioplasty, actually reduces the incidence of heart attack or prolongs life, except in selected subgroups of patients.[32]

The large, in-depth Coronary Artery Surgery Study (CASS) reported that regardless of whether one, two or more of the major coronary arteries were blocked—patients progressed very well without surgery, having the low fatality rate of 1.6% per year and a corresponding survival rate of 98.4%. During the same time period, those receiving bypass surgery had a fatality rate of slightly over 10%, or about one death for every 10 operations. This study—the most sophisticated of its kind ever done—shows that bypass surgery is at least five times as fatal as the disease it's intended to cure.[33] With the exception of a small subset of patients, those choosing not to undergo the operation live just as long or longer than those who have surgery.[34]

That small subset who may benefit from bypass surgery includes those whose major vessels are badly damaged; those whose left main coronary artery is blocked; and those who have extensive blockage of multiple major coronary arteries in conjunction with inefficient pumping capacity.

The *most* critical factor in determining whether or not a person will benefit from coronary bypass surgery seems not to be the number or extent of blockages, but rather how well the left ventricular pump is functioning. This is assessed by measuring the total amount of blood pumped with each beat, known as the *ejection fraction*. A healthy heart generally has an ejection fraction of 50% or greater. Studies have shown that almost 90% of all bypass surgeries are performed on patients whose ejection fraction is over 50%.[35]

Cardiac bypass procedures are not without repercussions in addition to possible long-term cognitive brain impairment. Because bypass surgery alters arterial blood flow, that portion of the artery upstream from the bypass graft site accumulates plaque at 10 times the rate of an ungrafted artery.[36] Also, the elderly have a very poor prognosis as recipients of this procedure. Up to one third of those over 80 years old die within one year following coronary bypass surgery.[37]

Many of the problems associated with conventional bypass surgery are caused because the heart is stopped for up to two hours while connected to a heart-lung machine which assumes the role of oxygenating the blood. If after understanding the above potential consequences of bypass surgery you still require the operation, inquire about the technique *off-pump bypass*, a procedure in which the heart is not stopped during the operation. To learn more about the dark side of bypass surgery, read Dr. Julian Whitaker's book *Reversing Heart Disease*.

Before the advent of modern surgery, man used plant-derived substances to treat cardiovascular disorders. The beneficial effects of G-strophanthin have been known for over a century, while the cardiovascular benefits of arjuna have been known for over two thousand years.

Many simple, natural, effective methods for combating the various faces of cardiovascular disease are discussed below. Although this section is divided into several sub-categories, e.g., hypertension, stroke, etc., many of the treatments discussed are applicable to more than one sub-category. Therefore, reading the entire **Cardiovascular Disease** section will ensure you've reviewed all information relevant to a particular topic.

Homosysteine & C-Reactive Protein Reduction
■ *Folic Acid, Vitamins B$_6$ and B$_{12}$, and Trimethylglycine*. Abnormally high levels of homocysteine are effectively treated by the daily oral intake of several nutrients including folic acid, vitamin B$_6$, vitamin B$_{12}$, and trimethylglycine (TMG; TMG

converts homocysteine into the energy booster dimethylglyceine, DMG.) Effective levels of these nutrients vary from person to person. To determine if your treatment regimen is effective, re-test regularly to assess homocysteine levels.

Persons with moderate homocysteine elevation may find the following daily regimen effective: 800 mcg of folic acid; 100 mg of vitamin B$_6$; 600 mcg of vitamin B$_{12}$; 500 mg of TMG. Older individuals and/or those with significantly elevated levels may require higher daily dosages, particularly of B$_6$, TMG and/or B$_{12}$, as follows: 250-1000 mg of vitamin B$_6$ and/or 1,500-3,000 mg of TMG and/or 1-2 mg of B$_{12}$. A weekly injection of 1 mg of vitamin B$_{12}$ offers increased effectiveness compared to oral intake in persons with malabsorption. Otherwise, oral intake has been shown to be equally effective. An increased dosage of folic acid beyond a base level may not provide added benefits.[38] (Daily intake of 2,000-4,000 mg of vitamin B$_6$ for extended periods may cause peripheral nerve damage).

■ *Cyruta Plus® and Curcumin*. Cyruta Plus is very effective in eliminating high levels of C-reactive protein, hence the detrimental inflammation which underlies plaque formation and growth. It is an extract of buckwheat that is high in vitamin C, inositol, and a rutin bioflavonoid complex. At a daily dosage of 6-15 tablets for 30-60 days, the results can be seen by a re-test. To purchase this product, visit www.totaldiscountvitamins.com.

Another powerful natural anti-inflammatory is the phenolic compound *curcumin*, a product of the yellow-colored spice turmeric, used as a medicament by the ancient Egyptian pharaohs as well as traditional Ayurvedic medical practitioners of India dating back some 6,000 years. Curcumin has been shown to be up to 75% more effective than cortisone as an anti-inflammatory.[39] This product should be purchased as *curcuminoids*, available in health food stores or on the internet. The treatment dosage is 300 mg three times per day. (The trademarked ingredient BCM-95® has been shown to be several times more bioavailable than other 95% curcuminoid compounds).

■ *Antibiotics*. If infective microbes do, in fact, prove to be a cause of cardiovascular disease, other antibiotics such as doxycycline may prove effective. Because of doxycycline's effectiveness against mycoplasma, as discussed under *Gulf War Syndrome*, it's logical this would be one of the next antibiotics to investigate clinically. Due to their broad-spectrum effectiveness, *Olive Leaf Extract* and *Sodium Chlorite*, discussed under **General Treatment Methods**, could also prove effective.

Dietary Factors

It is well known that dietary factors play a significant role in the cause, treatment and prevention of cardiovascular disease. Their influence cannot be underestimated.

■ *The Mediterranean Diet.* Within the past several years, articles in many prestigious journals have reported telling information about dietary factors which are responsible for much of the incidence of cardiovascular disease in the Western world. Furthermore, they have pointed out that changes in these harmful dietary practices could eliminate much-to-most of the incidence of this top killer of humans in the Western world. Sadly, very few physicians, including cardiologists, are aware of this information—not to mention an almost total lack of understanding of these facts by the general public. Stated another way, it is now known that by altering dietary practices in favor of certain health-giving and preventive foods, the prevalence of this disease could be drastically reduced.

In 1994, the *Lancet* reported the results of the Lyon Diet Heart Study, a study which was to evaluate the reason(s) for the low incidence of cardiovascular disease in the countries bordering the Mediterranean as compared to countries of northern Europe. The study was planned to continue for five years, but was terminated after only 27 months by its Scientific and Ethics Committee because of the striking benefits experienced in the experimental group, which consumed a diet known as the Mediterranean diet—an increase in vegetables and the monounsaturated fat olive oil. Those who followed the diet experienced a *70% reduction in both fatal and non-fatal incidents of coronary heart disease.*[40]

The Mediterranean diet, simply stated, is a diet focusing on whole grains and legumes, lean protein, fresh fruits and vegetables, and high in omega-3 polyunsaturated fatty acids (PUFAs) [eicosapentaenoic acid (EPA), docosahexaenoic acid (DHA) and alpha-linolenic acid (ALA)] and low in carbohydrates, saturated fats (common in junk foods) and omega-6 PUFAs (linoleic acid, common in most vegetable oils). Omega-3s are found in various foods including concentrates of free fatty acids of fish oils (cold-water fish such as bluefish, cod, herring, mackerel, salmon and sardines), soybean oil (~7%), Canola oil (~10%), and flax seed oil (~50%). To learn more, read Dr. Michael Ozner's book *The Miami Mediterranean Diet*.

Harvard Medical School's Dr. Alexander Leaf, writing in the journal *Circulation* in 1999, discusses the Lyon Diet Heart Study, elucidating some important conclusions, as follows:[41]

❖ Relatively simple dietary changes achieve greater reductions in risk of all-cause coronary heart disease mortality than cholesterol reduction.

❖ This reduction in the risk of CHD was not associated with differences in total cholesterol levels.

❖ Because of the high costs and invasive procedures that are the mainstay of CHD treatment, promotion of the Mediterranean diet could lead to a considerable reduction of health costs.

❖ Because there has been considerable disease and death caused by pharmaceutical drugs and invasive surgical treatment of CHD, these adverse effects could largely be avoided by dietary changes, particularly by adopting the Mediterranean diet.

❖ Research has demonstrated the prevention of fatal ventricular arrhythmias in rats, marmosets, and dogs by omega-3 consumption. This suggests that omega-3 fatty acids may prevent sudden cardiac arrest in humans.

■ *Fish & Fish Oil.* Marine sources provide all three of the important omega-3 fatty acids—EPA, DHA and ALA. Cold-water fish and high-quality fish oil are good sources of the omega-3s. Compared to fish oil, however, Neptune Krill Oil (NKO) is less subject to toxic contamination, better absorbed, and almost 50 times as potent an antioxidant.

■ *Flax Seed.* Either flax seed meal (ground flax seeds) or flax seed oil is a readily-available food source which is very high in omega-3 polyunsaturated fatty acids, specifically ALA. Although the process is slow and probably varies according to age and other factors, the body can convert ALA into EPA and DHA. Borage, hemp, and perilla are additional plant oils with considerable fatty acid content. By supplementing daily with omega-3s, a major step is taken in the prevention of cardiovascular disease, including sudden cardiac arrest.

Fats that are liquid at room temperature are referred to as oils. *Lipids*, or fats and oils as they are commonly called, are necessary for life. These substances are utilized by the body as an energy source, and represent the body's main source of stored energy. However, there are both healthy and unhealthy fats. Essential fatty acids (EFAs), which are unsaturated, are a special type of fat required by the body to maintain health. "Essential" means the body does not self-produce these substances. They must be acquired from the diet.

Hydrogenated oils interfere and compete with the assimilation of health-giving EFAs. It has been estimated, in fact, that up to 80% of the Western world, and especially Americans, consume insufficient quantities of EFAs in their diets, partially as the result of consuming too much hydrogenated oil. Some experts believe the introduction of processed oils into the marketplace has all but eliminated EFAs from the average American's diet, and also from the diets of many throughout the Western world.

Foods that typically contain either totally or partially hydrogenated (saturated) oils are processed foods such as snack foods—cakes, cookies, candies, chips, crackers—and processed foods such as meats, dairy and fried foods. Many grocery store oils also are hydrogenated and contain mostly omega-6s, e.g., canola, corn, safflower, and sunflower.

Leading lipid biochemist Dr. Mary Enig reported[42] the consumption of hydrogenated oils and *trans* fatty acids are linked to a long list of physical maladies including low sperm and testosterone levels in men; EFA deficiencies; heart disease; increased levels of LDL; low birth weight infants; low volume and quality of breast milk; prostate disease; and suppressed immune function. Additional information on EFAs is given under **Nutrition: Detoxification & Deficiencies** and Chia, in the section on **General Treatment Methods.**

■ *Magnesium*. Calcium intake into the heart muscle cells is regulated by magnesium, the 11th most abundant mineral in the human body. This helps maintain healthy blood pressure levels. Adequate intake of magnesium also helps reduce angina symptoms; increases the oxygen-carrying capacity of the blood; inhibits platelet stickiness, thereby helping to reduce abnormal blood clotting which can lead to a heart attack; increases heart efficiency; and improves overall healthy heart function. Additionally, magnesium is a cofactor necessary for the proper functioning of more than 300 enzymes.

Although magnesium is present in many foods including most nuts; dark-green, leafy vegetables; and many grains, people are often deficient in the mineral. The recommended daily dosage is 800-1,000 mg. Magnesium given intravenously is known to be a safe and effective treatment for cardiac arrhythmias.

Cholesterol Reducing Agents

There are many cholesterol-reducing agents in the marketplace—both pharmaceutical drugs and dietary (nutritional) supplements. It should be understood from the above discussion, however, that focusing merely on cholesterol reduction is a short-sighted and incomplete strategy. In fact, many medical experts now believe that so-called "high" cholesterol levels are a total non-issue. To learn more about this subject, visit the International Network of Cholesterol Skeptics at www.thincs.org.

■ *Statins and NSAIDs.* Aspirin has been shown to reduce inflammation and lower C-reactive protein. Also, the statin pharmaceuticals mentioned above are known to lower C-reactive protein. NSAIDs also inhibit inflammation. However, they also have significant potential side-effects that do not accompany the equally-effective, natural supplements such as those described in this section.

Although statin drugs such as Lipitor,® Zocor,® Pravachol,® Lescol,® Zetia,® Vytorin,® Crestor,® and Mevacor® are often well tolerated, about 10-15% of persons taking these drugs experience one or more of an array of harmful side-effects including liver and kidney toxicity; a serious breakdown of muscle cells (rhabdomyolysis); muscle weakness; impotence; cognitive impairment including memory loss; nerve damage—often irreversible—leading to peripheral neuropathy (tingling and pain in the hands and feet); a diminishing of psychomotor skills including difficulty walking; depression (resulting from lower cholesterol levels); and others.

[In 2008, news about Zetia and Vytorin (a combination of Zocor and Zetia) came to light when company-sponsored research withheld from the public by the manufacturers showed the drugs provide no health benefits for healthy people.]

Also, it is now well known that statin drugs inhibit the production of coenzyme Q10. CoQ10 deficiencies are associated with many disease states including cardiovascular disease—specifically heart failure—and should be a matter of serious concern to those using these drugs. Oddly, virtually all patients with heart failure are placed on statin drugs, even those with low cholesterol levels.

The statin class of prescription drugs is the best-selling medicines in history, used by more than 13 million Americans with an additional 12 million users world wide. Sales for the drugs in 2006 totaled nearly $28 billion. Notwithstanding their ubiquitous presence on television and the variety of celebrities who convincingly endorse them, the question remains: How effective are statins in preventing disease and death? A 2007 article in the well-respected journal the *Lancet* sheds some much- needed light on "the rest of the statin story."

To determine whether statins perform "as advertised," one must evaluate on whom they are used. To measure their true degree of usefulness, it's helpful to assess their effects on various groups of people: 1) those with no evidence of existing heart disease—so-called primary prevention use, 2) those showing no evidence of heart disease, but having multiple risk factors, and 3) those with diagnosed cardiovascular disease—secondary prevention use.

In the *Lancet* article,[43] authors Dr. John Abramson of Harvard Medical School and Dr. Jim Wright of the University of British Columbia report on their review of eight primary prevention trials of statin drugs. They conclude that for primary prevention, i.e., persons with no evidence of heart disease, statin therapy was not effective in reducing the overall risk of death (although the risk of cardiovascular events such as heart attacks and strokes was reduced by slightly over 1%). For secondary prevention, statins do reduce the risk of cardiovascular events such as heart attacks and strokes.

The remaining group, those with multiple risk factors but with no evidence of disease, was a specific group of people addressed by the famed Robert Jarvik, Ph.D., inventor of the artificial heart, in a series of television and print ads for Lipitor—the best-selling drug in the world, with 2008 sales of USD $14.4 billion. According to a Lipitor newspaper campaign featuring Jarvik, the drug "reduces the risk of heart attack by 36%...in patients with multiple risk factors for heart disease." The Jarvik ads were finally removed by government regulators, but not before his endorsement accrued millions for Pfizer, Lipitor's manufacturer.

But is it true that Lipitor reduces the risk of heart attacks by 36% in patients with multiple risk factors for but with no evidence of heart disease? Pfizer's ads claimed Lipitor reduces the risk of nonmortal heart attacks by 36%. However, in actuality, about three percent of patients taking an inactive placebo pill experienced a heart attack in comparison to two percent taking the statin drug—only one percent less for Lipitor than the placebo group. This, in a particularly biased way of looking at the result (one percent is 33% of three percent), produces the so-called 30-plus percent risk reduction. But in *real* numbers the reduction from three percent to two percent is only one percent—a much less significant-sounding result for Lipitor which likely would have resulted in less profitability for Pfizer—and the good Dr. Jarvik.

This example of spin is reminiscent of the apocryphal story of a once-upon-a-time race between an American race car and a Russian race car. The American car won the race, but the next day's headline in the Russian newspapers read, "Russian Car Comes in Second, while American Car Comes in Next to Last." Is this wrong? Not really. But it isn't right either. It would be a diplomatic understatement to say that Pfizer's reporting of the Lipitor statistic as a 36% risk reduction is disingenuous.

In summary, the two groups that comprise the bulk of Lipitor users—primary prevention users and high-risk users with no evidence of heart disease—obtain little if any health benefits from Lipitor use. Because the prevalence of side-effects is so high and potentially so serious, it can be assumed—as is concluded by Drs. Abramson and Wright in their *Lancet* article—that the risks of taking Lipitor for these two groups outweigh the benefits.

Especially because there are safer means of combating cholesterol, it will be up to the individual to educate him/herself as to which form(s) of treatment to seek. If cholesterol reduction is the goal, several side-effect free methods are available.

■ *Policosanol*. Continuing the discussion of cholesterol lowering—notwithstanding the fact that under most circumstances this should not be one's major focus, as discussed—another product deserves mention. Extracted from the wax of sugar cane (and bees wax), *policosanol* consists of octacosanol and several other long-chain fatty alcohol molecules. Cuban researchers and others have studied policosanol's cholesterol-lowering abilities on tens of thousands of people over many years. The studies document that at the level of 10-20 mg daily in divided doses, policosanol lowers total cholesterol by about 15%, lowers LDL-C (a dangerous form of LDL) by about 20%, and lowers triglycerides by about 15%, while at the same time increasing HDL-C ("good" cholesterol) levels by about 15%. After studying over 25,000 people, only three tenths of one percent experienced any side-effects, with weight loss being the most frequent. These results compare favorably to the most effective statins, without adverse side-effects. The daily dosage ranges from 5-20 mg, with 20 mg being the most effective. Policosanol can interact with blood-thinning drugs. To learn more, visit www.lef.org/mag azine/mag2001/june2001_cover_policosanol.html.

■ *Red Yeast Rice Extract*. An Asian and Indonesian dietary staple and food additive, red yeast rice is a natural, whole food product that is produced by fermenting cooked, nonglutinous rice with the red yeast filamentous fungus known botanically as *Monascus purpureus*. Therapeutic amounts of the compound *mevinolin* are yielded as a result of the natural fermentation process. Interestingly, mevinolin is the active compound contained within the original statin drug lovastatin (Mevacor®). This, in fact, led to an FDA ban on red yeast rice in 1998 because of its chemical similarity to the prescription drug and as such, according to the FDA, the (natural) product should be strictly regulated. Patent issues also were involved. These problems have now been resolved, and the product once again is on the shelves of most health food stores.

In addition to mevinolin, red yeast rice extract contains other powerful ingredients, including beta-sitosterol, campesterol, fiber, isoflavones, stigmasterol, trace elements, and unsaturated fatty acids. This synergistic combination of compounds has been found to have powerful cholesterol-lowering properties which surpass the use of mevinolin alone. Many studies have documented the ability of red yeast rice to lower triglicerides and LDL levels while either raising HDL levels or leaving them unaffected. Both U.S. and Chinese studies report levels of LDL being lowered by 18-32% in an eight week period. Because red yeast rice contains the statin-type compound mevinolin, it may reduce CoQ10 levels. Therefore, anyone taking this product should supplement with 200-300 mg of CoQ10 daily.

■ *Niacin*. Even traditionally-trained doctors recognize that vitamin B3, niacin—but *not* the "no-flush" versions such as niacinamide—is one of the most effective means of reducing triglycerides; lipoprotein a; LDL including VLDLs; fibrinogen; and the frequency and intensity of angina attacks. It's also effective in elevating HDL. Begin slowly with 500 mg twice daily with meals, and build to a level of 2,000-3,000 mg daily in divided doses after two weeks. Taking niacin at bedtime, with meals, or in a sustained-release form reduces the common "flushing" sensation. Persons taking these levels should have their cholesterol, triglycerides, and liver enzymes tested about every three months.

Angina Pectoris

Caused by insufficient oxygenation of the heart muscle (ischemia) most often as the result of blood vessel narrowing or blockage, *angina* is a relatively brief occurrence of chest pain of varying intensities—from bothersome to suffocating. It is typically experienced as pressure, fullness, squeezing, or pain in the center of the chest, but can also occur as pain in the arm, shoulder, neck, back, or jaw. Chest pain unrelated to but sometimes mistaken for angina can be caused by indigestion (heartburn), inflammation, a lung infection, or a broken or misaligned rib. If the pain goes away after shifting positions, drinking or eating, taking a deep breath, or if it lasts less than 30 seconds, it's not likely angina.

Although there are many more natural approaches discussed below, traditional medicine's approach to angina includes pharmaceutical drugs such as *nitroglycerin*, a vasodilator that improves blood flow and therefore the oxygen supply. Nitroglycerin is used in the following ways:

☞ To relieve symptoms of an in-progress attack

☞ To prevent an attack by taking it just prior to when the attack might be expected (stress, etc.)

☞ To prevent attacks by long-term use

"Nitro" is sometimes accompanied by a long list of less-than-dynamite side-effects including blurred vision; dry mouth; severe and/or prolonged headaches; skin rash; extreme dizziness or fainting; sensations of extreme pressure in the head; weak and fast heartbeat; fever; or convulsions. Also, nitroglycerin is known to lose its effectiveness following prolonged use. Other drugs include *beta-blockers* and *calcium antagonists*, each with their own set of potential side-effects. These drugs slow the heart rate in an attempt to decrease the heart's workload and need for oxygen.

■ **_Zinc_**. Relatively high doses of zinc taken for a short period of time totally eliminate severe angina in many/most individuals. This inexpensive yet effective angina treatment was reported in the medical literature during the early 1960s—and subsequently ignored—but was accidentally "rediscovered" by American physician Dr. William Halcomb and researcher George Eby in the 1980s—when it was further ignored. Treatments using a common substance such as a mineral are unpatentable and, therefore, have difficulty gaining traction within establishment medicine. Nevertheless, popularity of a treatment method isn't a good indicator of its effectiveness, or lack thereof.

Research by Halcomb and Eby has shown that, for most people, 60 mg three times daily with meals of zinc acetate, chloride, gluconate, glycinate, histidinate, or sulfate (the biologically active forms) for seven to a maximum of 14 days is sufficient to stop angina symptoms. Treatment should be stopped as soon as symptoms remit, which occurs for most people within seven days. Because high zinc intake can deplete the body's stores of copper—which could cause additional health problems—it is recommended a daily dose of 4-6 mg of copper chloride, lactate, malate, succinate, or sulfate (no other forms) be taken for two weeks prior to beginning the high-dose zinc treatment. For a more thorough understanding of the Halcomb/Eby protocol, read the expanded explanation and precautions for high-dose zinc administration at http://george-eby-research.com/html/angina.html.

■ **_Terminalia arjuna_**. India is a country whose medical tradition goes back thousands of years. One of the most ancient medicines in this tradition is a derivative of the *Terminalia arjuna* tree, whose bark has been used for treating heart conditions for over 2,500 years.

In a three-month study,[44] researchers at the Kasturba Medical College in Mangalore, India compared the effectiveness of arjuna to isosorbide nitrate, a nitroglycerin-based pharmaceutical commonly used for angina pain. The arjuna-treated group experienced a 30% reduction in angina, while the ISMN-group had a 27% reduction. Although the results are similar, those taking arjuna reported no side-effects, while the nitroglycerin group experienced the side-effects discussed above.

In a 1995 study reported in the *International Journal of Cardiology*,[45] a 50% reduction in angina episodes was experienced by 15 stable angina sufferers. Participants also experienced reduced systolic blood pressure as well as reduced body weight. LDL cholesterol levels also decreased. Arjuna improves congestive heart failure,[46] offers protection against ischemic heart disease,[47] raises HDL cholesterol,[48] helps prevent atherosclerosis,[49] combats some cancers,[50] and is antibacterial.[51] To learn more about *T. arjuna*, visit www.himalayausa.com.

■ **_G-strophanthin_**. The chief botanist on the David Livingstone Expedition ("Dr. Livingstone, I presume?") was the first to discover the beneficial heart activity of the West African plant *Strophanthus gratus*, and brought the plant to Europe in 1862. It was used to treat heart disease in Germany as early as 1906.[52] Early on, many German physicians recognized the powerful beneficial effects of this plant medicine, which is now referred to as *g-strophanthin* (stro-FAN-thin*)* and its byproduct *ouabain*. Unfortunately, because of Germany's political and scientific segregation before and during WWII, this valuable heart medicine became isolated from the rest of the world.

Strophanthin has a chemical structure similar to *digitalis*, a commonly-prescribed heart medication derived from the foxglove plant (*D. purpurea*).

While both medications strengthen the heart, one important pharmacological difference is that strophanthin has a deacidifying effect on the heart muscle—which makes it extremely effective both in preventing heart attacks and stopping a heart attack already in progress.[53]

German physician Dr. Berthold Kern reported the results of his clinical practice between 1947-1968 involving more than 15,000 cardiac patients treated with g-strophanthin. These patients included many who previously had heart attacks. In this group, there were no fatal heart attacks, and only 20 non-fatal attacks. In contrast, government statistics for the same time period would have predicted 120 fatal heart attacks and over 400 non-fatal attacks for a group of this size.[54]

In a double-blind, randomized, placebo-controlled study[55] of oral g-strophanthin in the treatment of angina sufferers, after 14 days of treatment 81% of the participants experienced a reduction in attacks, while the placebo-control group experienced a 72% *increase* in angina attacks.

Another German study of 150 patients with severe heart disease, who collectively had experienced 254 heart attacks, demonstrated an 85% success rate in preventing further attacks. The study coordinator remarked, "A positive result was registered when the severe heart attack abated within five minutes after the g-strophanthin capsule was bitten through, and after ten minutes at the latest, they disappeared completely."[56] (The symptoms, not the patients).

At present, there are approximately 5,000 German physicians using and prescribing oral strophanthin. A recent booklet (available in German only) gives the results of a survey of 3,645 German physicians who offered statements on their use of strophanthin between the years 1976-1983. Of the doctors interviewed, 3,552 offered exclusively positive testimony with no reservations. None of the physicians gave a negative response.[57]

The cost of strophanthin, which is currently available to German physicians and their patients, is about USD $30 per month. It is possible to obtain this product from Germany with a prescription from a physician in your country. For those living outside of Germany, there are several strategies for obtaining strophantin, depending upon where you live. A German pharmacy (Apotheke)

can be located through an international telephone operator. Call the pharmacy to arrange delivery by mail. Also, through a travel agency, arrange for someone traveling to Germany to bring back the drug. Be sure your country's customs permit these arrangements.

■ **_Capsaicin_**. Medical practitioners both ancient and contemporary have touted the medicinal properties of a variety of hot peppers such as bird, cayenne, chilli, and Tabasco. *Capsaicin* is one of seven capsaicinoid compounds present in peppers, and is the primary compound responsible for the hot sensation of the pepper fruit, as well as its medicinal benefits. It has long been claimed that cayenne, due to its high capsaicin content, is useful in stopping a heart attack in under three minutes, without damaging the heart muscle. A similar claim is made of capsaicin's ability to abort an in-progress stroke.

The late pioneer herbalist Dr. John Christopher recommended a glass of cayenne tea be given every 15 minutes until the medical crisis passed. Alternatively, it is said that a teaspoon of cayenne tincture (Google: Christopher's Original Formula Cayenne Extract™) every 15 minutes is equally effective. Dr. Christopher wrote,

> In 35 years of practice, and working with the people and teaching, I have never on house calls lost one heart attack patient...if they are still breathing, I pour down them a cup of cayenne tea (a teaspoon of cayenne in a cup of hot water), and within minutes they are up and around...The warm tea is faster working than tablets, capsules, cold tea, because the warm tea opens up the cell structure...and it goes directly to the heart, through the artery system...Cayenne is a certain remedy for heart attack; as a stimulant, it can start the heart into action again, and as it facilitates blood flow throughout the body, it will keep the heart going.[58]

In the September 2009 edition of the journal *Circulation*, Keith Jones, Ph.D. and a group of researchers from the Department of Pharmacology and Cell Biophysics at the University of Cincinnati announced findings which shed new light on capsaicin's relationship to heart function. This information gives credence to Dr. Christopher's anecdotal reporting, and takes capsaicin's near-miraculous effects to the level of evidence-based medicine.

The University researchers found that an over-the-counter pain salve containing capsaicin rubbed on the skin during a heart attack is a cardio-protectant which can prevent or reduce heart damage while other interventions are administered. Dr. Jones' team found that applying capsaicin to the stomachs of mice caused sensory nerves in the skin to trigger signals in the nervous system which activate cellular "pro-survival" pathways in the heart, reducing cardiac cell death by 85%. Apparently skin—the largest organ of the human body and its main sensor—has evolved to protect animals, including humans, in a variety of ways. The researchers also found that a small incision made on the abdomen triggered an 81% reduction in cell death. Said the researchers,

> Topical capsaicin has no known serious adverse effects and could be easily applied in an ambulance or emergency room setting [or by anyone present including the victim] well in advance of coronary tissue death. If proven effective in humans, this therapy has the potential to reduce injury and/or death in the event of a coronary blockage, thereby reducing the extent and consequences of heart attack.

> Both this and the capsaicin effect are shown to work through similar neurological mechanisms. These are the most powerful cardio-protective effects recorded to date...This is a form of remote cardioprotection, using a skin stimulus that activates cardioprotection long before the blocked coronary artery is opened... All of the current interventions require the vessel to be opened before doctors can act, and since it takes time to elicit protection, tissue dies...This treatment will protect the heart before the vessel is opened while producing a strong protective effect that is already active when we open the vessel.

> By activating these sensors in the nervous system, via skin, we think that a response to preserve and protect the heart is triggered...We think that this technique is fooling the body into sending out protective signals...This may be similar to the way certain acupuncture treatments work; there may be a neurological basis. In a broad sense, this work may provide a 'Rosetta stone' for translating alternative medicine techniques like acupuncture to Western medicine. Perhaps we can understand the biological mechanisms of how alternative treatments may be successful for patients...This could help create favorable outcomes for those

who are experiencing stroke, shock or are in need of an organ transplant, and the best part is that it is done non-invasively and is relatively inexpensive.[59]

In addition to alleviating tissue damage from a stroke by the above neurological signaling mechanism, capsaicin is an anti-hemorrhagic agent. The use of cayenne tea or tincture, as described above, equalizes blood pressure and induces clotting action. Dr. Christopher reported that for internal hemorrhaging of the lungs, stomach, uterus, or nose, cayenne tea or tincture will stop the bleeding. For lung hemorrhage, a warm cayenne vapor bath is also effective.

Blood Clots

Because a blood clot at any location in the cardiovascular system can obstruct blood flow to the extent of causing a heart attack or stroke, any therapy able to reduce this likelihood would be a health saver, and possibly a life saver.

■ *Nattokinase.* For centuries, the Japanese have consumed the boiled, fermented soybean product *natto.* A cheese-like product traditionally believed to promote cardiovascular health, the Japanese have prepared natto for over 1,000 years.[60] Interestingly, during the U.S. occupation of Japan following WWII, the Japanese were forbidden from preparing natto because of its pungent smell and misunderstood means of preparation.

While majoring in chemistry at the University of Chicago Medical School in 1980, Hiroyuki Sumi discovered that an enzyme extracted from natto has the amazing ability to dissolve blood clots (thrombi) and reduce blood viscosity (thickness). Of all the soy foods consumed by Asian people, only natto, he discovered, has this enzyme. He called the enzyme *nattokinase.* Because so many symptoms of cardiovascular disease are related to blood vessel blockage caused by blood clotting—for example, angina, cardiac arrest, heart attack, hypertension, intermittent claudication and stroke—the discovery of nattokinase is of great importance.

As the body's coagulation system becomes activated, the sticky substance *fibrin* is formed and deposited in the major vessels and capillaries of the vascular system. (Fibrin is a fibrous, filamentous protein formed from the plasma protein *fibrino-*

gen by the catalytic action of the enzyme *thrombin*.) At the same time, high fibrin levels within the blood increase the blood viscosity. These two factors lead to a corresponding decrease in blood flow throughout the entire body, producing anoxia (deficiency of oxygen) and nutrient deprivation to the cells. More seriously, blood clots are also formed.

When blood-clot-induced blockages occur in the heart, portions of the heart muscle can die due to lack of oxygen. Clots within the heart muscle can move through the bloodstream to the brain where they can cause cerebral infarction (stroke) or senility due to oxygen and nutrient deprivation to brain tissues. Independent of clots formed within the heart, clots can also form within the capillaries of the brain resulting in senility/dementia.

In the delicate balance of maintaining proper blood viscosity—not too thick, not too thin—the body manufactures several types of enzymes which induce clotting, i.e., the formation of thrombi. This would seem natural as an evolutionary means of preventing loss of blood. On the other hand, there is only one main endogenous enzyme for thinning blood and dissolving blood clots—*plasmin*. The biological properties and actions of nattokinase closely resemble those of plasmin.

Nattokinase is unique in that it functions in several beneficial ways. By simple oral supplementation, coagulation of the blood can be prevented. Also, nattokinase is able to dissolve fibrin directly, hence blood clots. It further is able to induce the body's own production of plasmin, and other clot-dissolving agents including *urokinase*.

Urokinase, *activase* and *streptokinase* are *tissue plasminogen activators* (tPAs), and are often administered to heart attack and stroke victims intravenously—but often fail because hardening of the arteries has surpassed the point of being treatable by any clot-dissolving agent. Nattokinase is useful in this regard in that it can prevent hardening of the arteries, known as *arteriosclerosis*, with a daily oral dose of about 100 mg.[61]

Also, medically-administered clot-dissolving agents are very expensive, in the range of USD $1,500 per dose, even though they are active only for minutes. Urokinase, for example, is active only for 4-20 minutes following administration. Nattokinase, on the other hand, has been shown to be active for 8-12 hours.[62] A recent article published in the *Biology Pharmacy Bulletin*[63] reported that the *in vivo* (within the body) thrombolytic (clot-dissolving) activity of nattokinase is stronger than that of either plasmin or elastase.

A stroke is referred to as *hemorrhagic* when there is bleeding in the brain. Otherwise, it is deemed *ischemic*, indicating a blockage of blood flow to a portion of the brain. Prior to tPA administration, a CT scan must be given to insure there's no bleeding present. Otherwise, tPA would worsen the condition. Current medical judgement is that tPA must be given within three hours following the onset of a stroke, as the risk of bleeding outweighs its potential benefits if administered subsequent to this window. These complications have made emergency room physicians reluctant to administer tPA, resulting in less than 5% of ischemic stroke victims in the U.S. receiving the treatment.

Thrombolytic enzymes are endogenously generated in the blood vessels of the endothelium in many areas of the body including the arteries, veins and lymphatic system. As the body ages, there is a decrease in production of these enzymes, rendering the blood more susceptible to clot formation. Regular administration of nattokinase significantly reduces the possibility of all the consequences related to cardiovascular disease and one of its major causative factors, abnormal blood coagulation. Dr. Martin Milner of the Center for Natural Medicine in Portland, Oregon remarked about nattokinase, "In all my years of research as a professor of cardiology and pulmonary medicine, natto and nattokinase represent the most exciting new development in the prevention and treatment of cardiovascular-related diseases..."[64]

In a research study published in 1990 Dr. Sumi, the discoverer of nattokinase, experimentally induced blood clots in a group of male dogs, followed by oral administration of four 250 mg capsules of nattokinase. X-ray angiograms of the blood vessels of the dogs were free of clots within five hours following treatment. The dogs receiving a placebo showed no sign of clot dissolving during an 18-hour follow-up examination.[65]

In a human study also reported in 1995, an extracted equivalent of 200 gm of natto food was given orally to five volunteers on four consecutive days. In four of the five participants, the systolic blood pressure (top figure) decreased an average of 10.9%, while the diastolic blood pressure decreased an average of 9.7%.[66]

In a study published in *Nutrition*[67] in 2003, researchers reported that 17 studies have evaluated the beneficial properties of nattokinase. Oral administration of the substance reduces blood pressure, suppresses thickening of the arteries, dissolves blot clots, and offers a protective function to the body's blood vessels. It is an important supplement for prevention and treatment of diseases of the heart and circulatory system.

The Japan BioSciences Laboratory has shown that nattokinase administered to rats at 700 times the recommended human dosage is safe and nontoxic. Moreover, the enzyme does not cause excessive bleeding as do the drugs heparin and Coumadin.[68] The only caution in taking natto or nattokinase is that it shouldn't be taken in conjunction with other blood-thinning agents such as antioxidants, aspirin, Coumadin, *Ginkgo biloba*, heparin, or with substances that affect platelet aggregation such as fish oil, garlic or vitamin E.

Several companies now market a nattokinase supplement some of which are available in health food stores, and all of which are available on the internet. Select a product which has 1,500-2,000 FUs per capsule, where FU is a fibrin unit, a standardized measurement of clot-dissolving activity.

Intermittent Claudication (IC)

Intermittent claudication is aching, burning, cramping, muscle fatigue, numbness or pain in the leg(s) and especially the calves which occurs when walking, and may disappear after resting a short time, but resumes after walking is resumed. The symptoms usually begin in the calf muscle(s), but can also be felt in the thighs, feet or buttocks. Walking uphill or at a faster pace can increase the severity of the symptoms. The seriousness of the disease is proportional to the distance one is able to walk before experiencing symptoms. Intermittent claudication is associated with an inadequate blood supply to one or both leg muscles, and is a symptom of *peripheral vascular disease* (PVD).

Peripheral Artery Disease (PAD) is a type of PVD, although sometimes the two terms are used interchangably. Slow-healing wounds (scratches, scrapes, sores, etc.) on the lower legs are also indicative of PVD/PAD. Those suffering from the disease may experience angina, among other typical signs of cardiovascular disease. By comparing blood pressure measurements at both the ankle and the arm—known as the *ankle-brachial index*—the risk of PVD can be assessed. Ankle blood pressure should be equal to or higher than arm blood pressure. If the pressure is lower, a narrowing or blockage may be present. In addition to the following remedies, see ***Varicose Veins***, and ***Photoluminescence*** under **General Treatment Methods**.

■ ***Padma 28***.® For centuries, Tibetan monasteries have been repositories of vast numbers of ancient healing techniques. Much of this knowledge has been destroyed over time the by invading Chinese armies. One special formulation—reported to be over 2,000 years old—was pirated out of Mongolia during the 1850s, and found its way to Switzerland sometime thereafter. The formulation, known as Padma 28, has been commercially available in Switzerland and other parts of Europe for the past 30 years. The designation "28" identifies the 28th formula in an ancient Tibetan medical textbook.

Padma 28 contains a mixture of 19 organically-grown dried and milled herbs and spices, together with natural camphor, calcium sulphate and a small quantity of the substance *aconite*. The formulation sold in the U.S. is identical with the exception that the U.S. product—called Padma Basic®—does not contain aconite due to FDA regulations.

Many scientific studies have evaluated the effectiveness of Padma for the treatment of many medical ailments including intermittent claudication, angina, restless leg syndrome, and others. In two German studies monitoring patients over a four month period, the average maximum walking distances of intermittent claudication sufferers increased by over 100%. In a 1998 study reported in the *Journal of Vascular Investigation*,[69] Padma decreased pain, significantly increased walking distances, and improved blood flow to the lower extremities. Dozens of other studies have confirmed these results. The product can be ordered from EcoNugenics by calling (800)308-5518.

■ ***Walking***. If PVD/PAD is in the early stages, walking can be an effective therapy. By walking to the point of pain, stopping to rest if severe, and then resuming walking—or even "walking through the pain"—collateral blood vessels can be caused to grow around occluded arteries. Walking two to three miles or more a day is hard work, but provides good therapy. Begin an exercise program slowly, and increase your walking distances over time.

Plaque Reduction and Removal
Because the presence of plaque within the arteries is so detrimental to good health and is, in fact, a principal causative factor for heart attack and stroke, treatments which reduce or eliminate plaque buildup are of major importance to the health and longevity of those persons with heart disease.

■ **Chelation Therapy.** The standard medical approach to intermittent claudication is surgery, or perhaps pharmaceutical drugs such as cilostazol or pentoxifylline, a preparation of questionable effectiveness which comes with a nasty set of potential side-effects including extreme dizziness and vomiting. One alternative medical approach is a technique known as *chelation* (key-LAY-shun) *therapy*. Developed during the 1950s to treat heavy-metal poisoning—mostly from lead and mercury—and various circulatory disorders such as atherosclerosis, chelation is thought to work by breaking up plaque within the arteries.

This, at least, was the initial proposed mechanism of action. An alternative explanation is that the lining of the arteries (endothelium) produces several substances that reduce blood flow resistance, including nitric oxide (NO), prostacyclin, and heparin. Heavy metals reduce the endothelium's ability to produce these substances. The removal of metals contributes to optimal blood circulation.[70] Chelation also thins the blood and encourages the formation of blood vessel growth around an occluded artery. Chelation therapy is approved by the FDA for treating lead toxicity.[71] It is an effective treatment for diabetes and cardiovascular disease, including intermittent claudication.

The word chelation is derived from the Greek word *chele*, meaning claw, which refers to the process by which organic molecules grip a mineral element. The agent typically used is *ethylenediaminetetraacetic acid*, or EDTA, a compound approved by the FDA as a food preservative. Other useful compounds include DMSA and DMPS [two mercury chelators; a transdermal DMPS lotion (TD-DMPS)

is available—see DMPS under **Autism**.], deferoxamine (for iron), and others. Chelation is administered via three modes: intravenously (IV), orally, and transdermally—either rectally via suppository or by application to other areas of the skin.

EDTA can be injected into a muscle, but is usually administered IV over a period of two to three hours, for a total of up to 20-30 treatments—one to three times weekly spanning several months, depending on the severity of the condition. A "short form" of chelation therapy is practiced by some physicians. Referred to as the "quick-push method" as pioneered by Swiss physician Dr. Walter Blumer, it is now viewed by some chelation therapists as being as effective as traditional EDTA.

An even less time consuming and less expensive oral (pill) version of the therapy is also available. The slow IV method of treatment costs ~USD $3500-$4000 for a course of 30 treatments, while the oral method costs about USD $60 per month. Research has shown that oral EDTA chelation is effective in toxic metal removal. The FDA has approved oral chelation for treating lead poisoning. Some practitioners use oral chelation in combination with the (slow or fast) IV methods. As of early 2010, it has not been convincingly demonstrated that oral EDTA is effective in plaque removal. The research literature supporting its effectiveness in this regard is minimal.

An oral chelation product not containing EDTA, DMPS, or DMSA is Chelorex.™ This product was formulated to work synergistically to mobilize toxic heavy metals and protect against heavy metal reabsorption and redistribution. Chelorex provides safe, gentle and effective mobilization of toxic metals by enhancing the natural mechanisms for excretion through the biliary tract, while avoiding the toxic overload associated with synthetic chelators, according to the manufacturer.

Chelorex has been shown to be effective in clinical testing for reduction of the entire spectrum of toxic metals: bismuth, cadmium, tin, lead, mercury, aluminum, nickel, antimony, arsenic, silver, beryllium, platinum, thallium, thorium, titanium, tungsten and uranium. This is important as the presence of multiple toxic metals significantly lowers the toxic threshold for each individual metal.

Chelorex contains both water-soluble and lipid-soluble agents, capable of penetrating the blood-brain barrier and the cell membrane so that CNS and intracellular metals can be mobilized. It can lower mercury levels safely in persons with amalgam fillings. Chelorex can be used before, during, and after amalgam replacement.

This product makes no claims of plaque removal. If heavy metal removal is, in fact, involved in plaque removal, Chelorex should aid in this. To learn more, visit www.scienceformulas.com.

The third method of administering EDTA chelation is rectally via suppository, a mode of administration that has shown considerable effectiveness. Some doctors report this method even surpasses the results obtained through IV administration. This is reasonable as the rectally-instilled EDTA is directly absorbed by the lining of the colon before moving into the bloodstream—initially bypassing the liver and kidneys; thus, the EDTA remains in the body longer than with IV administration.

Two rectally-administered EDTA products are Detoxamin® and Kelatox.® Detoxamin is available on the internet by doing a key word search for "detoxamin." It is available in 30-count boxes of individually-wrapped suppositories costing USD $250-$290, depending upon the source of purchase. Thirty Detoxamin suppositories, according to its manufacturer, are equal to 10 IV chelation sessions.

Kelatox is taken at night for approximately 30 days. There are 900 mg of EDTA per suppository, and a one-month supply is USD $199. For more information, visit www.kelatoxproducts.com.

■ **_Essential Phospholipids_** (EPL). While chelation therapy using EDTA (and other substances such as DMPS and DMSA) is effective in treating arterial plaque buildup, there is another effective treatment which focuses on removing (chelating) cholesterol and other fatty substances from atherosclerotic plaque deposits, the cardiovascular effects of which can be miraculous.

The treatment involves oral supplementation of lecithin, a lipid (fatty) material which is a major component of all cell membranes. It is also a major component of both HDL and LDL cholesterol molecules. Research has shown that with sufficient lecithin present in the bloodstream, cholesterol becomes soluble and breaks down into smaller molecules capable of passing through artery walls where it is thereafter absorbed by the body or pro-

cessed by the liver and excreted. Thus, lecithin is useful in removing years of arterial plaque buildup as well as lowering LDL and normalizing HDL. To achieve these benefits, supplement with lecithin capsules or add two tablespoons daily of non-GMO lecithin granules to either foods or beverages.

As effective as lecithin is in lowering LDL cholesterol and removing arterial plaque, a unique form of lecithin known as *essential phospholipids* (EPL) is four-to-five times more effective due in large part to its significantly higher content of phosphatidylcholine—the principal active ingredient in both substances. EPL has been shown to stop angina attacks in over 50% of patients in only one week, and reduce the severity of the remainder by as much as 90%. It also has been shown to reduce hardening of the arteries (arteriosclerosis), and halt intermittent claudication in over 85% of the patients in just six weeks when taken at the dosage of 1,500-1,800 mg daily[72]—even with no dietary changes.

For decades, an EPL product was available in Europe, marketed under the trade name LipoStabil. When its patent expired, LipoStabil was no longer marketed. The product has now been duplicated and is currently marketed under the name Plaquex,® which is administered intravenously.

A less expensive oral EPL formulation now being marketed by several companies often achieves similar results as Plaquex but without the higher expense of its IV counterpart. Both Plaquex and oral EPL often achieve results similar to EDTA chelation, and sometimes are effective even when EDTA chelation has failed. To learn more about EPL, visit www.life-enhancement.com/mediadisplayprint.aspx?ID=1575.

Oral EPL is available from several sources including Nutricology (800)545-9960 (LipoPhos Forte®) and International Research and Development Corporation (928)536-7646 (LipoFlow Forte®); www.lipoflow.com.

■ **_Linus Pauling Protocol_**. Linus Pauling, Ph.D. (1901-1994) was one of the most brilliant scientific minds of the 20th century. He was one of the first scientists to work in the fields of molecular biology, quantum chemistry, and orthomolecular medicine. Pauling was one of only four individuals ever to win two Nobel Prizes. He was also the only person ever to win a Nobel in two unrelated fields, and the only person ever to win each prize without sharing the award with another recipient. Pauling's doctorate was in the fields of physical chemistry and mathematical physics and, as such, his work focused on the nature of chemical bonds and the structure of molecules. Later in life, he turned his attention and vast base of knowledge toward the fields of health and medicine.

Pauling believed that cardiovascular disease has at its root a form of chronic pre-scurvy, caused by a long-term deficiency of vitamin C (ascorbic acid). This deficiency weakens blood vessels, making them susceptible to the formation of millions of tiny lesions/tears/stress fractures. The coronary arteries are particularly susceptible, as these vessels undergo the highest mechanical stresses as they open and are squeezed flat more than 100,000 times daily by the pumping action of the heart. After the damaged areas form, they begin to be coated by fatty deposits in an attempt to repair the weakened vessels. Over many years the repair process overcompensates and plaque deposits develop.

Several species including humans, other primates, the guinea pig, and the Indian fruit-eating bat don't endogenously manufacture vitamin C. Humans are one of only several animals that develops atherosclerotic plaque and has heart attacks. Sometime in the evolutionary past humans lost the ability to produce the vitamin. Until very recent historical times—about 100 years ago—this was of no consequence as man consumed a nutrient-rich, plant-based diet containing sufficient amounts of vitamin C not only to prevent outright scurvy but to stave off the deterioration of the arteries and the consequent formation of atherosclerotic plaque caused by the chronic presence of the disease.

The advent of the industrial and chemical farming revolutions, the development of modern farming methods, and the ascent of the fast food Western nations all have contributed to a food supply which is nutrient deficient in comparison to that of our ancestors. Thus, our current Western diet is sorely lacking in many nutrients including vitamin C. Seagoing wayfarers developed scurvy due to their inability to store a sufficient supply of vitamin C-containing foods such as fresh fruits and vegetables. In 1753 James Lind, a Scottish surgeon in the British Royal Navy, proved scurvy could be treated with vitamin C-containing citrus fruit. Although this

has been known for over 250 years, the understanding has never been applied to modern medicine's treatment of heart disease.

While plaque consists of a variety of substances—fibrinogen/fibrin; lipoproteins; cholesterol and other fatty particles, as mentioned—it is now known that the principal glue-like substance that initially binds to the arterial walls is *lipoprotein (a)*, abbreviated Lp(a)—a specific sub-type of lipoprotein. Lp(a) particles are particularly sticky due to *lysine and proline binding site receptors* on their surfaces. As the chronic state of scurvy progresses, continued deposition of fatty particles and liproproteins worsen the deteriorating atherosclerotic condition.

Dr. Pauling's simple but brilliant cure for heart disease is to supplement with high doses of *Lp(a) binding inhibitors*—the amino acids lysine and proline—and also vitamin C. These substances, when taken together, produce collagen, elastin, and other reinforcement molecules, thus strengthening and stabilizing the arterial walls. Further, lysine and proline fill the lysine and proline binding site receptors on the surfaces of Lp(a) molecules, neutralize their stickiness, and prevent them from contributing to further plaque buildup. They also release Lp(a) molecules from their anchor sites within the plaque, causing them to dissolve over time.

Even end-stage cardiovascular disease patients have reported results including cessation of angina pain, reduced blood pressure, and lipid normalization. Pauling found the effects of this therapy were so pronounced he doubted clinical studies would even be necessary.

Autopsies of soldiers from the Korean and Vietnam wars revealed that up to 75% of soldiers in their early 20s had already developed some form of atherosclerotic deposits. Therefore, we know that atherosclerosis isn't a disease affecting only those of advanced age. Further, Dr. Matthias Rath, a renowned German cardiologist and colleague of Dr. Pauling, discovered that—depending on lifestyle—atherosclerotic plaque formation can increase at an average rate of almost 50% each year. Because it's an aggressive disease which afflicts such a high percentage of Westerners, it would be prudent for most everyone to consider supplementing with the group of plaque-reversing nutrients discovered by Drs. Pauling and Rath.

Because atherosclerotic deposits form over the span of many years, it takes time for the vitamin C, lysine, and proline combination to halt and begin to reverse the disease. As reported in 1996 in the *Journal of Applied Nutrition*,[73] Dr. Rath and his colleagues discovered that in people with early stages of coronary artery disease, during the initial six month period the growth rate slowed, and essentially stopped during the second six months, as measured by EBCT scans. Thereafter, the deposits began to dissolve. More advanced atherosclerosis may take longer before the benefits are measurable. Despite these findings, Pauling noted that amazing symptom reversals in as little as 10-14 days are ordinary occurrences.

Dr. Pauling's dosage recommendations are: 1) Vitamin C as ascorbic acid—*not* other forms such as buffered vitamin C or Ester C®: 3-10 grams (gm; 3,000-10,000 mg) daily in divided doses for prevention; 10-18 gm daily for therapeutic treatment, to bowel tolerance. If diarrhea occurs, decrease the dosage slightly, 2) Lysine: 2-3 gm daily for prevention; 5-6 gm for therapeutic treatment, and 3) Proline: 250-500 mg daily for prevention; 2 gm daily for therapeutic treatment. The protocol is faster-acting when sugar (sucrose, fructose, etc.) is eliminated from the diet and omega-3 fatty acids are included. For more information, read Dr. Rath's books *The Heart* and *Why Animals Don't Get Heart Attacks—But People Do*, available as free downloads at www4.dr-rath-foundation.org. Also read *Practicing Medicine Without a License: The Story of the Linus Pauling Therapy for Heart Disease*.

■ ***Pomegranate***. A native of Afghanistan, Pakistan, India, and Iran, the pomegranate tree (*Punica granatum*) is a small, fruit-bearing tree cultivated in many semi-arid countries throughout the world and in California and Arizona. Steeped in history and romance, the pomegranate even holds a place in Greek mythology. The juice of its fruit is gaining wide publicity for its beneficial health effects.

In 2004, the journal *Clinical Nutrition*[74] reported the results of a three-year study of advanced atherosclerotic patients with carotid artery stenosis who consumed 50 mL (1.7 ounces) of pomegranate juice daily. After one year, the pomegranate juice drinkers experienced a 35% reduction in their CIMT scores, while those in the control group experienced a 9% increase. The pomegranate juice drinkers also showed a 44% improvement in carotid artery blood flow, a 21% decrease in systolic blood pressure, and a 130% increase in their blood serum total antioxidant status.

■ ***Serrapeptase***. Also known as Serratia peptadase, *Serrapeptase* is a proteolytic enzyme originally isolated in the late 1960s from the digestive tract of the Japanese silkworm—which uses the enzyme to dissolve its cocoon. Serrapeptase is currently produced commercially from Serratia E15 bacteria cultures. The German orthomolecular physician Dr. Hans Nieper used it to dissolve blood clots, cysts, and arterial plaque, as Serrapeptase digests non-living tissue. Dr. Nieper claimed Serrapeptase protects against ischemic strokes, and is both more effective and faster acting than EDTA chelation in removing arterial plaque. To learn more, read Robert Redfern's *The Miracle Enzyme*, or visit www.themiracleenzyme.info.

■ Two additional substances have been shown effective in significantly reducing atherosclerotic plaque. See Seanol,® and Iodo-niacin under ***Iodine***, both in the **General Treatment Methods** section.

Promoting Endothelial Health

Because healthy endothelial function is such an important aspect in the prevention and treatment of all aspects of cardiovascular disease, any means of promoting healthy endothelium is an important step in maintaining cardiovascular health.

■ ***Resveratrol***. A naturally-occurring compound, resveratrol is found in various food-stuffs and plants including berries, grapes, peanuts, pine trees, and some herbs. For use in dietary supplements, it is often extracted from the root of the *Polygonum cuspidatum* plant. Chemically, resveratrol is classified a *polyphenol*, a broad group of plant-derived compounds further subdivided into other categories including *flavonoids*, *tannins*, and *lignins*. First identified as recently as the early 1980s, there was no clinical interest in resveratrol until the 1990s when it was discovered that trans-resveratrol—the active component—is present in wine.

Harvard scientists have recently shown that resveratrol may prevent many of the detrimental health effects caused by overeating and obesity—including endothelial dysfunction—even without reducing the weight of the eater. Recent studies have shed light on this interesting phenomenon. When middle-aged mice were fed a high-calorie diet, they became obese and exhibited metabolic changes resembling diabetes, liver and heart damage, and suffered premature deaths. However, after about six months the mice fed resveratrol along with the high-calorie diet showed beneficial changes in their physiology similar to those fed a standard diet.

The resveratrol-fed mice on the high-calorie diet showed increased insulin sensitivity, lower blood sugar levels, enhanced mitochondrial energy production, and improved motor function. Non-resveratrol-fed mice on the high-calorie diet developed enlarged, fatty livers, while the resveratrol-fed mice did not. Further, heart disease and evidence of atherosclerosis were seen in mice fed the high-calorie diet without resveratrol, but not in the group that were also fed resveratrol. Resveratrol significantly increased survival, reducing the risk of death from the high-calorie diet by 31%. It also improved the animals' quality of life, as shown in their steady improvement in balance and coordination with age.

These benefits were experienced by the resveratrol-fed mice on a high-calorie diet even though they remained obese. This information offers powerful evidence that resveratrol may similarly protect humans from the harmful effects of a high-calorie diet. In fact, this could be a literal case "having your cake and eating it too." One product offering high levels of trans-resveratrol is Now Foods' Mega Potency Natural Resveratrol.

■ *Superoxide Dismutase*. *Superoxide radicals* are one of the most damaging *reactive oxygen species* (oxidants; free radicals) within cells. They compromise healthy endothelial function by inactivating nitric oxide, the chemical vasodilator of the blood vessels produced by the inner lining of the arteries. Quenching superoxide radicals in the arterial walls is associated with improved endothelial function and regression of atherosclerotic plaque. One of the body's most important and powerful antioxidants is *superoxide dismutase* (SOD). It is particularly effective in quenching superoxide radicals.

Until recently, it had been difficult for SOD to be effectively administered orally, as most forms of SOD supplements are deactivated in the digestive tract before entering the bloodstream. The French company Iocell SA has pioneered the development of a natural form of SOD called GliSODin.® The patented, plant-sourced product is available as an ingredient in various dietary supplement formulations marketed by several companies. Derived from cantaloupe melon, GliSODin is coated with the wheat protein extract gliadin, which protects it from degradation in the stomach's acidic environment and facilitates its intact absorption by the small intestines into the bloodstream.

In clinical trials, GliSODin raised levels of SOD by 49% and increased catalase by up to 170%. Supplementation for 18 months significantly reversed atherosclerotic plaque, as indicated by CIMT ultrasound. The investigators stated that GliSODin "improves, significantly, the antioxidant status and diminishes, remarkably, carotid artery IMT."[75]

■ *Cocoa*. Chocolate is derived from cocoa, the dried, fatty seed of the cocao tree. In recent years a specific form of cocoa has been shown to be one of the most effective substances in combating cardiovascular disease. Cocoa polyphenols are known to normalize platelet (blood-clotting) activation and enhance endothelial function by increasing nitric oxide levels. This in turn leads to a number of positive effects on the cardiovascular system including decreased blood pressure, reduced insulin resistance, reduced levels of oxidative stress, decreased LDL oxidation, increased HDL, and the general slowing down of the atherosclerotic process.

An example of these positive effects is a 2006 study reported in the journal *Heart*[76] which compared two groups of participants consuming chocolate. One group consumed dark chocolate while the other consumed white. The dark chocolate but not the white contained unique cocoa polyphenols shown to have positive health benefits in other studies. The dark chocolate but not the white chocolate group experienced a significant improvement in flow mediated dilation as measured by an ultrasound test of the brachial artery. Compared to baseline, flow mediated dilation in the dark chocolate group improved by 37% and the benefits persisted for about eight hours. Platelet activation—which has the dangerous effect of increasing blood viscosity—was reduced in the dark chocolate group

36% within two hours. The white chocolate group saw no alteration of platelet activity.

Although this and other studies clearly show very positive but short-term (short lasting—from hours to several days) effects from consuming cocoa in the form of chocolate candy (dark chocolate candy) and chocolate beverages, the benefits of continuous, long-term use of cocoa polyphenols are not gained by consuming many/most chocolate products in these forms, as these products contain hundreds of excess calories in the form of sugar and fats that counteract any positive benefits produced by the cocoa. One solution is to consume pill-form cocoa supplements that contain a standardized amount of cocoa polyphenols. Three such products are manufactured by the Life Extension Foundation: CocoaGold,™ Pomegranate Extract with CocoaGold,™ and Super Polyphenol Extracts with CocoaGold,™ all of which are available from sources listed in **Appendix A**.

■ *Wolfberry*. Known by its more common name goji berries, wolfberries (*Lycium barbarum*) have been used in Traditional Chinese Medicine for nearly 2,000 years as a general tonic, immune system enhancer, liver detoxifier, longevity promoter, and for many other purposes. The berries are available as dried berries, juice, or as a standardized extract. In one representative study,[77] when 64-80 year old patients were given wolfberry, they experienced a 48% increase in SOD levels in 10 days.

■ *Combination Formulations*. In addition to the three above-named products, the Life Extension Foundation markets two multi-formulation products focusing on enhanced endothelial function and arterial plaque reduction: SODzyme™ and Endothelial Defense.™ SODzyme contains GliSODin and wolfberry, while Endothelial Defense contains GliSODin, pomegranate extract, and cocoa extract.

Congestive Heart Failure

The leading cause of hospitalization in persons over 65, *heart failure* is an impairment in the ability of the heart to fill with blood or pump a sufficient amount of blood through the body. *Congestive heart failure* (CHF) implies an inadequate ability to pump blood. Many factors contribute to CHF, including diseases that weaken or stiffen the heart, past heart

attacks, and chronic hypertension. Symptoms can include fatigue; shortness of breath, particularly when lying horizontal; diminished exercise capacity; swelling of feet, ankles, legs or abdomen; and an increase in urination, particularly at night.

■ *Coenzyme Q10* (CoQ10). All living things contain enzymes, complex protein substances which initiate and accelerate chemical reactions either to create molecular structures or to produce the electrochemical energy which powers the organism's cellular engines. Enzymes are composed of at least two ingredients: a protein component and a cofactor component. The protein component consists of specific amino acids which are determined by the genetic code. The cofactor component consists either of mineral ions (e.g., magnesium, potassium, calcium or zinc), vitamins, or sometimes both. The vitamin component of the cofactor is typically referred to as a *coenzyme*.[78]

Discovered only in 1957, coenzyme Q10, abbreviated CoQ10, is a naturally-occurring molecule of critical importance to health and life itself. It's presence is essential for all of the body's cells, tissues and organs. CoQ10 is also called *ubiquinone*, formed from the word ubiquitous (everywhere present) and the coenzyme *quinone*. CoQ10 is similar in molecular structure to vitamin K.

There are presently 10 known CoQs—CoQ1 through CoQ10—various forms of which are contained in yeasts, bacteria, fungi, plants and animals, including humans. Human cells contain only CoQ10. Coenzymes from lower forms—plants and animals—can be converted into Q10 within the human body by the liver, but this ability declines with age. Deficiencies of CoQ10 greater than 50% have been observed in the elderly. As Q10 levels decline, there is a corresponding decrease in health and freedom from disease states.[79]

Dr. Karl Folkers of the University of Texas at Austin, recognized as the "father of CoQ research," was the first to identify CoQ10's crucial role in cell respiration and energy production. Folkers believes that overt disease states may appear at deficiency levels of 25-75%, and death may occur at deficiency levels of 75-100%.

The highest concentrations of Q10 are found within the organs that have the greatest energy requirements—the heart muscle, the liver and the cells of the immune system. A CoQ10 deficiency can result from impaired Q10 synthesis due to a nutritional deficiency; illness (infection or other suppression of the immune system); the aging process; a genetic or acquired defect; increased cellular requirements; or taking statin drugs.

CoQ10 has been found useful in the treatment of cardiovascular disease. It can prevent or reverse degenerative heart lesions caused by high blood pressure. It also can treat angina and congestive heart failure by supplying optimal cellular nutrition. Many recent studies conducted in the United States, Japan, and Italy have found CoQ10 extremely effective in treating congestive heart failure.

Cardiomyopathy is the deterioration of the actual heart muscle, the myocardium. Those with this disease have a reduced force of heart contraction and are at risk of arrhythmia and sudden cardiac death. The *Proceedings of the National Academy of Sciences* reported 89% of 80 treated patients with cardiomyopathy improved while taking 100 mg of CoQ10 for 12 weeks, maintained that improvement, but deteriorated when treatment was discontinued. Other studies have shown it to be an effective treatment in many ailments of the heart, including angina, arrhythmias, coronary artery bypass surgery, heart transplants, high blood pressure, hyperthyroid heart failure, mitral valve prolapse, and valve replacement.[80] Folkers stated,

> I am fully content to believe that a deficiency in CoQ10 may be a disease to be treated by oral administration... I believe it is quite possible that cardiovascular disease may be very significantly caused by a deficiency of CoQ10. ...patients in advanced cardiac failure, who had only a few months to live, under close medical care, have revealed almost 'miraculous' improvement after treatment with CoQ10.[81]

Various forms of CoQ10 are available, some better and more absorbable than others. The natural molecule is preferable to the synthetic. *Ubiquinol*, the reduced and more bioavailable form, is the most effective form of Coenzyme Q10.

■ *Enhanced External Counterpulsation*.® For those who appreciate a mechanical approach, Enhanced External Counterpulsation (EECP) is a non-invasive outpatient procedure shown by clinical trials to reduce or eliminate the frequency and in-

tensity of anginal symptoms by increasing blood flow to the heart, thereby decreasing the need for medication. EECP has also been used effectively in treating congestive heart failure (CHF).

EECP was pioneered by Vasomedical, Incorporated of Westbury, NY. The following description is excerpted from Vasomedical's website.

> EECP treatment uses unique equipment to inflate and deflate a series of pneumatic compressive...cuffs that are wrapped firmly, but comfortably around the patient's calves, lower thighs, and upper thighs, including the buttocks...While the heart is at rest the cuffs are inflated in rapid sequence from the calves upward, creating a pressure wave that increases diastolic blood pressure, coronary artery perfusion pressure, and blood flow to the heart muscle. This compression of the blood vessels in the legs also increases the volume of blood returned to the right side of the heart via the venous system. Instantaneous deflation of all cuffs at the onset of the heart's contraction lowers the resistance the heart must pump against, decreasing the heart's work load. This latter effect, when coupled with increased venous return, significantly raises cardiac output. The overall effect is to increase the oxygen supply of the heart, while decreasing its oxygen demand.[82]

It is believed that EECP creates new pathways around blocked arteries in the heart by expanding networks of tiny blood vessels that help increase blood flow to the heart muscle. This process is known as *collateral circulation*. EECP technology offers a treatment option for those who are unable (medically unsuitable) or unwilling to undergo the more invasive procedure of surgery. A course of treatments typically totals 35 hours, divided into one or two 60-minute sessions each day, five days a week, for four to six weeks.

In a three year follow-up study conducted at the State University of New York at Stony Brook, the majority of patients tested remained free of anginal symptoms, continued to improve on their heart scan monitoring, and experienced an increased ability to engage in routine daily activities.[83] To learn more, visit www.vasomedical.com.

■ *Testosterone*. It is known that heart muscle cells have testosterone receptors. It's not surprising to learn that aging men with CHF who supplement with bio-identical testosterone have shown dramatic improvement in their heart muscle function. To learn more, see Testosterone under **Diabetes**.

Hypertension

Abnormally high arterial blood pressure is referred to as *hypertension*, and its causes can include an inherited predisposition, poor nutrition, stress, excessive alcohol consumption, obesity, overuse of (regular table) salt, hormonal imbalances, and microbial infection, as discussed above. *Essential hypertension* describes the condition for the majority of cases (~95%) where no specific cause is isolated. In *secondary hypertension*, the cause is related to a specific medical condition (e.g., kidney, adrenal gland, etc.). A blood pressure measurement above 140/90 mm Hg is considered indicative of hypertension, and readings ranging from 120-129/80-89 are considered "prehypertension." About 25% of Americans have hypertension.

Hypertension is called a "silent killer" because its victims often experience no symptoms for years or possibly decades. By the time it is diagnosed, serious damage to critical organ systems may have occurred. Uncontrolled hypertension can lead to many additional complications, including damage to the blood vessels in the eye, kidney failure, and cardiovascular disease including stroke. The condition triples one's risk of death from a heart attack and increases by 700% one's risk of a stroke.

In addition to blood pressure, *pulse pressure* (PP) offers an indication of increased risk of heart disease. Pulse pressure is the numeric difference between the systolic (top figure) and the diastolic (bottom figure) pressures. For example, a blood pressure reading of 130/80 mm Hg (millimeters of mercury) yields a PP of 50. The most important causative factor of elevated PP is arteriosclerosis, or "hardening"—stiffness and reduced elasticity—of the arteries, which itself may be caused by hypertension or atherosclerosis.

Systolic blood pressure typically rises with age, while diastolic pressure often remains constant or declines. Especially in older adults, a pulse pressure reading over 60 is indicative of cardiovascular disease. The higher the number, the more damaged the vessels are believed to be. A 2000 article in the *Journal of the American College of Cardiology*[84] reported that for persons over age 65, for every 10 mm Hg increase in PP, the participants' heart disease risk increased by 12%; their risk of heart failure increased by 14%; and their risk of death increased by 6%. In a 20 year follow-up study of 6,539 adults reported in 2001 in the journal *Circulation*,[85] for persons under age 50 high diastolic pressure was the best predictor of heart disease; for persons aged 50-59, PP, systolic, and diastolic pressures were equally predictive of heart disease risk; and for persons aged 60-79, the strongest predictor of heart disease was high PP. Treating high blood pressure often reduces PP.

Many pharmaceutical drugs are available to treat hypertension, including *diuretics* [hydrochlorothiazide (Hydrodiuril®), furosemide (Lasix®), torsemide (Demadex®), metolazone (Zaroxolyn®)]; *alpha-blockers* [terazosin (Hytrin®), doxazosin (Cardura®), tamsulosin (Flomax®)]; *beta-blockers* [atenolol (Tenormin®), propranolol (Inderal®), metoprolol (Toprol®)]; *ACE inhibitors* [enalapril (Vasotec®), captopril (Capoten®), lisinopril (Zestril® and Prinivil®), benazepril (Lotensin®), quinapril (Accupril®)]; *alpha antagonists* [clonidine (Catapres®)]; and *vasodialators* [minoxidil (Loniten®)]. The often significant side-effects of these drugs include acute kidney failure; air passage swelling; dizziness; impotence; increased risk of heart attack; and worsening of congestive heart failure.

Side-effect-free treatments include the following, many of which are discussed in this section: 1) Coenzyme Q10, 2) Essential fatty acids (EFAs), 3) Essential phospholipids (EPL), 4) Melatonin, 5) Exercise (See **Nutrition: Detoxification and Deficiencies** under **General Treatment Methods**, 6) L-theanine (See **Stress**), 7) Nattokinase, 8) IR Sauna (See **Nutrition: Detoxification & Deficiencies** under **General Treatment Methods**), 9) Chelation Therapy, 10) Balance3 (Seven Chinese herbs; recommended by Dr. Julian Whitaker: "It lowers blood pressure rapidly and consistently." www.balance3.com), 11) RESPeRATE® (a mechanical device with FDA approval; www.resperate.com), 12) Fasting has been shown to have a dramatic effect on hypertension, with prolonged results. For more information, visit http://antiaging-europe.com/lists/96/diseases.html, and 13) HeartCare® by Himalaya USA is a multi-herb ayurvedic formula. 14) Carditone,® manufactured by Ayush

Herbs, has significantly reduced blood pressure in many hypertensive patients who were unsuccessful using any other method(s), including the above.

■ ___Zona Plus___.™ The Zona Plus is a hand-held device that is used to perform computer-regulated isometric hand exercises for 12 minutes a day, five days per week. When used as directed, it reduces blood pressure in non-medicated patients from five mm Hg (points) to 55 mm Hg, with an average drop of 25+ mm Hg. Individuals taking medication see an average drop of 19 mm Hg. A measurable drop in the resting systolic blood pressure (top number) will be seen after about four to five weeks. Maximum benefits are seen in six to eight weeks.

The discovery of the technology behind the Zona Plus was completely accidental. When the U.S. Air Force began deploying the F-16 fighter jet in the late 1960s, the difficult maneuverability of this aircraft led many fighter pilots to experience "G-force blackout," causing temporary loss of vision. The Air Force commissioned Dr. Ronald L. Wiley, a cardiopulmonary physiologist, to be part of a study to help increase G-tolerance. The study utilized extreme isometric handgrip efforts.

Dr. Wiley discovered over the 10 to 12 week test periods that not only was G-force tolerance increased, some test subjects with elevated blood pressure experienced a lowering of pressure. He realized he had discovered an exciting new therapy for treating hypertension. Over the next two decades, Dr. Wiley dedicated himself to researching isometric therapy protocols in various university laboratories to develop the ideal therapy to safely and effectively lower blood pressure. He then tested this therapy in numerous controlled studies conducted by physicians in private practice and in cardiac rehabilitation centers, and found it produced dramatic results in just weeks.

Clinical studies have consistently shown that Zona therapy, performed as recommended, is three to four times more effective in lowering blood pressure than 30 minutes of vigorous aerobic exercise performed three times per week—with greater ease and compliance capability. The price of the Zona Plus is reasonable when compared to long-term use of expensive and side-effect-producing blood pressure medication. It has been shown to reduce blood pressure equally effectively as a front-line anti-hy-

pertensive pharmaceutical. To learn more about the Zona Plus, visit www.zonaplus.com.

■ See ___Seanol___ under **General Treatment Methods**. This algal extract treats many aspects of CVD including lowering blood pressure significantly.

Rebuilding the Heart After a Heart Attack

It was believed at one time that atherosclerosis could not be reversed. We now know this is incorrect. Similarly, it was believed until recently that following a heart attack, damaged cells of the heart muscle couldn't be regenerated, and that damage was permanent. Researchers at New York Medical College and the Universities of Udine and Trieste, Italy, have now shed new light on this issue.

As reported in the *New England Journal of Medicine*[86] in 2001, the researchers microscopically examined portions of the heart muscles of 13 patients who had recently died of a heart attack. Cells were examined both in the locations of the dead tissue and in the unaffected areas. Several markers that signify cellular growth (mitosis)—key indicators of cell regeneration—were evaluated.

The researchers were surprised to find that in the area of damage, tissue regrowth was occurring at a rate of 4% compared to only 1% in areas of the healthy, undamaged tissue. In other words, tissue that had been damaged was regenerating 300% faster than the normal, healthy tissue. Even more surprising is the finding that the number of heart-muscle cells regenerating in the diseased hearts was 70 times higher in the zones bordering the necrotic tissue and 24 times higher in the remote myocardium in comparison to the control group's normal hearts.[87]

> Our results challenge the dogma that the adult heart is a postmitotic organ, and raise the possibility that the regeneration of myocytes may contribute to the increase in muscle mass of the myocardium.[88]

Dr. Claude Lenfant, Director of the National Heart, Lung and Blood Institute remarked, "With this landmark study, we have a new understanding of the heart that opens up the possibility of repairing heart muscle damage after a heart attack."[89]

Another conclusion of the researchers is that it is likely there are either stem cells or primitive stem-cell-like cells present in the human heart. This could be the mechanism that accounts for the dramatic self-regeneration of the damaged heart muscle. These cells might be able to be coaxed to migrate to the damaged area, and further assist regeneration.[90] It is known that injury to a target organ is sensed by distant stem cells which migrate to the damaged area, undergo differentiation, and assist in structural and functional repair. This is enabled by the high degree of stem cell plasticity.[91]

■ *Stem Cells*. When stem cells are injected into damaged myocardial tissue, regeneration is enhanced. As reported in *Nature*[92] in 2001, researchers from the National Institutes of Health injected bone marrow stem cells into the contracting wall bordering the necrotic myocardial tissue (dead heart cells) of infarcted mice. Within nine days, 68% of the dead portion of the ventricle was occupied by newly-formed myocardial tissue. See Stem Cells in the **Index** and in the Member's Area of *The Encyclopedia's* website.

■ *D-Ribose*. A naturally occurring substance used by the body to synthesize and rebuild energy in every cell, D-ribose is a five carbon sugar (monosaccharide)—unlike sucrose (ordinary table sugar), glucose, and fructose, which are six carbon sugars. Its use does not raise blood sugar levels as does ordinary sugar, and therefore would be appropriate for use by diabetics. In fact, ribose administered intravenously and by high-dose oral intake lowers blood sugar levels in a dose-dependent manner.

Ribose is the most basic building block of adenosine triphosphate (ATP), the principal energy source of every cell in the body, sometimes referred to as the "energy currency" of the cell. When blood flow to the heart is impeded (*ischemia*, a lack of oxygen to tissues), there is a substantial lowering of tissue energy due to a decrease in the level of ATP in the heart tissues. Ribose is the beginning point for the synthesis of energetic cellular components, and its availability determines the rate at which these components can be synthesized.

Many studies have shown that energy levels in the heart can be dramatically lowered by exercise or certain cardiac diseases. Depleted cardiac energy may be associated with increased cardiac stress, reduced blood flow to the periphery, fatigue, and decreased exercise tolerance. Ribose is a key nutrient for quickly restoring cardiac energy stores.

Clinical and laboratory studies on the hearts of both animals and humans have shown many positive benefits of ribose including increased ventricular function in patients with congestive heart failure; enhanced recovery of energy-carrying nucleotide levels following ischemia; increased ability to tolerate exercise in patients with stable coronary artery disease; and decreased recovery times following strenuous exercise.

Supplemental ribose provides many benefits to persons with congestive heart failure, cardiomyopathy, those having had a coronary artery bypass, and persons who have had a heart attack. Because ribose is so effective in boosting ATP levels within cells, its use is greatly beneficial in any instance of ischemia where the heart muscle is deprived of oxygen either by a decrease in blood flow (e.g., exercise or congestive heart failure) or cessation of blood flow that occurs during a heart attack.

Following a heart attack, damaged, blood-deprived cells have a limited window of time to regain their function before heart muscle damage occurs as the result of cell death. The delay in restoring blood—oxygen, nutrients, ATP, etc.—to the heart muscle subsequent to a heart attack (or cardiac bypass surgery), followed by the resumption of blood flow, causes *ischemia reperfusion injury*. Restoration of blood flow—reperfusion—produces inflammation and oxidative damage due to oxidative stress, and is known to be the major cause of long-term heart damage. Further, during reperfusion, cells require unusually high levels of ATP to address the damage caused by ischemia-induced oxidative damage. By quickly restoring ATP levels within the cells of the heart muscle, D-ribose is a powerful tool in rejuvenating and rebuilding the heart following reperfusion in cases of heart attacks and bypass surgery, as well as any other condition where the heart is deprived of adequate blood flow. Administration of ribose has been shown to restore post-infarction heart muscle ATP to normal or near-normal levels.

In one study, administration of ribose to the heart during bypass surgery in which blood flow was stopped for one hour showed significant improvement in heart function in comparison to the control group. The degree of improvement was related to heart levels of ATP.[93]

In another study published in 1991 in the *Journal of the American College of Cardiology*,[94] patients with coronary artery disease were subjected to a stress test of moderate exercise while their heart function was monitored using the radioactive tracer thallium viewed by a special imaging camera. One group of participants received a ribose infusion and were monitored four hours following the infusion. The control group received a placebo infusion and were monitored 24 hours thereafter. The ribose group showed 21 areas of defective (underperforming but still living) heart tissue that were not seen in the placebo group.

This remarkable result indicates that ribose awakened dormant or "hibernating" heart tissue—a result suggesting ribose's ability to improve healthy heart function following a heart attack. In addition, ribose's use enhances cardiologists' ability to access the true level of cardiac damage by differentiating necrotic (dead) from merely dormant cells.

Over time, researchers have determined the appropriate dosage recommendations for various health conditions, as follows:[95]

• Cardiovascular protection for healthy persons: 5 gm daily

• High-intensity exercise; persons with peripheral vascular disease; mild-to-moderate heart failure or other forms of ischemic cardiovascular disease; heart surgery or heart attack; stable angina: 10-15 gm daily in divided doses of 5 gm/dose.

• Frequent angina; advanced heart failure; heart transplant candidates; congestive cardiomyopathy; fibromyalgia or neuromuscular disease: 15-30 gm daily in divided doses of 5 gm/dose.

A full list of the cardiovascular benefits of ribose can be viewed at www.bioenergy.com/Ribose_Heart_Health.html. To purchase ribose, visit www.nutrabio.com/Products/ribose.htm.

■ *EWOT*. A powerful method of encouraging heart muscle growth following a heart attack is to increase the oxygen supply to the heart. A means of accomplishing this within the privacy of one's own home is EWOT, or Exercise with Oxygen Therapy. If one exercises while breathing pure oxygen, the body becomes super oxygenated. For those who have suffered a heart attack, this is a simple way to assist the heart in regenerating healthy cells. To learn more, see *Exercise With Oxygen Therapy* under **General Treatment Methods**, or read Dr. William C. Douglass' book, *Stop Aging or Slow the Process: Exercise with Oxygen Therapy (EWOT) Can Help.*

■ *Hyperbaric Oxygenation*. Another method of encouraging heart muscle regrowth following a heart attack also increases the oxygen supply to the heart. *Hyperbaric Oxygenation Therapy* (HBOT), discussed under **General Treatment Methods**, is an excellent tool to accomplish heart cell regrowth.

■ *Additional Strategies*. In addition to the various strategies discussed above, diet and lifestyle play a significant role in cardiovascular disease, including heart attacks. To treat the underlying cause and prevent further complications, changes in diet and lifestyle will be necessary. Adopt the Mediterranean diet, as discussed above. Walking at the leisurely pace of three miles per hour for 30 minutes five times per week (or shorter segments, as long as the segments are at least 10 minutes), both increases longevity and protects against cardiovascular events. Exercise regularly. Better yet, exercise with pure oxygen (EWOT). In addition, supplement with flax or chia (seeds and/or oil), coenzyme Q10, and a good multi-vitamin/mineral. Also control excess weight, stop smoking, and reduce your stress level.

Stroke

Within industrialized countries, stroke is the most frequent life-threatening neurological affliction. Caused by a rupture or obstruction (such as a clot) of an artery in the brain, a stroke results in diminished or loss of consciousness, speech or voluntary motion. Many techniques are discussed in this section which can help prevent a stroke from occurring—the most important of which is to maintain healthy blood pressure levels. If you have been an unfortunate victim, there are several methods that can assist in regaining lost function. HBO and EWOT are two important methods. Super oxygenating the blood, hence the brain, often leads to restoration of function in stroke victims.

■ *Constraint Induced Movement Therapy*. **(CIMT, or CI Therapy).** A technique offering much hope to stroke victims is being called an example of miracle medicine. Constraint Induced

Movement Therapy aims to assist brain-damaged individuals regain significant use of an affected limb when suffering from *hemiparesis*—total or partial paralysis of the limb or limbs of one side of the body which results from disease or injury to the motor centers of the brain. CI also appears to be effective in treating spinal cord injury, fractured hip, children with cerebral palsy, and musicians with focal hand dystonia (incoordination of the fingers).

During the initial period of limited mobility following an injury or other damage to the brain, a person learns not to attempt to use the affected limb(s), called "learned non-use." While efforts to use the affected limb are futile, painful and embarrassing, the motor area of the brain begins to atrophy as the result of non-use. This results in the person's continued inability to move the limb.

CI therapists believe that learned non-use can be overcome and reversed. The technique consists of constraining the unaffected (good) limb such as an arm or leg, while the affected limb receives intensive physical training six to seven hours per day for two to three weeks—referred to as "massed practice." The unaffected limb is immobilized either by bandages, a cast, a sling or a mitt, while the affected limb is exercised using routines such as drawing; playing chess or checkers; sweeping the floor; throwing a ball; or walking. The unaffected limb remains immobilized for 90% of the time.

Following brain injury, a certain number of brain cells die. However, many cells surrounding the area most severely affected are merely "stunned," and continue to live and have sufficient plasticity to recover, according to CI Therapies' underlying rationale. The goal of CI Therapy is to reawaken these stunned or partially-injured cells so that they take over the task of the totally nonfunctional cells. In effect, CI aids the brain in rewiring itself by triggering new connections, resulting in massive cortical reorganization.[96]

Of the several hundred patients who have received CI Therapy to date, the best results have been achieved in patients with mild to moderately-severe stroke—representing the upper 50-75% of the most severely-impaired. Virtually all patients benefit substantially, with most regaining much of their lost limb movement, even if begun years after the stroke occurs. Following two weeks of therapy, most patients begin using their affected limbs much more normally. Those with an affected hand or arm begin to dress themselves, brush their teeth—in fact, they reenter the world of the able bodied, and the results appear to be permanent.[97]

The routine of CI Therapy is fairly intensive. Those who most closely comply with the treatment guidelines receive the most benefit. Participants must have patience and a willingness to work hard, and must be continually encouraged that hard work will produce positive results.

There should be a span of several weeks between the initial injury/stroke and the initiation of therapy, as animal studies have shown that damage to the brain increases when the limb is used immediately following an experimentally-induced stroke.[98] Most of the studies have been done either at the University of Alabama or in Germany. Dr. Edward Taub is one of CI's leading proponents and administers it at the Taub Training Clinic in Birmingham. The cost ranges from USD $6,000-13,000, and is not covered by Medicare or other insurers. The CI Therapy Research Laboratory, also in Birmingham, carries out various therapy research projects for which treatment is free. To investigate clinical trial availability, visit www.strokecenter.org/trials/. To speak to the University of Alabama Taub Training Clinic, call (205)975-9799.

■ ***Nanotechnology***. It has been a challenge for neuroscientists to repair nerve damage, hence function, following traumatic damage such as that caused by a stroke. Nerve regeneration in the central nervous system—the brain and spinal cord—is problematic for several reasons, including the formation of scar tissue and the gaps which form in tissues as a result of the trauma. A novel approach to these problems has been studied by a team of scientists at two prestigious universities, the Massachusetts Institute of Technology and Hong Kong University, as reported in the *Proceedings of the National Academy of Sciences*[99] in 2006. The new approach focuses on nanotechnology—the branch of science dealing with the manipulation of the most basic physical elements, molecules and atoms.

The researchers mimicked the effects of traumatic brain injury by severing the optic nerve tract of hamsters, causing them to lose vision. The hamsters were thereafter injected at the site of injury with a solution containing synthetically-prepared, individual amino acids which create self-assembling peptide nanoparticles measuring five nanometers. Following the injection of the liquid—which looks exactly like water—the peptides spontaneously arrange into a scaffold-like criss-cross of nanofibers bridging the gap between the severed nerves.

In the study, the brain tissue knitted together across the molecular scaffolding, restoring vision and preventing scar tissue from forming. According to Dr. Rutledge Ellis-Behnke, a lead neuroscientist at MIT, "The first thing we saw was that the brain had started to heal itself in the first 24 hours. We had never seen that before—so that was very surprising."[100] After performing their task, the nanopeptides are quickly broken down by the body into a harmless substance and excreted in the urine.

The scientists studied both young hamsters with actively growing nerve cells, as well as adult hamsters whose nerve growth had stopped. They were surprised to find the nerves in both groups were able to regrow, restoring functional vision and orienting behavior to the animals without the need of providing cell growth factors.

During the researchers' study with the nanopeptide material, a remarkable discovery was made by accident. When the solution was applied directly to injured tissue, it stopped bleeding in less than 15 seconds. In further tests, it was found to stop the bleeding of skin, liver, lung, blood vessels, and a variety of other tissues. Although the exact mechanism(s) of this phenomenon are somewhat of a mystery, Ellis-Behnke has determined that clotting isn't taking place, as the constituents fibrin, thrombin, and platelets are not present as would be expected if clotting were the cause. Apparently, this nano-material can even be used to rebuild damaged tissue. It has been used successfully both internally and externally and may have important emergency medical and battlefield applications.[101]

■ *Music Therapy*. Researchers at the Cognitive Brain Research Unit of the University of Helsinki in Finland have shown that listening to music for a minimum of one hour daily soon after a stroke significantly increases recovery. In a research study,[102] the Helsinki scientists divided 60 stroke patients into three groups. One group listened to audio books of their choice. Another group listened to music CDs of their choice for a minimum of one

hour daily. The control group received only normal rehabilitation therapy.

The music group experienced significantly increased verbal memory, concentration/focus, and mood while experiencing significantly less confusion. Particularly in cases where the severity of the stroke prevents more active forms of rehabilitation during the early stages of recovery, listening to one to two hours of music daily can make a significant difference in a stroke victim's recovery rate.

■ *Caffeinol and Cooling*. In persons suffering a stroke, there is a short window of opportunity following the incident to apply treatment which aims to limit the potential damage caused by lack of blood flow to affected parts of the brain. As discussed earlier in this section, tPAs are given in less than 5% of ischemic stroke cases for fear of increasing the damage if given to a hemorrhagic stroke victim. Even so, tPAs must be administered by skilled physicians in a hospital setting.

One technique being used by a select group of enlightened physicians is generically referred to as *hypothermia*, or "thermo-cooling," where the body is rapidly cooled in an effort to limit the damage. Although this takes place in a hospital setting where the brain is cooled by two to three degrees Centigrade, the "at-home" version entails wrapping a wet towel around the stroke victim's head as soon after the onset of the stroke as possible—and keeping the towel in place on the way to the hospital. The evaporation of moisture from the wet towel causes a decrease in temperature, thus cooling the brain.

University of Texas neurologist James Grotta has developed a technique of treating ischemic strokes using a combination of caffeine and alcohol. The experimental drug, called caffeinol, has the equivalent potency of two to three cups of strong coffee and a shot of alcohol. When injected into rats within three hours of an artificially-stimulated stroke, brain damage was reduced by up to 80%.[103]

Grotta and colleagues have demonstrated the safety and neuroprotective effectiveness of caffeinol in a small group of ischemic stroke patients. A study[104] of 10 human patients found that 60% of caffeinol users had a complete recovery, compared to only 26% of those not treated by the caffeine/alcohol combination. In rat studies, neither caffeine nor alcohol alone offered protection. In fact, alcohol alone increased brain damage. Grotta postulates that caffeine blocks the release by the dying cells of the damaging chemical glutamate, and ethanol blocks the action of glutamate.

The "at-home" version of caffeinol would be to keep a stock of coffee and a good whiskey at your residence. At the first sign of a stroke, administer a combination of two to three cups of strong, black coffee and about two ounces of whiskey. (Some have observed this combination is a little whipped cream and sugar short of an Irish coffee.) Studies have determined that caffeinol can be used in combination with tPAs, so there is no conflict posed by using this potentially brain-saving technique at the earliest opportunity following a stroke.

■ *Ginkgo biloba.* The herb *Ginkgo biloba* offers a restorative function in seizure or stroke victims. The herb protects nerve tissue from damage, presumably by increasing the blood flow to damaged neurological sites. In Europe, where Gingko is a prescription drug, some physicians have had good success using the herb to treat stroke victims.

■ For immediate treatment of stroke, see also Capsaicin under Angina Pectoris, and Nattokinase under Blood Clots, both in this section.

■ See Omental Transposition, Laser Light, and DMSO under **Spinal Cord Injury**.

Erectile Dysfunction

Impotence is the general term used to describe the inability to achieve and maintain an erection. The term erectile dysfunction or ED connotes physiological involvement, although today the two terms are used almost synonymously. In the not-too-distant past, impotence was thought to have a strictly psychological rather than a physiological origin. It's now recognized either psychology and/or physiology can be important causative factors. Because the brain is intimately involved in human sexuality, psychological states such as anxiety, depression, guilt, and emotional stress often play a role in a man's ability to achieve and maintain an erection.

In 1994, the Massachusetts Male Aging Study[105] of 1,290 men aged 40-70 documented the high prevalence of ED in aging American men. Fifty percent of 50 year olds and 70% of 70 year olds were found to have ED. These statistics help ex-

plain the popularity of pharmaceutical drugs targeting ED such as Viagra,® Levitra,® and Cialis®—even though various of these medications have been shown to have serious potential side-effects including severe brain and eye damage including blindness. Implants, vacuum devices, suppositories, and gene therapy round out the current options.

There are many other common causes of impotence including certain prescription drugs, and non-prescription drugs such as alcohol and tobacco. Several disease states can lead to ED including hypogonadism, M.S., Parkinson's, Peyronie's disease, and prostate cancer. Healthy men experience involuntary erections during sleep—known as *nocturnal penile tumescence*—usually in the early morning hours. The absence of such erections implicates a physical rather than a psychological cause—although they may go unnoticed. Currently there is no standardized test to measure nocturnal erections.

A significant factor in many cases of ED is dysfunction and/or disease relating to the cardiovascular system. Such problems include atherosclerosis, diabetes, hypertension, and related physical concerns such as obesity and metabolic syndrome. ED and cardiovascular disease, specifically coronary artery disease, are intimately linked. A 2006 study[106] documented the connection between Italian men with severe heart disease and ED. Ninety-three percent experienced ED 24 months prior to a heart attack or heart disease symptoms.

Nitric oxide (NO), discussed earlier, is an important chemical produced by the inner lining of the arteries. It serves the critical function of dilating the arteries, causing an increase in blood flow. In the case of the erectile apparatus, it increases blood flow into the penile tissues. Without adequate production of NO in the penile arteries, blood flow is decreased and healthy, normal erections cannot occur. Any factor that reduces the production of NO decreases the dilation of penile arteries and interferes with healthy erections. Diabetes and a long list of cardiovascular-related abnormalities all have a deleterious effect on NO levels.

■ *L-Arginine.* Most ED remedies achieve their results by increasing NO levels either by increasing the production of NO or decreasing the level of chemicals interfering with NO production. One such remedy is the amino acid L-arginine. The body produces NO directly from the precursor raw material L-arginine. Even though 3,000 to 6,000 mg of L-arginine are consumed daily in the average Western diet in foods such as meats, dairy, nuts, seeds, and beans, supplementing with an additional 3,000 to 6,000 mg twice daily on an empty stomach over several months may decrease ED.

Dr. Romil Stanislavov of the Medical University of Sofia combined the pine bark extract Pycnogenol with L-arginine to produce more impressive results. Pycnogenol stimulates the enzyme that converts L-arginine to NO. Prelox,™ the patented formulation of these two ingredients, combines a daily dose of 1,700 mg of L-arginine with 120 mg of Pycnogenol. In Dr. Stanislavov's study,[107] 80% of the participants receiving Prelox experienced adequate erections within two months and 92.5% within three months. Prelox can be ordered online.

■ **Red Korean Ginseng**. It has been reported for centuries that Korean red ginseng has the "aphrodisiac" properties of enhancing sexual function and desire. Recent research suggests that a group of compounds known as *ginsenicides* relaxes the arteries, thus increasing blood flow. In one study,[108] 60 participants with ED were given 1,000 mg of Korean red ginseng three times daily for 12 weeks. Those taking ginseng experienced improvements in rigidity, penetration, and duration of the erection in comparison to the placebo group.

■ **Testosterone and DHEA**. Two important hormones known to drastically decrease with age are testosterone and DHEA (dehydroepiandrosterone). Testosterone supplementation—especially when applied topically or via injection—often successfully increases erectile function. In studies,[109] 40 to 60% of men with low-to-normal levels experienced improved erectile potency with testosterone supplementation. Success increased to as high as 65% when initial testosterone levels were low (300 ng/dL). Regarding DHEA, one study[110] reported that DHEA levels are closely related to erectile function. Another study[111] found that 50 mg of DHEA daily produced a much improved erectile response.

■ **L-Carnitine**. Carnitine—a naturally-occurring compound synthesized within the body from the amino acids lysine and methionine—enhances er-

rections as effectively as testosterone, according to an Italian study.[112] When taking a combination of two forms of carnitine daily—2,000 mg each of proprionyl-L-carnitine and acetyl-L-carnitine—participants experienced an improvement in erectile function slightly exceeding the benefit of oral testosterone administration and an improvement in mood and energy equal to testosterone. The supplement Magnum Drive, formulated by Dr. Jonathan Wright, uses this exact carnitine combination. To order, Google "magnum drive."

■ **Tongkat Ali**. Also known as Long Jack and botanically as *Eurycoma longfolia (Jack)*, tongkat ali has been used traditionally throughout Southeast Asia for a wide variety of ailments including arthritis, fatigue, headaches, and also as an aphrodisiac. Many studies[113] attest to its ability to increase libido, penile erections, and sexual performance. Although the specific mechanisms of actions are not fully understood, taking high levels of tongkat ali can increase testosterone levels as much as 400%. It's use is therefore not recommended for men having or suspected of having prostate cancer. The branded extract "LJ100"—featured in several supplement brands such as Tongkat Ali from Source Naturals—is a preferred, standardized product.

■ Several additional natural substances are beneficial in enhancing erectile function including the flavonoid plant extracts resveratrol, green tea EGCG, and Seanol®—an algal extract discussed under **General Treatment Methods**, which has been shown to equal or outperform Viagra.®

■ See Stem Cells, Omental Transposition and DMSO under **Spinal Cord Injury**. See also **Molecular Magnetic Energizer** under **General Treatment Methods**—which has shown effectiveness in treating stroke and congestive heart failure—and the Member's Area of *The Encyclopedia's* website.

CATARACTS

The lens of the eye, composed mostly of water and protein, is situated behind the pupil and iris. It functions much like a camera lens, focusing light on the retina—the light-sensitive inner lining at the back of the eye. When light strikes the retina, a biochemical reaction initiates electrical impulses which are transmitted to the brain, whereupon the signals are translated into visual images.

In a healthy eye, protein is arranged in a specific manner that enables the lens to be water clear. A cataract is a clouding of the eye's naturally-clear lens, and is painless except for the progressive loss of vision it can produce. Most are age related, with over 50% of Americans having had a cataract or cataract surgery by age 80.[1] The disease is a leading cause of blindness, robbing the sight of more than 17 million people worldwide.[2]

Most age-related cataracts form when proteins clump together, clouding the lens and reducing the amount of light reaching the retina. Also, as we age, the lens may acquire a yellow/brownish tint which, over time, may increase in saturation, thus making routine activities more difficult.

Age-related cataracts are classified as nuclear, cortical, or posterior subcapsular. Nuclear cataracts form in the nucleus, or center, of the lens as it hardens and yellows with age. Progression is slow, typically causing greater impairment of distance vision, known as nearsightedness or *myopia*. Some with nuclear cataracts are able to read without eyeglasses, referred to as "second sight."

Cortical cataracts form in the periphery of the lens, where the cloudiness begins near the outer edge and gradually extends to the center of the lens. A common symptom is glare from strong light sources such as automobile headlights. Diabetics are prone to developing cortical cataracts.

The cloudiness of a posterior subcapsular cataract begins at the back-most layer of the lens, and often occurs in younger people. Near vision is often more affected than vision at a distance. In addition to being caused by aging, subcapsular cataracts can result from trauma, radiation exposure, diabetes, and the use of corticosteroid drugs.

Although most cataracts are age related, they can form as the result of genetic factors. Congenital cataracts are present at birth in about one out of every 2,000 babies. They also can develop during childhood, often in both eyes. This type may be so small that vision remains unaffected.

Secondary cataracts can form as the result of surgery or other eye problems such as glaucoma. This type of cataract is often treated by laser surgery. Traumatic cataracts develop as a result of physical injury such as physical force, electrical contact, some types of radiation, or contact with chemicals. They may also form as the result of diabetes. Cataracts resulting from trauma can form immediately following the injury or years later.

The causes of cataracts are not fully known; however, researchers believe several factors play a prominent role. Avoiding the following factors are means of preventing the disease:

• Exposure to ultraviolet radiation produced by sunlight and other sources • Extensive use of certain pharmaceutical drugs such as steroids, diuretics, major tranquilizers, and acetaminophen[3] • Extensive use of alcohol • Cigarette smoke • Air pollution • Deficiencies in key substances including vitamins A and E; minerals zinc and selenium; and carotenoids lutein and zeaxanthin.

Western medicine recommends replacement of the lens when loss of vision begins to interfere with life's everyday activities such as driving and reading. Surgery may be suggested in other instances, e.g., when clouding interferes with the diagnosis and/or treatment of other eye diseases such as macular degeneration or diabetic retinopathy. The surgical technique most often used is *phacoemulsification* (or *phaco* for short), where a small incision is made in the cornea and a tiny ultrasound probe is inserted. The ultrasound waves break up the lens into smaller pieces, after which they are removed by suction. A clear, plastic interocular lens (IOL) is then inserted in place of the damaged, clouded lens and becomes a permanent part of the eye requiring no additional care.

Following a successful cataract operation, the new lens is neither seen nor felt. Several new types of IOL lenses are currently available, including one that allows its recipients to see at all distances, and another that blocks ultraviolet and blue wavelengths which are thought to damage retinal tissue.

Cataract surgery is one of the most frequently performed operations in the U.S., with over 1.5 million performed annually.[4] Because eyesight is one of our most valuable assets, surgery should not be taken lightly. Western medicine reports that cataract surgery is one of the safest and most effective operations performed, with about 90% of the cases resulting in improved vision. It logically follows, however, that 10% of the operations result in either no vision improvement or a worsening of vision. In addition, as with any surgery, the procedure is not without risk. In this case, there is a risk of infection, bleeding, inflammation, corneal edema, and retinal detachment. (Other eye diseases such as nearsightedness are known to increase the risk of retinal detachment following surgery.)

Even though the percentage of complications is low, because there are so many operations annually, there are thousands of complications. Although prompt medical attention often successfully treats most complications, they nevertheless can lead to double vision, abnormal eye pressure and even loss of vision. At times, the tissue covering the IOL becomes cloudy and causes blurred vision, known as *after-cataract* which can develop months to years after surgery. After-cataracts are typically treated with *YAG laser capsulotomy*, which may itself necessitate further surgery.

While surgery is successful for many, there are other, less invasive, inexpensive treatments that can be accomplished in the privacy of one's home. Even though the "failure" rate of cataract surgery is low, because the consequences can be so catastrophic, it is only reasonable to assume that trying a less invasive technique initially would be a prudent course to pursue.

■ *DMSO*. In the sections **Pain Relievers** and *Spinal Cord Injuries*, the wonder substance DMSO is discussed at considerable length. In yet another example of its usefulness and versatility, DMSO has been shown to be both an effective treatment and preventive for cataracts. Over time, use of an appropriate formulation often leads to a clearing of the lens. Such a formulation can be prepared by your local "compounding pharmacy" using medical grade DMSO at about 5% by volume. Some holistic physicians add additional eye nutrients, including vitamin C and glutathione—both in the range of 1.0% by volume— and vitamin A at 2000 units/cc. Upon applying the eye drops, a slight stinging sensation may be felt, which dissipates rapidly. Similar formulations have been used for decades.

It is important to use only products prepared by a professional compounding pharmacy. To locate one in your area, contact the Professional Compounding Centers of America (PCCA) at (800) 331-2498. The PCCA can further instruct you regarding a proper formulation.

■ *N-Acetylcarnosine*. In the early 1990s, Russian scientists at the Hemholtz Institute of Eye Disease developed a specific form of the amino acid carnosine for use in treating cataracts. The di-peptide (two amino acids linked together) is called *N-acetylcarnosine* (NAC; not to be confused with N-acetylcysteine, also denoted NAC, or L-carnosine).

According to the researchers, many forms of carnosine were evaluated before the correct formulation was settled upon and patented. Only N-alpha acetylcarnosine, the researchers maintain, has the purity and biological activity required for the effective treatment of cataracts. The method of producing this form of NAC has been patented by Innovative Vision Products, Inc. of Delaware, USA.

NAC has a very good clinical success rate within 3-12 months of treatment. The proprietary eye drops have been the subject of several clinical trials. In a recent study,[5] 96 participants aged 60 and above received two drops of 1% NAC twice daily for a six-month period. At the termination of the study, 90.1% of the participants were able to see more clearly, and 88.9% had improved sensitivity to glare. Among those with early-stage cataracts experiencing mild to moderate symptoms, 100% showed at least some improvement. Eighty percent of those having late-stage cataracts improved. No participants reported side-effects.

In a six to 24-month study[6] of 49 participants averaging age 65 with senile cataracts, half received treatment with 1% NAC eye drops while the control group received no treatment. All participants were evaluated at regular intervals. After six months of treatment, significant glare reduction was noted in 88.9% of the NAC-treated group; 41.5% of all eyes showed a significant improvement in clarity (transmissivity) of the lens; and 90% of all treated eyes showed improvement in visual acuity (focus). The control group showed little or no improvement in six months, and gradual deterioration in 12 to 24 months. With continued, daily use of NAC, those in the treatment group maintained their improvements at the 24 month study termination. NAC seems to function by its powerful antioxidant capability and its ability to reverse cross-linking proteins that lead to lens occlusion.

Several over-the-counter products use Innovative Vision Products Inc's proprietary NAC. Two such products are Nu-Eyes,® from BioNational

Pharmaceuticals [www.bionational.com/xcart/cat alog/variant/index.html, (702)368-5251] and Can-C.™ [www.can-c.net, (866)800-4677] Treatment dosage in the clinical trials was 1-2 drops in each eye 2-4 times daily for 3-6 months.

■ *Homeopathic Eye Drops.*[7] One additional possibility for non-invasively treating cataracts is a homeopathic formulation including the herb *Cineraria maritima.* India's Central Council for Research in Homeopathy, Ministry of Health and Family Welfare, states that tincture of Cineraria is the treatment of choice for prevention and possible reversal of cataracts. Cineraria increases intraocular and collateral circulation and normalizes metabolism. Clinical studies have shown that even in advanced stages of cataracts treated with Cineraria, beneficial results are obtained in roughly 20% of the cases. One such Cineraria product is Cineraria Cataract Eye Drops,® available online at www. naturaleyecare.com/store/detail.aspx? ID=1546.

CEREBRAL PALSY
See **Stem Cells**, **Magnetic Molecular Energizer** under **General Treatment Methods**, and the Member's Area of *The Encyclopedia's* website.

CHRONIC FATIGUE AND FIBROMYALGIA
The Western world is now plagued by relatively new pathological disorders of seeming unknown origins. Two of the most troubling are Chronic Fatigue Syndrome (CFS; also called Chronic Fatigue and Immune Deficiency Syndrome, CFIDS) and Fibromyalgia (FM). CFS is defined as,

> ...a group of symptoms of unknown cause including fatigue, cognitive dysfunction, and sometimes fever and lymphadenopathy [abnormal enlargement of the lymph nodes].[1]

Fibromyalgia is defined as,

> ...any of a group of nonarticular rheumatic disorders characterized by pain, tenderness, and stiffness of the muscles and associated connective tissue structures...[2]

The formal diagnosis of FM includes the identification of at least 11 of 18 specific "tender/trigger points" that are very painful when pressed. These points are located on the upper back and chest, lower back, inside of the elbows, and front of the knees.

Those suffering from FM often experience a combination of anxiety, constant pain, depression, headaches, irritable bowel, muscle stiffness, overwhelming fatigue, sleep disturbances, and weakness. While the definitive cause of FM is unknown, it has been associated with alterations in brain chemistry; anemia; hormone deficiency diseases (particularly thyroid disease); overexertion; parasites; tension; trama; and viral infection. Although much has been written in the popular press about FM, formal scientific research is largely lacking.

■ *Hypercoagulation.* In 1992, Dr. John Couvaras, an infertility specialist in Phoenix, Arizona, discovered that women who were infertile and/or who had recurrent spontaneous abortions, seemed to have one interesting physiological factor in common: their blood was abnormally viscous—cohesive and sticky. They suffered from *hypercoagulation*, an abnormally high tendency for blood to clot.[3] When Couvaras administered low dose *heparin*, a blood thinning drug, the infertility problems seemed to resolve. He also made another astounding observation; namely, that women receiving the injections reported their CF and FM symptoms were eliminated or diminished sharply.

Following these observations, 30 women with symptoms of chronic illness were tested, and all were determined to have coagulation system activation, or hypercoagulation of the blood. When heparin injections were given, their chronic symptoms diminished. This led to a major, multi-center, blinded study (neither patients nor physicians knew which patients received the medication), in which it was found that ill patients tested positive on at least two of the five blood assay tests that comprise a blood evaluation panel developed by Hemex Laboratories of Phoenix, AZ, called the Immune System Activation of Coagulation panel (ISAC).[4] Over 80% of CFS/FM sufferers test positive on two or more of these blood assay tests.[5]

As the body's coagulation system becomes abnormally activated—and does not automatically shut down as it normally should—the sticky substance *fibrin* is formed, and is deposited in the major vessels and capillaries of the vascular system. At the same time, abnormally-high fibrin levels increase blood viscosity. These two factors lead to a corresponding decrease in bodily blood flow, producing *anoxia* (deficiency of oxygen) and nutrient deprivation to the cells in various areas.[6] As an example of the process, if high fibrin levels accumulate in a muscle, a tender point may develop and be experienced as fibromyalgia.

Researchers have found that various pathogens (infective organisms) can activate the process of hypercoagulation by activating the immune system in response to infection. These pathogens include Epstein-Barr virus, cytomegalovirus, human herpes virus, chlamydia and mycoplasma. Patients having CFS/FM symptoms generally test positive for one to seven different pathogens. Additionally, other factors have been found to activate the immune system, and the coagulation response, including allergens; toxins such as metals and chemicals (including bio-warfare agents); parasites; physical trauma; and vaccinations.[7]

There also may be a genetic basis or predisposition to hypercoagulation. Another test developed by Hemex Labs is the Hereditary Thrombosis Risk Panel (HTRP), which evaluates eight different genetic abnormalities, any one or more of which may cause hypercoagulation.[8]

Evaluation for the presence of pathogens is done by the Polymerase Chain Reaction test (PCR). Evaluation for hypercoagulation and genetic factors related thereto (ISAC panel: USD ~$420, and HTRP: USD ~$705) is done by Hemex Laboratories, and is typically covered by medical insurance. For further details about these testing procedures (which involve shipping blood samples to Hemex), visit Hemex Laboratories at www.hemex.com.

■ *Ginkgo biloba.* As mentioned above, heparin injections are able to thin the blood, return it to normal viscosity, and often alleviate symptoms of chronic fatigue syndrome and fibromyalgia. Oral heparin is also effective, although injections are thought to be the most effective method of administration. In either case, heparin is a prescription medication. Alternatively, the herb *Ginkgo biloba* is known to have a blood-thinning effect. Although aspirin also thins the blood, it can cause serious side-effects such as internal bleeding in the stomach and intestines, even in doses as low as 75 mg.[9] In fact, many deaths have resulted from aspirin-induced gastrointestinal bleeding, as discussed under *Arthritis*.

■ *Nattokinase.* As discussed, excess fibrin can cause the blood to become abnormally viscous, blocking oxygen and nutrients to the cells. An extract from the traditional Japanese food natto—a cheese-like substance made from boiled, fermented soybeans—*nattokinase* has the amazing ability to quickly and safely thin the blood by directly reducing fibrin levels as well as increasing the production of endogenous (the body's own) anti-clotting agents. Nattokinase is inexpensive, powerfully effective, fast and long acting, and readily available without a prescription. It is suggested as the natural substance of choice for combating hypercoagulation, which often leads to symptoms of CFS. For a more detailed discussion, see Nattokinase under *Cardiovascular Disease*.

■ *Potassium & Magnesium Aspartate.* A simple, inexpensive approach to CFS has yielded positive results for many. During the 1950s-60s European researchers studied the beneficial effects of an unusual form of two minerals, potassium and magnesium aspartate (aspartic acid). Aspartic acid is an important, natural amino acid used by the brain to assist in transmitting nerve impulses, and by the body to produce energy from carbohydrates.

Researchers discovered that animals given this specific mineral compound experienced a dramatic increase in physical endurance.[10] In a human study of 80 patients who experienced post-surgical fatigue for over one year, more than 90% experienced complete relief in three days to two weeks, with an average time of seven days, while taking a dosage of one gram (1,000 mg) of potassium-magnesium aspartate twice daily.[11] Additional research involving thousands of patients experiencing fatigue due to a wide range of causes showed that 75-94% experienced significant improvement.[12]

Use only the aspartate form—that's what has been tested—*not* another form such as chloride, gluconate or oxide. One source of this product is Ecological Formulas, (800)888-4585.

■ *5-HTP.* Many FM sufferers have low blood levels of *serotonin*, an important brain neurotransmitter which plays a critical role in pain inhibition, sleep regulation and mood elevation. Conventional medicine relies heavily on Selective Serotonin Reuptake Inhibitors (SSRIs) such as Prozac to treat FM symptoms including pain and depression by increasing serotonin levels; however, these drugs have serious side-effects which include violent and destructive behavior including homicide and suicide.[13]

Alternatively, two natural products have demonstrated effectiveness in raising serotonin levels in the brain. The first of these is 5-hydroxytryptophan (5-HTP), a plant extract which is the immediate precursor of serotonin [chemically designated 5-hydroxytryptomine (5-HT)].

Not only is 5-HTP effective in treating depression, it is a proven, effective treatment for fibromyalgia. In a research study of 50 fibromyalgia patients given 100 mg of 5-HTP three times daily for three months, about half experienced significant reduction of anxiety, fatigue and pain, with an increased quality of sleep.[14]

■ **SAMe.** Another natural treatment for fibromyalgia is s-adenosyl methionine (SAMe; pronounced "sammy"). SAMe increases serotonin levels as well as having a balancing effect on other neurotransmitters. In a recent study reported in the *Scandanavian Journal of Rheumatology*,[15] patients experienced significant pain relief, enhanced mood and decreased morning stiffness when given 800 mg of SAMe per day for six weeks. See **Stress** for more information on 5-HTP and SAMe.

■ **HGH & DHEA.** Hormone deficiencies are common among FM sufferers. Recent studies have shown significant improvement in patients treated with injections of Human Growth Hormone (HGH) and *dehydroepiandrosterone* (DHEA), according to a recent article in the *American Journal of Medicine*.[16] Hormone administration should be monitored by a medical professional.

■ **Guaifenesin**. The active ingredient in many cough syrups, *guaifenesin* shows significant promise in the treatment of FM patients, according to Dr. R.P. St. Amand's book *What Your Doctor May Not Tell You About Fibromyalgia*.[17] Dr. St. Amand is Clinical Professor of Endocrinology at UCLA School of Medicine. The rationale is that guaifenesin assists in purging excess levels of the mineral phosphate from the muscles and other tissues. Excess phosphate interferes with the normal production of adenosine triphosphate (ATP), the body's

energy chemical—sometimes called the "energy currency" of the cell. Muscle fatigue and weakness are the result. Also, calcium combines with phosphate, causing muscle contractions and spasms. Dr. St. Amand reports high success rates with guaifenesin therapy. To learn more about his fascinating method of treating fibromyalgia, including details of the guaifenesin treatment protocol and the location of practitioners of this treatment in your area, visit www.fibromyalgiatreatment.com.

■ **D-Ribose**. Referred to chemically as a five carbon sugar (monosaccharide), D-ribose is a naturally occurring substance used to synthesize and rebuild energy in every cell of the body. It is the most basic building block of adenosine triphosphate (ATP), the principal energy source of all cells in the body. It is also a constituent of the building blocks that form DNA and RNA molecules. Ribose is the beginning point for the synthesis of the body's energetic cellular components. Its availability determines the rate at which these components can be synthesized by cells and tissues.

Those who suffer from FM and CFS often experience impaired cellular metabolism. In particular, muscles of FM and CFS sufferers are generally severely energy deficient. D-ribose has been found to increase the cellular energy of heart and skeletal muscles, thus restoring energy, preventing fatigue, and lessening the associated pain.

In a 2006 study reported in the *Journal of Alternative and Complementary Medicine*,[18] 41 patients diagnosed with FM and/or CFS received 5 grams of D-ribose three times daily for 19 days. Approximately 65% of the participants experienced significant improvements in all five categories measured: energy, sleep, mental clarity, pain intensity, and well-being. They experienced a 45% increase in energy and a 30% improvement in well-being.

D-ribose does not raise blood sugar levels as does ordinary table sugar (sucrose; a six carbon sugar), and therefore would be appropriate for diabetics. To purchase ribose, visit www.nutrabio.com/Products/ribose.htm.

■ **Chelation Therapy**. As discussed under **Cardiovascular Disease**, Chelation Therapy is often very effective in treating fibromyalgia. Another detoxification strategy is the IR Sauna, discussed in the section N*utrition: Detoxification & Deficiencies* under **General Treatment Methods.**

■ *Thymic Protein A* and *Del Immune V*, discussed under **General Treatment Methods**, are powerful immune boosters that have shown effectiveness. See also Cat's Claw under *Lyme Disease*.

■ See *Lyme Disease*. Some researchers believe Lyme is implicated in many cases of CFS/FM. See also **Pain Relievers**; *Photoluminescence*, *Sodium Chlorite*, and *Olive Leaf Extract* under **General Treatment Methods**; and CFS in the Member's Area of *The Encyclopedia's* website.

■ *NADH* (Nicotinamide Adenine Nucleotide) has been shown effective in treating CFS. To learn more, visit www.enadh.com/case_show.html.

CIRRHOSIS OF THE LIVER

The liver is the second largest organ of the human body—the skin being the largest—and the largest internal organ. It is also the largest gland in the body, normally weighing between three and four-and-a-half pounds. It performs numerous critical functions including 1) the production and excretion of bile, which aids digestion, 2) the storage of glucose (as glycogen) for use as needed, 3) blood plasma protein synthesis, 4) the regulation of a variety of biochemical reactions requiring specialized tissues, 5) the process of detoxifying the body of a range of substances including drugs, exogenous chemicals, as well as waste products generated by the body, 6) the decomposition of red blood cells, and, 7) the production of over 1,000 enzymes.

The Greek word for liver is *hepar*, hence medical terms relating to the organ often begin with *hepato* or *hepatic*. In all, the liver performs over 500 tasks. Although the artificial treatment of liver dialysis is capable of performing some of the liver's tasks, no man-made device is capable if simulating the myriad functions performed by this miraculous organ. It is one of the few organs capable of natural regeneration of damaged/lost tissue. Twenty-five percent of a remaining liver is capable of regenerating the entire organ.

Cirrhosis is characterized by certain cells in the liver producing collagen—a fibrous material that toughens skin and tendons—and replacing the nor-

mal tissue by fibrous scar tissue, also called *hepatic fibrosis*. The condition includes distinct architectural and structural changes of the organ with nodules of fibrosis that encapsulate *hepatocytes*, cells which make up between 70-80% of the mass of the liver. A lesser condition is known as *advanced fibrosis*, which lacks the architectural and structural changes characteristic of cirrhosis. Both conditions lead to progressive loss of liver function. The gold standard in diagnosing cirrhosis is a liver biopsy, but it is not viewed as necessary if clinical, laboratory and radiologic data indicate cirrhosis. Biopsies pose a small but significant risk of hemorrhage.

Cirrhosis is responsible for nearly 1.5 million deaths per year world wide. Its most common causes in the Western world are hepatitis C and alcoholism, although chronic hepatitis B and D can also play a role. Other potential causes include autoimmune conditions; exposure to toxic chemicals including both prescription and non-prescription drugs; the parasitic condition *schistosomiasis*; inherited diseases such as *hemochromatosis* (excess iron in the body); and Wilson's disease (a rare disease relating to inadequate copper metabolism).

The early stages of cirrhosis are symptom free, enabling damage to accumulate unnoticed. As the condition advances, symptoms can include fatigue; weakness; jaundice, a yellowing of the skin and eyes; enlarged liver; abdominal pain, fatty stools; itching; dry eyes and mouth; soft, yellow spots on the eyelid; fatty deposits under the skin; and hepatocellular carcinoma, liver cancer.

Traditional treatment of cirrhosis varies depending upon the cause. If alcohol induced, abstaining from alcohol is recommended. If infection is the cause, antibiotics are often administered. If hepatitis-related, various drugs are typically used such as interferon and corticosteroids. (See **Hepatitis** for additional treatment information.)

■ *Essential Phospholipids.* A unique form of lecithin known as *essential phospholipids* (EPL) has been shown to slow the progression of and actually halt both alcohol-induced and non-alcohol-induced liver damage before full-blown cirrhosis occurs.[1] EPL also has been shown to normalize liver enzymes, accellerate hepatocyte replacement, and reverse "fatty liver" when taken orally at the dosage of 1,500-1,800 mg daily.[2] For additional information including ordering, see Essential Phospholipids under **Cardiovascular Disease**.

■ **Kaprex**.™ Some assistance may be found in several natural products. Kaprex, a combination of herbs from Metagenics, works by reducing the negative actions of NF-kB. To learn more, visit www.metagenics.com.

■ **Cirrhotab**.™ Manufactured by Oslo Health Solutions of Oslo, Norway, Cirrhotab is a combination of six herbs and minerals. The product is based on the Greek Unani system of herbal medicine, and comes with a four month total satisfaction guarantee. Visit www.cirrhotab.com.

■ **Silymarin**. Also known as the milk thistle plant, studies have shown that silymarin supports healthy liver function. Preferably, take 400 mg of a standardized 80% milk thistle flavonoid product daily, such as Now Foods' Silymarin Milk Thistle Extract. To learn more, see Silymarin under **Hepatitis**.

■ **Liv-52**.® Another product that aids in liver recovery is sold throughout the world as Liv-52, also called Liver Care® in the U.S. Marketed by Himalaya USA since 1955, Liv-52—a combination of seven herbal ingredients—has been the subject of over 275 research studies and has been shown to improve both liver function and structure.

■ **Sulfasalazine**. The current medical wisdom is that cirrhosis is incurable, and the only treatment for the end-stage condition is a liver transplant. However, in 2006 a team at Newcastle University in the U.K. tested *sulfasalazine* in the laboratory and on animals with cirrhosis, and more recently in limited human trials. Sulfasalazine is approved for treating arthritis and inflammatory bowel disease, but hadn't heretofore been tested on cirrhosis. The researchers found the drug can stop the progression of cirrhosis and even reverse the condition to some extent. It does this by lowering or switching off the production of nuclear factor kappa beta (NF-kB), a protein complex involved in the development of fibrotic scar tissue. Human trials haven't been completed, but the animal studies give hope to those with this condition. A caveat is that sulfasalazine itself can cause liver toxicity.

A further bright star on the horizon is a manmade molecule developed by Dr. Yoshiro Niitsu and a group of researchers at the Sapporo Medical University School of Medicine in Japan. In 2008, the researchers reported that in a rat study these molecules were able to block collagen production and remove the fibrosis, allowing the liver to regenerate and thereby reverse the cirrhosis. Niitsu stated he was hopeful the molecules would provide a cure for cirrhosis in time, and that a drug will be available in a few years.

COLD SORES (Fever Blisters). See **Herpes**.

COLDS AND FLU

Viruses are infective particles smaller than any bacteria. In humans, they cause a number of familiar diseases including AIDS, Ebola, herpes, polio, smallpox, and many others. Both the common cold and influenza are respiratory infections caused by viruses. While symptoms of a cold include a runny nose, sneezing and sore throat, influenza—the flu—is typically more severe, with symptoms including fever; headache; aches and pains; lethargy; and fatigue and weakness that may last for days or weeks.

Both colds and flu viruses are transmitted by contacting respiratory secretions of an infected person (by shaking hands, touching an infected doorknob, etc., and then touching the mouth, eyes, or nose), or by breathing infective particles which can linger in the air for up to three hours.

There are several different types or "families" of viruses. The *Paramyxovirus* family includes the mumps virus, measles virus, and pathogens of the respiratory system called parainfluenza viruses. The *Picornavirus* family includes the so-called "rhinoviruses," often the cause of the common cold. The *Orthomyxovirus* family includes types A, B, and C, with type A being the most common and typically causing the most epidemics and severe illness.

The "Spanish Flu" pandemic of 1918 is perhaps the most well-known example of influenza's "worst case scenario," in which 20-50 million people world wide and more than 500,000 Americans perished in less than 12 months. The outbreak of Sudden Acute Respiratory Syndrome (SARS), "bird (avian) flu" viruses (including H5N1), and the so-called swine flu (H1N1) sends a chilling reminder that we've not yet defeated these formidable opponents of diminutive proportion.

That being said, the lethal flu strain responsible for the world-wide pandemic of 1918 would likely pose a much less significant threat to 21st Century humans. Most of the 1918 fatalities resulted not from the primary viral infection itself, but rather a secondary bacterial infection that today is more easily defeated. Also, sanitary and dietary standards are much improved, offering further barriers to infection and transmission.

Outside the body, viruses are metabolically inert, and said to be in a grey area between a living and non-living state. In order to multiply and be infective, viral particles must attach themselves to healthy (though often weakened) cells, take over their reproductive capabilities, and begin reproducing additional infective particles, called *virions*. Influenza viruses typically gain access to healthy host cells by means of spike-like protrusions projecting from their bodies.

Two glycoproteins on the outer surfaces of these spikes, *hemagglutinin* (HA) and *neuraminidase* (N), are known to have primary roles in how the viral particles attach to normal cells. HA is the glycoprotein that interacts with antibodies, and the specific antibody to HA prevents infection. Influenza A viruses are named according to their HA and N subtypes, and the location and year of the viruses' first isolation. For example, Influenza A/Hong Kong/68/H3N2 is the strain A of the H3N2 subtype first isolated in Hong Kong in 1968.

Agencies such as the CDC have publicized that roughly 35,000 Americans perish annually from so-called "seasonal" influenzas. However, according to the CDC's own publication *National Vital Statistics Reports*, only several hundred fatalities occur on an average year that are directly attributable to the influenza virus—mostly the elderly and those with preexisting conditions or weakened immunity. The remaining deaths are attributable to secondary bacterial infections such as pneumonia.

Over the past several years there has been much discussion in the media regarding new types of viruses that have the potential of spreading widely throughout the human population—SARS, bird flu, and the swine flu being the three most prominently discussed. Upon its outbreak, most of the world's press cast SARS as having the potential of causing a global pandemic; but in the end it caused less than 800 deaths worldwide, and not a single American death.

The bird flu virus is so named because it infects and is transmitted by birds. Although many human influenzas originate from an avian source, many avian flus never mutate to infect humans, even though they have existed throughout history.

The much-discussed H5N1 strain was first discovered in Scottish chickens in 1959, with the first bird-to-human case reported in 1997. Since its discovery, about 260 people have died of H5N1 worldwide, or about 60% of those infected as of winter 2010. The infections occur almost exclusively in persons who either eat infected meat or contact the blood, feces, saliva or mucus of infected birds. Although H5N1's high lethality rate is cause for concern, experts believe if its rate of transmission between humans increases, the severity of the illness will become significantly lessened.

H5N1 has been present in birds for over 50 years without becoming transmissible to humans—unless in close proximity to infected birds, or unless they are consumed. Nor does the virus appear to be easily transmitted from human-to-human. The fact that humans have been infected is most likely *not* a sign that H5N1 is mutating to become more infective to humans, but only that millions of birds throughout the world have been infected—which raises the probability of increased human contact and eventual infection. Some experts believe, in fact, that if the mutation causing human transmissibility has not yet occurred, it's unlikely to do so in the near term, if ever.

For years prior to the 2009 swine flu outbreak, some suggested a pandemic was overdue. Hudson Institute Senior Fellow Michael Fumento suggests there is no cycle or pattern to the three prior influenza pandemics, with 39 years between the first two, while the last two were separated by only 11 (1918-19, 1957-58, 1968-69). Fumento stated, "The idea that we are overdue...is mere superstition."[1]

Dr. Mark Siegel, Associate Professor of Medicine at New York University School of Medicine, came forward to help quell public fears of a bird flu (H5N1) epidemic. Said Siegel, "There is absolutely no indication that the transformation to mass killer is about to happen. The threat is theoretical."[2] Professor Siegel took a sabbatical from NYU to promote his 2005 book about the bird flu scare, *False Alarm: The Truth about the Epidemic of Fear.*

In basic agreement with Professor Siegel is Dr. Gary Butcher, an extension veterinarian specializing in avian diseases at the University of Florida's College of Veterinary Medicine. According to Butcher, who holds a Ph.D. in poultry virology,

> For it [H5N1] to become dangerous to humans, it has to go through a pretty significant genetic change. If you put this into perspective, it's not going to happen. For a person to be infected now, it appears that the exposure level has to be astronomical...Realistically, [H5N1] is not a threat to people, but everywhere you go, it has turned into a circus.[3]

Notwithstanding this fear-based circus atmosphere, many in the scientific community believe it so unlikely H5N1 will mutate to infect humans, some have suggested that if it does, it will likely be the result of human manipulation in the laboratory as opposed to a natural occurrence. A number of countries and politically-oriented organizations have the technical capability of modifying the virus to cause human infectivity and subsequent transmission. It's unfortunate to acknowledge that the potential for biological manipulation of naturally-occurring pathogens to achieve some military or social engineering purpose cannot be overlooked.[4] In fact, several prominent microbiologists have stated that, due to various unusual characteristics of the virus, the 2009 swine flu may have originated in a laboratory. In early May 2009, Dr. Adrian Gibbs, Professor Emeritus at the Australian National University and co-developer of Tamiflu, announced that the unusually rapid evolution of the gene clusters of swine flu points to possible man-made manipulation. Comprehensive, up-to-date information on the various flu strains is posted in the Member's Area of *The Encyclopedia's* website.

There are specific actions one must take in order to both prevent and treat flu viruses. Prevention is significantly aided by healthy diet and lifestyle choices (see **Nutrition: Detoxification and Deficiencies** under **General Treatment Methods**), as well as regular supplementation with immune-enhancing substances such as vitamin C and vitamin D3. The conventional approach to prevention is vaccination. Treatment involves either boosting immunity so that elements of the immune system

attack and kill the virus, or the use of antiviral substances which directly attack the virus. Some immune enhancers are also directly antiviral.

The Conventional Approach: Vaccination and Pharmaceutical Drugs. In the Western world, vaccination is one of the mainstay defenses against disease-causing pathogens, including influenza. Worldwide, vaccines are a $20+ billion business, with influenza vaccines probably the fastest-growing segment of the market—accounting for about 20% of total vaccine sales.[5] Although most lay persons consider vaccines safe and effective, both the safety and effectiveness of today's vaccinations are questioned by many medical authorities. Modern vaccines contain an abundance of potentially-toxic ingredients.

Among the list of troublesome ingredients are: thimerosal (a mercury-derived preservative which some believe contributes to autism and other diseases. Thimersol has now been removed from many vaccines, but not influenza vaccines); other heavy metals (including aluminum hydroxide and phosphate); preservatives (such as sorbitol and polysorbate); antibiotics (such as neomycin); formalin; formaldehyde (an embalming fluid); fetal bovine serum (used to nourish virtually all vaccines); foreign animal tissue containing genetic material (including RNA and DNA which can form latent proviruses that can activate at a future date); and dozens of other potentially-toxic ingredients that can be viewed at www.cdc.gov/vaccines/pubs/pink book/downloads/appendices/B/excipient-table-2.pdf. For an alternative listing of toxic ingredients, substitute "1.pdf" at the end of the preceding URL.

Hugh Fudenberg, M.D. is a world-renowned immunogeneticist. From 1970-1980, Dr. Fudenberg studied the connection between flu vaccinations and the incidence of Alzheimer's. According to Dr. Fudenberg, those who received five consecutive flu vaccinations during the 10 year span he investigated have a 10-fold increased risk of developing AD than those who received no shots, one shot or two shots. Fudenberg attributes this finding to both mercury and aluminum contained in influenza (and some other childhood) vaccinations.

Alzheimer's, autism, diabetes, and other serious ailments are associated with vaccinations. There is currently little question that vaccines bring with them much more than advertised. For additional general information on vaccines, see the **Index**, and visit www.nvic.org.

There is no current vaccine proven to confer protection against any type of flu. The annually-marketed, seasonal influenza vaccine contains three specific viral strains: two influenza A and one influenza B, based on the educated guesses of virus experts. It allegedly provides added protection against normal, yearly flus to those with weakened immune function, principally the elderly. The rationale is that by vaccinating not only the elderly but widely throughout the population, the elderly will be protected through "herd" immunity.

A 2005 *Lancet* article sheds new light on the effectiveness of the seasonal flu vaccine. In an historic study, researchers analyzed data on the worldwide performance of the vaccine over the past 37 years in people 65 years and older. According to lead researcher Dr. Tom Jefferson of the non-profit Rome, Italy-based Cochrane Vaccine Fields project,

> The runaway 100 percent effectiveness that's touted by proponents was nowhere to be seen...There is a wild overestimation of the impact of these vaccinations in the [elderly] community...In elderly individuals living in the community, vaccines were not significantly effective against influenza, influenza-like illnesses, or pneumonia...What you see is that marketing rules the response to influenza, and scientific evidence comes fourth or fifth ...Vaccines may have a role, but they appear to have a modest effect. The best strategy to prevent illness is to wash your hands.[6]

Jefferson and colleagues also found that vaccine effectiveness in long-term care facilities for the elderly—as opposed to individuals living in the community—was also non-significant. However, in both the elderly living in the community and in the group setting, a vaccine that is well-matched to the presently-infecting viral strain—which they seldom are—reduces complications such as pneumonia, and also hospital admissions.

In 2003, the intra-nasal vaccination FluMist® was introduced to the market by MedImmune. Wyeth pharmaceuticals, MedImmune's partner and distributor, intended to invest $100 million over three years in an advertising campaign to encourage physicians to promote the vaccine,[7] but it was not well-received in the marketplace. FluMist is approved for healthy individuals 5-49 years of age— the age group who least needs the protection.

The most common side-effects of FluMist are cough, runny nose, sore throat, chills, tiredness, weakness, abdominal pain, ear infection, diarrhea, and fever[8]—which is reminiscent of the old adage, "With friends like this, who needs enemies?" Meaning, why bother being treated when the treatment has nearly the same side-effects as those the vaccine is designed to prevent? At least persons receiving FluMist have the option of selecting the day and hour of infection, thereby eliminating the guesswork and stress of when one's illness will arrive.

Unlike injectable vaccines, FluMist is a live virus that has been "attenuated," or reduced in virulence/vitality. The living virus replicates within the nasal passages of the recipient, is shed via nasal secretions, and can be spread by sneezing. This opens the possibility of live virus being spread to those in close contact with a FluMist recipient in social settings such as work, school, church, and home.

Even though the live virus is attenuated, it could pose a danger to immuno-compromised individuals whose immune systems may not be capable of defending against even this low-level threat. According to the package insert, those using FluMist "should avoid close contact with immuno-compromised individuals for at least 21 days."[9] Whether it's infective viral particles in the air or nasal secretions on a doorknob, FluMist may be a threat to more than 50% of society, including those having weakened immune function due to ill health, advanced age, or chemical suppression.

Equally troubling, Rima Laibow, M.D., a graduate of Albert Einstein College of Medicine and Medical Director of the Natural Solutions Foundation, has stated,

> Each of the three viruses in FluMist can mutate and can cause mutations in the Avian Flu [H5N1]. Those mutations can supply the Avian Flu virus as it currently exists with the genetic sequences it needs to become a pandemic virus. The FluMist live virus nasal inoculation can assist the much feared Avian Flu virus to transform into the very pandemic we are being told to fear.[10]

■ ***Symmetrel***.® Amantadine (a-MAN-ta-deen), trade named Symmetrel, is used to treat Parkinson's disease and fatigue (especially in multiple sclerosis). It is a prescription drug which also has been used to treat certain type A influenzas. It is ineffective in treating colds, types of flu other than type A, and other types of viral infections. Amantadine and the chemically-related *rimantadine* (Flumadine®), known as adamantane derivatives, inhibit the influenza virus from reproducing.

As an antiviral, amantadine moderately reduces the transmission and symptoms/complications of influenza. It has been used to help control seasonal flu outbreaks in hospitals and nursing homes. There was initial hope this drug would serve as an inexpensive front-line tool in fighting dangerous viruses such as H5N1. However, its widespread use in the Chinese poultry industry since the late 1990s had led to H5N1 resistance.[11]

According to a 2005 *Lancet*[12] article, prior to 2000 virtually no virus was resistant to amantadine. By 2004, 15% of type A viruses collected in South Korea, 70% in Hong Kong, and 74% in China were resistant. During the first six months of 2004 in the U.S., about 2% of influenza-A viruses were amantadine resistant. One year later, 15% of the type As had developed resistance.

■ ***Tamiflu.***® Oseltamivir, known by its popular trade name *Tamiflu*, is an antiviral prescription pharmaceutical medication used to treat type A and B influenzas in adults, adolescents, and children older than one year. It is frequently prescribed, sometimes habitually, to treat common influenza. Tamiflu is most effective when begun within 48 hours of first symptoms. It's also used as a preventative, particularly in high-risk adolescent and other especially-susceptible populations. In December 2005, it was approved in the U.S. as a preventive in children older than one year. In accordance with FDA regulations, Tamiflu carries a "special warning;" namely, "its safety and effectiveness have not been determined in people with chronic heart or lung disease, kidney failure, or in people with high-risk underlying medical conditions."[13] Further, the safety and efficacy of multiple courses of treatment have not been established.[14]

Following recognition by the medical community that amantadine was becoming resistant to new flu strains including H5N1, it was hoped the much more expensive Tamiflu would fill the void left by amantadine's ineffectiveness. Unfortunately, H5N1

and other strains have begun to develop resistance to Tamiflu as well, at least in part the result of over prescribing the drug to treat common influenzas.

What is happening in the war of "antibiotics versus bacteria" is repeating itself on the battlefield of "antivirals versus viruses." These diminutive, infective microbes are proving to be formidable enemies in their seemingly never-ending ability to resist the best efforts of our best and brightest humans. Microbe against macrobe, survival is the name of the game in either world.

Regarding H5N1 and Tamiflu, the microbes appear to be gaining ground. As of early 2006, a Vietnamese strain of human H5N1 was exhibiting resistence to Tamiflu. This trend has increased as the virus continues to mutate and the use of Tamiflu increases. As of winter 2010, resistance to Tamiflu continues to increase in many countries. Indications are that it will not be effective against H5N1 (or many strains of H1N1).

Following the deaths of at least 18 Japanese children taking Tamiflu, Japan's Ministry of Health and Welfare warned doctors that Tamiflu should not be prescribed to teenagers between the ages of 10-19 for fear the drug leads to bizarre and self-destructive behavior including delusions, hallucinations, depression, panic attacks, convulsions, and suicide. The Japanese distributor of the drug was instructed to post a label warning disclosing these effects. Nearly 600 cases of psychiatric problems related to Tamiflu have been reported world wide, 75% of which have occurred in Japan. In the U.S., supplementary information on the label states:

> People with the flu, particularly children, may be at an increased risk of self-injury and confusion shortly after taking Tamiflu and should be closely monitored for...unusual behavior."[15]

■ ***Relenza.***® Zanamivir, trade-named Relenza, is prescribed for the treatment, but not the prevention, of influenza types A and B in persons seven years and older. It is available as an injectable or an inhaled powder. Similar to its chemical cousin Tamiflu, best results are achieved when given within 48 hours of onset of symptoms. Relenza is not effective against and may be a risk factor for persons with asthma, emphysema or chronic bronchitis.[16]

Although H5N1 resistance is not currently occurring, it may be only a matter of time/usage before Relenza meets a fate similar to that of other antivirals. Also, many people infected with influenza are most affected not by the virus itself, but by a secondary infection such as pneumonia. Because many of the new viral strains including SARS, H5N1, and H1N1 severely affect the respiratory tract, using a drug that may itself be a risk factor in these conditions is conditionally inadvisable.

Other, more natural treatments are available. Below are some of the most safe and effective.

■ ***Sambucol.***® Substances that interfere with the glycoproteins HA and N can be strongly antiviral, preventing viral particles from attaching to healthy cells. Sambucol works by interfering with HA and N on the coating of the viral spikes, thereby preventing adhesion to normal cells.

In 1980, Madeleine Mumcuoglu (Mum-SHOO-gloo) was a virology student at the Hadassah-Hebrew School of Medicine in Israel. While searching for an appropriate subject for her doctoral dissertation, Mumcuoglu's dissertation director, Dr. Jean Linderman, recommended she study the berries of the black elder tree called, appropriately enough, black elderberries. The Latin botanical name of the tree is *Sambucus nigra L.* Linderman knew that a rich folk history surrounds elderberries, having been used for more than 2,500 years for treating colds, flu and upper respiratory infections.

The initial trial of Sambucol was with patients of the Southern Israeli flu epidemic of 1992-93. Within the first 24 hours of infection, 20% of the Sambucol-treated patients showed dramatic improvements such as reduced fever, muscle aches and pains, and coughing. By day two, 73% were improved; and by the third day 90% reported dramatic improvement. In the untreated group, only 16% were improved after two days, and the majority didn't feel better for almost one week.[17]

Sambucol has been tested on at least seven different strains of influenza viruses including Hong Kong, Beijing, Singapore, Yamagata, Shangdong, Panama, Ann Arbor and Texas. In each case the treatment proved effective. If taken when symptoms first appear, Sambucol will relieve the major symptoms of flu viruses within 24 to 48 hours. If taken later in the course of the illness, it nevertheless will reduce symptoms dramatically.

Sambucol's manufacturer claims other elderberry products with similar-sounding names are imitation products using a different elderberry source and extraction method than the extensively-tested Sambucol. The original Sambucol is a front-line defense against any type of flu. To order, visit www.sambucolusa.com/where-to-buy-sambucol.htm.

■ ***Oscillococcinum.***® A homeopathic remedy that has proven itself over time is Oscillococcinum (awe-sill-o-COX-sin-um), or Oscillo for short. Packaged in the form of small pellets which are taken sublingually, Oscillo is pleasant tasting, safe, non-toxic, and well-suited for children and adults.

In a double-blind, placebo-controlled study reported in the *British Journal of Clinical Pharmacology*[18] in 1989, those participants who received treatment with Oscillo were significantly more likely to recover completely from influenza symptoms within 48 hours compared to those who received a placebo. The symptoms of fever, headache, stiffness, back pain, joint pain, and shivers were more likely ameliorated within two days compared to those not receiving treatment.

Another 1989 study[19] produced similar results. Compared to the placebo group, a 48-hour recovery from flu symptoms was significantly more likely in the Oscillo-treated group. While several participants in the placebo group experienced a worsening of symptoms, none of the Oscillo-treated group experienced such a worsening.

■ ***Vitamin C.*** This product is an old but powerfully-effective standby. Vitamin C is both antibacterial and antiviral and, as such, is effective in treating flu viruses and their bacterial complications, as well as cold viruses. Vitamin C works on several fronts. It energizes natural killer (NK) cells which attack pathogenic microbes even with no previous exposure to them. It also energizes macrophages, another of the immune systems front line of defenses against infection. Vitamin C also helps the body produce hydrogen peroxide, a tool used by immune cells against infectious microbes.

In the case of a bacterial or viral infection, high doses of vitamin C must be taken—in the range of at least 1,000-5,000 mg (1-5 grams) per hour. Treatment should begin immediately after onset—the sooner the better after symptoms are noticed. The only side-effect is slight diarrhea when bowel tolerance is exceeded. If the stool loosens, decrease the dosage slightly. When ill, greatly increased quantities of vitamin C are tolerated by the body before symptoms of diarrhea occur.

In one representative study, 700 college students were administered one gram of vitamin C per hour for the initial six hours following the onset of cold and/or flu symptoms, and three grams for several days thereafter. Both cold and flu symptoms were reduced by 85%.[20]

The *ascorbic acid* form of vitamin C rather than Ester C® or other buffered forms should be used orally—either as a pill or powder (crystals). One teaspoon of powder equals approximately four grams. Although the buffered forms of vitamin C avoid the possibility of diarrhea, they are much less effective in comparison to ascorbic acid. High-dose intravenous vitamin C is one of the most effective treatments for colds, flu, and even more virulent pathogens such as bird flu.

Pioneer vitamin C researcher Robert Cathcart, M.D. (1932-2007) used vitamin C to treat all types of flu including bird flu. He demonstrated that even potentially lethal cases of bird flu and other flus having serious lung involvement can be treated effectively with massive doses of vitamin C, either orally (as ascorbic acid powder) at the level of *12 grams every 15 minutes* (until diarrhea is produced—and then reduce the amount slightly), or preferably intravenously (as sodium ascorbate) by a qualified alternative/integrative physician at the level of *150-300 grams per each 24-hour period.*

The respiratory tract is the initial attack point of bird flu (H5N1) and some other flu strains. (See the discussion of the *cytokine storm,* below, for further information on this topic.) The damage inflicted upon the lungs is caused by the generation of high levels of free radicals. Vitamin C is the optimal treatment/antidote, as *it is the only substance/ antioxidant known* that can be taken in sufficiently large quantities—preferably intravenously but also orally, depending upon the severity of the condition—to counteract virtually any amount of free radical pathology produced by any disease state, including the high level of free radical pathology produced in the lungs by various strains of influenza. Because the body's tolerance to orally-ingested ascorbic acid increases in proportion to the degree

of toxicity of the illness, up to and beyond 200 grams per 24-hours of orally-ingested ascorbic acid can usually be tolerated without causing diarrhea.

In a world poised for the emergence of virulent strains of influenza and/or other infective pathogens, the vitamin C solution cannot be overlooked. To learn more, visit www.orthomed.com. Here you will find links to the influenza/bird flu treatment protocols, including instructions for physicians on the method of preparing vitamin C for IV injection. To locate a physician in your area capable of administering IV vitamin C, visit www.acam.org or www.icimed.com.

■ *Vitamin D.* Among the many vitamins that contribute to our good health, vitamin D is gaining recognition as a superstar. Vitamin D is unique in the vitamin world in that it is technically not a vitamin. It is the only known precursor of *calcitriol*—activated vitamin D—a powerful steroid hormone that regulates genetic expression in hundreds of genes.[21] Of the roughly 25,000 (protein-coding) genes in the human genome, as many as 10%—or 2,500 genes—are "activated" by vitamin D alone. As such, it is a master controller of a vast array of physical mechanisms throughout the body as it turns various genes "on" and "off." Vitamin D also stimulates the white blood cells to produce hundreds of *antimicrobial peptides,* substances known to attack bacteria, viruses, and fungi.[22] Chief among these is the *cathelicidin* group of peptides.

Vitamin D is naturally produced by the skin when exposed to the ultraviolet B radiation of sunlight. Doctors and government agencies have given warnings about the dangers of developing skin cancer resulting from overexposure to sunlight. This has led to an epidemic of vitamin D deficiencies in much of the world's non-equatorial populations. It is now recognized that a deficiency of vitamin D is a major factor in the pathology of many diseases and ailments including autoimmune diseases; birth defects; cancer (at least 17 types); cardiovascular disease; chronic pain; depression; diabetes; hypertension; multiple sclerosis; muscle wasting; muscle weakness; osteoarthritis; and periodontitis.[23]

It is recently understood that cold and flu seasons result largely from a deficiency of vitamin D caused by lack of sunlight in the months between the winter solstice—the shortest day of the year—

and the summer solstice—the longest day of the year.[24] Insuring adequate levels of vitamin D intake, especially during this low sunlight window, serves as a powerful preventive—what could be considered the ultimate natural oral "vaccine." Contrary to past understandings, vitamin D researchers now recommend adults obtain a minimum of 1,000-2,000 IU (International Units) daily of vitamin D3 during summer months—especially if one is receiving regular sun exposure—and double that amount during the late fall, winter, and early spring. Some have suggested the rule of thumb of 1,000 IU per 25 pounds body weight. Adequate levels can be achieved through one or a combination of: sunlight exposure; dietary intake of vitamin D-rich foods such as cod liver oil; or supplementation with D3—*cholecalciferol, not* D2, ergocalciferol. Pill-form or liquid D3 supplements are the simplest means of achieving the correct amount.

Daily amounts up to at least 10,000 IU are known to be safe, and some experts believe the non-toxic daily dose may be closer to 40,000 IU.[25] For treating colds or flu, some doctors now recommend 50,000-100,000 IU of cholecalciferol daily for several days only, up to the level of 1,000 IU per pound of body weight for three days. According to this protocol, a 200 pound person would take 200,000 IU for three days. To put these dosages into perspective, the skin produces 20,000 IU from 20-30 minutes of "unprotected," full-body summer sun exposure during hours where the shadow cast by the body is shorter than the body's height. An SPF 8-rated sun screen reduces vitamin D production by 95%. Optimal blood levels should be maintained from 50-80 ng/mL (nanograms per milliliter), as measured by the 25-hydroxyvitamin D test. To learn more, read the informative article at www.whale.to/a/cannell.html, or visit the Vitamin D Council's website, www.vitamindcouncil.org.

The Cytokine Storm. Respiratory viruses such as influenza sometimes cause the immune system to do more harm than good. Non-life-threatening influenza can escalate from a nuisance to a killer because the immune system responds too strongly to an attack by an infectious invader.

When the lungs are attacked by an infective microbe such as a virus, the immune system's T-cells are dispatched to the site. If the infection is not quickly cleared, the T-cells produce the mole-cule OX40, which signals them to remain in the lungs and continue combating the infection. At the same time, the immune system goes into overdrive, sending out a second wave of T-cells—resulting in what's referred to as a *cytokine storm.* It is this exaggerated immune response rather than the initial infection that is most damaging. Severe inflammation of the lung tissue and an overproduction of mucous potentially block air passages. Hemorrhaging of the lung tissue also can occur. This, in turn, blocks oxygen transfer to the blood which can result in labored breathing and even suffocation.

This exaggerated inflammation is an especially troubling symptom of SARS and H5N1 (and sometimes swine and other flu strains), and the principal cause of their lethality—pneumonia and acute respiratory distress. In November 2005, *Respiratory Research*[26] reported that 24-hours following infection with a human H5N1 strain, for example, there is a 10-fold increase in inflammatory cytokine levels compared to lung cells infected with regular influenza. Thus, in cases where the cytokine storm is present, once the infection is confirmed immune stimulation by agents such as medicinal mushrooms, beta glucan, echinacea, and other immune-enhancing substances should be avoided, and a course of one or a combination of immune regulators should be initiated.

Vitamin D3 is an immune system regulator which is capable of up-regulating or down-regulating immune function as necessary. In the case of an over-activated immune system which leads to a cytokine storm, vitamin D dampens immune system elements that produce inflammation. High levels of its intake—up to 1,000 IU per pound of body weight for three days (and several days longer if necessary)—should be a front-line treatment in cases of cytokine storm-producing influenza infection. Vitamin D is also useful in cases where the immune system requires up-regulation.

Thymic Protein A, discussed under **General Treatment Methods**, is also a powerful immune regulator, as is Samento,® a product discussed under **Lyme Disease**. High-grade fish oil with high levels of EPA (such as Cardiostat,® which is available at Kroger and Walgreens) is an immune depressant, and effective in dampening the cytokine storm.

As discussed, vitamin C at high dosages is effective in reducing the free radical damage and inflammation caused by the cytokine storm, as the electrons donated by vitamin C quell the free radical pathology, hence the inflammation and lung tissue damage. Lyprinol,® discussed under **Arthritis** and **Asthma**, is one of the most effective systemic anti-inflammatories known. It is used by marathon athletes to combat exercise-induced bronchial constriction resulting from inflammation. *Serrapeptase*, a proteolytic enzyme discussed under **Cardiovascular Disease**, is also an excellent systemic anti-inflammatory, as are *curcuminoids*—extracts of the spice turmeric. The most bio-active curcuminoid dietary supplements are those using the branded ingredient BCM-95,® such as Super Bio-Curcumin™ by the Life Extension Foundation. If the above immune regulators and anti-inflammatory agents would have been used to treat victims of SARS, H5N1, and the swine flu, it's likely there would have been many fewer deaths.

Capsaicin, discussed under **Cardiovascular Disease**, is the principal ingredient in hot peppers such as cayenne. It has been reported to have the ability of stopping hemmorhaging of the lungs.

■ *Allicin*. For centuries, garlic (*Allium sativum*) has been been used both medicinally and as a food ingredient. The (Codex) Ebers—an ancient Egyptian papyrus dating to circa 1550 B.C.—contains over 800 medicinal formulations, 22 of which contain garlic.

Allicin, a constituent of garlic, is the principal component that exerts powerful anti-microbial actions against a broad range of pathogens including bacteria, viruses, fungi, and parasites. As an antiviral, allicin as well as its condensation product *ajoene*, are active against cytomegalovirus, herpes simplex types I and II, HIV, influenza B, parainfluenza type III, and rhinovirus type II. Hence, garlic is useful for treating both colds and many strains of influenza viruses.[27]

When the garlic clove is crushed, allicin is formed by the interaction of the stable precursor compound *allinin* with the enzyme *allinase*. The allicin molecules thus produced are very reactive with other constituents within the clove, and have a very short half-life. For this reason, until recently garlic supplements contained only very small quantities of allicin, and liberated an unknown quantity when consumed. The branded ingredient Allisure®

(also called Allisure AC-23®) is produced by a patented process which insures a 100% allicin yield. A number of garlic supplements contain Allisure in their formulation, including Allimax® (180 mg of Allisure) and AlliUltra® (360 mg of Allisure). For use as an anti-microbial, products other than those containing Allisure are not recommended.

■ *Beta Glucan*. Most typically extracted from the cell wall of baker's (brewer's) yeast (*Saccharomyces cerevisiae*), *beta 1,3/1,6 D glucan* is a powerful immune system activator. The 1,3/1,6 "active linkages" (terminally-linked glucose molecules) of beta glucan bind to receptor sites on and activate *macrophages*, and also activate *neutrophils* and *natural killer cells*—immune system cells that defend against infection from many pathogens, including viruses.[28] Studies have shown that many/most commercially-available beta glucan products contain less-than-optimal levels of the 1,3/1,6 active linkages which are responsible for the desired anti-infective effects. Preferred products contain between 75-88% 1,3/1,6 linkages, with about 70-80% being the 1,3 linkage. Examples of such products include Beta Glucan #300® by Southeastern Pharmaceutical [www.beta-glucan.com; (800)479-5195]; Beta-1,3D Glucan® by Transfer Point [http://www.transferpoint.com/c-3-.aspx; (877)407-3999]; and Immune System Activator® (www.iherb.com). For more information, visit http://glucan.us/Glucan1-2007.pdf. Beta glucan is a front-line preventive and treatment for colds and flus.

■ Other natural substances effective against colds and flus include mushroom extracts such as AHCC® and MycoPhyto;® bovine byproducts such as colostrum and lactoferrin; hydrogen peroxide (H_2O_2); and colloidal silver (especially MesoSilver;® www.purestcolloids.com/mesosilver.htm), all of which are discussed in the Member's Area of *The Encyclopedia*.

See also **Del Immune V**,® **Olive Leaf Extract**, and **Sodium Chlorite** under **General Treatment Methods**. The mechanical techniques of Blood Electrification (discussed under **Herpes**)—which can be practiced "in-home"—and **Photoluminescence** (discussed under **General Treatment Methods**) are two of the most potent anti-infective technologies known.

DEPRESSION. See **Stress**.

DIABETES

Insulin, a familiar word to most, is a hormone secreted by the *Islets of Langerhans*—small clusters of cells within the pancreases of mammals. In addition to being a household name, insulin is one of the body's most important and studied chemicals. It is in our everyday vocabulary primarily because of its use in the treatment of diabetes, a disease of modern man characterized by inadequate utilization and/or secretion of insulin, which results in excessive sugar (glucose) in both blood and urine.

The Physiology of Insulin. The food we consume is converted into *glucose*, the typical form of sugar in which dietary protein and carbohydrates are assimilated in man and animals. Glucose is transported throughout the body via the vast "freeway to the cells," the bloodstream.

Insulin is secreted into the bloodstream by the pancreatic beta cells in direct response to an increase in blood glucose concentration. It is one of the primary functions of insulin to maintain the proper blood glucose level. It does this by allowing glucose to leave the bloodstream and enter the cells. Once glucose is cleared from the bloodstream, the pancreas is signaled to stop insulin production.

On the surface of most all mammalian cells are *insulin receptors*—chemical groups or molecules that have an affinity for insulin. Each cell in the body has between 100 to 100,000 insulin receptors,[1] and it is rare that cells have no receptors at all. As insulin molecules circulate throughout the body via the bloodstream, they attach to the receptor structures largely on cell surfaces.

It is this attachment of the insulin molecules to the cells via the receptors that allows the glucose within the blood to pass into the cells, thus providing cellular nourishment. Insulin is the "gatekeeper" of the cells, as it facilitates the diffusion (transport) of glucose across the membranes of the body's many different types of cells. It is the key which fits into the receptor sites' locks to unlock the cells and allow the cellular fuel to gain entry. In addition to the receptor-specific transfer of glucose, it is believed that insulin has a general tendency to "permeablize" the cell membranes. When insufficient insulin is produced and/or insulin receptors become insensitive to insulin molecules, the result

is diabetes, a hallmark of which is *hyperglycemia*—an excess of glucose within the blood plasma.

Incidence and types. Over six percent of the entire U.S. population has diabetes, or approximately 20 million people. At least nine percent of all Americans over the age of 20 and over 20% over the age of 65 have diabetes. However, as many as half of all diabetics, or almost 10 million people, are unaware they have the disease.[2] Roughly 65% of all diabetics die either from heart disease or stroke.[3] Reuters Health news has reported that over 30% of Americans are pre-diabetic,[4] a condition in which blood glucose levels are elevated but not enough to be classified diabetic.

The risk of premature death for a diabetic is about double that of a person without the disease.[5] Observing the rapid age progression of diabetics has been likened to watching the normal human aging process on fast-forward. Diabetes is becoming more common among African Americans, Native Americans, and Hispanics in comparison to Caucasians. In the U.S., the direct costs of the disease surpass $90 billion, while the indirect costs, including disability, loss of work and premature death, are over $40 billion.[6]

There are two major types of diabetes, referred to as Type I and Type II. Type I diabetes, which inflicts fewer than two million Americans, usually occurs in children or young adults under the age of 30, is also known as juvenile-onset diabetes and Insulin-Dependent Diabetes Mellitus (IDDM). Although the Western medical community suggests the cause of Type I diabetes is unknown or not totally understood, they maintain a genetic factor as well as auto-immune disorders are suspected to play a role. According to the auto-immune theory, pancreatic beta cells are attacked by the immune system's T-cells, and are damaged or destroyed.

Other medical practitioners who are willing to take a stand against the entrenched industrial influences of our modern world have suggested a range or other possible causes. It has been suggested that Type I diabetes is strongly influenced by: pasteurized cow's milk (at least two proteins contained in cow's milk can trigger an auto-immune attack on the beta cells); artificial sweeteners such as corn syrup; and chlorine—which is generally ingested into the body either by drinking it in tap water or through showering. Chlorine depletes vitamin E and combines with vitamin E complexes to form *alloxan*, a chemical toxic to beta cells. Research has shown that children who develop Type I diabetes generally have been breast fed for less than three months, and consumed either cow's milk or solid food within the first few months of life. One study showed that children not consuming cow's milk during the first three months had a 40% reduced incidence of diabetes compared to those who consumed cow's milk.[7] About 75% of those who develop Type I diabetes have immune system antibodies which attack the pancreas.

John Classen, M.D., has published over 20 scientific articles on the subject of vaccine-induced Type I diabetes. According to Dr. Classen, at least 80% of children with Type I diabetes acquired the disease as a direct result of receiving a vaccination. In one 1999 study reported in the *British Journal of Medicine*,[8] Classen showed that in Finland, the *Haemophilus influenzae* type b (Hib) vaccine caused three times as many cases of potentially-lethal Type I diabetes as the number of cases of brain damage it may have prevented. New Zealand witnessed a 61% rise in Type I diabetes following an aggressive hepatitis B vaccine campaign. Denmark, England, Italy, Sweden and other European countries, once having had stable levels of Type I, all experienced a significant rise in the disease following the introduction of new childhood vaccines.[9]

Type I accounts for only 5-10% of all diabetics. In Type I, the pancreatic beta cells produce too little insulin to effectively regulate blood glucose levels. Even though there is "food" within the blood, the cells starve due to the lack of insulin which would otherwise allow glucose to enter the cells. Type I diabetics require an external source of insulin, such as that received from daily hypodermic injections or an insulin pump.

Type II diabetes—referred to as adult-onset diabetes and Non-Insulin-Dependent Diabetes Mellitus (NIDDM)—is characterized by the inefficient production and/or utilization of insulin. It is related to obesity, high cholesterol, high blood pressure, and insulin resistance. *Metabolic syndrome*, also called *Syndrome X*—a group of risk factors relating to blood sugar metabolism—is closely associated with *insulin resistance syndrome* (IRS).

Those with metabolic syndrome are twice as likely to suffer a heart attack or stroke, and are three times more likely to die prematurely as a result. IRS is characterized by the inability of insulin molecules to attach properly to receptor sites, thus preventing or decreasing glucose transfer into the cells. This produces the hyperglycemic excess of sugar within the blood. (Low blood sugar is referred to as *hypo*glycemia.) When IRS is present, much of the food is stored as fat in the stomach area. Additionally, in an attempt to compensate for the cells' inability to utilize insulin efficiently in insulin-resistant individuals, the pancreas secretes additional insulin into the blood, causing further damage.

Some of the common symptoms of diabetes include frequent urination; excessive thirst; extreme hunger; unusual weight loss; weakness and fatigue; irritability; blurred vision; difficult-to-heal skin and gum lesions; tingling or numbness in the hands and/or feet; and itchy skin.

Food, Insulin & Blood Sugar. When food is consumed, the blood glucose (sugar) levels rise. Insulin allows the glucose to enter and fuel the cells. In a diabetic if the levels rise too high because of insulin resistance or too much insulin being secreted, insulin remains in the bloodstream causing irritation and constriction of the arterial vessels which is damaging to the entire cardiovascular system and organs, including the heart and brain. (It is one of the liver's tasks to remove insulin from the blood, but excess insulin causes fatty deposits in the liver, interfering with this ability.) This process gives rise to a host of specific physical problems that can occur over time, including blindness, burning foot syndrome, deafness, high blood pressure, insufficient blood circulation (especially to the lower extremities), kidney failure, nervous system diseases, periodontal (gum) disease, stroke, and a host of other complications. Diabetics are at risk of developing other illnesses and if they do, their prognosis is worse than a non-diabetic. Diabetes is the leading cause of blindness, heart attacks, kidney failure, and leg amputations.

Glucose levels rise more rapidly in diabetics, and remain elevated longer in comparison to non-diabetics. This unchecked overabundance of glucose within the blood so characteristic in both diabetics and pre-diabetics facilitates the binding of and cross-linking with glucose-metabolic intermediates (sugar-derived substances) with proteins throughout the entire body, including DNA—the material that contains the genetic instructions for the body's proper development and functioning. This is the complex chemical process of *glycation*, and further results in a group of harmful byproducts collectively labeled **advanced glycation end products** (AGEs). The similar chemical process of *lipoxidation* occurs when sugars cross-link with lipids (fats), producing **advanced lipoxidation end products** (ALEs). Both the brain and heart—as well as other tissues and organs—can be severely impacted as both organs have a high lipid content, the brain being composed mostly of fatty acids.

Once proteins and lipids become cross-linked, they become severely degraded and marginally functional. Glycated tissues produce 50 times more free radicals than their non-glycated counterparts. As these processes continue unchecked and the affected proteins and lipids accumulate, they emit signals which cause the production of inflammatory *cytokines*, cell-signaling chemicals which themselves emit further messages to increase the inflammatory cascade. This is one of the principal causes of the inflammatory process which is so common in aging people, especially aging diabetics.

Proteins of the blood vessel linings, nerve cells, kidney, and retina are particularly vulnerable to glycation, and are typically the first to be damaged. Glycation, AGEs, lipoxidation, and ALEs are associated with all of the detrimental physical maladies discussed above, and most age-related diseases including arthritis; abnormal DNA formation (that can lead to cancer); cataracts; early aging (including wrinkling of the skin); fatigue; kidney and blood vessel damage; neurological diseases such as Alzheimer's disease and Parkinson's disease; and vision loss.[10] These processes are linked so closely that some researchers are now referring to Alzheimer's disease as Type III diabetes—although what is being called Type III diabetes affects brain levels of insulin that are actually produced in the brain—a recent finding—and isn't believed to affect blood sugar. Post mortem biopsies show Alzheimer's victims' brains have higher accumulations of AGEs compared to those dying from other causes.

Many critical cells throughout the body—including cells of the kidneys, liver, lungs, and pancreas—have on their surfaces **R**eceptors for **A**dvanced **G**lycation **E**nd Products (RAGEs). As AGEs from both external (food cooked at high temperatures and for long durations) and internal sources (diabetes, for example) dock with RAGEs on these vital organs, cells degrade and dysfunction and disease manifest. Free radicals and a decrease in antioxidant levels are mediating factors.

In addition to AGE chemistry, the related chemical process *carbonylation* is the origin of the "browning" effect on foods such as roasted chicken and the browning of bread into toast. Carbonylation is the result of protein oxidation and reactions of proteins with sugars, aldehydes, and products of lipid peroxidation.[11] Over time, as the affected proteins accumulate in vital organs, they become progressively more damaged, causing organ dysfunction. Carbonylated proteins are visible in the aging skin as the darkened pigmented spots known as "aging spots" *(lipofucin* deposits), and as cataracts, the clouding of the normally-clear lens of the eye. The carbonylation "browning" process within the human body has been likened to a low temperature oven with a 65-75 year cooking cycle.

Carbonylated proteins are responsible for many age-related conditions including cardiovascular disease and neurodegenerative disorders. It is theorized that damaged proteins interfere with the cells' ability to detect damaged DNA, thereby preventing the cellular repair of this vital material which contains the body's genetic instructions. Additionally, damage occurs to the program which monitors orderly cell death, or *apoptosis*, causing damaged cells to survive and reproduce, leading to progressive chromosomal instability—which is a precursor to the development of cancerous states. As we age, about 30% of the body's proteins become damaged by carbonylation. Clearly, glycation and carbonylation of proteins and lipids are two of the principal causes of premature aging and premature death. Diabetes accelerates the formation and accumulation of AGEs and ALEs.

Diagnosis and Monitoring. Although a urine test may provide some indication of excess glucose, urine testing is inaccurate in comparison to blood tests. In fact, elevated glucose levels may not appear in the urine even in a person having high blood sugar levels. Several types of blood tests are used to diagnose and monitor diabetes. The most accurate results for both diagnosis and monitoring are obtained by using a combination of a *blood glucose test* [called a *fasting plasma glucose* (FPG) if done following a fast] and the *hemoglobin A1c* (HbA1c) test. Another test sometimes used is the *oral glucose tolerance test* (OGTT).

The blood glucose test provides a measure of what the blood glucose levels are at the time of testing. Using this test, a person is able to monitor what environmental changes affect their blood sugar levels—types of food eaten, exercise, medication, etc. These readings, which can be done at home using a blood glucose meter, enable a person to monitor glucose levels from hour-to-hour.

A fasting blood plasma glucose test is the preferred way to diagnose diabetes. A person fasts overnight and is tested before the morning meal. According to the American Diabetes Association, a "normal" (healthy) fasting plasma glucose level is less than 110 milligrams per deciliter (mg/dl). Two or more tests giving a reading greater than 126 mg/dl on different days is considered indicative of having diabetes. A range of 110-126 mg/dl is considered a "pre-diabetic state."[12]

On the other hand, a 1999 a study published in *Diabetes Care*[13] reported that men having an FPG reading above 85 mg/dl have a 40% higher risk of dying from cardiovascular disease than those whose FPG measures 85 mg/dl or below.

While the blood glucose test measures the levels of glucose in the blood at the time of measurement, it isn't able to assess whether or not cells are being damaged, and if so to what extent. The HbA1c test measures how much sugar is actually sticking to the cells. Because sugar molecules bind irreversibly to hemoglobin, and because red blood cell-containing hemoglobin has a life span of only several months, the HbA1c provides an historical indication (index) of the degree of blood sugar involvement over a period of 60-120 days, measured as a percentage. A percentage of seven (7%) or lower is considered to be average.[14] Eight percent or greater is considered in the high range.

A simple test for home use accurately measures HbA1c. The disposable device analyses one drop of blood with laboratory-like accuracy, according to its manufacturer QuickMedical. To learn more, visit www.quickmedical.com/metrika or call QuickMedical at (888)345-4858.

The oral glucose tolerance test (OGTT) is administered following an overnight fast of at least eight but not more than 16 hours. Initially, the fasting plasma glucose is tested, followed by consuming a very sweet drink containing 75 gm of glucose (100 gm for pregnant women). Thereafter, blood glucose levels are measured at 30 minutes, one hour, and then at one hour intervals for up to six hours. In order for the test to be reliable, the recipient must be in good health, normally active, and not taking medications that could affect blood glucose levels. For three days prior to the test, the recipient should eat a diet high in carbohydrates. Additionally, no coffee should be consumed or cigarettes smoked the morning of the test.

Blood sugar levels rise and fall quickly in persons who are non-diabetic. In diabetics, the blood sugar levels rise higher than normal and remain abnormally elevated. A normal response is indicated when the 2-hour glucose level is less than 140 mg/dl, and all values between 0 and 2 hours are less than 200 mg/dl. Impaired glucose tolerance (IGT) is indicated when the FPG is less than 126 mg/dl and the 2-hour glucose level is between 140-199 mg/dl. Diabetes is present when the glucose levels are greater than 200 mg/dl.

It's inspiring to know that when it comes to blood glucose levels—unlike dieting—a small decrease in the numbers produces very beneficial results. According to the Diabetes Control and Complications Trial, even a small 2% decrease in blood glucose levels was associated with a 75% reduced risk of developing eye disease, a 60% risk reduction of nerve disease, and a 50% reduced risk of developing kidney disease.

■ *Scout DS*.™ A new, high tech device for noninvasively assessing the presence of diabetes and pre-diabetes has been developed by researchers at the New Mexico firm VeraLight. Called the Scout DS,™ the device projects light of various wavelengths into the skin of the inside (palm-side) of the forearm where it measures the presence and extent of advanced glycation endproducts by *fluorescence spectroscopy*. The Scout has the appearance of a drugstore blood pressure monitor, weighs 10 pounds, and takes 60 seconds to deliver a result.

Other methods of diabetes detection can be problematic for many. Tests such as the OGTT, FPG and HbA1c require blood to be taken, which is a barrier to many patients because of the inconvenience and pain involved. The most widely used screening test is the FPG, which involves overnight fasting. FPG also suffers from a lack of sensitivity (40-60%) in its diagnostic capability, contributing to a late diagnosis of many who already have the disease. As many as 50% of diabetics, in fact, are not diagnosed with the disease until it's well advanced, often with irreversible complications.

In a study of 351 participants, the Scout was evaluated in a head-to-head comparison with FPG and HbA1c. The new noninvasive device was found to identify 28.8% more diabetic individuals than the FPG and 17.1% more than the HbA1c. As of mid-2008, the Scout is being tested in several hospitals across the U.S., and is considered an experimental device—with the hope that it will soon be widely available. For more information, to determine the status of its availability, and to view a picture of the Scout, visit www.veralight.com.

Pharmaceutical Treatments. While Type I diabetics are treated by insulin injection or with an insulin pump, Type II diabetics are often able to control their symptoms and physical complications effectively by healthy lifestyle changes including diet and exercise. However, the degree of benefit is a function of the extent of insulin resistance (insensitivity) and/or insulin underproduction. Pharmaceutical medications are given if diet and exercise are ineffective, or if the diabetic won't comply with the diet and exercise regimen.

Because of the high prevalence of diabetes, there is no lack of pharmaceutical drugs available to treat the illness. Several classifications of pill-form drugs are available, but these drugs are ineffective for many. Studies indicate that less than half of those prescribed pharmaceuticals are able to achieve and maintain healthy blood sugar levels following three months at treatment dosages.[15]

Beyond being ineffective for many, sometimes these drugs are dangerous. In March 2001, Pfizer's diabetes drug Rezulin was removed from the market after causing 63 confirmed deaths, with the death toll possibly being 10 times higher than the number of confirmed fatalities. The FDA has estimated that one out of every 1,800 Rezulin users could expect to suffer liver damage.[16] Despite these realities, the largely-unknowing public has made diabetes drugs one of the best-selling classifications of pharmaceuticals on the market today.

Because diabetes drugs affect the body in different ways, they are often used in combination. This practice sometimes medically benefits the patient, always costs more, increases the possibility of side-effects, and fills the pharmaceutical companies' coffers with a lot more ducats.

Those who take these drugs are cautioned to tell their doctors if they have kidney, liver or thyroid disease—meaning they're probably not helpful to these organs, diplomatically speaking. Patients are advised to discuss with their doctors the risks versus benefits of taking these drugs—and they should hope their docs give them the entire picture, including the potential downside that accompanies their use. This counseling is something that too often doesn't occur.

■ ***Cloned Antibodies.*** Jeffrey Bluestone, Ph. D., of the University of California at San Francisco Diabetes Center, has discovered a method which holds promise for the treatment of Type I diabetes. It is believed that one of the causes of Type I diabetes is the attack of the insulin-producing beta cells by the body's own immune system. Based on this understanding, Dr. Bluestone and colleagues tested a new approach using cloned antibodies to target and deactivate the damaging immune cells. The approach, used effectively on only a small group of patients to date, seeks to retrain the immune system without requiring the need for long-term therapy.[17] Bluestone's work is ongoing, and holds promise for Type I diabetics.

Treatment Alternatives. In contrast to pharmaceutical drugs, there are a number of more natural treatment approaches that have been shown to be side-effect free. In the long term, these approaches are often more effective than pharmaceuticals in increasing cell sensitivity to insulin, as well as possibly increasing insulin production via repair and/or regeneration of pancreatic beta cells.

■ ***Benfotiamine*** (**S-benzyolthiamine O-monophosphate**). Developed in Japan in the late 1950s to treat alcoholic and diabetic neuropathy and other nerve disorders including sciatica, *benfotiamine* has been marketed in Japan since 1962, in Europe since 1992 and in the U.S. since 2005. It is a slightly altered derivative of vitamin B_1, thiamine, and is present in trace amounts in roasted, crushed garlic, onions, shallots and leeks. Benfotiamine's supplemental use has been shown to significantly decrease the unpleasant physical symptoms of diabetes such as burning, tingling, prickling, or loss of sensation in the feet and hands. Its use may also lessen the more serious complications previously mentioned, which include deafness, loss of vision, high blood pressure and stroke. Due to its unique chemical actions, benfotiamine may also help repair and regenerate diabetes-induced damaged cells throughout the body[18]—including nerve cells in the extremities and cells of the small capillaries of the eyes (retina) and kidneys (glomeruli), thus restoring some function to these organs.

Ironically, while the characteristic underproduction of insulin and/or the lack of cells' sensitivity to it prevents glucose from entering many of the body's trillions of cells, excess glucose within the blood floods into blood vessel cells, causing great damage to both cellular structure and function.

In contrast to most of the other substances used to treat diabetes (described below)—which work either by increasing the quantity of insulin and/or increasing the cells' sensitivity to it—benfotiamine eliminates excess levels of potentially-damaging glucose metabolites (triosephosphates) from within the blood vessel cells. It accomplishes this cellular purging by increasing the activity of the enzyme *transketolase* by 300-400%, allowing glucose to be processed through an alternate metabolic pathway, thus normalizing glucose levels and metabolism within the affected cells.[19] Interestingly, benfotiamine's benefits are *not* the result of a drop in blood sugar levels—as measured by fasting plasma or HbA1c—but rather its unique ability to balance cellular glucose metabolism. By this means, it helps prevent glycation and AGEs.

Recent studies have shown benfotiamine may be helpful in treating many neurological conditions including Alzheimer's, Bell's palsy, herpes simplex, Parkinson's, sciatica, shingles, tinnitus, tooth hypersensitivity, and Tourette's syndrome. Other ailments which may benefit are AIDS, end stage kidney disease, and liver diseases including hepatitis. Benfotiamine has no known drug interactions or side-effects at treatment dosages. The basic treatment level is 600-900 mg daily in divided doses, with a maintenance dosage of 150 mg. However, this may vary depending upon the severity of the condition and the patient's subjective experience. Up to 1,200 mg/day has been used safely. To learn more, visit www.benfotiamine.org.

■ ***Carnosine.*** Carnosine, also called L-carnosine, is a naturally-occurring dipeptide—a combination of the two amino acids beta-alanine and histidine. Although it was discovered in Russia in 1900, carnosine has only recently been rediscovered by Western scientists. It has anti-glycation, antioxidative, neurotransmitter, and other properties, and is concentrated in the long-lived tissues of the body, the brain, and cardiac and skeletal muscles.

Orally ingested, carnosine is a very effective natural inhibitor of protein carbonylation. It reacts (bonds) with and removes the carbonyl groups in glycated proteins that are imbedded within cellular membranes. Moreover, carnosine suppresses the multiple pathways that lead to protein carbonylation."[20] It significantly inhibits the protein (inter- and intra-molecular) cross-linking of the glycation process and especially reduces the formation of advanced glycation end products. Thus, carnosine both prevents the damaging cross-linking of proteins, while it also neutralizes and eliminates them after they have formed, thereby restoring normal cellular function.

The high concentrations of carnosine found in the brain are used to protect this sensitive organ from oxidation, glycation, carbonylation, and the effects of excitotoxins. It is also a powerful chelator of copper and zinc (and heavy metals in general), which have been shown to contribute to the formation of amyloid beta deposits present in Alzheimer's patients. Carnosine also protects the brain against lipid oxidation and the harmful byproducts of alcohol metabolism.[21]

The primary dietary source of carnosine is meat. Of the few substances lacking in the diets of vegetarians, carnosine is one of them—which represents a significant vulnerability to this group of people. Also, carnosine levels decline with age. The 63% decrease of carnosine levels in human muscle which occurs between ages 10 to 70 may account for the reduction in muscle mass, strength, and function so typically evident in aging adults. Carnosine muscle levels in animals correlate with their maximum lifespans. Stress, infection, and trauma in humans also decrease its levels. Because carnosine levels decrease with age, daily supplementation is required to maintain its continued benefits. Carnosine is likely many times more potent an antiglycating agent than *aminoguanidine*, a European drug available as a dietary supplement in the U.S.

■ *EWOT*. Supplemental oxygen at 10 liters per minute while exercising helps reverse both the symptoms and the damage caused by diabetic neuropathy and retinopathy.[22] A particularly effective form of supplemental oxygen therapy is EWOT—Exercise with Oxygen Therapy. See EWOT under **General Treatment Methods**.

■ *The ReBuilder*.® ReBuilder Medical, Inc. of Charles Town, WV offers a small, battery-operated electrical device that promises to reduce or eliminate the pain, numbness, burning sensations, and tingling so common to peripheral neuropathy. The ReBuilder sends healing, non-painful electrical signals to the feet (or hands) which wake up dormant nerves and restore blood flow, hence oxygen, to the extremities. Patients begin by using the device once per day for about 30 minutes. As symptoms subside, frequency of use can be decreased to two or three treatments per week.

According to the company, patients average a 95% reduction in pain and burning and an 83% reduction in numbness. Even those who've been told "nothing else can be done, the nerves are dead" may find relief using this device. David Phillips, Ph.D., inventor of the ReBuilder, is also the inventor of the GST® Breast Cancer Detection System, and was given the Inventor of the Year award in 1986 for his development of the infrared ear thermometer, a well-known household item. To learn more about The ReBuilder, various models of which sell for USD$399-$699, visit http://rebuildermedical.com.

■ *Diet and Exercise*. Those who are pre-diabetic often can forestall the onset of Type II diabetes with lifestyle changes focusing on diet and exercise. For both men and women of all ages and ethnic backgrounds, these two lifestyle modifications reduce the development of diabetes by 40-60%.[23] Persons with Type II diabetes often are able to significantly control the disease symptoms using these methods.

Regular physical activity of moderate intensity is recommended—such as brisk walking for a total of several hours each week. According to a person's physical capabilities, other exercise regimens such as bicycling, swimming, and weight lifting may be appropriate. Exercise induces cells—especially muscle cells—to become more responsive to insulin, i.e., it reduces insulin resistance.

The "Don'ts." The Glycemic Index (GI) is a ranking of foods based on their immediate effect on blood glucose levels. Foods with lower GI values produce a smaller rise in post-meal glucose levels. Foods with GI values of less than 55 are considered low glycemic foods. It is prudent for diabetics and pre-diabetics to avoid foods that produce a high rise in blood sugar, including all products made with refined flour, such as store-bought bagels, bread, cereals, cookies, crackers, macaroni, rolls, spaghetti—all pastas. Refined carbohydrates made from refined flour cause a blood sugar spike almost as high as pure table sugar (which has a GI value of 100; honey has a GI value of 67). Complex carbohydrates, on the other hand, are the form found in unprocessed vegetables and other "natural" foods. Fiber contained in these foods slows the digestion of the plant sugars and starches (the chief form of stored carbohydrates in plants), eliminating the dangerous glucose spike.

Other problemed foods include refined corn products, white rice, high fat-containing foods, and all sugar-added products. This would include many/most/all fast foods and store-bought processed foods—foods which come packaged or canned. Some of the names associated with sugars added to processed foods include corn sweeteners, dextrose, glucose, high dextrose and fructose corn syrup, and others. If you have a sweet tooth, try *xylitol*, a sugar alcohol discussed in more depth in the section on *Asthma*. Xylitol is as sweet as sugar, but doesn't cause an exaggerated glucose spike due to its low glycemic index of 7. Xylitol is available in many health food stores. It can be ordered at a discount at www.emeraldforestxylitol.com or www.iherb.com, or by searching online for "xylitol." The herb *stevia* and extracts of the Lo Han Kuo fruit are also healthy sugar substitutes.

The founder of the U.S. Food and Drug Administration, then called the Bureau of Chemistry, was Harvey W. Wiley, M.D. Dr. Wiley was nobly concerned with the purity of the American food supply and those whose task it was to protect it from contamination. He was the architect of the nation's first Pure Food and Drug Law enacted in 1906, also referred to as The Wiley Act. Dr. Wiley's intention was to reform certain aspects of the food manufacturing industry. He led the fight against food additives, and among many other reforms sought to declare refined and bleached flour products and artificial sweeteners (specifically corn sweeteners) as adulterated foods and thereby prohibited from interstate transport. It was known almost 100 years ago that corn syrup causes diabetes in animals.

Dr. Wiley resigned in disgust in 1912 due to pressures brought by the food and pharmaceutical industries. He was so concerned about the potential dangers of these two industries that in 1929 he published his memoirs entitled *The History of a Crime Against the Food Law: The Amazing Story of the National Food and Drug Law Intended to Protect the Health of the People, Perverted to Protect Adulteration of Foods and Drugs.* Dr. Wiley died less than a year after his book was published, and within weeks the book "vanished from libraries and bookshops around the nation."[24] Dr. Wiley wrote:

> There is a distinct tendency to put regulations and rules for the enforcement of law into the hands of industries engaged in food and drug activities...I consider this one of the most pernicious threats to pure foods and drugs. Business is making rapid strides in the control of all our affairs. When we permit business in general to regulate the quality and character of our food and drug supplies, we are treading upon very dangerous ground.[25]

It has been found that kidney damage occurs in diabetics who consume too much protein.[26] Therefore, chicken, eggs and meats should be restricted. Fruits and root vegetables (beets, carrots, potatoes, etc.), which can cause a spike in blood sugar levels, should be eaten only with other foods— so that the sugar is more slowly metabolized, and the high blood glucose spike is reduced and delayed.

The "Dos." Replace refined carbohydrates with unrefined whole grains. The focus should be whole grains, vegetables, fruit (with meals only), beans, seeds and nuts. In a 1997 study published in the *American Journal of Clinical Nutrition,*[27] it was shown that eating mono- and polyunsaturated fats from vegetables, and omega-3 fatty acids in fish and flax seeds (and oil), reduce insulin requirements.

■ ***Chromium Picolinate.*** The body requires the mineral chromium for the efficient functioning of insulin. This mineral has been shown to have a significant influence on the reduction of insulin resistance, i.e., it increases cellular sensitivity to insulin. In particular, *chromium picolinate* seems to be the form of chromium that's most effective in reducing insulin resistance, as demonstrated by many studies published in peer-reviewed journals.

In 1997, a placebo-controlled study was reported in the journal *Diabetes*[28] in which 180 Type II diabetics were given a daily dosage of either 200 micrograms (mcg) or 1,000 mcg (one milligram) of chromium picolinate, or a placebo. The study concluded that persons with Type II diabetes experienced a dramatic reduction in both blood glucose and insulin levels. Especially in those individuals receiving 1,000 mcg daily, significant, sustained reductions in diabetic symptoms were noted.

Another study reported in the *Journal of Trace Elements in Experimental Medicine*[29] in 1999 found that 833 people with Type II diabetes who consumed 500 mcg of chromium picolinate per day experienced a significant decrease in their fasting and after-meal blood glucose levels. In more than 90% of the participants, blood glucose levels were significantly reduced after only one month of supplementation, with levels remaining reduced for at least one year. They also experienced significant long-term reduction in their diabetic symptoms, while 85% reported a reduction in fatigue, frequency of urination, and excessive thirst.

In 1999, the U.S. Department of Agriculture's Dr. Richard Anderson conducted a literature review of more than 30 years of clinical studies using chromium supplementation for the treatment of Type II diabetes. Anderson concluded that of the various forms evaluated, chromium picolinate was more effective than any other for improving the blood variables (glucose and insulin) associated with diabetes. Improvements were shown in those using as little as 200 mcg daily, but more pronounced benefits were seen at the daily level of 1,000 mcg.[30]

■ ***Bitter Melon.*** Also known as bitter gourd and balsam pear, bitter melon has been and even today is the most widely used Ayurvedic treatment for diabetic conditions. There's also some impressive science to back up the ancients' observations and prescriptive practices. Recently, the hypoglycemic peptide *polypeptide-p* has been isolated from its fruit, seeds and skin. *Cerasee*, a specific variety of bitter melon, has been shown to reduce blood sugar levels by 50% within five hours in diabetic mice.[31] Scientists at the Sri Venkateswara University in India published findings that after only 15 days, bitter melon significantly reduced fasting blood glucose levels in diabetic rats, and also reduced cholesterol and triglyceride levels.[32]

■ **Cinnamon**. The well-known spice cinnamon has been found very effective in combating high blood glucose levels. The ancient spice both imitates insulin and potentiates its effects. Supplementing with one gram (about one-fourth teaspoon) twice daily for 40 days reduced fasting glucose levels 18-29%, triglycerides 23-30%, and LDL cholesterol 7-27%. Increased levels of cinnamon, up to six grams, had no greater effect. When participants stopped taking cinnamon, the beneficial effects continued for about three weeks, after which their blood glucose levels began to increase to previous levels.[33] Use one-quarter to one-half teaspoon twice daily in tea or coffee, or take a pill-form supplement such as Cinnulin PF,® a 20:1 water-soluble concentrate (extract) that's been shown effective in clinical trials. For more information, visit www.cinnulin.com.

■ **Gymnema sylvestre**. Also called gurmar, *Gymnema sylvestre* is yet another herb used in the Ayurvedic tradition. Recent research has shown this herb decreases fasting blood sugar levels, lowers insulin requirements, and increases the pancreatic production of insulin. These benefits result from Gymnema's ability to repair the insulin producing beta cells, regenerate them, or both. The herb also seems to increase cell permeability to insulin. In one study performed on autopsied diabetic rats, the pancreas weight increased almost 30% following Gymnema administration. The number of beta cells increased by more than 100%. In the control group of non-diabetic rats, Gymnema did not alter insulin levels.[34] In fact, in healthy non-diabetic persons, Gymnema has no effect on blood sugar levels. In animals whose pancreases have been removed, the herb has absolutely no effect.

In a study[35] of 22 Type II diabetic patients who took 400 mg of *Gymnema sylvestre* extract daily

for 15-18 months along with conventional anti-diabetic drugs, a significant reduction in blood glucose was noted, and conventional drug dosage could be decreased. Five of the participants were able to discontinue the drugs completely, and maintain normal blood sugar levels with Gymnema alone. In another study,[36] 27 Type I diabetics who were taking insulin were given a Gymnema extract. Participants experienced a drop in fasting glucose levels and insulin requirements, and there was a general improvement in blood sugar control.

Available in health food stores, *Gymnema sylvestre* is safe to use and is accompanied by no side-effects. The preferred dosage is 400 mg daily. An excellent product formulated according to the Ayurvedic tradition is GlucoCare,® marketed by Himalaya USA. Also marketed as GlucoSim® to medical professionals and Diabecon® to non-U.S. residents, GlucoCare contains a proprietary formulation of several herbs which have been demonstrated effective in diabetes control, including bitter melon, *Gymnema slyvestre*, pitasara, and *Eugenia jambolana*. To review over 25 research papers on GlucoCare, visit www.himalayahealthcare.com/researchpaper/diabecon.htm.

■ **Niacinamide**. Researchers have known since 1950 that *niacinamide*, a water-soluble form of the B_3 vitamin niacin, confers protection against the onset of diabetes.[37] This research has gone relatively unnoticed—especially in the U.S.—in favor of treatment by means of pharmaceutical drugs. In many other countries, especially European countries including Germany and Italy, as well as Canada, Israel and New Zealand, there is ongoing research on using niacinamide to prevent and treat diabetes.

Niacinamide, also called *nicotinamide*, acts against diabetes on several levels. On the one hand, it inhibits components of the immune system which attack pancreatic beta cells,[38] and restores the activity of the insulin-producing beta cells and/or deters beta cell destruction.[39] It also stimulates production of insulin and increases the sensitivity of cells to insulin.[40]

Niacinamide shows promise in preventing high-risk children from developing diabetes. In one study, 14 children were given niacinamide while eight children in the control group were not. All of the untreated children developed diabetes at some future time, while only one who received niacinamide developed the disease.

Niacinamide works best either as a preventive or during the initial stages (first five years) of the disease. Some newly-diagnosed Type I diabetics have totally resolved the disease through the use of this vitamin. The recommended daily dosage is 25 mg for each kilogram of body weight.

■ *Conjugated Linoleic Acid* (CLA). It has been shown in both animal and human studies that CLA is effective in controlling the symptoms of Type II diabetes. CLA facilitates the uptake of glucose by increasing insulin sensitivity. In a 2003 article published in the *Journal of Nutrition*,[41] patients treated with CLA experienced a five-fold (500%) decrease in fasting blood glucose levels compared to the control group not receiving CLA. Lead researcher Dr. Martha Belury, Associate Professor of Human Nutrition at Ohio State University, stated that CLA is known to delay the onset of diabetes in rats, and assists in managing Type II diabetes in humans. It also has been shown to reduce body (including stomach) fat and increase lean muscle mass. Tonalin® CLA is a preferred product at a dosage of three grams daily.

■ *Banaba*. Known botanically as *Lagerstroemia speciosa*, banaba is a time-tested medicinal plant that grows in India, Southeast Asia, and the Philippines. It has been used traditionally to treat diabetes and other ailments. Extracts of banaba activate the transport of glucose across cell membranes exerting an action similar to that of insulin in controlling blood sugar levels. Banaba's principal active ingredient is *corosolic acid*, although other constituent elements are likely active.

Animal studies and human clinical trials have shown corosolic acid is both safe and effective in significantly reducing blood glucose levels with short term use—within four weeks. Even a one-time use leaves a "memory effect" for blood glucose control lasting several days. In rabbits, orally administered corosolic acid has been shown to act similarly to insulin injections. Therefore, corosolic acid is seen as a phyto-insulin or insulin-like plant extract. Its effectiveness is dose dependent, i.e., the higher the dose, the larger the drop in blood sugar levels. Persons using a corosolic acid supplement report the

absence of symptoms associated with adult onset diabetes, such as frequent thirst and urination. A slight loss of weight is also common.

To learn more, visit www.banabaherb.com/links.htm. Most banaba supplements are standardized to 1% corosolic acid. The Now Foods product GlucoFit,™ standardized to 18% corosolic acid, is one of the best products currently available.

■ *Salacia Oblonga*. An herb native to India and Sri Lanka, *Salacia oblonga* is used in traditional Ayurvedic medicine to lower blood sugar and insulin levels in a manner similar to prescription drugs—but safer than synthesized chemicals. In a study of 39 healthy adults, one gram decreased insulin levels by 29% and post-meal glucose levels by 23%. Dr. Steve Hertzler, co-author of the study, remarked "These kinds of reductions are similar to what we might see with prescription oral medications for people with diabetes."[42] One to five grams can be taken either with food, beverage, or in pill-form. *Salacia oblonga* is available on the internet.

■ *Vanadyl Sulfate*. Vanadyl sulfate is a form of the mineral vanadium, and has been shown effective in reducing the level of insulin requirements in diabetics. In larger doses, the mineral mimics the effects of insulin. Although there has been much speculation regarding why this is so, it has yet to be determined. Animal studies have shown vanadyl sulfate has permanently eliminated diabetes, even after its use is stopped. Begin slowly and gradually work up to an effective daily dosage of 50-100 mg daily. Persons taking these high levels of vanadium should be monitored frequently by a physician.

■ *Resveratrol*. A naturally-occurring compound, resveratrol is found in various food-stuffs and plants including berries, grapes, peanuts, pine trees, and some herbs. For use in dietary supplements, it is often extracted from the root of the *Polygonum cuspidatum* plant. Chemically, resveratrol is classified a *polyphenol*, a broad group of plant-derived compounds further subdivided into other categories including *flavonoids, tannins*, and *lignins*. First identified as recently as the early 1980s, there was no clinical interest in resveratrol until the 1990s when it was discovered that trans-resveratrol—the active component—is present in wine.

Harvard scientists have recently shown that resveratrol may prevent many of the detrimental health effects caused by over-eating and obesity— even without reducing the weight of the eater. In a 2006 study published in *Nature*,[43] middle-aged mice that were fed a high-calorie diet became obese and exhibited metabolic changes resembling diabetes, liver and heart damage, and suffered premature deaths. However, after about six months the mice fed resveratrol in conjunction with the high-calorie diet showed beneficial changes, and their physiology became similar to those fed a standard diet.

The resveratrol-fed mice on the high-calorie diet showed increased insulin sensitivity, lower blood sugar levels, enhanced mitochondrial energy production, and improved motor function. Non-resveratrol-fed mice on the high-calorie diet developed enlarged, fatty livers, while the resveratrol-fed mice did not. Further, heart disease and evidence of atherosclerosis were seen in mice fed the high-calorie diet without resveratrol, but not in the group that was also fed resveratrol. Resveratrol significantly increased survival, reducing the risk of death from the high-calorie diet by 31%. It also improved the animals' quality of life, as shown by their steady improvement in balance and coordination with age. These benefits were experienced by the resveratrol-fed mice on a high-calorie diet even though they remained obese.

This study offers powerful evidence that resveratrol may similarly protect humans from the harmful effects of a high-calorie diet. Could this be a literal case "having your cake and eating it too?" A product offering high levels of resveratrol is Now Foods' Mega Potency Natural Resveratrol.™

The Harvard researchers concluded,

> These data demonstrate that resveratrol can alleviate the negative impact of a high-calorie diet on overall health and life span. The ability of resveratrol to prevent the deleterious effects of excess caloric intake and modulate known longevity pathways suggests that resveratrol and molecules with similar properties might be valuable tools in the search for key regulators of energy balance, health, and longevity.[44]

■ *__Testosterone__*. The term *andropause* describes the male counterpart of the female-related condition menopause. It is the age-related dramatic decline of testosterone levels which begins in men in their thirties to early forties. The decline in free testosterone has been measured to decline at the rate of 0.5 to 1.6% yearly, while 25% of men over 60 are considered to have *hypogonadism*—the failure of the testes to produce sufficient testosterone. A number of symptoms are related to andropause including loss of lean body mass (weight gain), muscle mass, and strength; decreased bone mineral density; reduced sexual desire/erectile quality; fatigue; and increased anxiety and irritability.

Decreasing testosterone is also related to diabetes. Many enlightened physicians are currently aware that supplementation in aging men with bio-identical testosterone in the range of 50-100 mg weekly helps increase the quality of life in many ways, in part by helping to prevent many serious disease states such as heart disease (heart muscle cells have testosterone receptors), osteoporosis, and diabetes—and also by treating these conditions. (Bio-identical hormones are those having an identical chemical structure to those naturally produced.) Testosterone can be obtained in the form of a transdermal cream or gel supplied by a local compounding pharmacy rather than purchasing an expensive brand name pharmaceutical such as the Androderm® patch. It is also available as an intramuscular injectable and an implanted, time-release pellet. All forms of testosterone require a prescription.

According to Edward Lichten, M.D., a physician with over 35 years experience and a pioneer in the field of testosterone therapy, testosterone supplementation leads to improved long-term blood sugar control and lower required insulin levels in diabetics. Almost every diabetic man he tests has low testosterone levels. Harvard researcher Eric Ding also has shown that low testosterone is associated with an increased risk of diabetes.[45] Although many traditional physicians may not be aware, many studies have demonstrated diabetic men supplementing with testosterone show significant improvement in hemoglobin A1c, insulin sensitivity, fasting blood glucose levels, blood lipid levels, and weight reduction (waist circumference).[46]

Dr. Lichten believes testosterone is an important treatment for aging diabetic men, as well as an effective preventive. It's his view that inexpensive testosterone supplementation is such an important and beneficial treatment for aging men, if it were used more widely, healthcare costs—including prescription drug use—would be reduced by up to 75%.

A competent physician will monitor testosterone levels, both total and free, before and after supplementation. Use of testosterone with those having a PSA (prostate specific antigen) over 2.0 is contraindicated. Therefore, before beginning supplementation, a PSA test is advisable. For a further discussion of this issue, see www.peenuts.com/learning_center_testosterone.html.

According to Dr. Lichten, the use of bio-identical hormones in aging individuals would make obsolete most prescription medications for cholesterol reduction, insomnia, menopause, migraine headaches, and osteoporosis. To learn more, read Dr. Lichten's book *The Diabetes Conspiracy*, and visit his website www.foundthecure.com.

■ *The Gabriel Cousins' Protocol*. Well-known holistic physician Dr. Gabriel Cousins is reversing/curing 90-95% of those with Type II diabetes and markedly improving Type I diabetics in two weeks to three months at his Tree of Life Rejuvenation Center in Patagonia, Arizona. By "cure," Cousins means "off of all diabetes-related medications and a Hemoglobin A1c of six or less." At the heart of his treatment is a low-fat, vegan, raw food diet consisting mainly of raw fruits and vegetables, seeds, sprouted seeds, and nuts. For diabetics taking medication, his protocol requires supervision by a health professional. However, those not on medication can practice the protocol on their own. For more information, read Dr. Cousins' 2008 book *There Is A Cure For Diabetes*, or watch the video *Simply Raw: Reversing Diabetes in 30 Days* at www.rawfor30days.com. Another informative book is Mike Adams' *How to Halt Diabetes in 25 Days*.

■ *Capsaicin*. It has been well accepted throughout the medical community that the beta cells of Type I diabetics are severely damaged or dead—hence the diminished production of insulin. A group of physicians at Toronto's Hospital for Sick Children seems to have found a surprising caveat to this long-held belief, and published their findings in the journal *Cell*.[47] Hans-Michael Dosch, M.D.,

Ph.D., had noted from earlier research the presence of a great number of nerves surrounding the insulin-producing islets. Suspecting a link between the two, Dosch and pain specialist Dr. Michael Slater injected capsaicin—the active ingredient in chili peppers—directly into the arteries feeding the pancreases of mice prone to having Type I diabetes in order to kill the nerves and eliminate their activity.

The results shocked even the doctors. Virtually overnight, the mice no longer had the disease. "I couldn't believe it," remarked Dr. Slater. "Mice with diabetes suddenly didn't have diabetes anymore."[48] The islet cells began producing normal levels of insulin almost immediately, and some of the mice continued to produce normal levels for up to four months following a single injection.

Apparently, in certain situations which may include many/most/all of Type I diabetes cases, the pain neurons surrounding the dormant but still living beta cells signal the pancreas to stop producing insulin. At least in mice, once the mis-signaling nerves are disrupted with capsaicin, the islets begin producing normally. The researchers further discovered their capsaicin treatment also curbed insulin resistance of Type II diabetes. The results of Dr. Dosch's mouse study have been confirmed by other laboratories. Since these studies, Dosch's level of confidence has grown regarding transferring the research to humans.

Human studies were to have begun in 2008. Although further investigation is necessary to confirm these results in humans, it is believed this discovery may lead to both a cure and prevention of diabetes. In the absence of this confirmational research, supplementing with capsaicin may be helpful in cases of both types of diabetes.

■ *Stem Cells*. Recent research confirms stem cell therapy is able to reverse Type I Diabetes in many persons for an average of two years. See **Stem Cells** in the **Index** and the Member's Area of *The Encyclopedia's* website.

■ *Seanol*. Discussed under **General Treatment Methods**, Seanol is effective in treating neuropathy as well as benefitting diabetes in other ways.

■ *Myskin® Bandages*.[49] Professors Sheila MacNeill and Robert Short of the University of Sheffield,

England, have developed a "living bandage" made from the patient's own skin cells. The product comprises a flexible polymer coated with a special nutrient polymeric film that supports the growth of skin cells. Upon this substrate are affixed new skin cells grown from the patient's own skin—usually taken as a small skin biopsy from the patient's thigh. The Myskin bandage is placed directly on the wound site, after which the bandage releases the cultured skin cells into the wound, prompting new layers of skin growth. According to CellTran, the British manufacturer, the cells delivered to the wound site have a high proliferative capacity and accelerate healing significantly. After the cells have migrated into the wound, the bandage is removed.

Myskin has been used successfully on diabetic foot ulcers and venous leg ulcers. In one clinical trial, Myskin led to a complete healing of six out of nine neuropathic foot ulcers, and a reduction in size of another. Large wounds require contiguous applications. To learn more, visit www.celltran.com, or call CellTran at +44(0)114 2220980.

■ ***Diabetic Lesion Massage.*** Several decades ago the American physician Dr. J.B. Dawson developed a simple, inexpensive treatment for diabetic lesions.[50] One of the main problems with diabetic ulcerations is the slowness of healing due to inadequate circulation. Dr. Dawson developed a technique of massaging the ulcers to help restore blood flow, and thus speed healing. Ulcerations typically develop in a circular pattern resembling a bull's eye of concentric circles. The center of the inner circle is the inflamed and injured tissue. Surrounding the outside of the red, innermost section is usually a pus-filled area surrounded by swollen tissue.

Dr. Dawson begins by massaging the red center of the ulceration once a day in a circular motion. To reduce the associated pain, he applies a mixture of a two percent lidocaine ointment and an antibacterial ointment, although raw honey can be substituted in place of the antibacterial. (A further discussion of honey is found in the section on **Burns**; lidocaine should be available from your local pharmacy.) After several days of massaging in this manner, the firmness of the massage is increased and the outer rim area is also massaged. With continued massaging, the bull's eye border begins to heal which, according to Dr. Dawson, is

the key to the healing process. Within a period of one week or longer, ulcerations as large as three centimeters can heal completely. It's best to leave the ulcers uncovered and exposed to the air, with only a thin coating of vegetable oil or honey.

■ ***Honey***. Discussed in the **Burns** section, certain medicinal honeys are effective treatments for lesions.

■ See also Fiber in the section **Nutrition: Detoxification and Deficiencies** and ***Del Immune V*** under **General Treatment Methods**.

CAUTION: Diabetes is a serious, potentially life-threatening illness. Do not discontinue insulin and/or pharmaceutical treatment in favor of any of the above remedies unless under a doctor's care.

DIARRHEA. See ***Irritable Bowel Syndrome*** and ***Indigestion***.

DRUG INTERACTIONS

Pharmaceutical medications often cause health problems—even death—when taken in combination with other drugs or certain nutritional/dietary supplements. On the other hand, they may interact beneficially with one another. Furthermore, drugs and supplements affect our nutritional status, both beneficially and detrimentally. Certain foods also interact both positively and negatively with drugs and supplements. A list of these interactions is so voluminous it can't reasonably be known or remembered by health professionals.

A unique software program now enables both health professionals and non-professionals to track all of these potential interactions with a few clicks of a mouse. Developed by Leo Galland, M.D., president of Applied Nutrition, Inc. and former professor at several esteemed universities, the software program is called The Drug Supplement Workshop. To use the software, one simply selects all of the drugs and supplements currently being taken using a drop down menu. By clicking the "Find Interactions" button, the computer program searches the extensive data base, creates an individualized profile on one page, and displays all of the critical information. At the website www.nutritionwork shop.com, the software can be purchased or used free of charge for five log-in sessions.

EMPHYSEMA

Oxygen is absorbed into the bloodstream through *alveoli,* tiny air sacs in the lungs. Emphysema, a type of *Chronic Obstructive Pulmonary Disease* (COPD), is a progressive disease of the lungs that occurs when the alveoli become damaged and do not allow spent air to properly exit the lungs or fresh air to be uptaken, causing a depletion of oxygen to all cells of the body—with many attendant health problems including fatigue, weight loss, and even death. Although emphysema usually affects older people as the result of long-term lung damage caused by smoking, it also affects people employed in industries such as mining.

■ *Retinoic Acid.* According to a recent article published in the *European Respiratory Journal,*[1] researchers at the Medical Research Council's Centre for Developmental Neurobiology at King's College London have been able to restore the function of the alveoli in mice by administering (an *all trans* form of) *retinoic acid,* a derivative of vitamin A which is also used to treat severe acne. This raises hope the treatment will also be effective in humans. In this study, the retinoic acid was delivered via an intraperitoneal (abdominal) injection. The researchers suggested that retinoic acid works by triggering key genes which enable the alveoli to recover.

■ *Nebulized Glutathione.* The level of the master antioxidant *glutathione* plays a role in several lung diseases. Healthy persons maintain a high concentration of glutathione in the lungs, while its deficiency is related to lung diseases including COPD, *acute respiratory distress syndrome* (ARDS), and neonatal lung damage. In the lungs of smokers, glutathione concentration in alveolar fluid is inversely associated with the extent of inflammation.

As reported in *Alternative Medicine Review,*[2] the inhalation of nebulized (vaporized liquid; aerosolized) reduced glutathione has been used very successfully in the treatment of COPD, including emphysema and chronic bronchitis. The study authors conclude that "this treatment be considered for wide-spread use."[3] Up to 600 mg twice daily has been shown safe. Nebulizers can be purchased in drugstores or on the internet. In the U.S., glutathione is available from compounding pharmacies with a prescription. To locate such a pharmacy, contact the Professional Compounding Centers of America at (800)331-2498 or (281)933-6948.

■ *Hydrogen Peroxide* (H_2O_2). Integrative physicians have reported significant improvements in emphysema patients treated with intravenous food-grade hydrogen peroxide. To locate a physician familiar with this technique, contact the American College for Advancement in Medicine at (800)532-3688 or visit www.acam.com.

Cigarette smokers will also be helped by supplementing with anti-inflammatory *curcuminoids,* an extract of the herb turmeric. Also, the flavonoids *quercetin* (onions) and naringenin (grapefruit juice; six ounces three times daily) deactivate the liver enzyme CYP1A2, which activates certain cancer-inducing chemicals present within cigarette smoke.

ERECTILE DYSFUNCTION. See *Erectile Dysfunction* under **Cardiovascular Disease**.

FATIGUE. See *Chronic Fatigue Syndrome*.

FEET

One unique solution to tired and aching feet also provides relief for plantar fasciitis, flat feet, heel pain, and foot-related knee and lower back pain. Developed by podiatrist Dr. Ivar Roth—for five years the Medical Director of the California ballet company Ballet Pacifica—the product is called FABS,® Foot Arch Band Support. To stabilize the feet some athletes, including dancers, resort to a time-consuming taping process. Although this is effective, it often requires two people: one person to supply the feet, while the other does the taping.

FABS is the convenient alternative. Consisting of arch support pads mounted on a thin band that fastens via Velcro strips, the appliance is lightweight and can be worn with most shoes, either over or under socks, or even barefoot for added support. Foot Arch Band Support can be ordered online by searching for "fabs feet." To view a video about a simple surgical technique which permanently corrects flat feet, visit www.wellnesshour.com. Enter "ivarroth" in the search box. Click on "Ivar E. Roth, D.P.M., M.P.H." For a discussion of a diversity of foot-related conditions, visit www.drroths.com/ndex.cfm?fuseaction=conditions.all.

FIBROMYALGIA. See *Chronic Fatigue Syndrome*.

FOOD POISONING

Food poisoning is caused either by toxins such as pesticides; poisonous foods such as poisonous mushrooms; or by pathogenic organisms such as viruses, bacteria, or parasites. Viruses known to cause food poisoning include hepatitis A, noroviruses, and rotaviruses. More commonly, food poisoning is caused by infection from bacteria such as *Campylobacter jejuni*, *Clostridium botulinum*, *Bacillus cereus*, *Escherichia coli*, *Salmonella enteriditis*, and *Shigella*. In the Western world, parasites seldom infect food.

Common medical practice is *not* to treat food poisoning with pharmaceutical antibiotics unless the infection is blood-borne, as they are ineffective against viruses and often produce potentially harmful, long-lasting effects when administered against food-borne bacteria. There are many effective, non-pharmaceutical antibiotics that do not cause these harmful effects. As soon as symptoms are noticed, a course of one or more of these natural antibiotics can be initiated in an effort to eliminate the source of the infection: grapefruit seed extract, olive leaf extract, sodium chlorite, and high-dose oral or intravenous vitamin C—a discussion of all of which can be located in the **Index**.

GALLBLADDER

The gallbladder is a membranous, muscular sac in which bile from the liver is stored. It is located at the upper-right quadrant of the stomach, just under the rib cage. The liver and gallbladder comprise a system that works together to aid in fat digestion. For various reasons—typically an unhealthful diet and sedentary lifestyle—the bile can thicken and clog up the bile ducts of the gallbladder in much the same way that an automobile's engine or septic tank becomes sludged up and functions inefficiently.

If persistent pain occurs, the standard medical approach is surgical removal of the gallbladder, one of the most commonly-performed operations in the U.S.—over 500,000 each year, with an additional 300,000 hospitalizations that don't result in surgery. Surgery can cause side-effects and should be avoided when possible, especially in older individuals whose health often degrades dramatically following the procedure.

■ ***Diet.*** A high-fiber diet including ample fruits and vegetables is important in both the prevention and elimination of gallstones. Certain foods are known to contribute to gallbladder symptoms. Ranging in the order of those having the most pronounced negative effects, these foods include eggs, pork, onions, fowl, milk, coffee, citrus, corn, beans, and nuts.[1] In studies performed as long ago as 1968, it was found that adding eggs to the diet caused a gallbladder attack among a high percentage of participants.[2]

■ ***Beets & Apple Juice.*** Eating copious amounts of beets and beet leaves, as well as drinking copious amounts of apple juice, is also recommended as a gallbladder de-sludger. Naturally, organically-grown foods and juices are recommended. Beets can be baked or broiled, much as baked potatoes are traditionally prepared. Beet leaves can be liquified in a blender and added to tomato juice to taste. Some alternative-minded physicians have reported that half a glass of red beet leaf juice (mixed with another juice to taste) per meal will stop a gallbladder attack in most persons in less than 48 hours.

■ ***A-F Betafood.*** A-F Betafood, a product of Standard Process, Inc.—founded in 1929 by the famous Dr. Royal Lee—is a natural beet-derived tonic that helps thin the bile and return it to its normal consistency. This product is highly recommended to those with gallbladder pain. To purchase this product, visit www.totalhealthvitamins.net. (Note: A-F Betafood contains animal byproducts.)

■ ***Gallbladder Flush.*** An alternative to surgery—where surgery isn't an absolute requirement—is what's known as a *gallbladder flush*, a simple, safe and painless procedure. There's a wealth of information about this technique available on the internet, and various practitioners use slightly different variations of the same technique. Although the procedure can be accomplished on one's own, it's probably best carried out under the supervision of a holistic medical professional such as a naturopathic physician. If you are having persistent pain, inquire about this simple technique with your alternative health professional. You can also learn more by searching online for "gallbladder flush."

The general technique follows. However, as mentioned, your medical practitioner may have his/her own variation which should be adhered to. Before bedtime, mix 4-6 ounces of extra-virgin olive oil with two cups of fresh lemon juice warmed to body temperature. Slowly ingest this before retiring. Typically, you will have a bowel movement the following morning before breakfast. Inspect the contents for small green balls. These are gallstones that have been flushed out by this process.

■ *Water.* Drinking 1-2 quarts of pure (not tap) water daily can be effective in both prevention and elimination of gallstones.

■ *Taurine.* The amino acid taurine, at 500-1,000 mg per day, also helps thin the bile.

■ *Lecithin.* Vegetable lecithin, at the level of 1,000 milligrams daily, helps prevent the formation of gallstones by dissolving cholesterol within the bile. See Lecithin under **Cardiovascular Disease**.

■ *Chanca Piedra .* The herb *chanca piedra*, translated as "stone breaker," is often effective in treating gallbladder disorders. See **Kidney Stones** for a description of its use.

■ *Milk Thistle.* Silymarin, the primary active component of milk thistle, has been shown to increase the solubility of bile dramatically.[3] The recommended dosage is 100 mg three times daily. See Silymarin under **Hepatitis.**

■ *Bile Salts.* Following gallbladder removal, supplementing with bile salts is often beneficial. See Gallbladder in the Member's Area of *The Encyclopedia's* website for a discussion of this subject.

GASTROESOPHOGEAL REFLUX DISEASE. See *Indigestion.*

GLAUCOMA

The optic nerve, also called the *second cranial nerve*, is a bundle of more than one million nerve fibers that transmit visual stimuli from the retina to the brain. *Glaucoma* is a disease of the eye that damages the optic nerve primarily as the result of in-creased pressure within the eye. When damage to the optic nerve exists, glaucoma is said to be present. However, an increase of pressure within the eye without associated nerve damage is not defined as glaucoma. Increased eye pressure does not necessarily lead to glaucoma, but is an indication of increased risk of the disease.[1] Today, about two million Americans have glaucoma.

A clear fluid continuously flows in and out of the *anterior chamber* located at the front of the eye, nourishing nearby tissue. The fluid exits the chamber through a spongy meshwork of tissues at the open angle juncture where the iris and cornea meet. The most common form—affecting about 90% of those with the disease—is *open-angle glaucoma*, where the fluid flows too slowly through the meshwork causing a fluid buildup and associated pressure within the eye. *Low-tension* or *normal-tension* glaucoma exists when the optic nerve becomes damaged even under relatively normal eye pressures.

Initially, those with open-angle glaucoma experience no symptoms and the disease goes undetected. As it progresses, peripheral vision becomes affected where objects at the sides of the visual field are lost, as if looking through a tunnel. Eventually, even straight-ahead vision may be lost.

The causes of glaucoma are often individual and multifactorial, and can include infection, injury, eye tumors, stress, dietary imbalances, eye surgery and an hereditary factor.[2] Pharmaceutical medications are high on the list of causative factors as well. According to Leonard Levine, Ph. D., the Physicians' Desk Reference (PDR) lists 94 prescription medications that can cause glaucoma, including antihypertensives (blood pressure medications such as digoxin), steroids (anti-inflammatory drugs such as Prednisone®), antidepressants, and antihistamines (anti-allergy drugs).[3]

Orthodox treatments for glaucoma include prescription eye drops and oral medications the goal of which is to decrease the interocular pressure. These medications are often accompanied by systemic side-effects including unexplained dizziness.[4] *Laser trabeculoplasty surgery* may offer temporary relief by draining fluid from the eye. Conventional surgery, often performed when other treatments have failed, forms a new opening for fluid to be released. According to the National Institutes of Health, conventional surgery is 60-80%

effective in reducing intraocular pressure, but can cause serious side-effects including a buildup of fluid at the back of the eye; cataracts; corneal problems; a decrease in visual acuity; and inflammation and infection within the eye.[5] Due to the extraordinarily delicate visual mechanisms, however, surgical complications are common, and even "successful" surgeries can alter the subtle functions of a healthy eye.[6] Other, more natural therapies are available.

■ *Ginkgo biloba*. The Ginkgo tree is one of the oldest trees known to man, having grown on Earth for over 50 million years. Of the various species, only the *Ginkgo biloba* tree survives to this day. The extract of the *Ginkgo biloba* leaf is the most widely sold phyto- (plant) medicine in Europe, and one of the best-selling herbal medicines in the U.S. The European designation of the standardized product is EGb761, while in the U.S. the herb is sold as a dietary supplement. Standardized Ginkgo contains 24% ginkgo flavonoid glycosides, 6% terpene lactones, and not more than 5 ppm ginkgolic acids. Ginkgold,® Ginkoba,® and Ginkai® are three standardized products that have been used in clinical trials. *Ginkgo biloba* has been the subject of more than 100 clinical studies, mostly European.

Professor and Chief of Glaucoma Treatment at the New York Eye and Ear Infirmary, Dr. Robert Ritch has stated that *Ginkgo biloba* extract (GBE) might interrupt some of the suspected causes of nerve damage which could result in vision loss in people with glaucoma. It is proposed that GBE acts by increasing ocular blood flow and boosting the immune system.[7]

Over the past 20 years, upward of two billion individual doses of Ginkgo have been sold with only minor side-effects noted, the most significant being the potential problem of blood thinning. As such, *Ginkgo biloba* should not be used in conjunction with other blood thinning agents such as aspirin, warfarin (Coumadin®), and blood-thinning herbs such as dong Quai, feverfew, garlic, ginseng, and red clover. To prevent the possibility of postoperative bleeding, discontinue use one week before surgery. Standardized Ginkgo is available in health food stores in the U.S., and on the internet.

■ *Vitamin C*. Many studies have shown that near-normal pressure levels can be achieved by supplementing with high levels of vitamin C.[8] At the dosage of 500 mg per kilogram (2.2 lb) body weight daily, intraocular pressure is decreased significantly. A person weighing 150 pounds, for example, would take about 34 grams per day to achieve the results obtained in the studies. (150 lb ÷ 2.2 = 68 X .5 gm = 34 gm.) Pressure reduction is maintained as long as supplementation is continued. Intravenous use of vitamin C causes a more rapid initial reduction of eye pressure.

■ *Diet*. Nutrition is a major factor in maintaining good vision. Glaucoma, cataracts, and macular degeneration are linked to nutritional deficiencies.[9] Foods that are implicated in eye disease and vision impairment include alcohol, coffee, dairy products, eggs, fats, fried foods, processed foods, sugar, and tobacco.[10] A diet including many unrefined, natural foods—along with proper nutritional supplements—offers protection against most eye ailments. For more information about specific eye nutrients, see **Cataracts** and **Macular Degeneration**. See also **Nutrition: Detoxification and Deficiencies** under **General Treatment Methods**.

■ *Optic Nerve Regeneration*. For those who have had optic nerve damage, there is hope on the horizon. Although regeneration of a damaged optic nerve is not presently possible, recent animal studies indicate this possibility is not far away. By adding growth factors, stimulating natural growth factors (such as stem cells), and eliminating substances that prevent regeneration, within the next few years researchers hope to be able to restore function to a damaged optic nerve.[11] These techniques have already shown some success in animals.

GOUT. See *Arthritis*.

GRIEF. See Eye-Movement Desensitization and Reprocessing (EMDR) under *Stress*.

GULF WAR SYNDROME
The 1990 100-hour ground war known as Operation Desert Storm incurred only 147 KIA (killed in action) and 457 WIA (wounded in action). Although at first blush these figures are astoundingly low, most are unaware of the rest of the story. In addition to the 147 direct battlefield fatalities, since

the end of Desert Storm an additional 8,000 plus Gulf War veterans have died, over 400,000 of the 697,000 who deployed have some type of medical problem, and over 200,000 vets have filed claims for medical and compensation benefits, according to an April 2002 report by the Department of Veterans Affairs.[1] These numbers are very high, and some researchers maintain they are attributable at least in part to infective pathogens believed to be a cause of various illnesses collectively labeled Gulf War Syndrome. The recent Iraq war will only swell the number of those affected.

Many people suffering from Gulf War Syndrome have been found to have hypercoagulation of the blood,[2] as discussed under **Chronic Fatigue Syndrome/Fibromyalgia**. Similar to CFS and FM, anticoagulation therapy is the course of treatment. Also, about 50% of the sufferers of Gulf War Syndrome test positive for the infective pathogen *Mycoplasma fermentans incognitus*, a microbe whose genetic sequence appears to have been altered by human manipulation—probably the result of biowarfare genetic engineering.[3]

This, at any rate, is the conclusion of Dr. Garth Nicolson, currently the Chief Scientific Officer and Research Professor at the Institute for Molecular Medicine in Huntington Beach, California (www.immed.org), and the editor of two respected medical journals, *Clinical & Experimental Metastasis* and the *Journal of Cellular Biochemistry*. Dr. Nicolson is formerly Professor and Chairman of the Department of Tumor Biology at the University of Texas, M.D. Anderson Cancer Center, Houston, Texas. He was also a Professor of Internal Medicine, Pathology and Laboratory Medicine at the University of Texas Medical School, and has over 550 scientific and medical papers to his credit.

[Interestingly, it has been pointed out by various researchers that *Mycoplasma fermentans incognitus* is the subject of U.S. Patent 5,242,820, "Pathogenic Mycoplasma." Dr. Shyh-Ching Lo, working under a grant from the U.S. Department of the Army in the late 1980s, isolated from the tissues of AIDS patients the biologically pure mycoplasma denoted *Mycoplasma fermentans incognitus* (American Tissue Culture Collection ATCC 53949). The significance of this remains unclear.]

Dr. Nicolson has found that antibiotic treatment of *Mycoplasma fermentans incognitus* is the treatment of choice—particularly with the antibiotic *doxycycline*. To learn more about the antibiotic treatment of this pathogen, do a key word search for "garth nicolson mycoplasma." Another good resource is www.gulfwarvets.com. To be tested for the presence of mycoplasma, contact Medical Diagnostic Laboratories at (877)269-0090; www.medlab.com. See also **Sodium Chlorite** and **Del Immune V** under **General Treatment Methods**.

It is now known that *squalene*, an adjuvant contained in the military's mandatory anthrax vaccination, is also a contributing factor to the Gulf War Syndrome.

HAIR LOSS (Alopecia)

Although hair loss is enough to make balding men and women exclaim, "I could just die," no one has ever lost their life as the result of baldness. Especially for contemporary Western men (*and* men from many cultures throughout history), having a full head of hair is often related to self esteem and sexual prowess. In most cases hair loss, referred to as *alopecia*, is medically insignificant even though it is often quite psychologically significant.

There are several hypotheses regarding the cause(s) of hair loss. Insufficient blood supply to the scalp is one contributing factor. Excess sebum, a fatty lubricant substance secreted by the sabeceous glands of the skin, can clog up scalp conduits and cause malnutrition of the hair and hair follicle. The presence of excessive 5a-**dih**ydrotestosterone (DHT, the result of testosterone being transformed by the enzyme 5 alpha-reductase) is related to the shrinking of the hair follicle. Poor nutrition also is recognized as being a contributing factor.

Secondary alopecia can develop as the result of external factors such as chemotherapy. A host of prescription medications can contribute to the ailment, including various (but not all) drugs within the following categories: anabolic steroids, antiarthritics, anticoagulants, anticonvulsants, antidepressants, antihypertensives, antithyroid agents, and blood thinners.[1] There is no doubt a genetic component—a baldness gene—which leads to roughly 50% of men in the industrialized Western world to develop male pattern baldness (MPB), *alopecia androgenetica* (also called *alopecia hereditaria*). Female alopecia androgenetica is referred to as *female pattern baldness* (FPB).

The underlying cause of at least several types of hair loss is an autoimmune attack on the hair follicle, an explanation put forth by many researchers of considerable repute, including scientists at the Ronald O. Perelman Department of Dermatology at the New York University Medical Center, and the St. John's Institute of Dermatology at the St. Thomas' Hospital in London.[2] According to this belief, the immune system identifies "self" as "non-self," and launches an attack on various hair structures. Especially in *alopecia areata*, where there are well-defined round or oval bald patches on the scalp or other areas of the body, autoimmunity is believed to play a significant role.[3]

In both the past and present there have been many lotions, potions, and devices designed to treat alopecia—including wigs, wires, rugs, and plugs—most delivering less than satisfactory results. Perhaps the best known of these is minoxidil (Rogaine®), a topical treatment which the U.S. FDA approved for use in 1998. (The heavily marketed Avacor® lotion contains minoxidil.)

About 30% of Rogaine users grow mostly immature "baby hair"[4]—a result which, despite the advertising claims, is unsatisfactory for many. Rogaine must be used on a regular basis for the remainder of one's life to maintain any new regrowth that may have occurred. If treatments are terminated, any regrown hair is lost. Side-effects include irritation, itch, dermatitis, hives, swelling, and sensitivity.[5]

Taken orally, the synthetic compound *finasteride* (Propecia®, Proscar®) is an inhibitor of Type II 5a-reductase, the enzyme that converts testosterone into DHT. About 60% of men studied were at least somewhat successful using finasteride. Less than 2% had sexual side-effects including reduced sex drive; difficulty achieving and maintaining an erection; a decreased volume of semen; headaches; rash; abdominal pain; back pain; and breast enlargement and tenderness.[6] In the U.S., finasteride was approved in 1997 for use only by men.

Because over 50% of all men in the Western world are afflicted with alopecia, there is a huge market for hair loss medications/devices. Consequently, there is no dearth of products in the marketplace. While most bring more hype than hair, there are a few products that stand out because they have withstood the scrutiny of formal clinical trials, and have been shown to offer true value to the consumer.

■ ***Thymu-Skin.***® Of all the anti-alopecia formulas on the market, Thymu-Skin is one of the most thoroughly researched, effective hair regrowth product available today. It was jointly developed during the late 1980s and early 1990s by a group of nine well-respected German dermatologists and other specialists, including Professor Manfred Hagedorn, M.D., Medical Director, Dermatology Department of the Municipal Clinics of Darmstadt, Germany, and Chief of the Dermatology Department at the University of Frankfurt; Professor Benno Runnebaum, Medical Director of the Department of Gynecology and Endocrinology at the University of Heidelberg, Germany; and Professor Thomas Rabe, M.D., of the Department of Gynecology and Endocrinology at the University of Heidelberg, Germany. Thymu-Skin has been the subject of at least eight clinical trials at university medical centers throughout Germany and Austria.

Thymu-Skin is a topically-applied formula consisting of several ingredients. Initially, the product's main active ingredient was *thymus protein* extracted from young calves. The protein consisted essentially of short-chain peptides having molecular weights ranging from 300-1,000 daltons. Currently, a nature-identical *synthetic* analog (duplicate) of calf thymus is used which, according to the manufacturer, is far superior to the original animal-sourced product in both its consistency of ingredients and performance. Other ingredients include vitamins, minerals, enzymes, and free amino acids which become intermixed with the thymus extract.

In cases of both alopecia areata and alopecia androgenetica, Thymu-Skin successfully stops hair loss, and often regrows new hair, particularly in individuals who have been bald for less than five years. After balding has progressed past this point, most of the hair roots are no longer living, significantly decreasing the possibility of any further hair regrowth. Although the specific modes of action are not totally understood, Thymu-Skin functions by boosting the user's overall immunity. It also neutralizes the autoimmune attacks on hair follicles.[7] (See ***Thymic Protein A*** under **General Treatment Methods** for a more thorough discussion of the thymus gland and its relation to the immune system.)

Clinical studies on Thymu-Skin have shown that in about 95% of women and 70% of men with pattern baldness—which accounts for over 90% of baldness cases—hair loss stops. Depending upon many factors including how long a person has been balding and loss of hair due to advanced age, hair regrowth can range from no growth at all on the one hand, to growth of a full head of hair.[8] In cases of hair loss due to chemotherapy, the hair retention success rate is nearly 95% compared to a 78% success rate of the placebo group (who also retained their hair), representing a 16% reduced frequency of hair loss compared to the control group.[9]

Of the various hair loss products currently available, Thymu-Skin is likely the most effective. It appears to be the most thoroughly researched of the products discussed. Even significant hair regrowth is not unusual when using this product for six months to one year. To learn more about Thymu-Skin, read Dr. Morton Walker's 1998 book *Bald No More*, or visit www.biotechneusa.com.

Of the several products available in the Thymu-Skin product line, the Shampoo and Hair Treatment Revitalizer are the two essential products—the ones that were used in the clinical trials. The other products include a Conditioner Creme Rinse, Gel, and Hair Mask. All products are imported from Mannheim, Germany and are distributed throughout North America and some other countries by Biotechne Complex, Inc. of Gainesville, Georgia, (800)214-8631, (770)297-9811, www.biotechne usa.com.

■ **Curetage.**® Curetage is a topically-applied, all-natural product line (shampoo, conditioner, and scalp treatment) consisting of 15 herbs and six vitamins. The herbs are aloe vera, balm mint, buckthorn, burdock, cayenne, chamomile, comfrey, ginger, hops, horsetail, jojoba, nettles, rosemary, sage, saw palmetto, thyme, yarrow, and yucca. The six vitamins are A, C, D, E, F, and H. According to the manufacturer, excessive hair loss stops within two to three weeks and new hair growth can begin within 8-12 weeks.

Although there have been some small clinical studies using Curetage, they don't appear to have been published in peer-reviewed journals. One small study was done at Emory University. Our main reason for including this product is that it is recommended by the respected Dr. Julian Whitaker.

To learn more about Curetage, manufactured by Age Less Products of Albemarle, NC, visit www.curetage.com. Orders can be placed from their web site or by calling (800)273-4246.

■ **ElectroTrichoGenesis.**® A patent held by the Vancouver, BC company Current Technology Corporation protects the technology that underlies the ElectroTrichoGenesis electrical stimulation device. The person receiving treatment sits with the upper portion of the head inside an apparatus resembling a salon-style hair dryer. Treatments are administered once per week, with each treatment lasting 12 minutes. The ElectroTrichoGenesis equipment demonstrates this electromagnetic technology is capable of both stopping hair loss and regrowing new hair, with no known side-effects.

Two peer-reviewed published studies support the efficacy of this technology. There have been articles on the device in *Financial World*, the *Mexico City Times*, and in the *Rochester Democrat and Chronicle*. In one of the articles published in 1990 in the *International Journal of Dermatology*,[10] 30 men aged 19-49 experiencing male pattern baldness received one treatment per week for 36 weeks. At the termination of the study, 83.3% of the treated participants showed increased hair growth, and 96.7% experienced either increased growth or no further loss.

ElectroTrichoGenesis treatment is available in many countries throughout the world, including Australia, Canada, Mexico, New Zealand, and South Korea. It is not available in the U.S. For more information, call Current Technology Corporation at (800)661-4247, (604)684-2727, or visit www. hairsite.com/alt-etg.htm.

■ **Stem Cell Therapy.** One solution that's close on the horizon is growing new hair using stem cells. Stem cells are the master cells of the body. They are undifferentiated cells that give rise to the body's many varieties of specialized (differentiated) cells. They are, in effect, the precursors of specialized cells. The unique function of stem cells is that they can grow into virtually any other type of cell, as needed. It has been shown that stem cell therapy has successfully grown new heart tissue, new photosensitive light receptor cells in the retina of the eye, and even new teeth. It is only a matter of time until hair will be grown using either stem cell implantation or by somehow coaxing "on-site" stem cells to grow into hair follicles.

■ *Abrasion & Wound Healing*. While adult mammals—including humans—are efficient at repairing most types of bodily injury, unlike some other animals such as salamanders and newts, they lack the ability to regenerate lost parts, such as limbs. Until recently, it was also not believed possible to regenerate hair follicles. Researchers at the University of Pennsylvania-Philadelphia have now proved that assumption incorrect. As published in 2007 in the journal *Nature*,[11] the technique focuses on reawakening/reactivating dormant genes used during embryonic development.

Half a century ago in an experiment on rabbits, it was claimed that wounding (abrading) of the skin causes regeneration of hair follicles—but the research was viewed as unconvincing and was discounted. This new research demonstrates the effect is indeed real, and results from a molecular signal related to the protein "wnt." Following wounding of the skin, the signal regenerates hair follicles. By increasing wnt, in fact, the researchers found they could not only regenerate the follicles, but double their number. According to lead researcher Dr. George Cotsarelis, wound healing triggers an embryonic state in the skin which makes it receptive to receiving instructions from wnt proteins. It was found that even minor wounding also results in the mobilization of follicle stem cells to generate daughter cells that quickly move into the wound area.

Previous to this research, it was believed the number of hair follicles is set at birth, and would only decrease thereafter. Hair follicle development, it was believed, was limited to early developmental processes in the embryo. It is now known that under the conditions peculiar to the wound healing environment, hair follicles can be regenerated from apparently unremarkable cells of the healing skin and its underlying dermis. To date, the hair regrown by this technique did not have pigment.

■ *Additional Products*. There are so many additional hair loss products on the market it's difficult to sort the helpful from the hypefull. This is true primarily because most of these products are backed by very little research, even though they are often accompanied by stellar promises and glowing testimonials, not to mention big advertising dollars. Even though many of the manufacturers claim their products are backed by clinical studies, there is a lack of research on most of these products appearing in reputable scientific journals—unlike other products such as Thymu-Skin.

Some other products you may want to investigate include the following. To learn more about any of them, do a key word search for its name: Cell-wave Therapy, Fabio 101,® HairGenesis,® Hair Max LaserComb,® Loesch Laboratory, Luxor of Paris,® New Generation,® Nisim,® Nioxin,® Pelon Hair Growth,® Procerin,® Shen Min,® and Zhang-Guang 101.® For more hairy ideas, visit www.regrowth.com.

HEADACHES. See *Migraines*.

HEART ATTACKS. See *Cardiovascular Disease*.

HEARTBURN. See *Indigestion*.

HEMORRHOIDS (Piles)

Varicose veins are knotted, abnormally-swollen blood vessels close to the skin's surface. Any vein can become varicose, but the most commonly affected are superficial veins in the legs and feet. When veins in and around the rectal area become varicose, they are called hemorrhoids.

■ *Cryotherapy*. Cryotherapy is the therapeutic use of cold temperatures applied to the body. It is standard medical practice to use cryotherapy in the treatment of inflammatory conditions due to its vaso-constrictive properties. Cold temperatures applied to the body are known to decrease edema (swelling caused by excess accumulation of fluid) and hemorrhaging. Cold also produces analgesia, the reduction of pain.

With these facts in mind, Cryotherapy Pain Relief Products of Pembroke Pines, Florida has developed a device for the natural, non-invasive, drug-free treatment for hemorrhoids. Called Anuice,® the device is a small, probe-type instrument which is inserted inside the rectum. It is constructed of medical-grade plactic filled with a special coolant. After the device is placed in the freezer and the coolant becomes frozen, it then can be inserted into the rectum with the aid of a water-based lubricant supplied with the product. Due to the design of Anuice (somewhat T-shaped), its surface area contacts the skin inside and outside of the orifice, thereby coming in contact with both internal and external hemorrhoidal tissues wherever present. Different configurations of the applicator are possible so that the patient is able to select the one that is most personally effective. The patented device provides four applicators in one unit.

Anuice stays cold for 5-8 minutes, and can be cleaned and reused as needed. The manufacturer suggests the device be used as often as possible to obtain the fastest relief from pain, itching, inflammation, burning and bleeding. However, relief is often provided with the initial application. Four to five applications per day with a single applicator (5-8 minutes each with one applicator), or two to three applications per day using two applicators (used consecutively; 10-16 minutes each session) for a five day period is sufficient to reduce inflammation in most cases, according to the manufacturer. The device is also recommended for promoting post-surgical healing. Anuice produces no harmful side-effects. To learn more about Anuice or to place an order, visit www.anuice.com, or call (866)750-3230.

■ See also *Varicose Veins,* the Rectal/Vaginal Heater under *Prostate,* and the **Index.**

HEPATITIS

Any inflammation (itis) of the liver (hepa) is referred to as hepatitis. Its can be caused by a viral pathogen, or due to other factors including excessive alcohol consumption; various pharmaceutical medications such as acetaminophen (Tylenol®); environmental toxins such as inhaling or otherwise ingesting toxic chemicals; or autoimmune disorders. To date, at least seven viral strains have been identified: A, B, C, D, E, F, and G. Only these viral forms of hepatitis can be spread from person to person.

Hepatitis A (HAV) is primarily acquired through fecal contamination of food or water, although it also can be acquired through poor hygiene or by eating shellfish harvested from contaminated waters. HAV is not a blood-borne disease. Over 30% of Americans are estimated to have been infected with HAV at some point during their lifetimes. Ten to 40 days after exposure, flu-like symptoms generally develop, including aches, low-grade fever, and mild abdominal pain. Most of those infected completely recover on their own, even without treatment. Once recovered, a life-long immunity to the disease is developed.[1] Rarely, severe HAV infections may lead to liver failure and the need for transplantation. Good hygiene reduces the risk of contracting HAV, such as hand washing with soap and warm water after using the toilet or changing diapers. A vaccination is available to protect against acquiring HAV.

According to the U.S. Centers for Disease Control, about 1.25 million Americans are infected with hepatitis B (HBV). This strain of the virus can be transmitted through contaminated blood or blood products, sexual contact, or from mother to child during pregnancy or childbirth. Although about 30% of those with HBV have no symptoms, those who do experience flu-like symptoms such as aches, low-grade fever, and mild abdominal pain. Most individuals with a healthy immune system recover from HBV within six months, although if left untreated up to 10% develop chronic (long-term) infection which may lead to serious complications such as cirrhosis, liver cancer, or liver failure.[2] Those infected may experience fatigue, malaise, jaundice, or no symptoms at all. The CDC is currently supporting mandatory childhood HBV vaccinations. Diagnosis of hepatitis is made by the ELISA III (Enzyme Linked Immunosorbant Assay) or the RIBA (Recombinent Immunoblot Assay) tests, both of which measure antibodies to the virus. The Polymerase Chain Reaction (PCR) test offers a more accurate diagnosis, as it is a direct measure of viral load.

The most common chronic blood-borne disease in the U.S. is hepatitis C (HCV), with 4-5 million Americans infected, up to nearly a quarter million new U.S. cases annually, and 8,000-10,000 Americans succumbing to the disease each year, according to the CDC.[3] World wide, some 200 million people are infected, with up to 15 million cases in Western Europe and an even higher prevalence in Eastern Europe.[4] The disease is called a "silent epidemic" because most people with HCV have no symptoms for 10-20 years following infection. If symptoms manifest, they usually take the form of abdominal discomfort, extreme tiredness and weakness, jaundice, loss of appetite, unexplained weight loss, and vomiting/nausea. HCV is one of the most common causes of liver transplants in the U.S. It can be contracted from many sources including accidental needle sticks; blood transfusions before 1992 (after which more stringent blood screening was enforced); organ transplants; contaminated needles from recreational drug use; tattoos or body piercings; and unprotected sex.

Unlike hepatitis A and B, HCV is not easily cleared from the body, and 80% of those who contract it progress to the chronic stage of the disease where it may continue its liver damage for 10-30 years. Untreated, HCV can result in cirrhosis, liver cancer, liver failure, and death.

The main orthodox medical treatment for hepatitis C is a 24-48 month course of one or a combination of pharmaceutical drugs. The most commonly used drugs include (synthetic, injectable) interferon (interferon alfa-2b or peginterferon alfa-2b) and ribavirin (Copegus® and Rebetal®). Best results are obtained by taking a combination (Pegylated Combo) of pegylated interferon and ribavirin. According to the orthodox view, this combination may offer the only hope of eliminating the hepatitis virus from the body, although the results of this therapy are inconsistent. Some patients are in remission for long periods, while others regularly relapse. Unfortunately, the side-effects of these medicines are considerable.

The side-effects of synthetic interferon include difficulty breathing; chest pain; depression and/or suicidal behavior; fatigue; headaches; high fever; muscle pain; new or worsening mental health problems; nausea; unusual bleeding or bruising; vision changes; and worsening psoriasis.[5] Some of the more common side-effects of ribavirin include acid or sour stomach; belching; birth defects and/or death of an unborn child; discouragement; dizziness; feeling sad or empty; feeling unusually cold; heartburn; indigestion; irritability; itching skin; lack

of appetite; loss of interest or pleasure; lack or loss of strength; shivering; stomach discomfort, upset, or pain; tiredness; trouble concentrating; and trouble sleeping. Less common side-effects include change in taste; cough; crying; depersonalization; difficulty in moving; dysphoria; euphoria; fatigue; fever; gastrointestinal effects; headache; insomnia; joint pain; mental depression; muscle aching or cramping; muscle pains or stiffness ; nervousness; pain or tenderness around eyes and cheekbones; paranoia; quick to react or overreact emotionally; rapidly changing moods; rash; shortness of breath; stuffy or runny nose; swollen joints; and vomiting.[6]

A number of less toxic treatments are useful in helping hepatitis patients, some of the most effective of which include the following:

■ **_Vitamin C_**. Robert Cathcart III, M.D. was a pioneer in vitamin C research and treatment protocols. He reported vitamin C is useful in treating all forms of both acute and chronic hepatitis, but is especially useful in acute cases.[7] Cathcart explained that in severe cases vitamin C should be taken intravenously in large doses, from 40 gm to over 150 gm daily. Alternatively, high oral intake is often useful. High doses help quench the proliferation of free radicals produced by hepatitis.

According to Cathcart, hepatitis "is one of the easiest diseases for ascorbic acid [vitamin C] to cure."[8] He reported that in cases of acute hepatitis, significant improvement can be seen in 2-4 days, and that jaundice clears in about six days.[9] One study[10] showed that taking more that 1.5 gm per day offers significant protection from acquiring hepatitis B during hospitalization. For more information on the benefits of vitamin C in treating hepatitis, visit www.doctoryourself.com/hepatitis.html.

■ **_Thymic Protein A_**. Since the discovery of the importance of the thymus to proper immune functioning, many attempts have been made to produce thymus extracts to boost the immune capability. These preparations are generally whole animal thymus which is ground, dried, strained, and prepared as a liquid or in capsules. Many such preparations have been only marginally successful because they contain only fragments of the total complex of molecules responsible for the many critical immune functions governed by the thymus.

One product that has achieved success[11] in the treatment both acute and chronic hepatitis is Immune Strong WellnessBooster Plus,® another product from Enzymatic Therapy. This product includes a proprietary thymus polypeptide fraction/glandular complex consisting of thymus polypeptide fractions, freeze-dried spleen extract, thymus extract, freeze-dried lymphatic extract, bromelain, trypsin, and papain. It is available in health food stores and on the internet. For those who are concerned about possible Mad Cow (bovine spongiforn encephalopathy) contamination through the use of animal extracts, another thymus product would appear to all but eliminate that possibility.

In the early 1980s, after eight years of intensive research, immunologist Terry Beardsley, Ph. D., was able to isolate the thymus' master molecule that produces the mixture of regulatory proteins from the thymus. Rather than extracted fragments of molecules, Beardsley isolated a substance which he named Thymic Protein A (TPA), a complete protein comprising a 500 amino acid chain. Both the isolation and manufacturing processes are protected by U.S. patent 5,616,554: "Immune-enhancing Agent for Therapeutic Use in Immunocompromised Hosts." By supplementing with Thymic Protein A, one is provided with a continuous source of pure, native biomolecules identical to those produced by an optimally-functioning thymus gland.

Thymic Protein A is not derived from live animals, but is grown in cell cultures in only one laboratory in the world. The growth process was initially seeded from a single U.S. calf raised specifically for this purpose. All other proteins and fragments are filtered out, leaving only highly-purified TPA. As such, its potential to contain infective contaminants (including prions; see **Mad Cow Disease**) is virtually nonexistent, which cannot easily be said about other thymic extracts. One packet of product contains four micrograms (12 trillion active molecules) of freeze-dried TPA in a base of maltodextrin. The product is taken sublingually for both prevention and treatment. No adverse side-effects have ever been reported.

TPA is sold as ProBoost [(877)776-8496; www.proboostmed.com], and T-Cellerate [(800) 422-5518; www.theharmonyco.com]. To learn more about Thymic Protein A, see **Thymic Protein A** under **General Treatment Methods**.

■ **Intravenous Glutathione.** Glutathione is the liver's primary antioxidant. Because free radical pathology plays a significant role in tissue damage caused by hepatitis, glutathione replenishment is helpful in maintaining and increasing healthy liver function. More information about glutathione's role in maintaining a healthy liver is available in the section **Nutrition: Detoxification & Deficiencies**, under **General Treatment Methods**.

■ **Silymarin.** Also known as St. Mary's Thistle, Holy Thistle, and Blessed Thistle, the Milk Thistle plant has been used for over 2,000 years in the treatment of liver dysfunction. Milk Thistle is known botanically as *Silybum marianum*, and in the 1960s German researchers found it contains a group of active constituents including silybinin, isosilybinin, silychristin, and silydianin. Collectively, this group of active ingredients is called *silymarin*, and its source is primarily from the seeds of the plant. Many studies have shown that silymarin is effective in the treatment of both acute and chronic viral and non-viral (alcohol, chemotherapy, prescription drugs, etc.) induced hepatitis, cirrhosis, and fatty infiltration of the liver.[12] Even the extreme liver toxicant of the poisonous Deathcap mushroom, *Amanita phalloides*, can be neutralized by an injection of silymarin.[13]

Silymarin works in several ways[14] in support of maintaining normal, healthy liver function. It blocks the absorption of toxins into the liver cells by beneficially altering liver cell membrane structure. It increases the intracellular concentration of glutathione, one of the body's master antioxidants and the primary antioxidant of the liver. It also is a stand-alone antioxidant of considerable potency. Milk Thistle has been shown to stimulate the production of new liver cells.

One of the most effective Milk Thistle products is Super Milk Thistle, manufactured by Enzymatic Therapy. Several studies have shown that by binding silymarin to *phosphytidylcholine*, a principal constituent of soy lecithin, improved absorption and therapeutic action are achieved.[15] Super Milk Thistle is available in health food stores and can be purchased on the internet.

■ **_Selenium._** The mineral selenium, in appropriate dosages, produces many health benefits in the body. It is an antioxidant that helps combat free radicals, and has been shown to inhibit the replication of the hepatitis C virus, thus reducing total viral load.[16] Well-known holistic practitioner Dr. Julian Whitaker recommends selenium at 400 mcg daily.

■ **_Lipoic Acid._** Because of the wide range of benefits it offers, lipoic acid is sometimes called the "universal" antioxidant. It is a broad-spectrum antioxidant that functions in both lipid (fat) and aqueous (watery) environments. Lipoic acid is a powerful antioxidant with a potent electron-donating capacity that fights free radicals. Supplementing with lipoic acid has been shown to be an effective means of glutathione replenishment. When taken orally, it has been shown to raise glutathione levels in HIV patients, while being extremely safe and well tolerated.[17] R-lipoic acid is the most bioavailable and effective form of this substance.

Las Cruces, New Mexico physician Burton Berkson, M.D., Ph.D., has reported astounding success in treating hepatitis C with the three-antioxidant combination alpha lipoic acid (600 mg daily in two divided doses), silymarin (900 mg dialy in three divided doses), and selenomethionine (400 mcg in two divided doses). To learn more, visit http://curezone.com/forum/fm.asp?i=897753.

■ See Blood Electrification under **_Herpes_**, and **_Del Immune V_**, **_Insulin Potentiation Therapy_**, **_Olive Leaf Extract_**, **_Photoluminescence_**, and **_Sodium Chlorite_** under **General Treatment Methods**.

■ See also **_Cirrhosis_**, and the Member's Area of *The Encyclopedia's* website.

HERPES

Man's infection with the herpes virus is as old as recorded history. The word "herpes" is derived from the Greek word *herpein*, which means "to creep" or "to crawl." The ancient Greeks spoke this word themselves, as the disease was common within their culture over 2,500 years ago. More than eighty different strains of the virus have now been identified, of which only eight are believed to infect humans. The most common and well-known of these are Herpes Simplex virus 1 (HSV-1) and Herpes Simplex virus 2 (HSV-2), both of which appear identical when viewed under a microscope (but can be identified by laboratory processes), and either of which can infect the genitals *or* other areas such as the mouth. HSV-1 is usually associated with *cold sores* or *fever blisters*, and HSV-2 is typically associated with infection of the genitals. Chickenpox and shingles are caused by Herpes zoster, another well-known herpes virus.

From 60-90% of those infected with genital herpes have recurrent outbreaks, while 20-40% of cold sore sufferers have recurrences.[1] It is estimated that up to 99% of the adult population of Western countries may be infected with at least one variety of herpes. Because the herpes virus sequesters itself in the spinal ganglia, unfortunately it is likely it can't be eliminated from the body with any method known to current-day medicine. Therefore, any treatments are merely temporary and palliative, and are probably unable to root out the basic cause of the symptoms. That being said, the first treatment method discussed, Blood Electrification & Magnetic Pulsing, has at least the potential to rid the body of the herpes virus.

The pharmaceutical approach to the treatment of herpes is with acyclovir (Zorivax®), a drug that often takes three to seven days to become active. Acyclovir is commonly prescribed to help manage the symptoms of herpes outbreaks. Several strains of the virus are now acyclovir resistant, and prolonged use of the drug may encourage the proliferation of additional drug-resistant strains of herpes.[2] Also, the use of acyclovir may be accompanied by side effects including diarrhea, headaches, nausea, seizures, vomiting, and more seriously, coma, kidney and liver damage.

The following methods offer a safer and more sensible approach to herpes treatment.

■ **_Blood Electrification & Magnetic Pulsing._** This method of treatment is not backed by a large amount of published clinical research data. It is, on the other hand, backed by a United States patent issued to a physician from a prestigious university. This by itself does not validate the method as effective; however, it does indicate a considerable amount of research was conducted by the physician and his team of researchers in preparation for filing the patent application.

Furthermore, the U.S. Patent and Trademark Office (USPTO) is obliged to carefully review the private research data submitted along with the application provided by the medical researchers as documentation of their claims. If in the process of examination the Patent Office has unresolvable, unanswered questions about the data—questioning their accuracy or validity—the patent is not granted, i.e, it is not allowed to issue. When a patent issues, it is assumed the data are authentic, accurate and believable.

Additionally, there is a considerable amount of anecdotal evidence which helps substantiate this technique. Nevertheless, this type of information is considerably less rigorous than data published in peer-reviewed medical journals. Why hasn't there been research conducted and data published in such journals? Yogi Berra may have had the answer to this one. Could it be "*déja vu* all over again," in the same way that many other effective yet relatively obscure medical treatments have had their struggles in achieving recognition? You be the judge. The evidence is herewith submitted for your thoughtful consideration.

Background. Since time immemorial, man has understood that electricity exerts powerful effects on living organisms. For over one hundred years so-called "modern science" has known that electromagnetic forces exert a powerful and potentially-deadly effect on organisms, especially small ones such as bacteria and viruses. We can track this knowledge not only throughout the annals of the scientific literature, but also as the result of our modern-day method of registering new discoveries via the legal mechanism of patenting new inventions. Each and every patent serves as a benchmark along the path of discovery.

In 1893, Mr. Henry Roeska of Philadelphia, PA received a patent on the technique of purifying water using electrical forces—U.S. Patent 501,732, *Method of and Apparatus for Purifying Water*.[3] Over the next several years other inventors perfected various means of using electricity to purify water and other liquids as well as meat and other foodstuffs—U.S. Patent 592,735 to Jones, *Apparatus for Electrically Treating Liquids*, 1897;[4] U.S. 824,320 to Weitzmann, *Process of Refining and Cleansing Coffee*, 1906;[5] and U.S. 1,044,201 to Lin-coln, *Process of Preserving* [Meat], 1912,[6] represent only a few. Over the ensuing decades, many researchers continued to explore the effects of electricity on biological systems. Progressively, more knowledge was acquired relating to the beneficial uses and effects of electromagnetism.

Decades ago researchers discovered additional ways of using electromagnetic forces for the benefit of humanity. In 1968, U.S. Patent 3,368,155 —*Apparatus for Producing Radiation Penetrating Living Tissue*[7]—was issued regarding the therapeutic treatment of humans. In 1969, the Westinghouse Corporation experimented with the use of high magnetic fields on biological systems—U.S. Patent 3,467,076, *High Magnetic Flux Experimental Apparatus*[8]. In 1982, Corning Glass was granted U.S. Patent 4,323,056—*Radio Frequency Induced Hyperthermia for Tumor Therapy*.[9] In 1987 U.S. 4,665,898 was issued to Costa, et al—*Malignancy Treatment*. Disclosed in the patent is a simple, pulsed magnetic field (which is neither seen, felt nor heard by humans) which "selectively inactivates and/or destroys malignant cells with relatively little damage to normal tissues as compared to conventional radiation therapy procedures."[10]

Most relevant to the present discussion is the work of Dr. Steven Kaali of the Albert Einstein College of Medicine. In the early 1980s Dr. Kaali began experimenting with electricity as a means of deactivating human sperm. In 1986, he was granted U.S. Patent 4,616,640—*Birth Control Method and Device Employing Electric Forces*.[11] In 1990, he was issued another patent relating to an electrical means of birth control—U.S. Patent 4,932,421, *Electrified Intrauterine Device*.[12] In the text of the document Kaali states, "It is believed that the electrified IUD also serves an antibacterial, an antifungal and antiviral function."

The *piece de résistance* occurred in 1993 when Kaali was granted yet another patent—U.S Patent 5,188,738, *Alternating Current Supplied Electrically Conductive Method and System for Treatment of Blood and/or Other Body Fluids and/or Synthetic Fluids with Electric Forces*. In this document Dr. Kaali states that:

> ...the present invention has been devised to attenuate [kill] any bacteria, virus (including the AIDS/HIV virus) [and the herpes virus], parasites and/or fungus contained in the blood

contributed by a donor to the point that any such contaminant is rendered ineffective for infecting a normally healthy cell, but does not make the blood biologically unfit for use.[13]

The Albert Einstein College of Medicine research was reported in the March 30, 1991 edition of *Science News*: "Shocking Treatment Proposed for AIDS." The article described how tiny microvoltages, comparable in strength to the voltage produced by a cardiac pacemaker, can reduce the infectivity of the AID/HIV virus, and other viruses and bacteria present in the blood. The electrically-treated viruses lose their ability to manufacture an enzyme necessary for reproduction. Also, the treatment prevents white blood cells from clumping together as they do under heavy viral load.[14]

In 1992, *Longevity* magazine reported on Kaali's research in an article entitled "Electrocuting the AIDS Virus: A Safer-Yet Blood Supply." The article reported that:

> At the Albert Einstein College of Medicine in New York City, Steven Kaali, M.D., has found that most of the AIDS viruses in a blood sample will lose their infectious capability after being zapped by a very low-level current. Repeated exposure appears to leave blood virtually free of HIV, as well as hepatitis—without harming blood cells. Kaali cautions that it will take years of testing before a virus-electrocuting device is ready for use.[15]

After learning of Dr. Kaali's research, and the fact that Kaali suggested years would likely pass before a treatment apparatus could be adequately tested, this provoked Bob Beck, D.Sc., a former physics professor at the University of Southern California and a man fairly well known throughout the alternative health world. Bob Beck was an expert in the field of electrical apparatuses. He quickly realized he could modify the Kaali technique so that an inexpensive "in-home" device could be used to effectively accomplish the same goal—inactivation of pathogenic microbes within the blood. Beck set about to perfect such a piece of equipment, the end result being a small, inexpensive apparatus which he claimed offers similar results as Kaali.

Whereas Dr. Kaali's device withdraws blood outside the body into a holding vessel where it is electrified, Dr. Beck's device simply attaches two electrodes externally to arteries on the forearm, the blood being electrified as it passes the electrodes.

Beck carefully calculated the required strength of the electric signal at the point of the blood inside the artery to insure adequate electrification of the blood is occurring.

For those familiar with measurements of electricity, a typical comfortable input to the skin surface is in the range of 3 mA (milliamperes), and the typical maximum tolerable limit is in the range of 7mA. As the electrical current passes through the various layers of skin, it decreases to the appropriate blood electrification treatment level of about 50-100 uA (microamperes).

About the same time as the emergence of the Kaali invention, it was becoming understood that the AIDS virus "hides" in certain areas of the body which can be resistant to the blood electrification technique, e.g., in the lymph. It is also known that other viruses hide in an attempt to evade the body's immune forces. The herpes virus is known to lie dormant in the *trigeminal ganglion* and *sacral ganglion*, areas at the top and base of the spine, respectively. Beck knew that in order to treat these areas, another device would have to be developed in addition to the blood electrification unit.

Bob Beck happened to be the initial patent holder of the photographic flash unit, i.e., the flash bulb-type apparatus that generates a quick burst of energy that produces the photographic flash. He reasoned the flash unit could be redesigned to send powerful but imperceptible electrical impulses deep within living tissue. In this way the hiding viruses could be deactivated. The Costa invention mentioned above supports this idea. Dr. Beck believed his blood electrification unit in conjunction with the pulsed electromagnetic unit is the "poor man's solution" to many illnesses and diseases.

Therapeutic Results. Beck claimed to have personally funded clinical research to test the effectiveness of his two devices on a significant number of AIDS patients. Anecdotal feedback was also obtained from many cancer patients. He announced that the devices were often miraculously effective in the treatment of both of these conditions, with many AIDS patients being totally relieved of all symptoms and many cancer patients making full recoveries. Unfortunately, he never made his research public for reasons that remain unclear. After all, his inventions are not "medically approved" by any government agency for the general treatment of the public, and fear of reprisal may have loomed large in his mind. As Dr. Beck clearly pointed out, however, people in the U.S. can use these devices on themselves for "research purposes," so long as they don't attempt to treat others.

Dr. Beck didn't treat herpes sufferers *per se*, but given the patents of Dr. Steven Kaali and the claimed results of Dr. Beck regarding the effective treatment of AIDS with the use of both blood electrification and magnetic pulsing of the "hiding" HIV virus, it is logical to conclude these apparatuses hold the possibility of permanently eradicating the herpes virus from the body by ridding the virus from the blood and spinal ganglia. Also, in an alternative approach, other treatment methods discussed in this writing could be used to rid the virus from the blood, while using the magnetic pulser to treat the top (trigeminal ganglion) and bottom (sacral ganglion) of the spine where the virus lies dormant.

Equipment Availability. Both the blood electrification and magnetic pulse units, as approved by Dr. Beck himself, are marketed by Sota Instruments of Penticton, BC, Canada. The blood electrification unit is called The Silver Pulser, and the pulsed magnetic unit is called The Magnetic Pulser. To learn more about both of these devices, visit Sota at www.sotainstruments.com. To place an order, call Sota at (800)224-0242.

■ *Hydrogen Peroxide & DMSO*. An additional technique that many have found effective is the application of 3% hydrogen peroxide (H_2O_2) and DMSO (dimethyl sulfoxide) to the outbreak site or potential site in the same manner as described for using the Cold Sore Inhibitor (below). Hydrogen peroxide, as described by the well-known alternative physician Dr. William Campbell Douglass, is nothing short of a wonder molecule. The body's own cells produce H_2O_2 as a front-line defense against bacteria, viruses, parasites and other infective microorganisms—attacking them with an oxidative burst of H_2O_2.[16]

DMSO is another wonder substance, with many unique and beneficial properties. Medical researchers believe DMSO is able to dissolve viruses' protein coat, leaving it unprotected for further attack by the body's immune system.[17] A more detailed discussion of DMSO is found in the section on **Pain Relievers**.

Be careful to dilute the DMSO before applying so that stinging or burning doesn't occur. Experiment before applying to a large area, especially if you're using it on the genital area. It's perhaps best to start with a DMSO gel containing aloe, which is available in health food stores. Dab the DMSO on the skin, as opposed to rubbing. Three percent hydrogen peroxide can be sprayed or carefully dabbed on the affected area or potential outbreak site. Also, some have found that mixing DMSO with powdered vitamin C (crystals) is very effective in the treatment of the genital variety.[18]

Because DMSO is such a powerful skin penetrant—and at the same time able to carry other substances along with it—it takes only a short leap of logic to deduce that DMSO in combination with anti-viral agents would be effective in treating herpes. Olive leaf extract, discussed below under **General Treatment Methods**, combined with DMSO could deliver a powerful blow to viruses, including herpes. DMSO + H_2O_2 + vitamin C powder + olive leaf extract could be a winner.

Stopping Viral Migration Through the Skin. It has been estimated that over 60 million people in the U.S.—one in five adults over the age of 12—are infected with genital herpes, yet roughly 85% or over 50 million of these people are undiagnosed and don't realize they are infected. Although this may seem odd, the partial explanation is that some sufferers mistake an outbreak for other ailments such as jock itch, yeast infections, allergic reactions, etc. Another explanation is that many people who harbor the virus have never had an outbreak. What could be responsible for some infected people having multiple outbreaks and some having none? If this question could be answered, it might point to a possible long-term solution for preventing any further outbreaks.

Cell Movement Within the Body. The following material relating to the theory of and treatment methods for infectious cell migration is applicable to the spread of cells of other diseases, including cancer cells. In the case of both herpes, cancer and other infectious diseases, pathogens move through the body in a similar manner.

The human body is intricately composed of tens of trillions of individual basic living units—the cells. Each cell functions as a miniature biological factory contributing to the body's overall functioning. Cells are diverse and highly complex structures which differ in their physical characteristics and internal composition in relation to the various functions they perform. Healthy cells extract and convert energy from their environments and are thus empowered to maintain themselves, grow, reproduce and perform their vital functions. All of the body's healthy cells work in harmony to perform the complex and intricate symphony of life itself.

Cells are not static. Most cells are capable of changing their positions relative to one another, i.e., they are able to move within their environments. Blood cells simply traverse the highway of the blood stream to remote destinations where they accomplish their vital tasks. However, most all of the body's other cells are also capable of movement in quite another way.

Other than by traveling in the bloodstream, in order to change their positions and move through the body, cells must be capable of temporarily dissolving the tissue which surrounds them. This is true of any cell, whether it is a normal cell or an infective cell such as a cancer cell or herpes virus cell. Cells accomplish this movement by means of manufacturing and excreting protein-digesting enzymes which temporarily dissolve and weaken the surrounding tissue which is composed of elastic fibers (elastin) and collagen—the primary constituents of connective tissue. These enzymes are known as *collagen-dissolving enzymes*, which are themselves proteins. Cells are also able to secrete activating substances which catalyze (vitalize) dormant enzymes residing outside themselves. These vitalized enzymes assist in digesting and further weakening the surrounding collagen. The connective tissue then closes behind the migrating cell(s) by means of other mechanisms that repair the tissue.[19]

A healthy body's normal physiological functions often require cells to move through surrounding tissue. This occurs normally in many situations, such as during growth, the restructuring of certain organs (as in pregnancy), and in various metabolic pathways. The immune system utilizes this mechanism to accomplish many tasks. Monocytes, for example—one of the immune system's white blood cell warriors—are cells often on the move.[20]

In pursuit of infective microbes, monocytes are first transported via the bloodstream to a location near the invading, pathogenic microbes. They must then move through the blood vessel wall and toward the infection by secreting collagen-dissolving enzymes which allow them to move through the dense surrounding tissue similar to an explorer hacking his way through a thicket of underbrush. But in this case, the tissue closes behind the monocytes as they travel toward the pathogens.

Infectious disease cells, such as the cells of the herpes virus, travel within the body by using this same mechanism. Viral particles commandeer healthy cells and signal them to reproduce into more viral particles which are then released into the surrounding tissue. Commandeered host cells are also ordered to produce collagen-dissolving enzymes so that the virus is able to travel to the skin's outermost layer where the painful eruptions occur.

Picture this process as a football game where two teams confront each other on the playing field at the line of scrimmage. On one side of the line is the defensive team, whose job it is to hold ground and stop the progress of the football. On the other side of the line of scrimmage is the offensive team whose task is to advance the football through the defensive line all the way to the goal. In the case of the spreading herpes virus, the defensive team is the healthy cells of the body trying to hold back the spreading virus. The offensive team—the team with the football—is represented by the viral particles, but in this case there are multiple footballs, each representing a potential outbreak.

In order for the offensive team to be stopped short of the goal line, in this case the skin's surface, either of two things, or both of them, must occur. Either the defense must stand their ground and not permit the continued movement of the offense, and/or somehow the offense—irrespective of the state of the defensive team—must be caused not to perform. In the real battleground within the body, this points to two possibilities.

Somehow the defensive cellular structures must be strengthened so that they prevent the offensive viral particles from progressing, and/or the offensive viral particles must be affected in some manner that causes them not to advance. Fortunately, there are ways of effecting both of these means of prevention.

The Defense. The defensive means of preventing viral progress has to do with the integrity of cell membranes and connective tissues, and the way they are structured and positioned within the skin. The integrity of skin cells is maintained by structures called *desmosomes*, physiological structures—attachment sights—which anchor contiguous cells together. Desmosomes are the glue, as it were, that attach the skin cells to one another.

■ *Calcium, Vitamins D & F, and Magnesium.*
The desmosomes themselves are maintained by the presence of calcium, and their strength and cohesiveness is a function of the amount of calcium they contain. The more calcium available to the desmosomes, the higher their integrity, and vice versa.[21] When herpes is present and there is a calcium deficiency within the cells, the weakness or lack of cohesiveness of the desmosomes allows the viral particles to travel to the skin's surface and erupt in the formation of fluid-filled herpes blisters.

Most people have an adequate supply of calcium within the blood, especially if they eat dairy products such as milk, cheese, and yogurt. (These foods have their own problems, about which you can learn more by visiting www.notmilk.com.) More healthful sources of calcium are greens, broccoli, beans, peas and tofu. For many, the problem isn't the lack of calcium within the blood, *it's the lack of calcium within the tissues—which is caused by a deficiency of vitamins D, F, and the mineral magnesium.*[22]

The body is able to manufacture vitamin D if it's exposed to sufficient sunshine—20-30 minutes a couple of times per week. Alternatively, multivitamins contain vitamin D, but often in insufficient quantities to make a difference. Taking vitamin D_3 (cholecalciferol) at the level of about 5,000 IU daily (in divided doses with meals) is recommended, instead of the several hundred IU found in the typical vitamin pill.

Vitamin F is the simple name for unsaturated fatty acids—arachidonic, linoleic and linolenic acids. These substances are found in abundance in *flax oil*. We suggest organic, cold-pressed flax oil from either Barlean's Organic Oils or Omega Nutrition—preferably with a high lignan content, at the level of 2-4 tablespoons daily with meals. Most people eating the typical Western diet consume high quantities of saturated fats which are contained in animal foods, supermarket oils and processed foods.

Saturated fats compete with the more healthful unsaturated fats, which multiplies the problem by interfering with the assimilation of healthful fatty acids. (A more detailed discussion of fats and oils is given in the ***Cardiovascular Disease*** section.)

Magnesium should be taken at the level of 500-1,000 mg daily, with meals. Most good multivitamin-mineral supplements supply this quantity. If you want to take a calcium supplement, calcium *lactate* is an easily absorbable form. Despite the word "lactate," calcium lactate is not sourced from dairy. If you supplement with one or two specific minerals, it's best to take a multi-mineral as well, as various minerals compete with one another for absorption and block each other's actions.

■ *Vitamin C, Lysine and Proline.*
Another critical component of the defensive strategy is collagen, the main ingredient that composes connective tissues. In order for the progress of the migrating viral cells to be deterred, collagen must have its optimal biological structure. Collagen molecules, which wind around each other in triplicate like a twisted rope, can't achieve their optimal physiological structure, activity and stability without the *optimal* presence of three key substances: vitamin C, lysine and proline.[23]

[The use of vitamin C and lysine in the treatment of herpes has been known since the early 1970s.[24] However, it has been reported that lysine is effective because it is absorbed and utilized by viruses instead of the structurally similar arginine which is required by viruses for replication. Also, lysine and arginine compete for transport through the intestinal wall, and excess lysine reduces the uptake of arginine.[25] The present discussion, however, focuses on a very different method of action of these substances—namely, their use as defenses against collagen-dissolving enzymes.]

Added to vitamin C and lysine is the use of the amino acid proline. This method of treatment as well as its newly proposed method of action is put forth by the world renowned physician Dr. Mathias Rath. The addition of proline to the treatment regimen, according to Dr. Rath, is critical. He explains that a treatment capability is only as strong as its weakest link, and that when proline is absent from the treatment protocol, optimally-effective results cannot be expected.[26]

Vitamin C controls the production of collagen from within the collagen molecules' nuclei. Only the presence of *optimal levels* of vitamin C will ensure the optimal production of collagen and the elastic fiber molecules that produce *optimally-strong* connective tissues. The operative word here is *optimal*. Again, picture the offense—the team with the football(s)—not as your local high school or college team. These herpes viruses are professionals, take their job seriously and come ready to exert maximal effort to score touchdowns—outbreaks. If they win, you will have outbreaks. Therefore, the defensive strategy can't be slack. It must be at its optimal level of performance.

Similar to vitamin C, lysine and proline are two key ingredients that contribute to the strength of collagen and the elastic fibers that make up the structure of connective tissue. They are both amino acid building blocks of longer chains of amino acids that form the collagen fibers. About 25% of the collagen molecule is composed of lysine and proline. Between 25-33% of the collagen "reinforcement rods" are made up of proline.[27] When supplementing, as mentioned, there can't be a "weakest link" in the line of defense. All key elements must be present at optimal levels. Otherwise, the virus will exploit the presence of the weakest link and run for multiple touchdowns.

While proline is manufactured within the body at minimal levels (which may be easily depleted where there is a disease condition[28]), the body produces no lysine. Every molecule of lysine, an essential amino acid, must be supplied by the diet or through supplementation. Optimal levels of these two amino acids are required.

What constitutes optimal levels of vitamin C, lysine and proline? For vitamin C, the level differs from person to person, depending on one's individual genetic makeup and present state of health. The simplest way to determine your individual optimal level is by a step-by-step method of increasing the dosage until "bowel tolerance" is exceeded. At this point, mild diarrhea occurs. For healthy individuals, 8-10 grams (8,000-10,000 mg) daily is a ballpark figure to achieve. For persons with a compromised immune system, disease, etc., optimal levels could be substantially higher.[29] Ascorbic acid either in pill form or in a powdered, crystalline form is the product of choice, preferably complexed with

antioxidant bioflavonoids. One teaspoon of powdered vitamin C equals roughly four grams.

To achieve an optimal level, increase the vitamin C intake at the rate of one gram per day until the stool loosens. Then, reduce the intake by one or two grams until no sign of diarrhea is present. This is your optimal level of vitamin C intake. As mentioned, the level for healthy individuals will be in the range of 8-10 grams daily, taken in divided doses with meals. Eight grams would be approximately two teaspoons of powdered vitamin C. Less healthy individuals have been known to take 40-60 grams daily without experiencing diarrhea, because their individual need is so much greater. Alternative cancer clinics treat advanced cancers with up to 200-300 gm per day, given intravenously. Excess vitamin C is excreted in the urine.[30]

The level of the human need for lysine ranges widely, depending upon the body's state of health. Dr. Rath recommends high levels of this amino acid—from four to eight grams per day. Taking large quantities of lysine should not cause adverse effects, as the body simply excretes the molecules that are unused.[31] At the same time, arginine-rich foods should be avoided. Such foods include cereal grains (including whole wheat), carob, chocolate, coconut, gelatin, nuts, seeds, soybeans, and wheat germ.

Conventional medicine erroneously believes the body manufactures as much proline as needed.[32] According to Rath, this could be the weak link that leads to ineffective results. Take one to two grams daily in divided doses.

Once you begin this regimen, you may not see immediate results. After all, it's taken your body years to arrive at its deficient state, and it may take some time to strengthen your desmosomes and connective tissues. Physicians who promote this method of herpes treatment believe that your control of herpes outbreaks is not a matter of "if," but "when." This protocol is recommended for treating cold sores, genital herpes and shingles.

If the dosages suggested above provide relief from further outbreaks, by reducing the quantities of vitamin C, lysine and proline you will be able to determine the minimal amounts necessary to prevent outbreaks. However, your primary concern should not be discovering the minimal necessary amounts, but rather what dosages provide relief from future outbreaks.

Crippling The Offense. The means of defeating the offense, or the movement of the virus through the skin irrespective of the state of the desmosomes and connective tissue, is *by blocking the anchor sites within the connective tissue which are used by the collagen-digesting enzymes to attach themselves to the tissue.* Though infected cells may still produce high levels of collagen-dissolving enzymes, without the ability of attaching to connective tissue, the enzymes are rendered ineffective.[33]

The body has intrinsic means of blocking enzymes in this manner. However, when this fails because the body's reserves have been exhausted—indicated by continued outbreaks—another method of blocking becomes necessary. Lysine, in addition to being a key building block of collagen, is the key substance able to block the anchor sites used by the collagen-digesting enzymes to make their attachments to collagen molecules.[34]

In terms of our football team analogy, this would be the equivalent of locking the hips of the offensive players so that they are rendered immobile. They still have multiple footballs, but they're simply incapable of advancing against the defense, regardless of the status of the defense, i.e., independent of the condition of the connective tissue. Nevertheless, by using this two-pronged approach, the task is accomplished more effectively.

■ *Cold Sore Inhibitor.*® Among the many potions and lotions and prescription medications available for treating cold sore outbreaks, one new method has been shown to provide shockingly-good results. A device known as the Cold Sore Inhibitor® is a recent entry into the marketplace. About half the size of a pack of cigarettes, the Cold Sore Inhibitor provides an almost imperceptible low voltage electrical signal to the potential site of the cold sore. When the first sign of an outbreak is felt—typically experienced as a tingling, burning or itching sensation in the area of the lip—the two small electrodes on the device are placed on either side of the site of the potential outbreak, and treatment is initiated for 10-20 seconds, after which the polarity of the electrical impulse is reversed for an additional 10-20 seconds of continued treatment.

If treatment is begun within the first hour after experiencing the initial tingling or burning sensations, the lesion (sore) will not form, according

to the manufacturer.[35] To insure that the lesion doesn't form, during the first six hours following the initial symptoms the treatment should be applied whenever the tingling/burning/itching sensation manifests, with a minimum of at least one treatment per hour. If treatment is initiated after the lesion forms, the visible outbreak will disappear within 24-hours after treatment.[36] The device is equally effective on both HSV-1 and HVS-2, i.e., it can be used to treat both cold sores and genital herpes. The Cold Sore Inhibitor works by 1) penetrating the protein envelope of the virus with a weak electrical current, 2) breaking up the polypeptide structure of the virus core, and 3) stimulating the cells' capacitance via the increase in mitochondrial function, thus returning the cells to a normal state.[37]

To learn more, visit www.eliminatecoldsores.com. To place an order, call (800)680-7246. A similar device is the Cold Sore Eliminator,® available at www.siminator.com.

■ *Auto-Hemotherapy.* In his book *Medicine of Hope: Insulin-Cellular Therapy* (1994), the Canadian physician and medical pioneer Dr. Jean-Claude Paquette relates his experiences in treating herpes. So unusual is Dr. Paquette's recounting that it leaves us speechless to comment further.

> A few years before the discovery of the antiviral drug zovirax (acyclovir) in 1973 or 1974, for which a subsidy of $17 million was paid, I developed by myself a treatment for labial herpes which does not cost anything and which has absolutely no side effect nor contraindication.
>
> A lady about thirty had been consulting me for the last 12 years for labial herpes. Three dermatologists and an allergist had not found any solutions for her problem. Eager to help this patient, I pondered about it for a long time when the idea came to me that her blood contained antigens...By injecting antigens, the system would probably produce antibodies.
>
> I remembered having heard about hemotherapy, which consists in treating someone with his own blood, but I was completely unfamiliar with the technique. I then began with 1cc, then 2, then 4 cc, and I finally adopted the dose of 10 cc in my practice with spectacular results. I was drawing 10 cc of blood from a vein in the arm and injecting it back intra-muscularly in the gluteus muscle (buttocks), noth-

ing else. [Alternatively, the blood could be re-injected into the thigh muscle]. The lesions dried out within 2 or 3 days and the pain disappeared usually the very same day. I have treated over a hundred cases.

As for acyclovir, an expensive drug with so extraordinary predictions, it has not solved the problem as anticipated. It does nothing but diminish it without ever solving it. The prescription is to be repeated monthly and it will be necessary to take it for life.

Occasionally, I meet former patients that I treated twenty or more years ago. They are very proud to tell me that they never had any recurrences. This is how discoveries are made. I do not have enough experience on a sufficient number of genital herpes cases to affirm whether or not auto-hemotherapy is effective, but I have the feeling it will.[38]

■ See **Shingles.** See also ***Del Immune V, Hyperbaric Oxygenation Therapy***, ***Olive Leaf Extract***, ***Photoluminescence*** and ***Sodium Chlorite*** under **General Treatment Methods**. See also Herpes in the Member's Area of *The Encyclopedia's* website.

High Blood Pressure. See Hypertension under *Cardiovascular Disease*.

Hot Flashes

Also called hot flushes, hot flashes are flushing sensations of heat caused by dilation of skin capillaries. These symptoms are usually associated with menopausal endocrine imbalances. Although they are not medically significant, women experiencing these symptoms find them quite bothersome, stress producing and even sleep depriving.

■ ***Indium Sulfate.*** Indium sulfate has been reported to offer relief from hot flashes associated with hormonal imbalances. Indium is a trace mineral occurring at very low levels in some foods—less than 8 micrograms (0.008 gm) per day in the average diet.[1] Indium sulfate is the only chemical form of the mineral that is generally recognized as safe (GRAS) by the U.S. FDA.[2]

Although the means by which indium achieves its beneficial results have not been established, it is theorized the mineral provides enhancement to the pituitary gland and hypothalamus, thereby helping to maintain optimal hormonal function.[3] It also may

function by regulating the "master gland" (hypophysis-hypothalamus) feedback loop which controls the production of over 30 hormones.[4]

A further mode of action was put forth by Henry A. Schroeder, M.D., an expert in trace minerals whose work on removing lead from gasoline is well known. Schroeder's work indicated that indium triggers the body's uptake of other beneficial metals (minerals) including copper, chromium, manganese, and zinc.[5]

No clinical trials have been performed on indium, primarily because it is a non-patentable, naturally-occurring element. The beneficial qualities of the mineral, however, have been reported by many consumers.

For more information, refer to *Indium: The Missing Trace Element* by Dr. Robert Lyons, or *Indium: The Age-Reversing Trace Element* by Dr. Morton Walker. To purchase indium sulfate, visit www.vital-nutrients.com/indium.htm, or www.eastparkresearch.com.

■ ***Hypothyroidism.*** One possible cause of hot flashes is *hypothyroidism*, which is characterized by a sluggish or underactive thyroid gland producing inadequate levels of thyroid hormones. The thyroid gland is part of the endocrine (hormonal) system, and is located in the front of the neck just below the Adam's apple. The thyroid produces the two master metabolism hormones T-4 (thyroxin) and T-3 (tri-iodothyronine), which regulate the rate of metabolism and the functioning of many additional systems throughout the body. As such, the thyroid plays a role in virtually every bodily function.

The interaction between thyroid hormones and many other hormones including cortisol, insulin, and the sex hormones explains why an improperly-functioning thyroid is associated with such a broad range of symptoms and diseases. Auto-immune diseases, chronic fatigue syndrome, fibromyalgia, depression, heart disease, IBS, and many other conditions could indicate an under-active thyroid. Symptoms include intolerance to cold; cold hands and feet; constipation; dry skin; fluid retention; frequent urination; memory problems; physical fatigue; recurring infections; slow pulse; weakness; and weight gain, as well as many additional symptoms.

More than 10% of the adult American population and 20% of American women over the age of 60 have at least sub-clinical hypothyroidism, where no symptoms are yet noticed. Approximately half of these people are never diagnosed; and of those who are, many make only a partial recovery due to inadequate treatment. Hypothyroidism is often difficult to diagnose as many of the symptoms are vague and overlap with other disorders. Nutritional imbalances, environmental toxins, lack of exercise, and stress are contributing factors.

A simple test can be performed to help evaluate whether or not a thyroid problem exists. The test was pioneered by Broda O. Barnes, M.D., Ph.D., author of the 1976 classic *Hypothyroidism: The Unsuspected Illness*. The test is called the Basal Temperature Test (BTT), and is sometimes referred to as the Barnes Thyroid Test. The BTT can indicate thyroid deficiency even when blood tests such as Free T-3, Free T-4 and *thyroid stimulating hormone* (TSH) show normal thyroid function.

The BTT is performed by taking the underarm temperature in the morning immediately upon awakening. Have a thermometer handy by the bedside, already shaken down (if mercury), so that you don't have to move around before taking the test—or use a digital thermometer. Place the thermometer securely in the armpit for three to five minutes. Follow this procedure for 10 mornings in a row to obtain an average of readings. (Menstruating women should perform the test during the first two weeks of their cycle.)[6] According to Barnes, if the temperature averages 97.6 degrees Fahrenheit or lower, a possible thyroid deficiency should be suspected, especially if many of the above-described symptoms are being experienced.

TSH is produced by the pituitary gland in response to signals from *thyroid releasing hormone* (TRH), which is produced in the hypothalamus. TSH in turn signals the thyroid to produce and release T-4 and T-3, which control the metabolism of all cells in the body. In the past and even currently, many/most physicians believe the level of TSH is the only important indicator of thyroid function, and if TSH is within the "normal" range of 0.3 to 3.04, there is no thyroid problem. However, physicians are discovering that the TSH value is grossly unreliable for diagnosing hypothyroidism (although many recognize that a TSH over 1.5 is indicative of a potential problem), and that Free T-3 and Free T-4 values are critical in making an ac-

curate diagnosis and proper prescription for treatment. In reality, TSH, Free T-4, Free T-3, and the BTT are all important diagnostic measurements which in combination should be evaluated on a person-to-person basis.

Another simple test which can be performed "in-home" gives an indication of the body's need for iodine, which is required to manufacture thyroid hormones. If hypothyroidism is present, supplementation with iodine can be helpful in reducing or eliminating symptoms.[7] With a Q-Tip, paint a two inch by two inch square of 2% iodine tincture (use only this form of iodine) on your stomach (near the navel) or inner thigh. If the iodine stain can be seen 24-hours later, your body is not likely iodine deficient. If your body is deficient in iodine, it will uptake the iodine and the stain will disappear in under 24-hours. If this is the case, iodine supplementation can reduce the deficiency.

Iosol,® Lugol's® solution, and SSKI (potassium iodide) are beneficial oral, liquid iodine supplements that can help increase iodine levels. To purchase these, Google "iosol," "lugol," and "SSKI." Pill-form Iodoral® is also effective. DO NOT take iodine tincture internally. Whatever type of supplementation is used, the iodine test can be repeated until the iodine stain remains visible 24-hours after application. For additional information, see *Iodine* under **General Treatment Methods**.

Prescription medications are also available. Synthroid® is a synthetic preparation designed to simulate natural thyroid substances. However, many physicians observe that the "natural" thyroid treatments, consisting of extracts from a porcine (pig) source, are often more effective than their synthetic counterparts. One beneficial over-the-counter bovine thyroid supplement is Thytrophin PMG,® manufactured by Standard Process. To order, visit www.totaldiscountvitamins.com. On the other hand, even though there are several prescription alternatives available, natural thyroid supplements such as Armour,® Natur-Throid,® and Bio Throid® are often the most effective, and are those that are most prescribed by alternative-minded physicians. For a directory of physicians knowledgeable about the intricacies of thyroid function and who are aware of non-synthetic, more natural prescription remedies, visit www.thyroid-info.com/topdrs/index.htm. To evaluate your potential for having hypothyroidism, answer a questionnaire at http://thyroid.about.com/library/hypoquiz/blhypoquiz.htm.

■ *Flax.* Supplementation with either ground flax seeds or high-lignin flax oil has been shown to significantly reduce the incidence of hot flashes. See flax seed in the **Index** for more information.

■ *MenopauEase,*® *MindEase,*® *& PMX.*® Three products based on traditional oriental herbal medicine that are often effective in quelling hot flashes as well as general menopausal symptoms are MenopauEase,® MindEase,® and PMX.® MenopauEase is based on the traditional Kampo formula tokishakuyaku-san, while MindEase and PMX are based on the Chinese formula jia-wei-xiao-yao-san. Either can be ordered from: Willner Chemists, (800)633-1106, www.willner.com; or BenSalem Naturals, Inc., (215)638-0627, www.bnatural.com/honso.htm. Order PMX from Ormed, (707)575-7070.

■ *Red Clover.* The herb red clover is used in Chinese medicine to reduce the incidence of menopausal symptoms. Many women find the herb useful in reducing the incidence and severity of hot flashes. Red clover contains high quantities of the compound *isoflavones*, a type of phyto- (plant) estrogen that closely resembles the estrogen molecule produced by the human body.[8] It is believed that phytoestrogens produce their effects by using the estrogen receptors.

In a 2002 double-blind, placebo-controlled study conducted in Amsterdam, Holland, 15 menopausal women ages 49-65 received a daily dosage of 80 mg of red clover extract (Promensil®) for three months. All participants removed from their diets any foods containing isoflavones, e.g., cabbage, grains, soy, etc. At the termination of the study, women in the placebo group experienced no change in the frequency of their hot flashes, whereas the women taking red clover extract experienced a 44% reduction at about eight weeks into the study, and was maintained for the remainder of the study.[9]

A July 2003 study reported in the *Journal of the American Medical Association*[10] found virtually the same beneficial effect from the use of red clover extract (Promensil) on quelling hot flashes (41%); however, the placebo group experienced a

36% decrease in incidence. This is somewhat confusing considering the Amsterdam study which reported no improvement for the placebo group. One possible explanation is that the placebo used in this latter study may not have been "inert." That is, it may have contained ingredients which actually did produce some active, beneficial effect. The contents of the placebo preparation were not disclosed—and this brings up an interesting issue.

According to the National Institutes of Health, the placebo effect is defined as "desirable physiological or psychological effects attributable to the use of inert medications," where inert means a substance having *no active physiological or psychological properties*. In fact, placebos, the pills against which substances being tested are evaluated, are assumed to be a sugar pill, or some similar substance having no active properties.

Traditionally, inert placebos have been used to measure the true effects, including side-effects, of a drug or supplement by comparing the substance being tested against a substance known to cause no effect—a placebo. Recently, however, new light has been shed on questionable practices of the drug industry related to their use of *non*-inert placebos.

According to Beatrice Golomb, M.D., Ph. D., Associate Professor of Medicine at the University of California San Diego, pharmaceutical companies often use placebos containing *active* ingredients. The drug companies often know before the clinical trial begins that the substance to be tested produces certain side-effects. The placebos are then formulated—by these same drug companies—to mimic the side-effects of the drugs being tested.[11]

The rationale of the drug companies is that in order for the clinical trial to be double blinded, where neither the test subjects (patients) nor the researchers knows the true identity of the substance being tested—active medication or placebo—the placebo has to be designed so that it mimics the side-effects of the active substance.[12] If you are a person who enjoys this type of circuitous logic, try this one on for size: "Nothing would be what it is. Because everything would be what it isn't. And contrary-wise, what it is, it wouldn't be. And what it wouldn't be, it would. You see?" Alice (in Wonderland) had an excuse for using the logic of a blithering idiot. She was young, in a strange environment, and was probably quite stressed out. What are the excuses of the M.D.s and Ph.D.s who design these drug trials?

While using a non-inert placebo may help insure the true double-blind status of the research study, does it not seriously jeopardize the true evaluation of the drug being tested—especially in terms of getting an accurate measure of the drug's true level of side-effects? Then, after the study is concluded, the results may be stated that the drug being evaluated produced no more side-effects than did the placebo—which was assumed to be a harmless substance having no effect. In the red clover study cited above, if an active, *non*-inert placebo was the cause of the placebo group having such a high level of positive effect, almost as high as the red clover, this would tend to discredit red clover as being a beneficial substance.

Dr. Golomb has been fighting the pharmaceutical companies' assertions that placebos are inactive substances. She has suggested that 1) drug companies make public all placebo ingredients, and 2) a standardized set of placebos be developed whose side-effects would be predictable.[13]

There are two possible cautions for women taking red clover extract. Because red clover may thin the blood, caution should be observed when combining it with blood-thinning agents (anticoagulants) such as Coumadin® (warfarin), *Ginkgo biloba* or aspirin. Also, because estrogenic activity is stimulated by isoflavones, caution should be observed in persons with hormone-sensitive diseases such as thyroid dysfunction.

■ *Progesterone Cream.* Many women report relief from hot flashes, as well as other menopausal symptoms, by using a cream containing natural phytosterols derived from the Mexican wild yam, natural progesterone, and synergistic herbs (such as black cohosh, burdock root, chamomile and ginseng) that aid in the formulation's effectiveness. To learn more about this treatment, visit www.johnleemd.com, or read Dr. John Lee's books *What Your Doctor May Not Tell You About Menopause: The Breakthrough Book on Natural Progesterone* (earlier work) and *What Your Doctor May Not Tell You About Premenopause*—a more recent work which is the more highly recommended of the two books. Additionally, for women or men wanting to evaluate their hormone levels, a mail-in saliva test can be ordered by visiting www.heranswer.com/hormonetest.asp, or www.salivatest.com.

There are two strategies regarding the use of a progesterone cream. One approach suggests that more isn't necessarily better, and that many women experience benefits from using a product that contains about 10 mg of natural progesterone (not synthetic progestin) per 2-ounce jar. The other approach, recommended by Dr. John Lee, is to begin treatment using a cream containing about 1,000 mg of natural progesterone per 2-ounce jar, and reduce the number of applications until determining the minimal dosage that produces the desired result. *As long as the user follows the recommendation of locating the minimal effective dosage*, this second approach would bring symptom reduction more quickly, and for this reason if nothing else would be the preferred approach for most women.

■ *Bioidentical Hormone Replacement.* Replacing decreasing levels of hormones with natural, so-called bioidentical hormones as opposed to synthetic ones, offers many benefits to aging women. To learn more, see Menopause in the Member's Area of *The Encyclopedia's* website.

HUMAN IMMUNODEFICIENCY VIRUS. See *Acquired Immune Deficiency Syndrome.*

HYPERTENSION. See *Cardiovascular Disease.*

HYPOTHYROIDISM. See Hypothyroidism under *Hot Flashes.*

INDIGESTION
Multiple millions of people following the Western lifestyle and diet, including millions of Americans, suffer from what is currently called GERD, **G**astro-**E**sophageal **R**eflux **D**isease, the most common symptom of which is heartburn, or indigestion. In fact, approximately 40% of the adult U.S. population suffers from GERD, with 60 million Americans experiencing heartburn at least once per month while 25 million experience painful symptoms on a daily basis. The pain resulting from GERD ranges from mild to severe, with some sufferers experiencing such intense pain they rush to the hospital mistaking the pain for a possible heart attack. More than $8 billion is spent annually by Americans on medications to treat heartburn.

The *esophagus* is the tube that carries foods and liquids to the stomach. GERD occurs when the sphincter muscle, acting as a one-way valve at the lower end of the esophagus, doesn't close properly and fails to prevent stomach contents from regurgitating (refluxing) into the esophagus. It is commonly believed that the regurgitated components consist solely of stomach acid, whereas they also consist of imbibed foods and liquids, bile, and pancreatic enzymes. The tissues which line the esophagus are delicate relative to the more resistant stomach lining and can become damaged in such a harsh environment. The chronic refluxing of harsh digestive components increases the risk of cancers of the esophagus, larnyx, and pharynx, and has led to an epidemic of esophageal cancer in the Western world.

Several factors contribute to reflux, including 1) the consumption of certain types of foods (including black pepper, chocolate, fatty foods, garlic, peppermint, raw onions, spicy foods, and vinegar), 2) the consumption of certain types of drinks (including alcoholic, caffeinated, and carbonated beverages), 3) overeating, and 4) lying down within three hours after consuming a meal. Acid reflux symptoms are labeled GERD when they occur two or more times per week and are difficult to control. Other causes of GERD include *hiatal hernia*—a condition in which a portion of the stomach abnormally protrudes into the diaphram—and *esophageal stricture*, a narrowing of the esophagus.

The typical orthodox medical strategy for treating this ailment is to attack what is seen as the main culprit, stomach acid, by either neutralizing it or reducing its production. The "solutions" have familiar names such as the antacids Maalox® and Tums,® and the so-called H2 antagonists Tagamet,® Zantac,® Pepcid,® and Axid,® as well as the proton pump inhibitors (PPIs) such as Prilosec,® Prevacid,® Aciphex,® and the best-seller Nexium® which, as mentioned, made it to the marketplace just in time to take over the duties of Prilosec—just when Prilosec's patent protection was about to expire.

Does the standard medical approach work, i.e., are pills like Prilosec and Nexium effective in reducing or stopping the production of acid? In a word, yes—so much so that some physicians have referred to Prilosec and Nexium as "purple crack." Are there any problems caused by the use of these

pills that interrupt the normal cycle of stomach acid production? In another word, yes. Here's the issue. The stomach is lined with a mucus membrane layer called *stomach mucosa*. It is this thick mucus membrane that protects the stomach lining from the powerful digestive acids. When food enters the stomach, the mucosa secretes *gastric juice* (commonly called stomach acid), which consists of hydrochloric (gastric) acid (HCl) and other substances (including pepsinogen, intrinsic factor, gastrin and mucus). A delicate balance exists within the stomach, and imbalances cause problems that are experienced as stomach upset, e.g., indigestion.

On the face of it, the use of antacids seems logical. If acid is burning the stomach lining (and esophagus), stop the production of the acid and voila!, you've got relief! Unfortunately, the story isn't quite so simple. For example, in some cases the antacid neutralizes the acid already present and changes the pH (acidity-alkalinity) of the stomach contents. Sensing this, the body "rebounds" by producing *more* acid, and a painful cycle ensues.

Chronic indigestion can lead to peptic ulcers and, as mentioned, damage to the esophagus, larynx, pharynx, and promote related cancers. Another difficulty is that proton pump inhibitors such as Prilosec, Prevacid, and Nexium only inhibit stomach acid, leaving the esophagus vulnerable to the remaining digestive components. Yet a further problem with both H2 blockers and PPIs is that they can impair the absorption of vital nutrients such as beta-carotine, calcium, folic acid, iron, sodium, thiamine, vitamin B_{12}, and zinc.

Stopping or decreasing the production of stomach acid causes inadequate digestion of the nutrients our bodies need in order to maintain good health, and can place an unnecessary burden on the liver and kidneys.[1] Furthermore, stomach acid functions to kill pathogens that may enter the body via the foods we eat. Without adequate acid levels, we become more subject to infection as the pathogens reproduce in the low-acid environment.[2]

If not purple, then what are the solutions to GERD, indigestion, heartburn, gas, bloating, etc? Several well-established remedies exist that are essentially side-effect free.

■ *Hydrochloric Acid*. By age 50, many persons produce only 15% of the hydrochloric acid produced by 25 year olds, and over 35% of everyone over 65 produce no HCl. Because indigestion is sometimes worsened by the underproduction of stomach acid, increasing the level of HCl is often a remedy. By supplementing with *betaine hydrochloride*—an acidic form of the vitamin-like substance betaine—increased stomach acid levels can be achieved. Persons who have no indications of stomach ulcers should begin with 10 grains/650 mg. To determine the correct level, increase the dose by one capsule (or tablet) with each meal until a warm sensation is felt in the upper part of the stomach. Thereafter, reduce the dose by one capsule. If no warm sensation is experienced taking five capsules, continue at this level. Under no circumstances should more than five capsules be taken at a single meal. Also, take the capsules following the meal so that the stomach naturally produces as much acid as it's able. Betaine HCl is sold online and in health-food stores.

■ **Zinc & L-carnosine.** The Japanese have pioneered an effective treatment consisting of the combination of two powerful antioxidants: zinc and L-carnosine. The trace mineral zinc promotes wound healing by increasing tissue cell production. The amino acid complex L-carnosine, known to protect and rejuvenate cells, assists zinc in adhering to the stomach lining. In a human trial of 44 gastric ulcer patients taking 75 mg of zinc-carno-sine twice daily, moderate to significant improvement was noted in 80% of the participants. When examined by endoscopy, nearly 60% of the patients' ulcers had healed. Ninety percent of both the doctors and patients rated the product as useful to extremely useful. No adverse side-effects were noted.[3]

The mechanisms of action of the zinc-carnosine combination are not totally understood, although it is thought the promotion of cell growth and tissue healing is an important factor. Additionally, researchers at the Akita University School of Medicine have discovered that the zinc-carnosine combination promotes re-balancing of the GI system by promoting the expression of the protein HSP72 (heat shock protein) which enhances the protective ability of mucous membranes.[4]

Lane Laboratories manufactures Nature's Lining,® an analog of the zinc-carnosine combination studied in Japan.

■ **Potter's Acidosis.** Another effective remedy for indigestion and acid reflux has been sold in the United Kingdom since 1812. The product is Potter's Acidosis, which is a combination of the herb meadowsweet, the rhubarb plant and charcoal. Meadowsweet has been shown to have anti-ulcerative properties. Rhubarb is used in traditional Chinese medicine (TCM) to treat gastric disorders including bleeding ulcers. Charcoal is effective in reducing gas in the stomach and intestines.

Meadowsweet contains heparin, and therefore should not be used in combination with other blood thinners such as Coumadin® (warfarin), *Ginkgo biloba*, aspirin or heparin. Also, because charcoal can reduce the absorption of nutrients, minerals, and other medications, Potter's Acidosis should be taken on an empty stomach. It can be ordered on the internet at www.herbal-direct.com, or www.academyhealth.com (Click on "herbals." Scroll down to Potter's Herbal Medicines).

■ **Protexid.**™ Brazilian physician Dr. Ricardo Pereira has developed and tested a combination of readily-available dietary supplement ingredients which appear to eliminate heartburn and other symptoms of GERD completely. Dr. Pereira calls this product Protexid, and it contains the following ingredients in these daily dosages: melatonin (6 mg), L-tryptophan (200 mg), vitamin B6 (25 mg), folic acid (10 mg), vitamin B12 (50 mcg), methionine (100 mg), and betaine (100 mg). Melatonin is known to inhibit gastric acid secretion. It also inhibits nitric oxide (NO) production. NO causes relaxation of the sphincter muscle that protects the esophagus from stomach acid. By inhibiting NO, stomach acid is thereby prevented from entering the esophagus. The other ingredients have anti-inflammatory and pain-reducing effects.

As published in the *Journal of Pineal Research*[5] in 2006, Dr. Pereira tracked 351 patients who experienced symptoms of severe heartburn or regurgitation at least weekly. Patients ranged in age from 18 to 88 years, 60% of whom were women. One hundred seventy-five patients received Dr. Pereira's supplement formulation, while 176 received 20 mg daily of the popular proton pump (gastric acid) inhibitor omeprazole (Prilosec). Following seven days of treatment, the participants taking Protexid reported some relief of symptoms, while after nine days the Prilosec group experienced marked improvement. After 40 days however, only 65.7% of the Prilosec group reported elimination of their symptoms, another 2.3% obtained partial relief, while the remaining 32% experienced no relief at all. On the other hand, 100% of the Protexid group reported total elimination of their symptoms following 40 days of treatment. Every single one of the 175 participants taking Protexid for 40 days stated that all their GERD symptoms disappeared.

As is common with pharmaceutical drugs, side-effects in the Prilosec group were more pronounced than in the Protexid group. Two participants in the Prilosec group withdrew from the study due to persistent headaches. Ninety percent of the Protexid group experienced sleepiness, but none complained because they experienced improved sleep, which was a benefit. This effect was no doubt caused by the melatonin and tryptophan, and can be eliminated by taking Protexid at bedtime. To purchase Protexid, visit www.protexid.com.

■ ***D-Limonene***. Derived from orange peel oil, d-limonene has shown an impressive ability to treat heartburn and other symptoms of GERD. Most people taking just one 1,000 mg capsule either every day or every other day for 20 days have reduced or eliminated symptoms for at least six months.

Although the means by which d-limonene achieves its spectacular results has not yet been established, several mechanisms of action have been proposed.[6] 1) It may promote a more rapid transit of the digestive contents out of the stomach, 2) It may inhibit bacterial infection by providing a barrier to the stomach and esophagus, 3) It may reduce the amount of gastric components refluxed into the esophagus, and 4) According to Joe Wilkins, the Houston-based developer of the treatment, the small amount of burping experienced by those taking d-limonene coats the esophagus and protects it from the reflux of harsh digestive components.

In a trial evaluating d-limonene's effectiveness, 19 participants rated the severity of their heartburn symptoms at a level of 8 and the frequency of occurrence at 8.3 on a scale of 1 to 10, with 10 being the most severe and frequent. Following the consumption of a single 1,000 mg gelcap either every day or every other day, 86% of the participants reported a score of 1 or 2 on the severity index, while

92% of those taking the same amount of d-limonene every other day experienced the same result.[7]

In a double-blind study of 22 participants randomized to take either 1,000 mg of d-limonene or a placebo, 83% of those taking d-limonene for 14 days reported a score no higher than 2 on the 1-10 severity test, compared to only 30% of the placebo group. After 20 days, 75% of the d-limonene group reported relief from symptoms, while only 20% of the placebo group shared these results. Participants who experienced relief maintained this state for at least two weeks after discontinued use of d-limonene, while nearly 50% of the participants maintained relief for at least six months.[8]

Although none of the participants reported any adverse side-effects, d-limonene should not be taken by pregnant or lactating women or those who have or suspect they have stomach ulcers. Two effective products are Enzymatic Therapy's Heartburn Free with ROH10,™ and Life Extension Foundation's Natural EsophaGuard with ROH10.™

■ The remedies DGL (deglycyrrhizinated licorice) tablets and digestive enzymes are often effective in relieving the symptoms of indigestion. See also ***Irritable Bowel Syndrome.***

INSOMNIA. See ***Stress***.

INTERMITTENT CLAUDICATION. See ***Cardiovascular Disease***, ***Ultraviolet Blood Irradiation*** under **General Treatment Methods**, and the Member's area of *The Encyclopedia's* website.

IRRITABLE BOWEL SYNDROME (IBS)
Also called irritable colon, spastic colon, and nervous indigestion, IBS is characterized by symptoms which may include abdominal pain, bloating, constipation, cramping, diarrhea, and gas. The cause of IBS is debated, little understood, and at least to some extent probably differs somewhat from person to person. At one time IBS was thought to have a psychosomatic origin, but today most enlightened practitioners recognize the disease as having a physiological basis. Whatever the cause(s)—viral, bacterial, system imbalance, stress related, etc.—IBS affects tens of millions of people throughout the Western world. Closely related to IBS is Inflammatory Bowel Disease (IBD), an inflammatory dis-

ease of the bowel generally categorized as either Crohn's disease or ulcerative colitis, depending on disease criteria and location of the inflammation.

■ *DiarCare*.® Traditional Ayurvedic medicine offers a clinically evaluated solution to the symptoms of IBS. The treatment consists of the product DiarCare®—a formulation composed of the following traditional Ayurvedic herbs: bael tree fruit, conessi tree, guduchi stem, and pomegranate fruit.

In one study,[1] 45 participants who suffered from at least moderate diarrhea (loose stools 4-5 times daily, some 8-10 times daily) took one tablet three times daily for five days. Most of the participants began to respond by the second day, and diarrhea was "completely controlled" from the second to third day of treatment. All participants were monitored for at least three weeks, with no recurrence of symptoms or negative side-effects.

A second study[2] was conducted at Banaras Hindu University Hospital in Varanasi, India. Twenty-four percent of the 50 participants had chronic diarrhea for one month or longer; the remaining participants experienced acute symptoms—symptoms present for 7-14 days. Frequency of bowel movements for all participants was at least three times daily, with about 25% of the group having a frequency of more than 10 times daily. The dosage was two tablets three times per day for 10 days (chronic group) and two tablets three times per day for three days followed by one tablet three times daily for an additional two days (acute group). Seventy percent of all participants had the frequency of bowel movements reduced to 2-3 per day, with only one participant remaining at 7-10 per day. Most participants had reduced pain, gas, and abdominal discomfort with improved stool consistency.

In a third study,[3] 49 patients formally diagnosed with IBS took two tablets three times daily for 10 days, followed by three tablets two times daily for the next 50 days. Over 60% of the participants experienced 3-6 bowel movements before the study, with some as many as 10 or more. At the termination of the study, the frequency of bowel movements for more than 80% of the participants was reduced to 2-3 per day. Relief in other areas included decreased abdominal pain and weight loss.

Whether you suffer from chronic or acute symptoms of diarrhea or IBS, DiarCare is a po-

tent, all-natural remedy offering hope for those in need. To order DiarCare, contact Himalaya USA at (800)869-4640, or access www.himalayausa .com.

■ *Seacure*.® Another product that has benefitted many IBS sufferers is Seacure,® a dietary protein made from the fillets of deep-ocean white fish. Seacure emerged out of a global research effort to develop a marine protein source to supplement the diets of malnourished children in third world countries. According to a patented process, the fish protein is pre-digested into small peptides and amino acids by means of an enzymatic process incorporating natural fermentation. All of the vital nutrients in fresh fish, including the omega-3 fatty acids, are retained. The viscous liquid is dried into a fine powder and encapsulated for ease of use.

Several clinical studies have evaluated Seacure, and demonstrated its efficacy in supporting the cells of the GI tract as well as regulating bowel function in IBS patients.[4] For more information and to purchase Seacure, visit www.merc-buyers.com/SEA CURE.htm#5.

■ *Artichoke Leaf Extract*. Artichoke leaf extract has been shown effective in the treatment of IBS. As reported in *Phytotherapy Research*,[5] United Kingdom researchers found that a group of IBS sufferers studied for six weeks had significant reductions in symptoms. The extract was well tolerated, and 96% of the participants rated the extract as equal to or better than any other product they had tried. Artichoke leaf extract is available from health food stores or can be purchased on the internet by doing a keyword search for "artichoke leaf extract."

■ *Food Allergies*. Certain foods are irritants to the GI tract, and may aggravate the symptoms of IBS. Among the most common are citrus, corn, dairy products, eggs, peanuts and wheat. Additionally, food allergies have been known to cause a host of other ailments, including acne, anxiety, arthritis, asthma, chronic fatigue, depression, diabetes, eczema, food/sugar cravings, frequent urination, hyperactivity/ADD, migraines, muscle aches, obesity, perennial rhinitis, and psoriasis.[6]

US BioTek Laboratories offers mail-in tests that can help determine which food may be causing symptoms. For more information on their food allergy panels for assessing specific food sensitivities, visit www.usbiotek.com/services/allergy.htm, or call them at (206)365-1256. Another food allergy test, the ALCAT test, is offered by the AMTL Corporation. More information can be obtained by visiting www.alcat.com, or calling the AMTL Corporation at (800)881-2685.

■ *Lactobacillus plantarum 299v*. Commonly referred to as a type of germ, bacteria are uni- (single-) cellular organisms having a wide range of shapes—such as rods, spirals, spheres, etc.—and are typically only a few micrometers (microns) in length. It is believed there are from a half-million to five million different bacterial strains inhabiting Earth, although to date scientists have identified only about 4,000. Approximately 10 times as many bacterial cells as human cells reside on and within the body, and scientists have identified about 400 different species living within the stomach and intestines, although there are probably twice that number—totaling roughly 50-100 trillion individual cells collectively weighing three to four pounds. Of these many different types, most potentially harmful strains are rendered harmless by the body's immune system, although some pathogenic strains can cause a variety of diseases such as anthrax, bubonic plague, cholera, syphilis, and tuberculosis.

The beneficial bacterial strains living within the stomach and intestines perform important functions such as the production of acid mixtures that aid digestion; the production of vitamins; breaking down food stuffs into smaller molecules; the control of pH (acid/alkalinity) within the gut; and the control of harmful bacterial strains. One such beneficial strain is *Lactobacillus plantarum* 299v (Lp299v), a member of the lactobacillus family of "friendly" micro-flora that populate the human gastrointestinal tract. Studies have shown that Lp299v may produce up to a 90% decrease in the severity and frequency of IBS symptoms. It is referred to as a *probiotic*, a term put forward in 1992 denoting living microorganisms which upon ingestion exert health benefits beyond inherent general nutrition.

Lp299v has been extensively researched as a treatment for digestive disorders, and IBS in particular. Lp299v colonizes the lining of the intestines and forms a protective barrier against pathogenic

strains, thereby preventing these harmful forms from taking hold and flourishing. The disproportion of pathogenic strains within the gastrointestinal tract in relation to beneficial strains such as Lp299v is believed to be a principal cause of IBS. Chronic use of some pharmaceutical drugs including antibiotics—as well as the use of sugar, alcohol, and processed foods—depletes the GI tract of friendly micro-flora, with negative consequences.

Friendly bacteria including Lp299v aid in the manufacture of short-chain fatty acids such as butyric acid, which helps support the epithelial cells lining the gastrointestinal wall. The production of short-chain fatty acids also assists in nurturing the growth of friendly bacteria by maintaining the proper pH level in the gut. Unlike Lp299v, which has shown an exceptional ability to transit the stomach intact, most strains do not survive the passage through the acidic environment of the stomach, and are therefore unable to populate the large intestine.

In one study reported in the *European Journal of Gastroenterology and Hepatology*,[7] 40 IBS patients were divided into two groups. One group was administered Lp299v daily for four weeks, while the other group received a placebo. All participants treated with Lp299v reported resolution of their abdominal pain compared to only 11 in the placebo group. In those participants who were constipated, six out of 10 in the Lp299v group experienced a trend toward the normalization of stool frequency, while only two of the 11 in the placebo group shared this result. Regarding all IBS symptoms, 95% of the Lp299v group noted improvement compared to only 15% of the placebo group.

The lactobacillus strain Lp299v is patent-protected by its manufacturer, the Swedish firm Probi AB. It is sold in various European countries under the product name Lactobacillus 299v. To view a list of stores marketing Lp299v in the U.K. and Ireland, visit www.lp299v.co.uk/stocklists. In France, the product is marketed as BION® Transit. In the U.S., it is marketed by the firm Metagenics as LactoFlamX.™ Visit www.metagenics.com. To learn more, visit www.lp299v.co.uk/home.

■ *Bacillus coagualans*. Sometimes called *Lactobacillus sporogenes*, *B. coagulans* is a spore-forming bacterium (probiotic) which, as Lp299v, has the exceptional ability of surviving the harsh stomach environment, whereupon it successfully colonizes and proliferates. It has been shown to be an effective treatment for IBS and Crohn's disease.

■ The following drugs can contribute to diarrheal symptoms: Aldomet,® Cleocin,® Dulcolax,® Doxidan,® Maalox,® Milk of Magnesia,® Peri-Colace,® Ser-Ap-Es,® and Sumycin.® These drugs may cause constipation: Benadryl,® Cogentin,® and Maalox.®

KIDNEY STONES

Kidney stones are small, hard, sand-like crystalline particles that separate from the urine and form on the inner surfaces of the kidneys. Normally, urine contains chemicals that prevent this formation. However, in some people, these chemicals are ineffective and allow stone formation. Diet can play a role in stone formation, as can chronic dehydration and deficient levels of certain minerals.

The most common type of kidney stones are made of calcium. Stones tend to form under two circumstances. When the body becomes too acidic due to a high protein and/or high fat diet, alkaline minerals such as calcium are pulled from the bones to neutralize the over-acidic blood. The calcium is subsequently removed through the urine. Similarly, a diet deficient in calcium can result in calcium being pulled from the bones to increase calcium blood levels. Excess calcium in these two circumstances may lead to the formation of kidney stones.

The initial symptom of a kidney stone is severe, sharp or dull cramping pain, usually experienced in the back (above the buttocks) or side (below the rib cage), but also may be felt in the lower abdomen. Blood in the urine may also be present, and sometimes nausea and/or vomiting occurs. Pain may later spread to the groin area. If the stone is small enough, it will (sometimes painfully) pass from the body during urination. Kidney stones are diagnosed via X-ray or ultrasound (sonogram). The problem occurs when a stone is too large to pass during urination, which could result in damage to or failure of the kidney. If a stone is too large, surgery if often employed, or a technique called *lithotripsy*, where the stones are crushed into smaller pieces by a high-intensity acoustic pulse.

■ *Chanca Piedra*. Kidney stones can often be treated by drinking from two to three quarts of pure water daily, which assists the stone on its pathway through the urinary system. If this is ineffective, short of surgery or lithotripsy, there is another effective, less invasive, less expensive measure. An herb imported from the Amazon rain forest, *Chanca piedra* (literally meaning the "stone breaker"), known botanically as *Phyllanthus niruri*, not only assists the body in expelling kidney stones in one-to-three weeks at treatment dosages, but also helps prevent them from forming. The herb is also known to be useful in preventing and eliminating gallstones.[1] *Chanca piedra* has been used in the ancient Ayurvedic tradition as well.

It functions by relaxing the smooth muscles of the urinary tract, expanding them so that the stones pass more easily. Many studies have shown the herb is very effective in treating kidney stones, as well as a host of other ailments too numerous to describe. Because of its abortive characteristics, it should not be used during pregnancy. For more information on *Chanca piedra*, access www.rain-tree.com/chanca-techreport.pdf. To order, visit www.rain-tree.com, or call Raintree Nutrition at (800)780-5902.

■ *Lemon Juice*. A simple home remedy is often effective in dissolving kidney stones. Drink eight ounces of fresh-squeezed lemon juice followed by one ounce of lemon juice mixed with a glass of water. Repeat every hour for 12 hours. Lemon juice contains citric acid which dissolves the stones. The ascorbic acid form of vitamin C taken orally to bowel tolerance levels (until stool loosens) is also effective. Begin with 1-2 grams per hour.

LEG CRAMPS

Leg cramps during the sleeping hours can occur in both the young and old, the healthy and unhealthy, for a variety of reasons including abnormal hormonal or mineral levels; obstructed blood (oxygen) flow to the leg muscle(s); or pinched nerves.[1] Some believe the most common cause of nighttime cramping is a harmless but painful exaggeration of a normal muscle reflex. Muscles contract when we toss and turn, and remain contracted.[2]

■ *Quinine*. Quinine sulfate, a derivative from the bark of the cinchona tree (and a treatment for malaria), has been used successfully in the prevention of nighttime leg cramps. It works by decreasing the excitability of the leg muscles and nerves. Meta-analyses published in peer-reviewed journals have substantiated quinine's effectiveness in reducing the incidence of leg cramps, but not their severity and duration.[3]

However, quinine has some fairly serious potential side-effects including asthma, chest pain, disturbed vision, headache, nausea and tinnitus (ringing in the ears). This caused the U.S. FDA to remove it from OTC sales in 1994. Prescription quinine is not allowed to be labeled for use in treating leg cramps, although a sympathetic physician can prescribe it for your personal use.

Alternatively, most tonic water contains quinine and can be used by anyone seeking a solution to their leg cramps. Begin with six ounces of tonic water at bedtime. Discontinue if you experience allergic reactions such as headache, itching, or runny nose. Also consider Leg Cramps with Quinine,® a homeopathic formulation by Hylands which may also provide relief.

■ ***Vitamin K and Magnesium.*** Leg cramps also may be caused by the body's inability to assimilate calcium. Vitamin K (the unsaturated fatty acids *arachidonic, linoleic* and *linolenic acids*) is one of the best substances to help the body assimilate calcium into the cells. One of the best natural sources of vitamin K is raw, cold-pressed flax seed oil—preferably with a high *lignan* content. Barlean's Organic Oils and Omega Nutrition manufacture some of the best flax seed oil, both of which are available in many health food stores. The mineral magnesium is also useful in helping the body assimilate calcium. It is also a muscle relaxant, and is very effective in relieving nighttime leg cramps (especially in older individuals and pregnant women) at the dose of 400 mg of powdered magnesium citrate in water 30 minutes before bedtime.

■ ***Muscle Stretch.*** There is a simple and effective exercise that prevents nighttime leg cramps for many by exhausting the stretch reflex of the calf muscles. Just before retiring, stand about 2-3 feet from a wall, and lean forward with both hands touching the wall until you feel the calf muscles stretch. Hold this position for about 10 seconds, relax, and then repeat the exercise one more time.

■ ***Methyl Sulfonyl Methane*** (MSM). Both muscle soreness and cramps, particularly leg and back cramps, are often relieved by supplementing with MSM. Some race horse trainers administer MSM both preceding a race to prevent soreness and stiffness and after the race to prevent cramping. See MSM under **Arthritis** for more information.

■ ***Vitamin E.*** The well-respected physician Robert Cathcart III, M.D. has reported that vitamin E is useful in preventing nighttime leg cramps. He believes it to be safer and more effective that quinine. At the dosage of 300 IU daily, Cathcart has reported that vitamin E is "almost universally effective" in treating nocturnal leg cramps of unknown origin.[4] The dosage of 300 IU was arrived at after considerable experimentation. Lesser quantities were found to be ineffective.

■ Leg muscle pain also can be caused by oxygen insufficiency resulting from cardiovascular disease. See ***Padma 28*** ® under ***Cardiovascular Disease***. See also **Pain Relievers**, and the Member's Area of *The Encyclopedia's* website.

LYME DISEASE

Symptoms of what is now known as Lyme disease were reported in the European medical literature as early as 1883,[1] although its diverse set of symptoms were not recognized as being caused by a single infectious agent until the mid-1970s. In 1977, the disease was dubbed "Lyme" following an outbreak of arthritis in a group of children clustered in and around Lyme, Connecticut.

In 1982, Swiss researcher Willy Burgdorfer, Ph. D., isolated a spirochete (SPY-row-keet; a bacterium) from the midgut of the adult black-legged deer tick *Ixodes scapularis*. The spirochete, called *Borrelia burgdorferi* (Bb), now bears the name of its discoverer. A spiral, corkscrew-shaped bacterium, the spirochete is able to swim its way through the blood and burrow itself deep within tissues of the brain, organs, muscles, tendons—literally anywhere in the body.

Conclusive evidence that *B. burgdorferi* causes the disease came in 1984 when spirochetes were cultured from the blood and cerebrospinal fluid of patients with Lyme symptoms.[2] While the official number of people in the U.S. having Lyme disease is less than 200,000, many other respected and knowledgeable researchers believe the true numbers are much higher.

The generally accepted position is that Lyme disease is transmitted to humans by the bite of either the black-legged deer tick *Ixodes scapularis* (in the northeast and north-central U.S.), *Ixodes pacificus* (on the West coast of the U.S.), or similar ticks in other parts of the world. The tick generally attaches to a creased or otherwise protected area such as the armpit, back of the knee, nape of the neck, navel, or groin. Researchers have determined the tick usually doesn't begin to transmit the infection until 36-48 hours after the initial bite.[3]

One of the hallmarks of Lyme disease is an expanding rash, *erythema migrans* (EM), which occurs in 60-80% of all cases. The rash appears either as a red, expanding rash or blotch, or a central spot surrounded by unaffected skin which is ringed by an expanding red rash, giving the appearance of a "bulls-eye." The rash may have a bruise-like appearance on dark-skinned people. (An allergic reaction to tick saliva may cause redness of the skin even in the absence of spirochete infection.)

The rash usually radiates from the site of the tick bite, but can occur in other locations. It appears from 3-30 days following disease transmission—usually within one or two weeks—and persists for 3-5 weeks; averages 5-6 inches in diameter, although the range is from two inches to two feet; and is usually not painful or itchy. There may be swelling of the lymph glands near the puncture site, headache, or general achiness.[4]

As the untreated disease progresses, there can be two or more rashes distant from the site of the bite; abnormal pulse; facial paralysis (similar to Bell's palsy); fever of 100-102° F; headache; multiple enlarged lymph glands; pain in the joints, muscles, and tendons; severe fatigue; sore throat; stiff, aching neck; tingling and/or numbness in the extremities; and visual changes. As the disease further progresses there may be arthritis in one or two large joints and disabling neurological disorders such as confusion, dizziness, lack of concentration, short-term memory loss, and "mental fog."[5]

According to the U.S. Centers for Disease Control, diagnosis following a recent tick bite should be made on the basis of symptoms and the evidence of a bite, and *not* on serological (blood)

tests which can give false results especially if given within the first month following infection. Thereafter, the CDC recommends the ELISA and Western-blot blood tests. However, if serious symptoms persist and Lyme infection is suspected but not detected by these two tests, the Polymerase Chain Reaction (PCR) test offers a more reliable assessment. Because the ELISA and Western-blot tests are not as accurate and reliable (test may incorrectly indicate no infection) as the PCR, a negative indication by either should not be considered a definitive indication of lack of infection.[6] A new, more accurate diagnostic technique is described below.

Treatments. Traditional treatment during the early stage of the disease consists of a 3-4 week course of the oral antibiotics doxycycline or amoxicillin. For persons who can't take penicillin or tetracyclines, cefuroxime, axetil or erythromycin is recommended.[7] According to an article in the *New England Journal of Medicine*,[8] a four-week course of oral doxycycline is just as effective in treating later stage Lyme as an intravenous course of ceftriaxone (Rocephin®). However, if neurological or severe cardiac abnormalities are present, later-stage Lyme may require one or more courses of IV treatment. A small percentage of late-stage Lyme patients are chronically treatment resistant—and may respond slowly or incompletely—with symptoms persisting for months or even years. For these patients, several courses of oral treatment are generally required, or IV treatment. A course of antibiotic IV treatment longer than 4-6 weeks is not typically recommended due to possible adverse side-effects.[9]

To this point in our discussion of Lyme, the "traditional" view of the disease has been presented. A growing number of researchers and clinicians world wide, however, are painting an altogether different picture of the disease, with important ramifications for both diagnosis and treatment. At the basis of their contentions are the following. Lyme disease, they believe, is:

❏ not just tick-borne

❏ easily transmissible via blood (insects, etc.)

❏ difficult to eradicate

❏ difficult to detect due to its stealth attributes

❏ more prevalent than currently believed

❏ associated with many other chronic diseases, including Alzheimer's, ALS, Parkinson's, and MS.

Having led the discussion on the alternative view of the nature of Lyme disease was Lida Mattman, Ph.D., Professor Emeritus of Biology at Wayne State University, and former Director of Research at the Laboratories of the United Nations. Dr. Mattman's contention was that *Borrelia burgdorferi* is a "stealthy" bacterium that is much more difficult to detect than previously believed. While most bacteria have cell walls as part of their physical structure—making them relatively easy to identify—certain forms of the Bb bacterium do not.

Bb is known as a *cell wall deficient* (CWD) form of pathogen. As such, it is both more difficult to detect and more difficult to treat. It is typically the presence of a pathogen's cell wall that evokes much of the body's immune response. If unrecognized by the immune system and not identified as a major threat, the pathogen evades the body's mechanisms which ordinarily offer protection against these foreign invaders. Also, Bb seems to be a *pleomorphic* organism; i.e., it is able to change its structural identity into multiple forms. There is reason to note Dr. Mattman's opinions, as it was she who wrote the book on this type of stealthy pathogen. Her book, *Cell Wall Deficient Forms: Stealth Pathogens*, is a monumental work of over 400 pages.

According to Dr. Mattman and others, the Bb bacterium is present in a much larger portion of the population than is currently believed, and is associated with many other diseases than is commonly recognized, including ADHD, Alzheimer's, arthritis, Bell's palsy, chronic fatigue syndrome, chronic pain, fibromyalgia, heart disease, irritable bowel syndrome (IBS), lupus, multiple sclerosis (MS), Parkinson's, schizophrenia, scleroderma, and a host of additional diseases.[10]

Dr. Mattman found live Bb spirochetes in blood and spinal fluid, and also in amniotic fluid, breast milk, semen, tears, urine, and vaginal secretions.[11] She's also found them in fleas and mosquitos. Accordingly, she believed the bacterium is not only transmitted by tick bites, but also may be transmitted from person to person via blood and saliva, and from insects (or other organisms) to humans.

As reported[12] in 1999, Mattman detected the live Bb spirochete in all eight Parkinson's patients tested, all 41 MS cases tested, all 21 cases of ALS, and in every case of Alzheimer's tested. Based on her findings, she believed Lyme is much more prevalent in society than is currently acknowledged. What this means is that the Lyme spirochete may be implicated—at least a contributing factor—in a variety of other degenerative illnesses without a suspected Lyme connection.

This view is supported by other Lyme researchers such as Dan Kinderlehrner, M.D., who told viewers of the June 10, 2002 *Today Show* that the true incidence of Lyme in the U.S. may be as high as 18 million cases, closer to 100 times the number reported by the CDC.[13] Still other investigators believe Lyme may be a contributing factor in at least 50% of all chronically-ill people.[14]

Fortunately, another researcher has discovered a new means of diagnosing Lyme disease that appears to be 100% accurate. Jo Anne Whitaker, M.D., former Director of Central Florida Research, Inc. in Winter Haven, Florida, developed a test to identify the bacterium itself (antigens) as opposed to detecting antibodies (immune response agents) as do the ELISA and Western Blot tests. The importance of this is that if Bb is in some way sequestered away from the immune system or the immune system isn't producing antibodies to the bacterium, the disease will go undetected.

The new diagnostic test, called the Rapid Identification of Borrelia burgdorferi (RIBb), uses a fluorescent molecule which is able to attach to both the spirochete and cell wall deficient forms of Bb. When a specimen is viewed microscopically under a fluorescent light source, Bb-positive structures are observed to fluoresce.[15] Dr. Whitaker also has developed a (titration serial dilution) method for quantizing the amount of Bb found in the blood. This enables a practitioner to assess the effectiveness of various treatment methods by determining the amount of pathogen destroyed. In addition to Lyme testing, Central Florida Research laboratory also tests for co-infections frequently associated with Lyme, including *Babesia microti* (a parasite of red blood cells) and *Ehrlichia phagocytophila* (a bacterium observed in white blood cells).

Working with Dr. Whitaker, Dr. Mattman cultured Bb in hundreds of blood samples evaluated as positive by the RIBb, thus confirming the accuracy of the RIBb test as virtually 100% sensitive to the Lyme microbe, with virtually no false positives (indicating infection when there is none) or false negatives (incorrectly indicating no infection).

At the present time, the RIBb test is available only through Central Florida Research. A blood sample can be mailed to their offices in Winter Haven, FL, with results being available in 24-hours. The cost of the test is USD $250. To contact the laboratory, call (863)299-3232 or visit http://centralfloridaresearch.com.

Concerning treatment, the antibiotics amoxicillin and Rocephin function by inhibiting the cell wall formation of bacteria. Because Bb may be present in forms other than those having a cell wall, these medications are likely to be less effective than desired. Doxycycline and clarithromycin, on the other hand, are protein inhibitors and may be more effective in treating cell wall deficient forms of the disease.[16] Mynocycline may also be effective in treating Lyme. It has been shown effective in treating rheumatoid arthritis, a disease linked to cell wall deficient forms of bacteria.

■ *Cat's Claw*. A new addition to the Lyme treatment armamentarium is a special form of the herbal product Cat's Claw, botanically identified as *Uncaria tomentosa*. Cat's Claw contains powerful alkaloid compounds including *tetracyclic oxindole alkaloids* (TOA) and *pentacyclic oxindole alkaloids* (POA). Most commercial Cat's Claw products contain both alkaloids. Many on the cutting edge of infectious disease treatment with natural compounds believe it is the POA constituents that are the true active agents, and that the presence of even a small percentage of TOA inhibits POA effectiveness. In fact, TOA-free Cat's Claw contains significant quantities of several *quinovic acid glycosides*, the active chemical basis of the popular quinolone antibiotics, of which ciprofloxacin (Cipro®) is the most well-known. This helps explain the herb's potent antibiotic (both viral and bacterial) effects.

These understandings have led to a TOA-free Cat's Claw product. Several small clinical studies as well as many anecdotal reports have found that TOA-free Cat's Claw brings symptom relief to a high percentage of Lyme sufferers, and works seeming miracles for others.[17] The herb *artemisinen* is sometimes used in combination with excellent results. To learn more, visit www.samento.com.ec/sciencelib/sammain.html.

Two companies marketing TOA-free Cat's Claw are Allergy Research Group (Nutricology)

and Nutramedix. Prima Una de Gato® is Allergy Research Group's product, and can be ordered by calling (800)545-9960 or by visiting www.nutricology.com. Nutramedix's product is called Samento,® and is available in both liquid and pill form. The one ounce bottle of liquid, according to the company, is equal to 20 bottles of Samento capsules at the price of only slightly higher than one bottle of capsules. Samento can be ordered by calling Nutramedix at (800)730-3130 or by visiting their website at www.nutramedix.com.

■ *Spiro*.™ A combination formula by Raintree Nutrition, Inc. of Carson City, NV offers hope to Lyme sufferers. Spiro consists of six herbs which traditionally have been used for a variety of ailments by many Indian tribes of the Amazon. Combined into a single formulation, Spiro has shown effectiveness in a limited, informal, non-placebo controlled study undertaken by Raintree Nutrition.

One hundred participants who tested positive for Lyme took Spiro twice daily for three months. Most of the participants suffered from chronic Lyme. At the end of the testing period, many of the participants anecdotally reported that Spiro had changed their lives for the better. Ten of the participants re-tested for the presence of Lyme. All 10 tested negative. Spiro is available as a concentrated liquid extract from Raintree Nutrition by calling (800)780-5902 or (775)841-4142, or by ordering at www.rain-tree.com.

■ *Sodium Chlorite*. A substance that has shown effectiveness in treating Lyme is sodium chlorite ($NaClO_2$). This substance offers hope for many conditions caused by microbial infection from viruses, bacteria, fungi, or parasites. Lyme is one such condition. To learn more about this powerful anti-infective, see **Sodium Chlorite** under **General Treatment Methods**. See also Lyme disease in the Member's Area of *The Encyclopedia's* website.

MACULAR DEGENERATION

The retina is the light-sensitive inner lining on the back surface of the inside of the eyeball. It contains an array of millions of light-sensitive cells called *rods* and *cones*. When light strikes the rods and cones of the retina, the biochemical reaction that occurs initiates electrical impulses which are transmitted to the brain. These signals communicate information about light intensity, color, and position, and are assembled, processed and interpreted within the brain into the perception of visual images.

The *macula* is a small area in the central portion of the retina about the size of this letter "O." It is located directly opposite the lens and is rich in cones, the photosensitive cells that enable detailed vision and the perception of color. Macular degeneration (MD) is a disease that causes the photosensitive cells of the macular portion of the retina to malfunction and at times may progress to a total loss of function. This results in a diminishing or loss of detailed vision and/or vision in the center of the field of perception (straight ahead vision).

Although there are forms of MD that are hereditary, known as Juvenile Macular Degeneration (including Best's disease, Sorsby's disease and Stargardt's disease), the most common form occurs in people over the age of 55, called Age-Related Macular Degeneration (AMD, or ARMD). ARMD is the leading cause of legal blindness (vision 20/200 or less with eyeglasses) in the developed world among those over the age of 65, with more than 17 million Americans having symptoms of the disease and over 500,000 new cases being diagnosed in the U.S. annually.[1] This disease affects just under 20% of Americans aged 55-64, 25% of Americans aged 65-74, one third of Americans 75 and older, and about 130 million people worldwide. The current understanding regarding the cause of MD is that it is likely influenced by both genetic factors (family history) and environmental factors including diabetes, head injury, infection, diet, and a history of light exposure.[2]

Symptoms of MD can vary from person to person, with only one or both eyes affected. Typical symptoms include 1) a blurry, dark area or "white-out" in the center of vision, 2) straight lines appear wavy or distorted. The center of vision may appear more distorted than the image toward the periphery, and 3) perception of color changes. [Floaters (moving "cob-webs" caused by floating debris), cataracts, and dry eye are not known to be related to MD.][3]

There are two forms of ARMD, known as the "dry" and "wet" forms. At least 70% of those with ARMD have the dry form, which is characterized by thinning of the macular tissues and the formation of *drusen* (fatty waste deposits) on the macula. The remainder have the wet form, which typically involves bleeding within or behind the retina, opaque deposits, and a progression toward the formation of scar tissue. Ninety percent of all cases of legal blindness are the result of the wet form of ARMD.[4]

Three stages of ARMD are typically defined:

❍ *Early ARMD*. One or both eyes contain either several small, yellow fatty drusen, or a few medium-sized drusen. No vision loss occurs during this stage.

❍ *Intermediate ARMD*. One or both eyes contain either many medium-sized drusen, or one or more large drusen. Little or no vision loss occurs during this stage.

❍ *Advanced ARMD*. The presence of drusen, and additionally a degradation of light-sensitive cells of the macula (dry), or leakage of fluid or bleeding from blood vessels under the retina (wet).

Several techniques are used to diagnose MD: 1) When viewing an *Amsler grid*, some of the grid lines appear wavy, and some portions of the grid appear blank or otherwise abnormal. To take the Amsler grid test, visit www.macular.org/chart.html, or do a key word search for "amsler grid," 2) Visual acuity, as measured by a standard Snellen eye chart, has declined to 20/80 or lower, 3) Fundus photographs of the retina indicate the presence of drusen spots in dry MD, 4) Angiography indicates a leakage of indicator dye from blood vessels behind the macula in wet MD, and 5) An electroretinogram of the macula indicates a weaker or absent electrical signal in comparison to a normal eye.

The progression of the disease may slow or stop for many years depending upon a number of factors including the nutritional status (diet) of the individual. Only one eye may be affected during its early stages. However, as the disease progresses it is not unusual for both eyes to become affected. Upon its diagnosis, several techniques are available that treat MD with varying degrees of success:

❒ In younger individuals with Juvenile Macular Degeneration, surgical removal of scar tissue is sometimes successful. In older individuals, however, this type of surgery is less successful.

❏ Laser surgery, called *photocoagulation*, is used with some success in individuals with wet MD whose vision is 20/70 or below. Photocoagulation does not improve vision, but often is able to reduce further loss of vision by coagulating (sealing) leaky blood vessels, thereby preventing or slowing further leakage. Only about 50% of those with wet ARMD are candidates for photocoagulation surgery, and it is effective in only 50% of these cases.[5]

❏ Low vision aids such as sophisticated magnifying devices help enable MD sufferers to adapt to the handicap.

❏ Several pharmaceutical companies are developing new drugs to treat MD, particularly wet MD. Most of these drugs are currently under development, and it remains to be seen how effective they may be, and whether they will be plagued by the unwanted side-effects that typically accompany pharmaceutical drugs. To view a list of drugs currently under development and/or enroll in a clinical trial, visit www.retinaconsultants.org/RC/Trials.htm. Other techniques offer true help for those suffering from MD.

■ *Micro-Current Stimulation*. Low intensity electrical stimulation of various parts of the body has been used for decades in treating a variety of ailments. For example, TENS units use electricity to control pain, as discussed under *Electricity* in the section on **Pain Relievers**. Small electrical currents applied to the head are used to treat stress and addiction, as discussed under **Stress**. Medical researchers now use electricity in treating MD.

Micro-current stimulation (MCS) has been shown to stop the progress of MD in some individuals, and actually reverse the disorder to a degree in others. Although it is effective on both the dry and wet forms, the consensus is that MCS is more effective in treating the dry form. Micro-current stimulation applies low intensity electrical signals to various specific points around the eye. The treatment is simple, painless, and takes only several minutes once or twice daily.

Several modes of action may explain MCS's effectiveness. It is known that those who suffer from MD have a significantly decreased blood flow to the retina—about a 30% lower volume compared to healthy eyes.[6] It is also known that low level electrical stimulation increases blood flow significantly, thereby increasing nutrient supply to the tissues and increasing the ease of cellular waste disposal. It is also theorized that the photoreceptor cells of the eye receive a boost in energy due to increased production of ATP, the energy chemical of the cells. Whatever physiological mechanisms are involved, MCS provides measurable vision improvement in about 60% of MD sufferers who use the device.

In 2002, the *Townsend Letter for Doctors & Patients*[7] reported on several studies of various eye disorders treated with MCS. A two year study of 114 subjects was conducted by Grace Halloran, Ph.D. during the years 1983-1985. Of the 18 patients with MD, 16 showed improvement following treatment. Sixty two of the 78 patients with Retinitis Pigmentosa improved; and 16 of the 18 persons with various retinopathies improved.

A 10 year clinical study of 400 eyes with MD resulted in 78% of the eyes showing from 1-9 lines of improvement in reading the visual acuity chart. Over 50% of the eyes studied improved from 2-9 lines. In a two-year preliminary study of 120 subjects by the Macular Degeneration Foundation, there was a 68% improvement over pre-treatment vision in those with dry MD, and a 58% improvement in subjects with the wet form of MD. Thirty percent of the participants with dry MD experienced a 100% or more improvement over pre-treatment vision, while nearly 17% gained 150% or more. (Because MCS effectively increases the blood/nutrient flow to the retina, an integral part of the treatment involves supplementing with specific antioxidant nutrients that are known to nourish the eye, as described later in this section under *Prevention Through Nutrition*.)

It is important to point out that MCS and TENS units may differ in certain important respects, and that the units cannot necessarily be used interchangeably. Appropriate MCS units use a chip that continually adjusts current levels according to the body's resistance. Several units are available for home use, but require a doctor's prescription. Ophthalmologist and pioneer MCS researcher Dr. Edward Kondrot's website is www.healingtheeye.com.

Because the U.S. FDA has not approved MCS devices for the specific treatment of eye disorders, including MD, no claims can be made in the U.S. by the equipment manufacturers as to their effectiveness. Their use in the U.S. for eye diseases is a legal, off-label use of the device, however. To learn more about MCS and macular degeneration, visit Dr. Edward Kondrot's website or read his book *Microcurrent Stimulation: Miracle Eye Cure?*

■ *Intravenous Glutathione.* In the June 2001 edition of *The Townsend Letter for Doctors & Patients*,[8] it was reported that intravenous administration of the master antioxidant *glutathione* is able to stop the progression of MD, and often reverse the condition to some extent. After glutathione is given, there is a noticeable reduction in the size of the *scotoma* (a blind or dark spot in the visual field), as measured by tests including a standard eye chart. Following glutathione administration, the size of the scotoma is often reduced by 50%, and patients are able to read one or two lines lower on the Snellen eye chart.

The lasting effects of visual improvement vary from person to person, but usually last weeks to months. A slight return to the original state may occur in some individuals. Treatments are sometimes given weekly, or multiple times per week, with additional treatments increasing the beneficial effects. Intravenous glutathione is effective in treating both the wet and dry forms of MD. Dr. Jonathan Wright of the Tahoma Clinic in Renton, WA and Dr. Stanley Covert of Elk, WA are specialists in this procedure.

Dr. Covert describes the procedure as follows: IV glutathione is obtained from a compounding pharmacy at the strength of 200 mg/cc. The typical starting dosage is 1,000 mg, and is sometimes increased to 1,500 mg. A 20cc syringe is used to withdraw the glutathione, the remainder of the syringe being filled with normal saline. The solution is given over a 15 minute period through a 25 gauge butterfly in the dorsum of the hand. No adverse reactions have been noted.

■ *Stem Cell Implantation.* One treatment that's close on the horizon is stem cell implantation. Stem cells are the master cells of the body. They are undifferentiated cells that give rise to the body's many varieties of specialized (differentiated) cells. They are, in effect, the precursors of specialized cells. The unique function of stem cells is that they can grow into virtually any other type of cell, as need-

ed. It has been shown that stem cells can in fact grow into photosensitive light receptor cells in the retina.

So-called *totipotential* cells can differentiate into virtually any other type of cell in any location of the body. Researchers have harvested these resting omnipotent cells and injected them into sites in the macula of persons with MD. After awakening the cells by various processes, these cells are then able to replace the defective, dying or dead retinal cells.

One organization currently treating MD (and several other eye diseases) with stem cell therapy is the XCell-Center. For more information, visit www.xcell-center.com.

■ *Retinal Transplantation.* Further out on the horizon is the actual transplantation of retinal tissue into the diseased eye. This approach is yet experimental, and will also likely take years to evaluate its safety and effectiveness.

Prevention Through Nutrition. The October 2001 edition of *Archives in Ophthalmology*[9] announced to the world that the risk of developing MD is significantly decreased in certain groups of people by taking a combination of antioxidants. Specifically, the combination consists of vitamin C (500 mg), vitamin E (400 IU), beta-carotene (15 mg), zinc (80 mg) and copper (2 mg).

The study, known as the Age-Related Eye Disease Study (AREDS; sponsored by the National Institutes of Health's National Eye Institute) which used 4,757 participants, concluded this combination of nutrients will delay the progression of advanced ARMD in persons at high risk for the disease—namely, those with intermediate ARMD in both eyes, or those with advanced ARMD in one eye. This group of people experienced a 25% reduction in disease progression and a 19% reduction in vision loss over a five year period. (Those participants having no ARMD or early ARMD received no apparent benefits.)

Previous research has suggested that persons who eat a diet rich in dark, green leafy vegetables are at lower risk of developing ARMD. However, the antioxidant levels used in the AREDS study would be difficult to attain through dietary intake alone.

Other antioxidant nutrients also provide protection against ARMD. Of the many carotenoids in the diet, the human retina accumulates only two: lutein (LOO-tea-in) and zeaxanthin (zee-uh-ZAN-thin). There is such a high concentration of these two carotenoids in the macula they are visible as a dark yellow spot (macular pigment). Zeaxanthin is known to absorb light of blue wavelengths, that portion of the spectrum which is harmful to human eyes. By so doing, photoreceptor cells—rods and cones—are prevented from injury or death.

The beneficial effects of these two carotenoids were first reported in 1994 in the *Journal of the American Medical Association*. Since that time, other studies have provided additional documentation.[10] (Both lutein and zeaxanthin were commercially unavailable at the time of the AREDS study.) While the antioxidant combination studied in AREDS is believed only to slow the progression of ARMD in high-risk groups, lutein and zeaxanthin are believed to retard its development.[11]

Other substances thought useful in the treatment and prevention of MD, and generally recognized as powerful eye nutrients, are bilberry extract, flavonoids, *Ginkgo biloba* extract, omega-3 fatty acids, N-acetyl-cysteine, riboflavin, selenium, and taurine.

MAD COW DISEASE

(Bovine Spongiform Encephalopathy; BSE)

Most people reading this book don't own cows. That's a privilege reserved for select groups of people—generally only dairy farmers and cattle ranchers. Excepting India, where cows are traditionally regarded as sacred, societies have relatively few uses for the beast outside of their agricultural value. Although you'd find they're nice enough creatures if you ever had the chance to spend some time with one, for most Westerners a cow is both too large an object and too large a liability to keep as a pet.

Many people, especially city-dwellers, have never even seen a cow up close and personal. To these people, for all they know, cows may not even really exist! But we know they do, because we see them on T.V., and unless this is *The Truman Show* all over again, cows probably really do exist.

We know that watching cows on T.V. can't harm a person—unless you watch too many of them—and that will only hurt your eyes. So what's

the problem if there's such limited contact between cows and the majority of people? The problem is that people really *do* come in contact with cattle—most of us on a daily basis. They're stretched over our feet, draped over our backs, and sat on while we drive our cars and watch T.V. And, well, we eat them, too. And therein lies the rub. Whatever happens to the cow, so it may very likely happen to us. You are what you eat. Get it?

Bovine (cow) Spongiform (sponge-like) Encephalopathy (brain disease), or BSE, popularly known as Mad Cow Disease, is bad news in a protein particle. It can be transferred to humans by various routes, which will be discussed. BSE is a particularly lethal disease against which little progress has been made. The disease has a human counterpart—called Creutzfeldt-Jakob (CROITS-felt YAW-cob) disease (CJD)—and the symptoms are similar to those observed in cattle. Some researchers believe BSE/CJD is so threatening it may one day eclipse AIDS as a killer of humans. If it is not already clear from reading the above material on diabetes, cardiovascular, and other diseases discussed in this writing, the present section will serve to further elucidate the reality that consuming animal flesh has serious potential drawbacks.

BSE was first observed in British cattle as early as 1985. The symptoms of the disease mimic those of the spongiform disease *scrapie* which is found in sheep, so named because infected animals tend to scrape themselves against fences, walls and other objects. Scrapie in sheep is a neurological disorder characterized by the "staggers" (lack of coordination), behavioral changes and, as the disease progresses, microscopic holes form in the brain giving it a sponge-like consistency.

Scrapie has been known for some 200 years, and has been present in the U.S. since 1947. In 1990, the U.S. Department of Agriculture (USDA) reported that 7,500 sheep in 39 states in the U.S. were infected.[1] In 1952 a voluntary eradication program was launched, but this was found to be ineffective. A compulsory eradication program was then enacted which some years later was discontinued by the USDA "because it would be perceived by the public that it [scrapie] was a threat to health."[2]

Although it is not conclusive scrapie is a public health threat, there is growing evidence that it could pose a more serious problem than once thought. At the least, it could be upsetting to a consumer to realize the animal upon which he is supping may have died from a disease that rotted the animal's brain and spinal cord.

The cause of both Mad Cow Disease and scrapie is believed by many/most BSE researchers to be an infectious version of a specific type of protein particle called a *prion*—rhymes with neon. The prion theory was originally proposed in 1982 by University of California San Francisco biochemist Dr. Stanley Prusiner, for which he was awarded a Nobel Prize. Even though infectious, the prion is neither a virus nor bacterium, but a protein particle gone awry. These proteins are bent abnormally (misshapen) and appear to be able to infect normal prions by bending them into a similar form. Misshapen prions accumulate in the brain, causing the formation of spongy gaps. These particles are assumed to be many times smaller than viruses.[3]

There are, however, other interesting theories regarding the origin of BSE put forth by scientists of considerable repute. One such theory is the brainchild of Anthony R. Parish, Ph. D., a Fellow of the New York Academy of Sciences, and a year before his death was selected for inclusion in *Who's Who in the World* (2001) in recognition of his many years as a leading medical researcher. Dr. Parish believed animals are being poisoned by industrial chemicals, and the poisons are further transmitted to the offspring. Prions, he believed, are merely symptoms of the underlying cause. You can read more about Dr. Parish's theory at www.gerry parish.co.uk/research/bse/.

Also on the chemical bandwagon is British organic farmer Mark Purdy. Purdy believes BSE was caused by the compulsory spraying of organophosphate pesticides such as phosmet to combat a British plague of Warble fly. These chemicals, in turn, activated a prion mutation in cattle. Purdy also believes the mineral manganese is a co-factor. He found that high levels of manganese were sprayed on British cattle along with the pesticides. He further discovered that infected clusters of U.S. deer and elk have an association with high levels of manganese. Also, he believes that radioactive minerals from the Chernobyl nuclear accident—including manganese—are part of the problem. Purdy's view is that because of the huge potential liability of the chemical companies involved, and the coverup of this aspect of the Chernobyl accident, the true causal agent(s) will never see the light of day.

The culprit particle, call it a prion or by any other name, appears to be a totally new infective agent having neither DNA nor RNA. Deadly nevertheless, the spongiform diseases caused by these agents can be transferred to other species both by injection and orally.[4] Their infectivity cannot be destroyed even at temperatures of 360 degrees Celsius, and they also appear to be resistant to radiation and most disinfectants, including bleach.[5] Infected animals have been buried for up to three years and upon exhumation, their remains are still infectious.[6]

The most infective parts of affected animals are referred to as the *offal* (appropriately pronounced "awful"), which consists of any tissues of the brain, spinal cord, intestines, lymph nodes, spleen, thymus, and tonsil. Blood also has been shown to be infective, as will be discussed. Other tissues also could transmit infection.

For decades, producers of food animals have incorporated the remains of sheep, chickens and cows into the animal feed of cattle as well as other animals. Many of the animals rendered into animal feed are diseased with infectious agents such as scrapie. It is now generally accepted (with certain notable exceptions, as mentioned) that Bovine Spongiform Encephalopathy, or Mad Cow Disease, originated as the result of cattle being fed scrapie-infected sheep, including the byproducts of infected sheep such as bone meal—which is often an ingredient in pet food. In an effort to avoid waste and inexpensively produce animals for human consumption, every bit of an animal is recycled for use. Dr. Raymond Burns, head of the alternative uses program of the Kansas Department of Agriculture told *The New York Times* in a 1996 interview, "We use everything but the squeal, the cluck, and the moo."[7] And in some cases, diseases are thrown in at no extra charge.

About four billion pounds per year of "inedible" parts from cows, chickens, pigs, road kill and other animals are ground down and recycled into animal feed in the form of meat, bone meal and blood meal.[8] Tallow and gelatin are also produced in this process. About 30% of the recycled product is used in pet food, 30% in chicken feed, 20% in pig feed and the remainder in beef and dairy cattle feed.[9] It's simply a matter of economics.

Also—and don't let Bowser or Buttercup read this—it's standard practice for some rendering plants to recycle house pets back into animal food. According to a 1997 *New York Times* article, each month the city of Los Angeles alone ships 200 tons of euthanized dogs and cats to rendering plants to be recycled back into animal food.[10] Additional reading on recycled house pets is found in Ann Martin's books *Food Pets Die For: Shocking Facts About Pet Food* (©2000), and *Protect Your Pet: More Shocking Facts* (©2001). Contact New Sage Press, (877) 695-2211; www.newsagepress.com

Disabled cattle that die from either known or unknown causes are called "downer" cows, and constitute a group known as 4-D animals: dead, dying, diseased and disabled, the majority of which are recycled into animal feed. Before the outbreak of Mad Cow Disease in Britain in the mid-1980s, the recycling of animals into animal feed was considered a trade secret of the feed companies.[11] Now, because of BSE, worldwide attention has been focused on the practice.

The lack of American media exposure to these important albeit controversial subjects should signal some cause for concern, particularly when issues involving public health go unreported or under reported. For two decades, Britain and Europe have been afire with the Mad Cow controversy and the human deaths believed to result from eating contaminated beef.

Although to date the human death toll has reached 150—most being permanent or temporary residents of Britain—Britain has slaughtered upward of five million cows infected or believed to be infected with BSE, at an expense of billions of dollars. In a gesture of helpfulness the Cambodian government suggested that, as an alternative to incinerating these millions of infected animals, they be used to detonate some of the 10 million land mines, about 140 mines per square mile, that remain following the Cambodian civil war.

Over 180,000 BSE cases have been documented in Britain to date, and more than 70 cases per week were being reported as of 1996.[12] After that time the incidence declined dramatically, with only 30 cases being reported throughout Europe in 1999. In the year 2000, however, the incidence surged slightly to more than 100 cases,[13] which once again caused concern. To date, BSE has spread to cattle

in more than two dozen countries, including Austria, Belgium, Denmark, France, Germany, Holland, Italy, Ireland, Poland, Portugal, Spain, Switzerland, Sweden, and Japan. Britain, however, remains the focal point of the outbreak.

When the disease first struck, England's top scientists were fearful of what the future could bring. Thames Valley University Professor of Food Policy Tim Lang stated,

> We are in a mass experiment which is killing us. Never before have diseased ruminants (sheep) been fed to other ruminants (cows) and then fed to humans. We have interfered with the whole process of nature and what is now happening is one of our worst nightmares. This is a tragedy on a massive scale. The Government has been so totally stupid. Even now they are still employing crisis management techniques and damage limitation exercises.[14]

Microbiologist Richard Lacey of Leeds University stated:

> ...we are now estimating that next [21st] century the typical number of...human cases will run at between 5,000 and 500,000 a year..The only logical approach for the human population in the U.K. is to avoid all beef products.[15]

Dr. Lacy's colleague, Dr. Stephan Dealler of Leeds University Medical School, believes that "no one who knows enough about this subject would feed their daughter a beef burger."[16] It is Dr. Dealler's opinion that those eating infected meat have a 50/50 chance of acquiring spongiform encephalopathy. In an article published in the *British Food Journal*, Dr. Dealler stated that by the year 2001, most adult British meat-eaters will have ingested a potentially fatal dose of BSE-infected beef,[17] which could be as small as one gram of infected meat.[18] (One gram is the approximate weight of half of one U.S. dime.) Other researchers believe that infection may be transmitted by as little as one or two infective molecules, depending on the state of a person's immune system.

It is unfortunate to note that during the years 1982 to 1992, roughly 13 tons of meat, bone meal and other meat-related by-products implicated in the British epidemic were imported by the U.S. from Britain.[19] It is humorous to note that after the news of the initial human spongiform cases in Britain, the burger giant McDonald's posted window signs advertising "veggie" burgers instead of beef[20]—such was the uproar about Mad Cow Disease and its potential to infect humans.

Contributing further to the uneasiness is the fact that over 100 cats in Britain have died from feline spongiform encephalopathy, presumably the result of eating contaminated pet food.[21] The spongiform disease also has infected mice and pigs, as well as zoo animals such as antelope, cheetah, eland, elk, kudu, marmoset, ocelot, ostrich and puma,[22] all presumably infected from contaminated feed.

In the U.S., a form of *transmissible spongiform encephalopathy* (TSE) is being found in other animal populations as well. Referred to as *chronic wasting disease* (CWD), it has been found in white-tailed deer, mule deer and elk in Colorado, New Mexico, Utah and Wyoming, and mule deer in Nebraska and Saskatchewan, Canada. CWD also has been found in captive elk herds in Colorado, Montana, Nebraska, Oklahoma, South Dakota, and Saskatchewan as well as in captive white-tailed deer in South Dakota. CWD is spreading quickly.

As mentioned, the human counterpart of BSE is Creutzfeldt-Jakob Disease, and the symptoms are similar to those observed in cattle. In addition to being caused by meat consumption, CJD is known to occur spontaneously at the annual rate of about one case per one million people, or roughly 300 cases per year in the U.S. This type of CJD, called sporadic CJD, has been known for decades prior to the discovery of BSE in the early 1980s. The cause of sporadic CJD is unknown. The variety of CJD caused by eating meat manifests with slightly different symptoms, and is labeled *new variant* CJD, or nvCJD (also called vCJD). There can be a long incubation period for either type of CJD, producing a latency period of as long as 10-40 years before symptoms manifest,[23] although symptoms typically manifest much sooner. vCJD tends to occur in younger people than sporadic CJD, and often produces more psychotic symptoms.

Now Americans are aware of Mad Cow Disease, although it has received surprisingly little press coverage in the U.S.—until the U.S.'s first mad cow was discovered just in time for Christmas, on December 24, 2003. Prior to this incident, Americans witnessed a brief display of bravado by the beef industry during the Oprah Winfrey trial, the culmination of a lawsuit brought by Texas cattlemen

against Ms. Winfrey. During her television program which aired April 16, 1996, after learning some of the facts surrounding Mad Cow Disease Oprah exclaimed, "It just stopped me cold from eating another burger."[24]

The trial did not provoke the U.S. press to engage in dialogue concerning the difficult questions surrounding BSE including its possible transmission to humans. Rather, the media side-stepped the issue in favor of vacuous nightly discussions of the trial in a manner characteristic of American journalism in the late 20th century.

Do Mad Cow Disease and CJD pose a threat to the health of Americans? Many related to the U.S. beef industry say, "No way!" The beef industry has always maintained, both preceding and even following the U.S.'s first mad cow incident, that the U.S. beef supply is not a threat to the Americans—or the countries who import U.S. beef. However, it may be wise to take a lesson from the Brits.

In 1988, the British established a prestigious committee of scientists to evaluate the potential health threat in England. The Southwood Committee reported that it is "most unlikely that BSE will have any implications for human health."[25] But British politicians and their scientific community quickly began whistling a different tune. In March of 1996, the government-convened Lord Phillips Inquiry stated as many as 136,000 people could lose their lives to vCJD. Since the time of that Inquiry, the Blair administration upped the estimate to as many as 250,000, and believes the worst case scenario is one out of every 250 British citizens dying from CJD. Various agencies continue to publish conflicting information on how many might be infected.

Noted scrapie specialist, the late Dr. R.F. Marsh of the School of Veterinary Medicine at the University of Wisconsin, stated for years that the U.S. already has its own form of Mad Cow Disease. Dr. Prusiner, the premier proponent of prions, agrees with Dr. Marsh.[26] Adding to this view Dr. Joseph Gibbs, a researcher at the U.S. National Institutes of Health, has stated, "I'm convinced that BSE has occurred here."[27] Most serious BSE researchers agree with Marsh, Prusiner, and Gibbs. In vehement disagreement with these views—insisting that BSE is not a problem in the U.S.—is the $40 + billion per year U.S. cattle industry which slaughters 35+ million cows annually.

The infection of U.S. cattle could be the result of recycling 4-D cows back into the food of living cows.[28] Dr. Marsh estimated that in Wisconsin alone, 35,000 downers per year have been shipped to renderers who supply the recycled protein product for use in animal feed and also possibly human foods such as ground beef (hamburger) and hot dogs.[29] In the U.S. there is an incidence of hundreds of thousands of downer cows in a given year—conservatively estimated to be about 200,000.[30] Some have estimated the incidence to be as high as 15,000 per day. It is further estimated that up to 400,000 people could be infected by a single infected animal entering the food chain.[31]

An incident that occurred in 1985 at a Stentsonville, Wisconsin mink ranch gives support to Dr. Marsh's beliefs concerning transmission of BSE via downer cows. All the minks at this ranch were destroyed as the result of Transmissible Mink Encephalopathy (TME) after consuming a diet consisting of more than 95% downer cows.[32] It is also known that spongiform encephalopathy has been transmitted to laboratory chimpanzees and pigs, and researchers believe there is the potential of crossing other species barriers.[33]

On numerous occasions, the U.S. Congress tried to enact a law to prevent the use of downer cows as human foods, but on each occasion the beef industry exerted sufficient pressure to scuttle such attempts. Fortunately for U.S. consumers, shortly after the detection of U.S. mad cow #1, the USDA announced the banning of all downer cows from use in human foods, dietary supplements and cosmetics. Under continued industry pressure, whether or not the ban will have legs strong enough on which to walk remains to be seen. This is an important issue, as shown by a 2001 German study which found that downer cows are up to 240 times more likely to be infected with BSE.[34] Even if the ban is enforced, however, potentially-infected downers are still allowed to be used in feed for pigs, chickens, and other animals, which then is allowed to be fed back to cattle—and humans.

Dr. Paul Brown, a leading CJD researcher at the U.S. National Institutes of Health, believes that humans may be able to contract BSE by eating either infected meat, meat byproducts or by contact with products containing infected animal ingredients. Products such as facial creams, moisturizers, shampoos, gelatin (including the gelatin used to encapsulate many nutritional supplements and pharmaceuticals) and even floor wax contain animal ingredients that are potentially infective, although there is no conclusive evidence that CJD can be acquired by these means.[35] On the other hand, correlational studies discussed below raise cause for concern. To view a list of hundreds of products made from bovine (and other animal) sources, see **Appendix C**.

On October 20, 2000, the United Kingdom Department of Health issued a recall notice for oral polio vaccines produced by the British manufacturer Medeva, near Liverpool. The Department of Health was concerned that Medeva used potentially-BSE-infected material from British cattle in 11 million doses of polio vaccine that have been administered to children and adults over the last decade. The problems surrounding the polio vaccine could be merely the tip of the iceberg. Medeva also manufactures vaccines for flu, tuberculosis, tetanus and hepatitis B. Medeva's Fluvirin® has been used by some 20 million unsuspecting Americans. U.K. Liberal Democrat Norman Baker stated:

> The Department of Health and the MCA [U.K. Medicines Control Agency] have completely failed to act in the interest of public health. In their desperate attempts not to undermine the vaccination program, they have tried to sweep all problems under the carpet. As a result, public confidence has been shattered. When will they learn that the answer is not to cover up, but to identify problems and deal with them immediately?[36]

Shortly thereafter, the Canadian Broadcasting Corporation announced the Canadian government is studying whether or not BSE could exist in products that contain beef byproducts such as vaccines and cosmetics. Several childhood vaccines, including diphtheria, tetanus and polio, contain bovine byproducts.[37] Virtually all vaccines (whether or not they are grown in tissue cultures that include tissue from bovine sources, which some are) are nourished (fed) with bovine fetal cells. Even the British Southwood committee admitted the greatest risk of human BSE infection would come from either contaminated vaccines or other injectable medications (insulin, hormone-based drugs, etc.; see **Appendix C**) prepared from infected bovine tissues.

The following is a short digression into the nature of vaccinations. In addition to the above-mentioned problem of BSE contamination, it is now widely recognized by many researchers that vaccines are plagued by contamination from other sources as well, including preservatives such as formaldehyde, mercury and polysorbate. Also, because of their intimate contact with animal material, vaccines often are contaminated with harmful microbes such as viruses. In addition, miscellaneous animal-sourced fragments of RNA and DNA can be contained within the finished vaccine, forming latent proviruses that can later become activated as diseases such as arthritis, cancer, and lupus.[38] Vaccinations also seem to play a significant role in the onset of autism and diabetes.

There is a further fact relating to vaccinations that is often overlooked—especially by the allopathic medical community, not to mention a large percentage of the unknowing public. Namely, the efficacy of vaccinations is seriously in question, despite all of the (largely-government-sponsored) advertising to the contrary. In other words, do vaccines really work? Are they able to confer immunity to humans against the diseases they are designed to combat?

The answer to this question is controversial, but many within the medical research community believe that vaccines are ineffective—in fact, they do not work as proposed (and advertised). In spite of the fact that vaccines are heavily promoted by trade organizations such as the American Medical Association, and government agencies such as the National Institutes of Health (NIH), the Centers for Disease Control (CDC), the Food and Drug Administration (FDA), and the World Health Organization, there are many reasons to believe they are ineffective, if not harmful.

Most people view vaccines as a modern wonder medicine that has rescued humanity from the ravages of many once-highly-feared diseases—including diphtheria, influenza, measles, pertussis (whooping cough), smallpox, and tetanus. A more thorough investigation paints a different picture altogether. If one examines the annual incidence from 1900 to present of the many diseases for which vaccines are available, a most revealing pattern jumps straight off the paper. All of the diseases, without exception, show a steady decline from 1900, continuing to decline directly through the years during which these vaccines were introduced, up to the present. In fact, by the time vaccines were introduced (mostly from the mid-1940s until the mid-1960s), the diseases they were designed to fight were almost nonexistent.

Improved nutrition and sanitary conditions are generally believed to be the reasons for this gradual but steady decline in the incidence of most diseases against which we continue to vaccinate. "Twenty shots by the age of two!" says Uncle Sam, whose activities help support a multi-billion dollar per year industry. Voicing an opposing opinion, in November 2000 members of the Association of American Physicians and Surgeons unanimously passed a resolution calling for an end to all government-mandated vaccination programs in the U.S.

For more information, contact the National Vaccine Information Center at (703)938-0342, or www.nvic.org; view Dr. Len Horowitz' CD *On Vaccines*. Good books include Alan Phillips' *Dispelling Vaccination Myths* and Neil Miller's *Immunization: Theory Versus Reality*.

Now, back to the beef. Of the roughly 300 people in the U.S. that die from sporatic CJD annually, there have been only several establishment-reported cases of CJD in the U.S. that "official sources" admit could have been caused by consuming infected beef. Researchers now believe that any form of CJD—both sporadic and vCJD—may be related to consuming infected meat. The sometimes 10-40 year incubation period before symptoms manifest probably masks the true incidence.

Many scientists world wide now believe CJD is being mistaken and misdiagnosed for other diseases such as multiple sclerosis; dementia; viral infections such as meningitis and encephalitis; and Alzheimer's disease. Today, about 10% of Americans over the age of 65 have Alzheimer's, and nearly 50% who live beyond 70 years will develop some form of dementia during their lifetimes. In July 1990, an editorial in the *Lancet* suggested that CJD is often misdiagnosed for Alzheimer's. The authors of the editorial propose that whereas 30-40 cases per year of CJD in Britain are documented, a more accurate figure would be 4,500.[39] The symptoms of CJD and Alzheimer's are similar—demented behavior and steadily increasing lack of coordination followed by death. Autopsied victims' brains are found to be shrunken and riddled with microscopic holes. Complicating the issue of monitoring and detection, in the U.S. fewer than 15% of corpses are autopsied. Furthermore, the CDC does not require reporting of CJD cases.

Presently there are four to five million cases of Alzheimer's in the U.S., with tens of thousands of new cases occurring each year. The disease claims 50,000 American lives annually, and the incidence of the disease is expected to more than triple by mid-century. This could mean that tens of thousands of people may be afflicted with and dying from an undetected meat-related spongiform disease each year. The incidence of CJD itself has been on the rise in several Western countries for the past 10-15 years. These are issues few discuss, especially politicians and members of the media.

In 1989, doctors at the Veterans Administration Hospital in Pittsburgh, Pennsylvania consecutively autopsied 54 patients who had been demented. They discovered three of these patients had been victims of CJD—a rate of about 1,000 times higher than expected.[40] Additionally, Gareth Roberts, an Alzheimer's and dementia expert for SmithKline Beecham Pharmaceuticals, reviewed brain samples of 1,000 patients collected from 1964 to 1990. Roberts found 19 CJD cases upon reexamination, whereas only 11 had been detected initially. This represents a 40% error in misdiagnosing CJD patients. Similar results have been found in other studies.[41]

For over a decade scientists, physicians, citizen's groups and even some government agencies recommended to the FDA and USDA that a ban be instituted on feeding ruminants to ruminants. In 1993, the Foundation for Economic Trends petitioned the FDA to stop the practice of feeding ruminant animal protein to animals. In 1994 the FDA seemed to agree that such a ban was necessary, and published a proposed ban in the Federal Register. However, the ban was shouted down by the rendering and livestock industries. The USDA's Animal and Plant Inspection Service explained that "the cost to the livestock and rendering industries would be substantial" and that a change in the present policy "could pose major problems for the U.S. livestock and rendering industries."[42]

In June of 1997, the U.S. FDA finally enacted a feed ban—of sorts. Most knowledgeable scientists from around the world have suggested the only way to stop the spread of BSE is a total ban preventing all mammalian protein from being used in animal feed. The new regulations put forth by the FDA came far short of that goal. In fact, the regulation is actually not a ban at all, but rather a labeling requirement stating that meat and bone meal from ruminants is to be labeled "Do Not Feed To Ruminants"—a wholly voluntary practice on the part of the meat industry.[43]

Even though the USDA maintains there is 99% compliance with this regulation, investigations by the General Accounting Office, the organization that carries out investigations for Congress, has shown the enforcement of the "ban" is lax. According to the 1997 regulation, cattle are not to be fed meat, bone meal, or other products of ruminants (cattle, deer, elk, goats, and sheep). However, in 2001 the FDA published the results of a national survey of rendering plants and feed mills, showing up to 25% of the plants in violation of the "ban."[44]

Many BSE experts, not to mention other humans who still maintain intact brains, believe the regulation as it is presently set forth—even if it were enforced—is a case of too little, too late. The ruling has serious shortcomings:[45]

♦ Cow tallow (solid fat) and cow blood are allowed to be fed to cattle. NIH Medical Director Dr. Paul Brown demonstrated in his laboratory that blood is a carrier of TSEs. Many other studies have confirmed this.[46] Yet, according to the 1997 FDA "ban," massive amounts of cattle blood are allowed to be fed to calves in milk replacer, "calf starter," and feed supplements [47] because it's an inexpensive source of protein. Dr. Prusiner has called this practice "stupid."[48] (In a partial attempt to deal with this issue following the U.S.'s mad cow discovery, in January 2004 the FDA proposed a rule preventing mammalian blood and blood products from being fed to other ruminants as a source of protein).

♦ Pigs, chickens, fish, horses and other animals are allowed to be fed to their own species.

♦ Pigs, chickens, fish, horses and other animals are allowed to be fed to cattle.

♦ Both healthy and known spongiform-infected animals, including cattle, are allowed to be used in feeds for pigs, chickens, horses, farmed fish as well as—look out Fido and Fluffy—pet food. These animals are then rendered and all of their parts fed to their own species and also to cattle. This creates a potentially-infectious "feeding loop" that can only serve to increase the incidence of spongiform diseases. Also, chicken and other animal manure is often used to fertilize human food crops, including organic crops. The potential ramifications are huge.

Before the U.S. ban was enacted, a National Institutes of Health Advisory Panel recommended to the FDA that a total ban on all mammalian protein in animal feed be instituted, as the European Union has put into place. Given the magnitude of the potential threat to large segments of the meat-eating population of the U.S.—and even vegetarians—the enactment of more stringent regulations for recycled meats would seem to be a no-brainer—which makes one wonder what kinds of foods our lawmakers have been eating.

An article in the March, 1998 *Seattle Weekly* newspaper concluded their treatise on Mad Cow Disease with the following words:

> For the time being, we'll dally with partial bans and uncertain risk reduction while the price of not being careful enough is slowly tallied in England. There, the unleashed prions are silently burrowing their way through the brains of an unknown number of future victims.[49]

And so it came to pass that as the U.S. dilly-dallied, and placated the interests of the big beef business by not enacting stricter bans on cattle feed—and not strictly enforcing such regulations as were enacted—the first case of U.S. BSE was detected. These lax practices will no doubt lead to other incidents and detections—provided that the overseeing monitoring agencies and institutions are "allowed" to report what is actually occurring in the field. Because such vast sums of money ride on the backs of the cattle herds, there's always room for slight of hand in matters such as these.

During the decade of the 1990s, while many industry analysts and scientists clearly saw the ensuing public health crisis, the cattle industry employed 143 lobbyists on Capitol Hill, 28 of whom were previous congressmen or congressional aids. The watchdog group Center for Public Integrity reported that the food industry "managed to kill every bill that has promised meaningful reform."[50] The power held and pressure exerted by industry forces are tremendous. During the 1990s, for ex-

ample, the U.S. meat industry spent $41 million financing the political campaigns of members of the U.S. Congress, with more than one third of the money going to House and Senate agriculture committee members—including such personages as Tom Daschle, Trent Lott, Newt Gingrich, and Dick Gephardt.[51]

Immediately following the announcement of America's first mad cow, high-level government and industry officials saturated the media assuring Americans that the U.S. food supply is the safest in the world—a tactic reminiscent of what occurred in England and other countries at the beginning of their mad cow problems. In late 1986 when the British government became aware of BSE, its initial internal memo warned the disease could bring "severe repercussions to the export trade and possibly also for humans." Because of this, the memo suggested, all news regarding BSE was to be kept "confidential."[52] In 1996, Agriculture Minister Douglass Hogg assured the British public they had nothing to fear from the disease, and that "British beef is wholly safe."[53] Three months later Health Minister Steven Dorrell broke the sad, mad news to the British Parliament.

Similar downplaying of the potential BSE problem also occurred in several other countries. In 2001, a French Senate investigation found their Agriculture Ministry minimized the potential threat of BSE, and "constantly sought to prevent or delay the introduction of precautionary measures" because such measures "might have had an adverse effect on the competitiveness of the agri-foodstuffs industry."[54] In 2002, a similar investigation accused the Japanese Agriculture Ministry of "serious maladministration" by siding too heavily with the meat-producing industry.[55]

In early 2004, U.S. Agriculture Secretary Ann Veneman assured the American public the U.S.'s first mad cow had been an isolated incident, and that all is well in beefdom—"we remain confident in the safety of our food supply." Even a cursory look beyond the media fanfare reveals a different and more complex story. One recent revelation is that Alisa Harrison, Secretary Veneman's spokeswoman, came to the USDA from the National Cattleman's Beef Association, where she occupied the position of Director of Public Relations. In this position she battled against the installation of government food safety regulations on behalf of her employer, the cattle industry's largest and most powerful trade group.[56] It has also come to light that Dale Moore, Secretary Veneman's Chief of Staff, was previously the chief lobbyist for that same organization.[57] Other high-level positions at the USDA are held by former meat-packing executives, and even a former president of the National Pork Producer's Council.[58] You can read more about this issue in **Appendix B** under The Revolving Door.

One of the assurances given by Secretary Veneman was that "muscle cuts"—including steaks and roasts—are no danger to the consumer since only brain and spinal cord tissue are infective. Not to confuse the issue with facts, but in 2002 Nobel laureate Stanley Prusiner published an article in the *Proceedings of the National Academy of Sciences*[59] revealing that high prion levels, including the disease-causing isoform (PrP^{Sc}), were found to be present in the skeletal muscles of experimental animals (mice), and that skeletal muscles allow active prion replication. In addition, it is well known that lymphatic tissues and fluid can contain high titers (concentrations) of prions. Prusiner stated these findings "raise the concern that humans consuming meat from prion-infected animals are at risk for acquiring infection."[60]

Boneless cuts also can be contaminated when the animal is cut in half with a band saw, a routine practice in meat processing. Such cuts are made down to the spinal cord, thereby aerosolizing the spinal cord and contaminating the surrounding meat. A recent European study revealed that meat from animals slaughtered in this manner showed a 100% level of contamination.[61]

Yet another part of the story that goes largely untold is a further method by which cattle are processed. In 1994, American meat processors began using a system called *advanced meat recovery*, or AMR, in order to "increase yields and profitability." The majority of U.S. meat processing plants currently use AMR, having invested $40 million on this technology since 1994. Although the brain and spinal cord are supposed to be removed before AMR is initiated, spinal cord remnants often remain intact. Even though the European Commission considers the removal of these parts as "the single biggest contribution that can be made to reducing the risk to humans,"[62] legislation to require

removal of the spinal cord before processing has been opposed by all of the major meat-producing industry groups including the National Cattleman's Beef Association, the National Meat Association, the National Renderer's Association, and others.

In 1997, when the consumer advocacy group Public Citizen obtained USDA inspection records through the Freedom of Information Act (FOIA), it was learned that a significant percentage of AMR samples were contaminated with brain and spinal cord tissue. The USDA responded by instructing the meat inspectors to continue testing the meat for possible contamination rather than requiring the spinal columns to be removed before being processed by the AMR system.[63] Over the next three years, from 1997 to 2000, the USDA took only 60 samples, some of which were contaminated with central nervous system (CNS) tissue.[64]

In 2001, researchers at Colorado State University published the first major study of AMR meat. They reported that "well over 50%" of samples tested from beef neck bones were contaminated with CNS tissue.[65] The researchers also visited seven major beef suppliers of prominent fast food chains across the U.S. Six of the seven sites inspected had CNS tissue in their hamburger patties.[66] When the USDA's inspection results were made public in 2002, 30 of the 34 meat processors tested (88%) were producing beef containing CNS tissue, and 96.5% of the samples contained potentially-infectious bone marrow.[67]

For those curious minds who want to know the answer to the proverbial question "Where's the (contaminated) beef?," the answer is that most AMR beef is found in beef jerky, ground beef (hamburger), hot dogs, and sausages, as well as pizza toppings, taco fillings, and beef bouillon and stock.[68]

One of Secretary Veneman's assurances was that measures would be taken to insure the removal of spinal cord material from the food supply. Given the fact that AMR technology is such an integral component of the U.S. meat processing industry, and that multiple tens of millions of dollars would be lost in the time-consuming task of totally removing spinal material from cattle prior to processing, skeptics have assumed a wait-and-see posture—knowing the American public does not follow these issues with great discernment. Also promised is a tracking system capable of tracking each and every cow throughout its life on planet Earth. Because of the possibilities of using this technology for tracking other (unnamed) animals, this part of the plan is likely to be put into place.

Meat mavens should also take note that other cuts of meat are potentially contaminated, notwithstanding Dr. Prusiner's research on muscle tissue contamination. The "T" in T-bone steak is actually a vertebra from the animal's spinal column and may contain a section of the spinal cord. Other potentially-contaminated cuts include bone-in rib steak; chuck blade roast and loin (if bone containing); porterhouse; prime rib with bone; and standing rib roast. These cuts may include spinal cord tissue and/or dorsal root ganglia which also have been shown to be potentially infectious.[69]

Bovine byproducts such as milk, and milk's byproducts such as cheese, ice cream, yogurt, etc., are also quite suspect. In December 2003, Britain's Secretary of Health announced that BSE had been passed from an infected blood donor to a human recipient. According to Dr. Robert Cohen (www.notmilk.com), an average quart of milk sold in the U.S. contains over 300 million dead white blood cells. Cohen reasons that if BSE can be passed through blood from human to human, it may also be passed from cow to human through aspects of blood contained within milk. That's enough to ruin anybody's hot fudge sundae.

Virgil Hulse, M.D., author of the 1996 groundbreaking classic *Mad Cows and Milkgate*, believes that consuming milk, even when pasturized—notwithstanding the possibility of BSE contamination—puts one at risk for Hodgkin's disease, leukemia, lymphoma, multiple myeloma, multiple sclerosis, and cancers of the breast, colon, and prostate. Got milk? Got medical insurance?

Even though the above information is damning, these facts may not cause many Americans to worry about their meat supply because of the rigorous inspection procedures in place which guard against defective and inferior cattle entering the U.S. from foreign countries such as Canada. Retired meat inspector Bill Lehman, who worked in the 1990s at the Sweetgrass, Montana port of entry for Canadian beef, quickly bursts that bubble.

After contaminated meat caused the *E. Coli* deaths of several children in the 1990s, Lehman went public with his observations. He stated that

he was allowed merely to walk to the back of the incoming trucks and observe. He was not allowed to touch animal carcasses or open boxed meat. He couldn't use a flashlight or walk into the truck. He was allowed only to observe what he could from the back of the tractor-trailer. He stated that he once inspected over 80,000 pounds of meat in under one minute—after which he stamped the paperwork "USDA Inspected and Passed."[70]

Lehman described some of the meat as containing,

> pus-filled abscesses, sticky layers of bacteria ...obvious fecal contamination, stains, metal shavings...chemical residues, salmonela, added substances, and advanced disease symptoms."[71]

When he saw it, he rejected it—up to 2.3 million pounds of beef imports annually. What USDA meat inspectors aren't allowed to see is served for lunch and dinner to unsuspecting Americans.

Whether originating from the U.S. or from another country, the next-to-the-last destination of the (non-dairy) cow is the meat packing plant. (The final destination, of course, is your stomach...) In the U.S., four meat packers control 85% of the market: ConAgra, Excel (a subsidiary of Cargill), IBP, and National Beef. As reported in his recent book *Been Brown So Long It Looked Like Green To Me*,[72] Jeffrey St. Clair describes a typical day at the Pasco, Washington IBP plant. The key to understanding the "success" of the operation is that the dangerous and complex network of conveyor belts and overhead chains and hooks runs as fast as possible. Time is money, and plant managers don't want the production line stopped for any reason.

If it's true that "haste makes waste," it's also true that haste makes for unhealthy beef. Workers are under extreme pressure to keep up with the production line as cows—some dead, some alive—go whizzing by. Workers often urinate on themselves for fear of being fired for taking a bathroom break. Meat is routinely contaminated with feces and human urine because workers don't have time to wash their hands. When meat falls on the floor, which is typically littered with unsavory entrails and other cow parts, it is often placed back on the production line without being washed. According to the workers at the plant, cutting tools and conveyor belts are regularly coated with pus from abscesses and tumors that time hasn't permitted to be properly excised from the carcasses. "They don't care about the cows or the cow shit on the meat. They've got quotas to meet," say the workers.[73]

Some cows survive the 200 mile-per-hour bolt that's either driven through their heads or impacted against them. Research has shown that regardless of which stunning technique is used, CNS material may become disbursed across the dressing environment of the slaughterhouse. Also, CNS material may enter the bloodstream of the animal, and can travel to the lungs or other parts of the body.[74] Often, according to the IBP workers, cows are not rendered unconsciousness before processing begins, and the animals frantically moo as they are dismembered and skinned alive.[75] All in all, not a very pretty picture for either man or beast.

Back to the bureaucrats. Dr. Prusiner is on record as having warned Secretary Veneman six weeks prior to the first U.S. mad cow discovery that it was "just a matter of time" before BSE was detected in the U.S.[76] Prusiner told *The New York Times* that he encouraged Veneman to begin immediate testing of every cow showing signs of illness, and eventually every cow upon slaughter.[77] Fast, accurate, and inexpensive tests are available, Prusiner told *The Times*, including one he patented through his university (UCSF).

In Japan and Europe, every adult cow is tested for BSE upon slaughter, and test results are known before the animal enters the food chain. France alone, having a fraction of the U.S. cattle population, tests more cows in one week than the U.S. tests in 10 years. In 2003, the European Union tested 10 million cattle for BSE, while the U.S. claimed to have tested 1-3% of its herds. Upon closer investigation, it was found that only about 20,000 cows were tested during each of the years 2002 and 2003, even though the USDA refused to make those records available to United Press International (UPI)—even upon threat of legal action.[78]

Retired USDA veterinarian Dr. Michael Schwochert told UPI he was always concerned that the U.S. never used the same rapid-testing procedure used in many other countries. Said Schwochert, "It was almost like they didn't want to find mad cow disease."[79] Supporting this notion is the fact that although the U.S. supplies about 25% of the world's beef, it was the 24th country to detect its first mad cow. With the average (non-dairy) cow being slaughtered by the age of two—far too young to display any outward signs of BSE—testing is the only means of evaluating the safety of cattle. Without a testing program, diseased animals will continue to slip by undetected.

Several U.S. beef producers have gone public stating they would like to test every animal at their own expense, only to be refused permission to do so by the bureaucrats at the FDA and Department of Agriculture—which brings to mind the ancient Chinese proverb which states that "if you don't look, you won't find what you're not looking for."

Another former USDA veterinarian, Dr. Lester Friedlander, pointed out that an outbreak of BSE within the U.S. would likely dwarf the outbreaks in Britain and other countries due to the size of the U.S. beef market both within and outside of the U.S. Billions of people world wide are at risk of potential exposure to infected meat.[80]

According to a 1997 FDA document,[81] *even if* a total feed ban were put in place immediately after the detection of the first mad cow in the U.S., 299,000 additional cases of infection would occur due to the long, invisible latency period of BSE and its spread via infected feed. "If a feed prohibition were not implemented at that time, the number of deaths would be much higher," said FDA officials.[82]

When one considers the precarious situation in its totality, it's clear that the beef business in the U.S. is a disaster in the making. Considering the high incidence of dementia in the U.S.—almost 50% of all people over the age of 85—it takes a brave individual to contemplate the possible BSE connection, and to consider the unthinkable. Interestingly, the committee which awarded Dr. Prusiner a Nobel Prize noted that his discovery of prions may eventually shed light on Alzheimer's disease. Only time will reveal how prophetic were these words.

Are Other Animals A Potential Threat? In 2001, French researchers discovered a strain of scrapie that caused brain damage closely resembling sporadic CJD in mice. Because there are several types of sporadic CJD and more than 20 strains of scrapie, it's been difficult to demonstrate a link between CJD and lamb consumption. However, the French researchers concluded that some cases of sporadic CJD may be caused by some strains of scrapie.[83] An article in the journal *Neuroepidemiol-*

ogy[84] agreed that some cases of sporadic CJD may be caused by eating infected sheep meat. Because scrapie occurs in epidemic proportions in the U.S., this should cause great concern to Americans.

Pigs are also a potential source on spongiform infection. Research has shown these animals are indeed susectable to spongiform encephalopathy.[85] In the U.S., slaughterhouse waste is allowed to be fed to pigs because no case of spongiform encephalopathy has ever been detected in their population. Because American pig farmers typically slaughter these animals at only five months of age—long before symptoms would be expected to manifest—detecting the presence of a spongiform disease in this population would be difficult.

According to a 2002 issue of the industry publication *National Hog Farmer*,[86] hundreds of thousands of downer pigs—crippled by injury or illness—are sold to slaughterhouses every year. Several epidemiological studies have confirmed a link between sporadic CJD and pork consumption. Consuming roast pork, pork chops, smoked pork, ham, hot dogs, and scrapple (pork pudding) may be a risk factor in developing CJD, according to the researchers. Those who include ham in their diet, for example, were 10 time more likely to develop CJD than those not eating ham.[87]

It is presently unclear whether or not consuming chicken meat poses a risk. Even if it were found that poultry is not susceptible to the disease, some researchers believe they are likely silent carriers. Dr. D. Carleton Gajdusek, a Nobel laureate for his research on prion diseases, told *Dateline NBC* in 1997 that "it's got to be in the pigs as well as the cattle. It's got to be passing through the chickens."[88]

In the U.S., slaughterhouse refuse including cow brains, eyes, spinal cords, intestines, manure, and blood are still allowed to be fed to chickens (and other poultry), pigs, and domestic house pets—which in turn can be re-fed to these animals. (In January 2004 the FDA stated it would ban the use of poultry litter in cattle feed.) Should it be surprising that sporadic CJD has been associated with weekly beef consumption,[89] and the consumption of roast lamb,[90] veal, venison,[91] and North American seafood?[92] Even though the Cattleman's Beef Association stated in the early 1990s that there are economically-feasible alternatives to using slaughterhouse waste as ingredients in animal feed,

it didn't want to set the precedent of being overly influenced by "activists."[93] Yet another example of unbiased, clear thinking.

Your Diet. Prudent persons may want to avoid dietary supplements containing animal glandular tissue and gelatin. Several companies offer meat that is specifically raised to avoid problems such as spongiform diseases. Applegate Farms deli meats, Beeler's and Sara Joe's Pork, Coleman meats, Diestel's Turkey, Oregon Country Beef, Ranger, Rocky Junior, and Rosie's Organic Chicken, have provided assurances the feed used for their livestock is free of all animal by-products.

Early Detection. Until recently, the only means of evaluating a patient for CJD was either to perform a brain biopsy, or examination of the brain following death. Recent breakthroughs offer other means of early detection.

■ ***Blood***. In early 2002, a patent was issued to the British biotech firm Proteome Sciences, Plc, for the detection of BSE in the blood of humans or animals. The test works by detecting changes in the prion proteins that accompany BSE infection. Several other biotech companies are also pursuing a BSE blood test. Dr. Adriano Aguzzi of the University Hospital in Switzerland also has developed a novel means of testing blood for infective prions, according to a recent article published in *Nature*.[94]

■ ***Magnetic Resonance Imaging*** (MRI). News of another detection model has recently been published.[95] Dr. Alan Coulthard, a radiologist at the Royal Victoria Infirmary in Newcastle, England, believes it likely that scarring of the brain of vCJD patients can be detected using standard brain scanning technology such as the MRI. In a small study, he compared the brain scans of three vCJD patients with scans of 14 patients without the disease. Coulthard found a higher intensity of "certain signals" in the scans of vCJD patients, compared to the controls. Although the differences are subtle, and it is yet uncertain how effective the scanning techniques may be, the technology holds the promise of providing a useful non-invasive test.

■ ***Gradiflow*™ *Technology***. One of the most promising diagnostic technologies has recently surfaced from a biosciences firm down under.[96] The

Australian company Gradipore has developed technology capable of detecting and removing infectious and/or non-infectious prions from the blood of animals, including humans. Gradiflow™ technology is the result of a collaborative effort between Gradipore and The Scottish National Blood Transfusion Service—a world leader in transfusion research—and Q-One Biotech, an authority in the design and implementation of validation testing.

A benchtop diagnostic unit is about the size of a TV set. When a blood sample is introduced, the unit sifts the prions through a wafer-like membrane either by electrical charge or by varying the size of the holes in the Gradiflow membrane.

Gradiflow technology provides a fast, sensitive, reliable and non-invasive diagnostic capability for use in both veterinary and human medicine. Accurate diagnosis of cattle will allow farmers to cull only the infected animals, instead of practicing "over-kill" to insure all diseased animals have been excised. Early detection could save lives and provide confidence to those who test negative.

The Scottish National Blood Transfusion Service is eyeing the technology for evaluating the blood supply as well as removing infected prions from the blood. The capability of removing infective (misshapen) prions from the blood suggests the possibility that the technology may one day be used for the treatment of transmissible prion diseases by reducing the burden of blood-borne prions through the Gradiflow filtration process.

Treatments. Several bright stars loom large on the horizon of possible treatment modalities. Reported in the March 6, 2003 edition of the British journal *Nature*, British researchers from the Imperial College London have demonstrated what could be a major breakthrough strategy in the treatment of prion diseases. They have successfully used monoclonal antibodies to treat laboratory animals (mice) infected with the prion disease scrapie. Other potential treatments are on the horizon.

■ ***Monoclonal Antibodies.*** *Antibodies* are high molecular weight proteins produced by the B-cells of the immune system in response to any substance within the body perceived as foreign. They serve an important front-line function of the immune system. *Monoclonal antibodies* are genetically engineered antibodies which are (theoretically) designed to mimic the body's own defense processes. The British researchers used two types of monoclonal antibodies with similar, positive results.

In the study,[97] one group of mice received monoclonal antibody injections twice a week beginning either seven or 60 days after being infected with scrapie prions, but before any disease symptoms had manifested. In both cases, the antibodies were found to inhibit the spread of prions. They appeared to work by inhibiting the replication of the disease-causing prions which brought about a substantial reduction of infective prion levels, even when the antibodies were first administered at a point of near maximal prion accumulation.

Mice treated with the antibodies survived for more than 500 days, more than twice as long as those in the untreated group. Furthermore, no clinical signs of scrapie or weight loss were observed in the treated mice. Studies are ongoing to determine whether prion infection in this group has been suppressed or totally eradicated. (The treatment was found ineffective if begun after the onset of the clinical symptoms of scrapie.)

Preventing Prion Conversion. According to a 2003 article published in *Science*,[98] an important new discovery regarding prion infectivity has been made. Heretofore it was believed that the mere presence of prions and the manner in which they clump together cause the symptoms of BSE and CJD. Scientists at the University College London have found that the presence of abnormal prions in and of itself doesn't seem to be the causative factor, but rather something related to the actual process of conversion from normal to misshapen prions seems to be at the root of the symptomology.

The researchers conclude there is a toxic intermediate stage that is the actual cause of prion-disease symptoms, without which no symptoms occur. They suggest the transition (conversion) might produce a toxic by-product, could cause nerve tissue to break down, or may deplete a factor crucial to brain cell survival and development. One strategy would be the development of a drug that binds to normal prions and causes their depletion.

Surgical Transmission. One problem that has developed relating to BSE/CJD is its transmission to otherwise healthy surgical patients. An example of this was reported in the *Montreal Gazette* newspaper. According to the *Gazette*,[99] seven former

New Brunswick hospital patients may have contracted CJD from contaminated surgical instruments following neurosurgery. The infective prions adhered to the surgical instruments and were not decontaminated by the processes ordinarily used.

More disturbing still, as reported in the *New England Journal of Medicine*[100] in November 2003, researchers at the Institute of Neuropathology in Zurich, Switzerland announced they had isolated infective prions in both spleen and muscle cells of CJD victims. The infective particles were found in 10 of 28 spleen and eight of 32 skeletal-muscle specimens. The researchers concluded they have new concern that CJD could be transmitted in surgical operations other than neurosurgery.

As mentioned, neither heat, detergents, UV radiation, nor chemicals are capable of destroying infective prions, including those that adhere to surgical instruments. In response to this potential catastrophic situation, scientists at the UK Health Protection Agency Laboratories of the famed biowarfare facility Porton Down recently announced they have developed a disinfectant that reduces the risk of transmitting infective prions during surgery.

A genetically-modified version of a naturally-occurring enzyme initially obtained from volcanic pools, the new enzyme-based disinfectant works by degrading the chemical bonds between the protein's amino acids. The disinfectant requires less than one hour at a temperature of 60°-70° Celsius to degrade the prions and reduce their infectivity about one million-fold.[101] It is hoped this new discovery will prevent the surgical transmission of CJD.

MENOPAUSE. See *Hot Flashes*, Testosterone under *Diabetes*, and Menopause in the **Index**.

METHICILLIN-RESISTANT STAPHYLOCOCCUS AUREUS (MRSA)

Approximately 10 times as many bacterial cells as human cells reside on and within the human body, and scientists have identified hundreds of different species living on the skin and within the stomach and intestines. Of these many different bacterial types, most potentially harmful strains are rendered harmless by the body's immune system.

Staphylococcus aureus is a category composed of various strains of bacteria carried long-term on the skin and in the nasal cavities of about 20% of the population. It is the most common cause of many infections, including acne, boils, infection of heart valves, pneumonia, and many others. As in the case of most potentially harmful bacteria, a healthy immune system typically prevents serious infection. Methicillin Resistant Staphylococcus Aureus, or MRSA (MUR-sa), is a strain of *S. aureus* that's resistant to a large number of the most powerful antibiotics including the penicillins and cephalosporins. As a result, it has become increasingly difficult to treat, even with the best of medicine's front-line arsenal of antibiotics. MRSA is one of a growing number of 21st Century "superbugs."

Two sub-categories of MRSA have been defined. Community-Associated MRSA (CA-MRSA) commonly spreads where there are groupings of people such as schools, prisons and athletic facilities such as gyms. It typically manifests as swollen and painful skin infections. Healthcare-Associated MRSA (HA-MRSA) is a serious problem in hospital settings where invasive medical devices, open wounds, and people with low immunity are commonplace. Under such conditions, the bacterium can enter the blood, become systemic, and infect internal organs. About 2.5 million Americans carry MRSA, and 5% of hospital patients are either infected with or carry the bacterium. It is three times more lethal than less drug-resistant strains.

■ *Honey*. As discussed in the section on *Burns*, certain medicinal honeys—specifically those with a UMF rating of 12 or higher—demonstrate powerful antimicrobial properties. Several studies have found these honeys effective in treating skin lesions caused by MRSA. It is ineffective, however, if the bacterium becomes blood-borne. Colloidal silver used topically is also suggested. Sovereign Silver Hydrosol™ is available in health food stores and OxySilver™ is available online.

■ *Phage Therapy*. Dr. Domenico Iannetti of the University of Naples in Italy has successfully used bacteria-killing viruses—known as *bacteriophages*, or *phages*—to attack and kill various strains of *S. aureus*, including MRSA. While harmless to humans, the phages are deadly to targeted bacteria and much less subject to the development of bacterial resistance than are antibiotics.

■ *Elecampane*. Also known as horseheal, wild sunflower scabwort, and botanically as *Inula helenium*, elecampane is used to kill intestinal parasites and respiratory infections including asthma and bronchitis. Researchers at the Cork Institute in Ireland have reported that elecampane is effective in killing over 300 varieties of staphylococcus, including MRSA. It is available in capsules, tinctures, and as a tea. Rasayana and Lipistat are two Ayurvadic products containing elecampane.

■ *French Green Clay*. Drs. Lynda Williams and Shelley Haydel of Arizona State University work with various antibacterial clays including Agricur, a green volcanic clay found near Massif Central, France. It is formed from ancient volcanic ash composed mostly of the minerals smectite and illite. The clay has been shown to kill MRSA, the flesh-eating disease *buruli*, and other harmful bacteria. French clays are available in healthfood stores.

■ *Silver Dihydrogen Citrate*. The hard-surface disinfectant Silver Dihydrogen Citrate by PURE Biosciences is being used by some correctional facilities to prevent the spread of MRSA. It is a broad spectrum anti-bacterial, antifungal, and antiviral.

■ *Light*. Researchers at the New York Institute of Technology have reported that blue LED light at the wavelength of 470 nm eradicates both the CA and HA types of MRSA with only several minutes of treatment. 470 nm LEDs are readily available.

■ Several natural remedies are recommended for the treatment of systemic/blood-bourne MRSA. *Hyperbaric Oxygen Therapy*, *Olive Leaf Extract*, *Photoluminescence*, and *Sodium Chlorite* are four such remedies, all of which are discussed under **General Treatment Methods**. A poultice of olive leaf extract or acidified sodium chlorite are appropriate for topical application. Used systemically, these treatments may also be effective against other superbugs including Vancomycin-resistant Enterococcus (VRE) and *Clostridium difficile*.

MIGRAINES

It is estimated that over 100 million people in the United States are affected with some type of chronic head pain. For many of these people the term "migraine" has become practically synonymous with

"headache." When frustrated, many people say, "I'm having a migraine." In reality, there are different types of headaches, each with their attendant causes, with some overlap. The general classification of headaches typically includes four specific types: tension, sinus/allergy, cluster and migraine. Even these categories are further broken down into more specific classifications too numerous to list. Some headaches are symptoms of serious disease processes or physical abnormalities such as a tumor, stroke or aneurysm. It is therefore important to receive an accurate diagnosis of the problem, for which the MRI and CAT Scan are often useful.

The various classifications of headaches have the following sets of symptoms, although not all headache sufferers experience identical symptomology or respond to the same treatments. There is some overlap of symptoms, sometimes making it difficult to achieve an accurate diagnosis:

❑ *Tension*: constant, dull, usually mild to moderate pain which is not incapacitating • often on both sides of the head • pain often accompanied by muscle tightness in shoulders and neck • often described as a band of pain around the head "like a vice" • may last from thirty minutes to one week • absence of certain symptoms including diarrhea, nausea, vomiting, migraine prodrome and aura • pain not usually intensified by physical activity • genetic predisposition to certain triggering events including anxiety, bright lights, cigarette smoke, lack of sleep, extreme hunger, stress • believed to be caused by muscle tension and changes in the central nervous system and blood vessels (initiated by triggers) • usually responds to ice packs, OTC medications, massage, meditation, and rest.

❑ *Sinus/Allergy*: generally mild to moderate pain • centered around sinuses, above and below eyes • pressure often makes teeth ache • may include feeling of pressure behind eyes • often relieved by decongestants, antihistamines, or other allergy medications • often seasonal.

❑ *Cluster*: severe, sharp, stabbing pain • usually on one side, centered around eye • almost always severely incapacitating • occurs in clusters of 1-4 episodes/day for several weeks • lasts 10 minutes to two hours each • may stop for months • on affected side, the eye tears and nose is often runny or stuffy, swelling or redness of eye, shrinkage of pupil, sweaty forehead or face • occurs most often in men, in spring or fall • probably not hereditary • believed to be caused by blood vessel swelling in head region from unknown triggers.

❑ *Migraine*: throbbing, intense pain usually moderate to severe • usually on one side, but can affect both sides or move from side to side • pain often near the eye • often disabling • may last hours, days or weeks • often accompanied by visual disturbances and/or sensitivity to light, sound or smell • may be preceded by warning symptoms called an "aura" • often consists of four phases: prodrome, aura, headache, postdrome • hereditary factor often involved • possible triggers include certain foods, change in barometric pressure, estrogen, extreme hunger, lack of sleep, medications (especially hormonal), stress, strong scents • cause is believed to be vascular in origin, produced by nerve excitation (irritation) as blood vessels expand and contract, or nerve irritation of muscular or other origin (initiated by triggers).

The standard medical approach to migraine headaches is treatment of the pain with pharmaceutical drugs ranging from the prescription drug codeine to OTC drugs such as aspirin and ibuprofen. Betablockers attempt to prevent the onset by dilating blood vessels which sometimes has the effect of actually increasing the severity of the pain. Betablockers also have serious potential side-effects which include depression, digestive disturbances, low blood pressure and muscle weakness.[1]

In actuality, it is estimated that up to 75% of all headaches are tension headaches. This type and also those of a more serious nature may receive help from the following remedies:

■ *Butterbur*. The herb butterbur, known botanically as *Petasites hybridus*, has been used for centuries to treat a variety of ailments including asthma, colds, fever, urinary complaints and whooping cough. Recently, it has increased in popularity as a non-narcotic analgesic in the treatment of migraine headaches, reducing their frequency of occurrence, duration, and pain.[2] It works by reducing muscle and tissue spasms and reducing inflammation of affected blood vessels.

In 1996, a double-blind study at the University of Munich evaluated the effectiveness over a three month period of the product Petadolex,® containing a 15% standardized extract of *petasin*, butterbur's key active ingredient. Prior to treatment, all study participants had experienced at least three migraines per month for over one year. Following treatment, participants experienced longer intervals between attacks and reduction in severity of the pain. The average number of migraines decreased from 3.4 to 1.3 per month.[3] Other European studies have confirmed the herb reduces the incidence of headaches by 50-62%.[4] No adverse side-effects were experienced by the participants.

Properly-prepared formulations of butterbur, including Petadolex, remove the alkaloid *pyrrolizidine*, a substance contained in native butterbur that is toxic to the liver and possibly carcinogenic. Petadolex by Enzymatic Therapy is available in health food stores, or can be ordered on the internet by doing a key word search for "petadolex."

■ *Food Triggers*. Many authorities consider certain foods to be triggers (precipitating factors) of headaches. Among the most common are caffeine, chocolate, citrus fruits, cola beverages, dairy products, eggs, grains (including barley, corn, oats, rye and wheat; gluten—a sticky mixture of protein found in wheat, rye and barley—can be a particular offender), sugar and (red) wine.[5] Elimination of some or all of these foods often can do wonders.

■ *MigraSpray*.® MigraSpray® has been shown to be an effective, fast-acting migraine treatment. Consisting of four traditional herbs—dandelion, feverfew, goldenseal and *Polyporous officinalis*—the product is sprayed under the tongue where it gains rapid absorption into the bloodstream. In 2001, the manufacturer of MigraSpray conducted a placebo-controlled study of 20 migraine sufferers. Sixty-six percent of the participants reported full recovery, while 88% reported some level of improvement. The average time between administration of MigraSpray and relief was just 6.5 minutes.[6] More information is available at www.migraspray.com. This product is available from many pharmacies, some health food stores, and on the internet.

■ *Peppermint Oil & Ethanol*. Researchers at the University of Kiel in Germany have stumbled upon a unique technique for treating migraine pain. When a mixture of peppermint oil and ethanol (ethyl alcohol) was dabbed onto the foreheads of 32 participants in a double-blind, placebo-controlled study, the participants experienced an almost immediate lessening of headache pain.[7] Peppermint oil is available in health food stores, and ethanol is available in liquor stores as pure grain alcohol. Mix the two together before applying to the skin.

■ *Plastic Surgery*. Dr. Bahman Guyuron recently discovered an unusual phenomenon while attending to his routine plastic surgery duties. After the surgical removal of the *corrugator supercilii muscles* that lie underneath the eyebrows—a routine procedure performed during a face lift—80% of his patients reported their migraines either disappeared or substantially lessened.

Following this observation, Dr. Guyuron performed a study of 22 patients reporting to have pre-operative migraine headaches. Fifty-five percent reported total elimination of further headache pain while pain of the remaining participants was substantially lessened. Of those whose headaches were not totally eliminated, the incidence dropped from five to less than one headache per month, and the pain was less severe.[8]

Before committing to surgery in a attempt to quell the pain of a migraine, a simple procedure can accurately predict the outcome of surgery. Dr. Guyuron refers prospective surgical patients to a neurologist for botox injections (botulinum toxin type A at the cost of ~USD $1,000) into the suspect muscles so that they are temporarily paralyzed. If the headaches are eliminated using this technique, it is reasonably certain the surgical procedure will bring long-lasting results (at the cost of ~USD $6,000). To learn more about this technique, Google "guyuron migraines," or call Dr. Guyuron's office in Ohio at (440)461-7999.

■ *Teeth Clenching*. Dr. Phillip Lamey, Professor of Oral Medicine at the Royal Hospital in Northern Ireland, has discovered that migraine sufferers have severely-elevated saliva peptide levels—between 50,000-60,000 units—while non-migraine sufferers have about 100 times less, or about 500 units. He further discovered the cause of this elevation of peptides seems to be nighttime teeth clenching. To prevent this behavior, Lamey had 19 sufferers wear an oral appliance while sleeping, preventing the upper and lower teeth from contacting.

The device used in the study was fashioned from two millimeter thick acrylic plastic. The saliva peptide levels dropped to the levels of non-migraine sufferers—around 500 units, with a corresponding drop in migraine attacks to about 40% of their previous levels. After wearing the device each night for one year, 70% of his patients no longer experienced migraines.

Lamey found his technique works best for people who experience at least two episodes per week, and particularly for those who have attacks upon awakening. Although Dr. Lamey's appliance isn't available in the U.S., it's quite similar to mouthpieces used in sports such as boxing and football. The most important factor seems to be that no upper and lower teeth make contact, including the wisdom teeth and molars. The thinner the appliance, the more comfortable the fit.

There is a device sold in the U.S. called the Doctor's® Night Guard. This just might fit the bill, and is available in pharmacies.

■ *Riboflavin*. Dr. Jean Schoenen and colleagues of the University of Liege in Belgium have found that mega-doses of riboflavin, vitamin B_2, are useful in preventing migraine headaches. Studying 55 mild-to-moderate migraine sufferers aged 18-65 whose pre-testing frequency ranged from two to eight episodes per month, those who took 400 milligrams of B_2 daily had 37% fewer attacks, with greatly-reduced severity of the continuing episodes. The riboflavin therapy was well tolerated, the only side-effect being diarrhea in one participant.[9]

Some experts suggest that supplementing for two to three months may be necessary before the positive benefits are seen. If supplementing with extra B_2, it's best also to supplement with a protocol containing all of the B-vitamins (B complex).

■ *Magnesium and HCL*. Alternative practitioner Dr. Joseph Mercola describes a technique for treating migraines which uses an intravenous injection of magnesium and hydrochloric acid. The treatment is administered over a period of five to 15 minutes, and has the ability to abort over 95% of migraines before the needle leaves the arm. The protocol can be seen at Dr. Mercola's comprehensive website http://articles.mercola.com/sites/articles/archive/2000/06/03/flu.aspx.

Oral magnesium supplementation at the level of 300-400 mg daily (in two divided doses with meals) also has been shown to prevent the onset of migraines. For some, the combination of oral magnesium and riboflavin is particularly effective.

■ See *Prolotherapy*, which has been shown to be ~90% effective in treating migraines. See also *Sphenopalatine Ganglion Block* under **Pain Relievers**, and Migraines in the Member's area of *The Encyclopedia's* website.

MULTIPLE SCLEROSIS

Diagnosed primarily in young adults, multiple sclerosis is a chronic disease affecting the white matter of the central nervous system (CNS). Inflammation occurs in seemingly random patches called *plaques* or lesions, followed by destruction of *myelin*, the soft, somewhat fatty material that forms a thick sheath of protection around nerve fibers of the brain and spinal cord. It is the presence of myelin that facilitates the high-speed transmission of electrochemical signals both internally between the brain and spinal cord, and also between the CNS and the nerves throughout the body. While MS is considered by many researchersto be an autoimmune disease, the definitive cause of the disease remains unknown.

Diagnosing MS is challenging. Although various tests including brain imaging techniques are used, diagnosis is often a process of eliminating other disorders. The symptoms and severity of the disease can vary greatly depending on the affected areas and the extent of damage to the myelin structures. Because lesions can occur in such varied locations throughout the CNS, those with MS can experience either partial or total loss of virtually any function or process associated with the brain or spinal cord. Because of this the course of the disease is largely unpredictable.

Most often MS progresses slowly, with few people experiencing the total array of possible symptoms. While 75% of MS sufferers don't require a wheelchair, as the disease progresses many require the use of a cane or similar walking aid. Still other sufferers experience only occasional, mild symptoms. Very few people die as a direct result of the disease. Typical symptoms can include, with varying degrees of severity: blindness; blurred or double vision; cognitive dysfunction; constipation; cramps; depression; difficulty breathing; fatigue; incontinence; loss of balance; muscle weakness; neuropathic symptoms such as numbness, tingling, and pins and needles; nausea; sexual dysfunction; spasticity; spasms; and speech and urinary dysfunction.[1]

Four main types of MS are typically defined:[2]
◆ Relapsing/Remitting (RRMS). Relapses, also called exacerbations, can occur during which old symptoms reappear or worsen, and new symptoms can manifest. Relapses are followed either by partial or total remission of the symptoms experienced during relapse. The length of relapses varies, and can range from days to months. The recovery period also varies from slow to gradual to almost instantaneous. Most people with MS are in the RRMS category—about twice as many women as men—and are typically diagnosed while in their 20s-30s.

◆ Secondary Progressive (SPMS). This stage marks a general progression of the disease. After about 10 years, roughly 50% of those with RRMS progress to this stage which is characterized by a gradual worsening of symptoms between relapses. After 20-30 years, about 90% progress to this stage.

◆ Progressive Relapsing (PRMS). This form of MS is characterized by a progressive course from the initial onset. Although significant recoveries may follow relapses, there is a gradual overall worsening of symptoms between relapses.

◆ Primary Progressive (PPMS). In this form of the disease there is a gradual progression from onset, with no remission of symptoms, although there are periods where symptoms level off. Onset of PPMS is typically in the late 30s to early 40s; men and women are equally likely to contract this form of MS; and the initial disease activity is focused in the spinal cord, after which it may migrate to the brain.

Risk factors include,[3] 1) A family history of MS. There is a 30% chance of MS if one identical twin has the disease. If a father, mother, or sibling has MS, there is a 1-3% chance of acquiring the disease; 2) A diet high in saturated fat and animal products; 3) Being Caucasian. Caucasians are at greater risk than African-Americans; 4) Living in high-altitude, temperate climates; 5) Being a recipient of vaccinations; 6) Cigarette smoking. A study of over 22,000 Norwegians found that male smokers had a 275% higher risk and women a 161% higher risk of developing MS.[4]

Treatments. There are several pharmaceutical treatments for MS. Treatment goals are threefold: 1) to prevent or lessen the number of relapses, 2) to hasten the recovery from attacks, and 3) to halt the progression of the disease. Because the diversity of possible symptoms is as broad as the various areas of the CNS that can be affected, a wide range of pharmaceutical drugs often are employed in an effort to control symptoms. These can range from immune-stimulating agents such as interferon (Capaxone® and Betaferon®) to the chemotherapeutic agents mitixantrone (Novantrone®) to corticosteroids such as methylprednisone (Depo-Medrol®). Also used are the anti-convulsants Neurontin,® Tegretol,® and Dilantin.®

Several non-pharmaceutical approaches are useful in treating MS, including:

■ *Hyperbaric Oxygen Therapy* (HBOT). This technique entails saturating the body with pure oxygen under higher-than-normal pressure—usually from 1.25-2.0 atmospheres. The body becomes super saturated with oxygen independent of the bloodstream, the body's normal oxygen source. It is now known that HBOT increases stem cell production by 800%.

Also, some have suggested an infective component is implicated in MS. If this is the case it would help explain the beneficial results of HBO, as it is known that oxygen compromises the integrity of most infectious pathogens.

In the United Kingdom, HBO is the leading treatment for MS. For more information, see *Hyperbaric Oxygen Therapy* under **General Treatment Methods**. Minocycline, a member of the tetracycline family of antibiotics, is often effective in treating relapsing M.S. A pathogenic origin of the disease would explain these results. See Minocycline in the **Index** and *Sodium Chlorite* under **General Treatment Methods**.

■ *Electromagnetic Therapy* (EMT). Pioneer researcher Reuven Sandyk, M.D., of NeuroCommunication Research Laboratories in Danbury, CT, believes the symptoms of MS are related to or

caused by the calcification of the pineal gland, a small body situated in the brain at the location of the "third eye." According to Sandyk, there is a calcification of the pineal gland in 100% of MS patients (although many people with pineal calcification don't experience MS symptoms).

Pineal calcification causes a reduction in serotonin levels in the brain, exacerbating MS symptoms. Sandyk has found that using magnets placed at the temples for 30 minutes "jump starts" the production of serotonin, causing a "marked improvement" in 60-70% of his MS patients.[5]

■ *The Liberation Treatment*. In November 2009, Canadian Television (CTV) broadcast the story of a newly-discovered possible cause of MS—and a treatment. Italian physician and professor at the University of Ferrara, Dr. Paolo Zamboni discovered that 100% of MS patients have stenosis (narrowing) of one or more jugular veins of the neck, and/or the azygos vein, one of a system of veins in the center of the chest that drains the thoracic and abdominal walls. Further, the severity of symptoms corresponds to the severity of the blockage. In normal people, or people with other diseases including neurological diseases, no narrowing of these veins is present. The venous strictures could be a congenital defect which triggers the onset of MS. Dr. Zamboni calls the condition Chronic Cerebro-Spinal Venous Insufficiency (CCSVI).

Stenosis of the veins leads to poor blood drainage from the brain, and even a reversal of venous blood flow. The presence of iron deposits (lesions) in the brain near veins that are responsible for cerebral drainage—a hallmark of MS—could be explained by this abnormal venous blood flow, as increased venous pressure pushes iron into brain tissues. The iron deposits cause inflammation, cell death, and immune dysfunction.

Zamboni's treatment is called *The Liberation Treatment*, which consists of correcting the abnormal venous narrowing(s), usually by balloon angioplasty, a technique commonly used to decrease coronary artery blockage. The earlier the patient is treated, the better the result. Following treatment, 73% of patients have no more MS attacks, and there is a drop in the number of new brain lesions. Renarrowing of the veins causes a relapse, which can then be re-treated. Some patients have regained much of their lost function following treatment, even if they have had MS for years.

As of November 2009, 120 patients have received Dr. Zamboni's treatment. As of winter 2010, The Liberation Treatment is not widely available. In the U.S., Dr. Robert Zivadinov at the University of Buffalo and professor Mark Haake of McMaster University in Hamilton, Ontario and Wayne State University in Detroit are working to confirm Zamboni's work. To view CTV's presentation on The Liberation Treatment, visit http://csvi-ms.net/en/content/ctv-w5-liberation-treatment-is-online.

■ *Prokarin.*® Developed by registered nurse Elaine DeLack, Prokarin is a topical preparation consisting of histamine, caffeine, and other ingredients. It replenishes depleted histamine levels which seems to improve demyelinated nerve fiber function and stimulates regrowth of myelin sheaths. Prokarin is available from compounding pharmacies, with a prescription. To learn more, visit www.msakc.org/Articles/Prokarin.htm, or www.edmsllc.com.

■ Stem cell therapy has been shown to reverse MS in some cases. See Stem Cells in the **Index** and MS in the Member's Area of *The Encyclopedia's* website. See also Robson Splint under *Sleep Apnea*, which has shown remarkable results in some MS cases. Other MS treatments include *Bowen Therapy* and *Photoluminescence* under **General Treatment Methods**; Padma-28 under *Cardiovascular Disease*; bee venom therapy; mega-doses of IV vitamin B; monoclonal antibodies; and oral myelin (e.g., bovine-sourced Sphingolin®).

■ A device that's shown some effectiveness in treating MS is the Magnetic Molecular Energizer (MME). The MME offers hope for many difficult-to-treat medical conditions, including MS. To learn more, see *Magnetic Molecular Energizer* under **General Treatment Methods**.

■ *Fat Elimination.* Dr. Roy Swank reported in his 1987 book *The Multiple Sclerosis Diet Book* that many of his MS patients significantly benefitted from eliminating all dietary animal fat.

■ Tremor due to MS often can be treated successfully by Deep Brain Stimulation. See Deep Brain Stimulation under *Parkinson's Disease*.

■ See also *Lyme Disease*. Some researchers believe Lyme is implicated in many cases of MS.

MUSCLE

The mineral magnesium is sometimes helpful in reducing muscle pain and soreness, particularly muscle cramps. Other useful treatments are discussed under **Leg Cramps** and **Pain Relievers**. See also vitamin D under **Osteoporosis**.

MUSCULAR DYSTROPHY

A device that's shown effectiveness in treating Muscular Dystrophy is the Magnetic Molecular Energizer (MME). The MME offers hope for many difficult-to-treat conditions, including MD. To learn more, see *Magnetic Molecular Energizer* under **General Treatment Methods**.

NECK

Many of the methods discussed in this book are applicable to neck pain, including acupuncture, Bowen therapy, chiropractic, Prolotherapy (see **Index**), and many treatments under **Pain Relievers**.

NEUROLOGICAL DISORDERS

A neurological disorder is any of a group of disorders involving the brain, spinal cord, nerves, or muscles. Although several hundred specific diagnoses comprise this group of ailments, more familiar neurological disorders include Alzheimer's disease, autism, back pain, herpes zoster, multiple sclerosis, muscular dystrophy, and Parkinson's disease—all of which are discussed separately.

■ *Creatine*. A natural substance manufactured in the liver, pancreas, and kidneys, creatine is supplied to muscles via the bloodstream. Supplemental creatine is being used effectively to increase muscle strength and enhance the daily activities of persons suffering from neurological disorders involving muscle wasting and weakness such as muscular dystrophy and Parkinson's. Five to 10 grams daily of creatine monohydrate are recommended.

NEUROPATHY

Neuropathy is an abnormal and usually degenerative state of nerve fibers, or the nervous system. It may also include muscular atrophy (wasting) as a result of the condition. In short, it is a malfunctioning of the nervous system that can produce symptoms anywhere in the body that are often referred to as *neuralgia* or *neuritis*.

The causes of neuropathy include 1) excessive glucose/insulin in the blood, 2) sciatic nerve entrapment (from sitting, aging trauma, etc.), 3) trauma caused by accidents, extended standing on hard surfaces, etc., 4) chemotherapy side-effects, 5) side-effects from prescription drugs, 6) toxic chemicals such as Agent Orange, solvents, etc., 7) complications from surgery, and 8) temporary inflammation in the lower back.

Oral pain medication blunts but typically does not eliminate the pain of neuropathy. The **Spheno-palatine Ganglion Block** discussed under **Pain Relievers** is often an effective remedy. At times, a localized procaine or similar analgesic injection is effective. This is sometimes given along with DMSO, a substance discussed in more detail under **Spinal Cord Injury** and **Pain Relievers**. Otherwise, many of the **Pain Relievers** and **General Treatment Methods** offer relief. See *Light* and *Electricity* under **Pain Relievers** and *Prolotherapy* and *Seanol* under **General Treatment Methods**. See Memantine under **Alzheimer's Disease**, which has been shown to reduce the pain of neuropathies. See Alpha Lipoic Acid under **Alzheimer's Disease** and Tamanu Oil under **Psoriasis**. See also Benfotiamine, EWOT, and The ReBuilder® under **Diabetes** for an expanded discussion of neuropathy.

OBESITY. See Weight Loss in the **Index**.

OSTEOPOROSIS

Referred to by the lay public as "thinning of the bones," osteoporosis is a systemic skeletal disease characterized by increased bone porosity and fragility with increased susceptibility to fracture. Although the disorder occurs mainly in postmenopausal women, a significant number of men are affected. In the Western world, roughly 15% of women aged 50, 30% aged 70, and 40% at the age of 80 will develop osteoporosis. One in 12 men will acquire the condition at some stage,[1] although women account for 90% of patients hospitalized.[2]

Undiagnosed and untreated, osteoporosis can progress silently and painlessly until it first becomes apparent when a bone breaks. Annually in the U.S., osteoporosis results in 700,000 spinal (compression) fractures, 300,000 hip fractures, 250,000 wrist fractures, and 300,000 fractures at other locations.

The probability of suffering a hip fracture by age 50 is 20% in women and 8% in men. The incidence of suffering a fracture of any type for a person aged 60 and over is 56% for women and 29% for men.[3] The mortality rate in the first year for persons having hip fractures is roughly 25%,[4] with men outnumbering women by nearly two-to-one, despite the higher incidence in women.[5] Deaths are most often the result of blood clots, infection, or pneumonia.[6] Only 25% of those suffering a broken hip attain a pre-injury level of activity.[7]

On the face of it, osteoporosis seems straightforward—the bones weaken and are subject to fracture. However, the more one investigates the subject, the more controversy raises its head. We know, for example, the mineral calcium is involved; but there are conflicting views regarding proper calcium intake and its role in osteoporosis.

It is here that the plot, if not the bones, thickens substantially. Some authorities believe the higher the calcium intake the better, as the bone mass (BMD, bone mineral density; BMD = mg of mineral per cm^2 of bone) can be built up "for a rainy day." The more calcium stored in the bones, the longer it will take to deplete them. On the other hand, there is evidence suggesting excessive calcium intake contributes to disease progression.

The following are a few facts that are known. People in countries whose populations consume the highest levels of milk and other dairy products have the highest average bone mineral density (BMD),[8] which is *usually assumed* to mean stronger, healthier bones. For example, in Australia, the U.S., Italy, Kuwait, Northern Europe, and the U.K., high levels of milk are consumed with a corresponding high average BMD of these residents.

Conversely in China, Japan, and Poland, where there is a low intake of milk, there are correspondingly lower levels of BMD in their citizens.[9] So far, so good. However, in those countries having the highest dairy (milk) consumption, there is also the highest incidence of osteoporosis (including hip fracture), and conversely in those countries having the lowest dairy (milk) consumption, there is also the lowest incidence of osteoporosis (including hip fracture),[10] and this is where the logic becomes as curdled as spoiled milk.

In China, for example, an average of eight kilograms of milk is consumed per year compared to 254 kg in the U.S., yet the incidence of hip fracture in China is six times lower than in the U.S.[11] If high milk consumption produces a higher BMD level—which is *assumed* to indicate strong, healthy bones—why does it also produce the highest incidence of osteoporosis, and vice versa?

Supporting these cross-cultural studies is a 12-year Harvard study by the famed Drs. Willett and Stampfer, as reported in 1997 in the *American Journal of Public Health*.[12] In the study of 78,000 women, those who drank milk three times daily suffered more broken bones than women who rarely drank milk. In a 1994 study of elderly Australian men and women, as reported in the *American Journal of Edipemiology*,[13] those persons consuming higher amounts of dairy products experienced an increased incidence of bone fracture.

In her book *Better Bones, Better Body*,[14] Susan Brown, Ph.D., CCN informs us that about half the people with low bone density never experience an osteoporotic fracture, while a significant number of people who test in the medium to high range of BMD unexpectedly suffer fractures. It is also known that in many countries having a low incidence of osteoporosis—such as China, Japan, Poland, and some African countries—the women also have a relatively lower average bone mass, irrespective of genetic differences.[15] *Clearly*, these data indicate that *something* about the relationship between calcium intake, BMD, and bone fracture incidence remains unclear, or at least not adequately explained by conventional concepts.

Osteoporosis is a condition of *premature* degeneration of the bones. It is assumed that most osteoporotic individuals had normal, strong bones earlier in life. What is it that causes the bones of osteoporotic persons to prematurely age and degenerate at a faster rate in comparison to healthy bones of persons of a similar age? What are the processes that accelerate premature bone aging?

One theory that may explain this—as well as some of the seeming contradictory data associated with this topic—suggests the answer lies in the fact that all cells within the body have a fixed number of times they are able to multiply/regenerate. Skin becomes wrinkled, for example, when old cells reach their limit of renewal and are unable to re-place the old, dehydrated cells. All organs of the body experience a similar process. If this were not the case, humans would be virtually immortal.

Within bones, the activity of calcium requires two types of specialized cells: *osteoblasts*, whose activity is required in calcium absorption and formation of bone matrix upon which calcium can precipitate, and *osteoclasts*, whose activity is required in deportation of calcium from the bones, known as *resorption*. The bones do not simply store calcium indefinitely, but are in a state of continuous turnover—a process of removal and replacement called *remodeling*. As we age, resorption overtakes replacement, and eventually bone loss occurs.

As this turnover progresses during a lifetime, osteoblasts die in the formation of new bone matrix. As more calcium is uptaken, more otosteoblasts die. If a person consumes high levels of calcium over a lifetime, osteoblasts help compose new bone matrix, and in so doing 50-70% die.[16]

Because there is a limited number of times a cell can be replaced, *the capacity to continue to form strong bones becomes reduced*. If large quantities of calcium are regularly consumed, the replacement capacity can become exhausted due to the lack of new osteoblasts. As this occurs, there is a lack of new bone matrix upon which the calcium precipitates to compose healthy bone. At the same time, bone is continuously being decomposed, resulting in the formation of unhealthy, porous bones.

The answer to the seeming dilemma of high BMD with an accompanying high incidence of osteoporosis may very well be that in osteoporosis, the supply of osteoblasts becomes exhausted due to high calcium intake over extended periods, resulting in the bones' inability to function normally because of loss of osteoblast activity, and the consequent formation of porous, brittle bones. Even though BMD can be increased by high calcium intake, by consuming calcium-rich foods or by supplementation, high calcium intake over extended periods leads to a premature exhaustion of the ability to form normal bone, according to this view.

Therefore, as has been observed, there can be either a low or high BMD in either strong or weakened bones, depending upon several factors. It follows that BMD in and of itself is not predictive of osteoporosis, and that low BMD due to low calcium intake over long periods of time is protective while low BMD due to high calcium intake over extended periods (causing an excessive turnover of osteoblasts) tends to accelerate osteoporosis.

These issues have continued to perplex the traditional Western medical community, at least for those who recognize the inconsistencies in the data. Otherwise, doctors continue to encourage their patients to consume high levels of calcium in an effort to increase the BMD, not realizing the issue of osteoporosis is a complex affair and many other factors are in operation.

For example, it is increasingly understood that bone can be sufficiently dense, yet at the same time quite brittle. This one understanding is a necessary component of anyone's comprehensive understanding of osteoporosis.

Several conventional pharmaceuticals, having questionable results and not-so-questionable side-effects, are offered by traditional practitioners.

■ *Contemporary Pharmaceutical Treatment.*
Fosamax® (alendronate; manufactured by Merck), a member of the bisphosphomate family of drugs, is prescribed to approximately 90% of all hospitalized U.S. osteoporosis patients.[17] Evista® (raloxifene; manufactured by Eli Lilly) is another popular pharmaceutical which is classified as a selective estrogen receptor modulator (SERM). Both of these popular drugs have significant drawbacks.

According to two 1998 studies funded by its manufacturer Merck, Fosamax was reported to prevent osteoporosis in young postmenopausal women as effectively as hormone therapy[18]—a method of treatment that has its own set of significant drawbacks, discussed below. Yet in an independent four year study of 4,000 patients published in 2000, Fosamax demonstrated no reduction in bone fracture risk.[19] In addition to the possibility of being ineffective, the drug may cause bone inflammation leading to potentially severe bone, joint, and muscle pain including serious-to-debilitating periodontal problems.[20] It has been shown that Fosamax damages the gastric lining when in the presence of an alkaline pH.[21] It also has been shown to cause ulceration of the esophagus.[22] Kidney failure, ocular damage and skin reactions also have been reported.[23] Other bisphophomates such as Actonel,® Aredia,® Boniva,® Didronel,® Reclast,® Skelid,® and Zometa® may have similar side-effects.

Evista also has been recommended for the prevention of bone loss especially in women who, for various medical reasons, cannot take estrogen—a hormone assumed to benefit osteoporosis, but with the significant trade-off of serious side-effects. However, a 2000 study[24] reported the results of a three year clinical trial which showed Evista increases the risk of blood vessel blockage caused by dislodging of a blood clot (thromboembolism), and also increases the risk of diabetes. It also may increase the risk of ovarian and breast cancer,[25] and of developing blood clots within the veins (venous thrombosis), abnormal particles such as air bubbles circulating with the blood vessels of the lungs (pulmonary emboli), and hot flashes.[26] In a 2001 edition of the *Journal of Clinical Endocrinology and Metabolism*,[27] Evista was shown to alter brain activation patterns in postmenopausal women, the meaning of which is not totally understood.

Causation, Treatment and Prevention. Generally, a deficiency of the following six substances can be considered causative, while their application can be considered treatments for those who have osteoporosis, and preventive measures for those who don't, with the possible exception of calcium.

■ *Calcium.* The most abundant mineral in the body, calcium is a principal constituent of bones. Ninety-nine percent of the body's calcium is stored in the bones and teeth, with the remaining one percent being present in body tissues and fluids where it is essential for cell metabolism, muscle contraction, and the transmission of nerve impulses. Its role in the genesis of osteoporosis is a deficiency in the bones themselves and not necessarily in the blood (diet). Most peoples' diets probably include sufficient quantities of calcium necessary for proper bone formation, as is seen in the cross-cultural studies discussed above. Calcium deficiencies within the bones are believed by many researchers to be related to inadequate amounts of other nutrients which assist in its absorption and utilization, as well as the excesses of other substances.

Other researchers believe many people don't consume enough calcium, either from the diet or through supplementation. If one chooses to supplement with calcium, it's best to insure that additional substances are taken along with it, as the deficiency of several dietary nutrients is believed to play a significant role in calcium absorption and utilization, principally the mineral magnesium and vitamin D,[28] as well as other nutrients.

Also, high stomach levels of hydrochloric acid (HCl) are necessary to properly digest calcium. By age 50, many persons produce only 15% of the HCl produced by a 25-year-old (*hypochlorhydria*), and over 35% of everyone over 65 produce no HCl (*achlorhydria*). Therefore, to aid in calcium digestion, supplemental *betaine hydrochloride* (begin with 10 grains/650 mg)—an acidic form of the vitamin-like substance betaine—should be considered when supplementing with calcium. See Hydrochloric Acid under **Indigestion**.

Even though calcium plays such a major role in bone structure, and that supplemental calcium has been shown to reduce the loss of bone mass, calcium's anomaly is that its use is questionable in reducing the incidence of bone fracture.[29]

■ **Magnesium.** The presence of magnesium assists calcium movement into the bones. However, excess calcium interferes with the absorption of magnesium, and an unproductive cycle is begun. Too much calcium within the blood may create unabsorbed calcium and/or a magnesium deficiency. Magnesium at the dosage of 500-1,000 mg daily is useful in the treatment of osteoporosis. Some doctors have pointed out that magnesium by injection is often able to provide dramatic, long-term relief from osteoporotic chronic back pain.

■ **Vitamin D.** The absorption of dietary calcium relies upon still other mechanisms. In the case of high calcium intake, the calcium is absorbed passively from the gut through the digestive process and into the bones—provided there are adequate levels of magnesium. However, with low levels of calcium intake, absorption relies upon an active transport system which is vitamin D dependent. Therefore, low calcium intake combined with low vitamin D intake results in lack of adequate calcium absorption and bone formation impairment.[30]

When studying a group of 1,500 women ages 45-80, Dr. Cees Vermeer of the University of Limburg in The Netherlands found that calcium loss through the urine could be reduced by as much as 50% by taking tiny amounts of vitamin D.[31] Some practitioners recommend 2,000-10,000 units daily

of vitamin D_3 (cholecalciferol) for persons over 60 years of age, especially during the winter months.

Researchers at the Mayo Clinic announced in 2003 there is a vital connection between vitamin D and body pain. In a study of 150 children and adults with unexplained muscle and bone pain, 93% were found to be severely deficient in vitamin D.[32]

■ **Vitamin K.** The lack of vitamin K indirectly contributes to osteoporosis. It assists the body in assimilating calcium into the bones and also prevents loss of bone calcium. Beef liver (preferably organic; see **Mad Cow Disease** regarding the problems associated with consuming animal foods), broccoli, lettuce, and turnip greens are additional sources of vitamin K. Also, it is available as an oral supplement, and can be administered via injection. Dr. Vermeer also has reported that in a placebo-controlled study of 200 postmenopausal women, daily administration of calcium + vitamin D + vitamin K retarded bone loss by 40% and sustained that result over three years. Calcium + vitamin D alone, on the other hand, had only a short-term, transient effect which dissipated after three years.[33]

It is well known that astronauts suffer significant bone loss while in space. Scientists from Jean Monnet University in Saint Etienne, France have reported that cosmonauts aboard the Mir space station were able to maintain proper bone strength when supplementing with vitamin K. When the supplement was discontinued, the problem promptly resumed.[34] Vitamin K2 is the preferred form, and should be taken as a pill-form supplement

■ **Boron.** Other factors contribute to the development of osteoporosis. Researchers at the Grand Forks Human Nutrition Research Center (GFHNRC), one of six human nutrition research centers operated by the Agricultural Research Service of the U.S. Department of Agriculture, have discovered some unusual properties of the mineral boron. Inadequate levels of boron exacerbate osteoporosis, and the presence of sufficient amounts provides several significant benefits. It maintains calcium levels in the body by preventing its excretion in the urine. Adequate levels of boron also increase the levels of estrogen in some post menopausal women equal to the levels found in women taking estrogen replacement therapy.[35]

GFHNRC researchers administered three milligrams of boron daily to a group of 12 postmenopausal women aged 48 to 82. After eight days of supplementation, calcium and magnesium excreted in the urine was reduced by 40% and 33%, respectively. The researchers also reported "markedly elevated" blood serum testosterone and estrogen levels. Toxicity of boron occurs only at levels that approach 40 mg per day for an adult.

■ *Strontium.* In the late 1700s near the small town of Strontian, Scotland, a new mineral element was isolated by Sir Humphry Davy. The pale yellow metallic element *strontium* takes its name from the town near which it was discovered.

Not to be confused with strontium 90, a radioactive isotope and byproduct of nuclear reaction, the naturally-occurring mineral strontium has electrochemical and other properties very similar to calcium, including the fact that it is concentrated within the body almost exclusively in the bones and teeth. As early as the 1950s, researchers were establishing the role of strontium in treating a variety of skeletal disorders. Throughout the decades, studies have indicated that strontium is useful in the treatment of osteoporosis, and may even reverse the disease. According to these studies, strontium 1) contributes to bone density, 2) is highly retained, 3) helps retain calcium, and 4) is able to be absorbed by the bone even when calcium has reached its maximum absorption level.

In a contemporary study reported in the *New England Journal of Medicine*[36] in 2004, researchers found that *strontium ranelate*, a synthetic (patentable) form of the mineral, is effective in significantly reducing the incidence of osteoporotic fractures. Participants were given strontium ranelate (along with vitamin D) daily for three years. Fractures were reduced by 49% in the first year, and 41% overall. BMD increased in the lumbar spine region by almost 15%, and slightly over 8% in the hip.

The journal didn't mention there are more natural forms of the mineral that are far less expensive while being equally effective. In fact, earlier studies used other forms such as strontium carbonate, citrate, gluconate and lactate. Advanced Orthomolecular Research manufactures the strontium citrate product Strontium Support,® available by calling (800) 387-0177 or by visiting www.aor .ca. Strontium is included as an ingredient in some multi-ingredient osteoporosis formulations.

■ *Exercise.* It is widely recognized that weight-bearing exercise is an effective preventive and treatment for osteoporosis, and a lack thereof may hasten its progression. Weight-bearing exercises include both free-weight lifting and isometrics (resistance), where strain is placed upon the bone with little movement. Any exercise stressing the bone produces a piezoelectric current that assists in the deposition of calcium and the formation of new bone.[37] The *British Medical Journal* reported regular exercise helps prevent bone loss in older adults[38] while lack of exercise leads to bone loss.[39]

In 2002, *the Journal of the American Medical Association*[40] published the results of a study of over 61,000 postmenopausal, non-osteoporotic registered nurses aged 40-77. The researchers noted that physical activity is known to reduce the risk of hip fractures, although the type and duration of the activity had not yet been determined. The purpose of the study was to shed light on these unknowns, and specifically to evaluate walking and leisure-time activity as a deterrent to bone fractures.

After controlling for body mass index, dietary intake, smoking, and use of postmenopausal hormones, several surprising results were discovered: 1) As the level of activity increased, the incidence of hip fracture decreased linearly in women not taking hormones, but not in women taking hormones, 2) A further reduction in hip fracture risk was noted even in women at lower risk due to higher body weight, 3) Women who walked at least eight hours (or equivalent) per week at an average pace experienced a 55% lower risk of hip fracture compared to sedentary women walking less than one hour, 4) Women who walked at least four hours per week with no other exercise experienced a 41% reduced risk of hip fracture compared to those who walked less than one hour, 5) The more time spent standing was associated with lower fracture risks, and 6) The researchers concluded that moderate levels of everyday activities, including walking, are associated with a substantially lower risk of postmenopausal hip fracture.

An exercise program should begin slowly and with caution, especially for older persons. In addition to walking, one of the best and safest ways for the elderly to exercise is with an OsteoBall.® Also described in the section on *Arthritis*, the OsteoBall was designed by the internationally recognized rheumatologist and Clinical Professor of Medicine at UCLA, Dr. Robert Swezey—an expert in back pain, arthritis and osteoporosis.

The OsteoBall is an inflatable, canvas-covered ball with attached straps that allow the user to perform a series of 10 isometric resistance exercises which target key muscle groups at the sites where they attach to the bone. This results in the strengthening of both muscles and bones. Each exercise takes only five seconds, and can be accomplished even by most people with physical limitations. The total time for the complete workout is 10 minutes, including warm up and cool down. The exercises can be done even while watching T.V. The Osteo-Ball deflates for easy travel. It comes complete with a user's manual and a detailed instructional video. To learn more about the OsteoBall or to place an order, visit www.bonefitness.com.

Whole-body Vibration Therapy is a unique form of exercise known to build bone strength and density. Learn more about this amazing method of exercise in the section on *Arthritis*.

■ *Flax*. One of the oldest continuously-cultivated plants in history is also one of nature's most perfect foods. Flax, which can be consumed either as an oil or as seeds (preferably ground into flax meal), is high in calcium, magnesium, omega-3 and -6 fatty acids, and phytoestrogens. Taken at the daily dosage of either 2-4 tablespoons of oil or four tablespoons of flax meal, flax has been shown to reduce bone loss. A 1998 article published in the *Journal of the American Nutriceutical Association*[41] found that, in postmenopausal women not taking HRT, the daily addition of about four tablespoons (~38 gm) of ground flax seeds significantly reduced the rate of bone loss. If supplementing with oil, the high lignan version is preferred.

■ *Xylitol*. Discussed at greater length in the section on *Asthma*, the sugar alcohol *xylitol*—in addition to preventing inner ear, nasal and sinus infections and reducing cavities, dental plaque, and gum disease—has been shown in animal studies to increase bone density. In 1994, a study from Finland found that rats who had their ovaries removed

were able to maintain and slightly increase bone density, while the bone density of the control group not receiving xylitol fell significantly.[42] The same Finnish researchers studied the effects of dietary xylitol on aging male rats. At the end of the 20 month study, there was a xylitol-induced bone density increase of almost 10%.[43] The human dosage of about three tablespoons daily equates to the effective treatment levels used in the animal studies. Xylitol is available in many health food stores, or can be ordered at a discount at www.emeraldforest xylitol.com or www.xylitolnow.com.

■ *OsteoKing*.® A 3,000-year-old Chinese bone-healing herbal formula has recently become available in the U.S. The subject of innumerable clinical trials in China, OsteoKing is not only able to increase BMD in osteoporotic subjects, but also aids in quickly healing fractured bones. A study of 60 cases of traumatic fracture showed a 98% improvement in fracture healing, a 95% reduction in swelling, and 98% effectiveness in reducing pain. Due to its long history of safe and effective use, this is one product that shouldn't be overlooked. OsteoKing can be ordered from Nature's Healing Solution at (800) 550-9285, www.osteoking.com.

■ *Magnetic Mattress*. In clinical trials, the unipolar magnetic mattress manufactured by the Canadian company Magnetico has been shown to maintain or increase bone density using the device over a period of only several months. For more information about this product, see *Magnets* in the section on **Pain Relievers**.

Hormones. Sex hormones are known to be important regulators of bone replacement and resorption. Hormones including *estrogen, progesterone, testosterone*, and *calcitonin* play a role in the prevention, formation, and treatment of osteoporosis. Although estrogen receptors are present on cell lines of both osteoblasts and osteoclasts, it appears to be mediated through local cytokine production [through changes in interleukin-1, interleukin-6, tumor necrosis factor (TNF-a) and granulocyte/ macrophage colony stimulation factor (GCSF)] rather than directly at the receptor sites.[44]

The important role of estrogen in the prevention and treatment of both pre- and postmenopausal women has been stressed by many traditional Western physicians. However, estrogen's role has increasingly been brought into question in terms of both its efficacy and safety.

For decades, hormone replacement therapy (HRT), either estrogens alone (ERT; known as "unopposed estrogens") or estrogen in combination with progestin, was touted as the first choice in therapy for the prevention of osteoporosis in postmenopausal women. With the recent, shocking exposés on the ineffectiveness of and tragedies caused by HRT, this treatment serves as a sad example of a treatment method highly recommended by mainstream medicine, only to discover decades after the fact that HRT can be extremely harmful.

It has been known since 1976 that ERT causes up to an 800% increase in uterine endometrial cancer.[45] It is now known that ERT, even in low potency such as 1-2 mg of oral estriol, significantly increases the risk of endometrial cancer. As reported in the Lancet[46] in 1999, postmenopausal women who had ever taken low-potency estrogen doubled the risk of endometrial cancer compared to those who had never taken the drug. The relative risk of developing the disease increased by 8% for each year ERT was taken in low dose.

As a result of these findings, over the ensuing decades estrogen/progestin combinations increased rapidly in popularity, assuming that adding progestin to estrogen would nullify the increased incidence of endometrial cancer. Because so much was at stake—the health and welfare of many nations' postmenopausal women—this should have been a case of "look before you leap." However, doctors wantonly prescribed women with concoctions of hormones that caused much suffering.

In a 2000 study published in the Journal of the National Cancer Institute,[47] it was reported that in addition to increasing the incidence of endometrial cancer, ERT also increases the incidence of breast cancer by 6% for every five years of use. Additionally, it was revealed that when progestin is added to the regimen, i.e., estrogen and progestin combined—the "gold standard" for HRT—five years of use increases the risk of breast cancer by 24%, almost four times as much as ERT alone.

It's hard to argue with statistics such as these which are published in the world's most prestigious medical journals, although the drug companies still do. They have tried to make a case for the continued use of HRT based on the claim that the benefits of the therapy—the decreased incidence of heart disease—outweigh the increased risks of endometrial and breast cancers. Recent research has called that bluff, and put it to serious rest.

According to a 1998 study of 2,763 postmenopausal women published in the Journal of the American Medical Association,[48] called the HERS study (Heart and Estrogen/Progestin Replacement Study), estrogen/progesterone HRT therapy "did not reduce the overall rate of CHD [coronary heart disease] in postmenopausal women with established coronary disease," and showed "a pattern of early increase in risk of CHD events," including heart attack (increased 29%), stroke (increased 41%) and blood clots (increased 200%). HRT also increased the risk of breast cancer by 65-85% in long-term users, and increased risk of gallbladder disease.

The study authors concluded,

> Here is another case where a medical assumption was made and presented to the public before a well-structured study was performed to prove out that assumption...People were told and placed on this medical regimen with everyone believing that they were preventing heart disease. In fact it did not, and unfortunately it increased venous thromboembolic events and gallbladder disease.[49]

Another nail in the HRT coffin was hammered by a 2003 study reported in the Journal of the American Medical Association[50] showing a link between dementia and estrogen/progestin HRT. In a group of women over 65, the risk of dimentia for those taking HRT was double the incidence of the control group of women not taking the drugs.

The drug companies are quick to point out that alternatives are available to the types of estrogens and progestins evaluated for safety and efficacy in the above-discussed research. There are synthetic conjugated estrogens and esterified estrogens, as well as ethinyl estradiol, estropipate, and estrone—all available in oral forms, by injection, as vaginal creams and transdermal patches, just in time for Christmas. At some point the female consumers of the Western world must begin making reasonable choices based on research data and relevant historical precedent, not merely by listening to the advertisements put forth by the pharmaceutical community. That time is far overdue.

It was once thought all women experience considerable bone loss following menopause as the result of decreased estrogen levels; thus, an estrogen deficiency was seen as the principal cause of the disease. Many researchers now believe the causal link is not so clear cut. Cross-cultural studies show, as discussed, that women of various cultures around the world experience a far lower incidence of postmenopausal osteoporosis than women in the U.S. and many other Western countries. In addition, all other factors being equal, it is known that 1) some women lose considerably more bone than others following menopause, 2) some women lose considerable bone before the onset of menopause, and 3) women lose bone at differing rates.

■ **_Progesterone_**. The research of Dr. Jerilynn Prior, Professor of Endocrinology at the University of British Columbia, points to another hormone that is central in the bone-building process, and a deficiency of which, she believes, serves a key role in the onset of osteoporosis. Dr. Prior's studies indicate there are progesterone receptors on osteoblast cells that mediate the formation of new bone. She has found that osteoporotic women often retain high levels of estrogen, while having low levels of progesterone.[51] As such, many women find that supplementation with natural, plant-derived progesterone, as described in the section on **Hot Flashes**, is an effective treatment.[52] Prescription-only progesterone products are also available.

■ **_Testosterone_**. Typically considered a male hormone, testosterone is also produced by the female ovaries. It is an important hormone for both men and women in the treatment and prevention of bone loss. Unlike estrogen, testosterone supplementation appears to be safe as well as effective. A 1999 study published in the *Journal of Endocrinology and Metabolism*[53] showed that supplementing with testosterone increased the bone mass of the lumbar spines of elderly men. Testosterone can be administered in many ways, including gels and by transdermal patch. See Testosterone under **Diabetes**.

■ **_Calcitonin_**. Another hormone playing a part in bone formation is calcitonin, a polypeptide hormone secreted from the thyroid gland. Calcitonin tends to lower calcium blood plasma levels by suppressing osteoclasts. It also promotes bone growth by stimulating osteoblasts.[54] Calcitonin can increase bone density and strength in osteoporotic women, with a corresponding decrease in the incidence of fractures.[55] It is often effective in relieving the pain of spinal compression fractures. Calcitonin is available as an injectable and as Miacalcin Nasal Spray,® both of which are effective forms of treatment.

■ **_Other Bone Builders_**. *Lactoferrin*, a glycoprotein derived from whey protein, and *ipriflavone*, a synthetic counterpart of a plant constituent of the same name, have been shown to inhibit bone breakdown, increase bone density, and boost overall bone health. The daily dosage recommendation is 300-900 mg of lactoferrin and 600 mg of ipriflavone.

Dietary Factors. The consideration of dietary factors brings the topic of osteoporosis more clearly into focus. Because cross-cultural studies have shown that people in certain cultures are significantly more subject to developing osteoporosis—independent of BMD levels—differences in dietary factors loom large as possible answers to its causes. Two principal factors are highly implicated in the origin of osteoporosis: the acidity/alkalinity levels of the body, and the intake of phosphorous/phosphates.

To maintain good health, the body must maintain a proper acidity/alkalinity balance, referred to as the pH balance. pH ranges from 0, the most acidic, to 14, the most alkaline, with 7 being neutral. Normal, healthy pH is *slightly alkaline* at a value of about 7.4—a figure which the body strives to maintain. Enzymes, those substances which catalyze the body's myriad chemical reactions, require an optimal range of pH in order to function properly. The body utilizes many systems such as the liver, lungs, pancreas, kidneys, and sweat glands to maintain optimal pH. When these systems aren't able to maintain a pH level of at least 7.38, acid-neutralizing minerals begin being robbed from the body's mineral storehouse—the bones and muscle tissue.

Dietary intake has a direct effect on body pH. When too many acid-producing foods are consumed and the body's normal acid-neutralizing systems aren't able to maintain proper pH, bone loss begins to occur. Drs. Anthony Sebastian and Deborah Sellmeyer of the University of California at San

Francisco analyzed data from more than 87 different studies which included the typical diets of people in 33 countries.[56] They reported that two thirds (~67%) of all hip fractures could be accounted for by diets rich in acid-producing foods. The remainder of the fractures, they believe, can be accounted for by factors such as lack of exercise, and secondary factors such as those discussed below.

Supporting this research are cross-cultural studies showing that countries such as South Africa and Singapore, whose citizens consume less that one third of the (U.S.) recommended daily amount of calcium while eating low acid-producing diets, have far fewer hip fractures than people of Western countries who consume high-calcium, high acid-producing diets.[57] Citizens of Germany and Sweden, where there is the highest consumption of acid-producing foods, have 40 times (4000%) the incidence of hip fractures compared to a country such as Thailand, whose citizens consume far more alkaline-producing foods and far less acid-producing ones.[58]

Animal protein, as opposed to vegetable protein, is heavily implicated as one of the most serious bodily acidifiers. Animal foods are predominantly rich in acid precursors, while protein from vegetable sources is accompanied by base (alkaline) precursors not found in animal protein. A net acid load is created which the University of California researchers believe causes bone degradation.[59] This helps to explain several other conflicting studies, some showing that high protein intake is related to osteoporosis, while others show the opposite.

Dr. Walter Willett of the Harvard School of Public Health has stated that he believes it is the high protein content of milk that tends to leach calcium from the bones. This helps explain why high milk-consuming countries have such a high prevalence of osteoporosis, a result that is opposite from that which is generally assumed and publicized. Got milk? Got osteoporosis?

Acid-forming foods include[60] all meats (including fish); alcoholic beverages; beans (most unsprouted varieties; when sprouted, they become alkaline-producing); breads (including cereals, crackers and pastries); grains (most grains including wheat and oat bran, corn, Kamut, oats, quinoa, all rice, rye, and spelt); butter and cheese; caffeinated drinks (coffee and soft drinks); drugs (almost

all pharmaceuticals); nuts (including Brasil, cashews, dried coconut, filberts, legumes, macadamias, peanuts, pecans, and walnuts); pastas; salt (refined table but not genuine sea salt); sweeteners (carob, corn syrup, and sugar); tobacco products; alcohol (including beer, wine, and hard liquor).

Alkaline-producing foods include[61] almost all vegetables and fruits (and their juices, including citrus fruits which produce alkaline-forming end products); beans (green, lima, snap, soy, and string; also tofu); eggs; grains (amaranth, barley, flax, millet); herbs (most); nuts (including almonds, chestnuts, and fresh coconuts); oils (most unprocessed, cold-pressed); spices (most); sweeteners (raw honey, Sucanat, stevia, brown rice syrup); teas (most herbal); bee pollen; lecithin.

There is an easy and accurate "litmus test" that can measure the body's pH level. The test uses acid/alkaline-measuring Hydrion Papers which are available from your local pharmacy, and should be performed between meals. To evaluate saliva, spit several times to generate fresh saliva, and lick the saliva onto the Hydrion test strip. A dark blue color correlates with a pH of 7.5, and medium blue to 7.0. If the tape turns light blue, blue-green or yellow, body fluids are overly acidic, indicating a probable state of calcium deficiency.

The second important dietary factor seriously implicated as causative for osteoporosis is the over-consumption of phosphorus/phosphates. Although phosphorus is an important mineral found in bones, teeth, and all living cells (as organic phosphates), excess phosphorus has a negative effect on osteoporosis. Calcium binds to phosphorus within the body, and is excreted when excess phosphorus is eliminated. In its continuous attempt to regulate the many varied processes, sensing lowered calcium levels in the blood, the body uses the parathyroid glands to adjust the blood-calcium levels by leaching calcium from the bones—the most readily-available source.

The modern Western diet is replete with sources of phosphorus. In addition to phosphorus within the foods, dozens of phosphorus-containing substances are used as food additives such as colorizers, emulsifiers, and humectants.[62] These as well as other phosphorus additives are used in the preparation of many common foods. Some phosphorus-enriched foods are baked goods, bread, cheeses, and processed meats. Foods containing naturally high levels of phosphorus include bran, cheeses, corn, ice cream and yogurt. High protein foods also contain high phosphorus levels. Milk is one such food, which again helps to explain the milk/osteoporosis connection.

One of the most egregious phosphorus offenders is carbonated beverages, especially soft drinks, aka soda pop, one of the Western world's—especially young people's—most favorite consumables. In the U.S., soft drink consumption surpassed water consumption over two decades ago. Fifty-six percent of eight-year-olds and one-third of teenaged boys drink at least three cans daily. Annual U.S. sales of soft drinks is over 15 billion gallons.[63] That's a daily average of at least one 12-ounce can for every man, woman and child living in the U.S.—more than 50 gallons annually per person.

[To help you wrap your head around how large "a billion" is, a billion seconds ago it was 1959; a billion minutes ago Jesus was alive; a billion hours ago our human ancestors were living in the Stone Age; and a billion dollars ago was only one third of one day ago (slightly more than eight hours), at the rate the U.S. government spends our tax dollars.]

Harvard researchers recently published two studies on the effects of carbonated soft drinks on the bones of teenaged girls.[64] Among over 400 physically active girls 14-15 years of age, carbonated beverages, and especially cola drinks, were shown to be highly associated with bone fractures. Although the mechanism(s) by which carbonated soft drinks are associated with the increased incidence of fractures was not determined by these studies, the researchers point out that as long ago as the 1800s it was known that exposure to phosphorus increases the rate of fractures. The phosphoric content of soft drinks could well be a causative factor.

Cross-cultural studies are telling, and clearly demonstrate that diet plays a significant role in the formation of osteoporosis. Boyd Eaton and Marjorie Shostak, authors of the 1988 book *The Paleolithic Prescription*,[65] point out that human genetics is rooted in ancient biochemistry and physiology which is fine-tuned to conditions of life that existed hundreds of thousands to millions of years ago. While 100,000 generations of our ancestors were hunter-gatherers sustained by whole foods, 500 generations were dependent on agriculture, and 10

generations lived since the beginning of the industrial revolution, only two generations have lived during a time when much-to-most of the diet consists of highly refined, processed foods.

Dr. Anthony Sebastian, one of the University of California scientists who researches the pH/osteoporosis link discussed above, has stated that "the paleolithic diet is my guiding principal... I try to get back to our roots..."[66] Clearly, the modern diet—high pH and high phosphorus foods, refined sugar, artificial sweeteners, refined (bleached) flour, processed salt, *trans* fats, artificial food additives—is heavily implicated not only in the formation of osteoporosis, but many other degenerative diseases.

Secondary Factors. There are other secondary, external factors that contribute to osteoporosis including endocrine gland abnormalities such as Cushing's syndrome; diabetes; hyperparathyroidism; hyperthyroidism; hypogonadism; involvement with drugs such as alcohol; aluminum-containing antacids; antibiotics; anticonvulsants; caffeine; chemotherapeutic agents; diuretics; glucocorticoids; heparin therapy; nicotine (cigarettes); oral contraceptives; neoplastic conditions such as bone metastasis and multiple myeloma; anorexia nervosa; celiac disease; and post gastrectomy.

To a degree, genetics is also implicated in osteoporosis. Most of the evidence to support this contention comes from the study of twins, either monozygotic (identical twins) or dizygotic (nonidentical twins). Even taking environmental factors into account, a genetic component seems to account for about 75% of the determinant of *peak bone mass*,[67] defined as the highest bone mass achieved during a lifetime, usually around the age of 30.

Testing for Osteoporosis. In addition to the simple pH saliva test described above, there are other tests which attempt to measure osteoporosis risk, some more effectively than others. The standard test for the measurement of BMD and BMC (bone mineral content) is *dual energy X-ray absorptiometry*, or DEXA, which uses low levels of ionizing radiation at the primary sites of the hips and vertebral bodies, and also secondarily at the wrist and heel. These findings are compared to DEXA values of a person of similar age, and also to the estimated peak bone density of a healthy young adult. Although viewed as the "industry standard" by most traditional physicians, DEXA has its drawbacks.

Some physicians believe it may be possible to test normal on one particular DEXA machine, while testing severely osteoporotic at another testing site. Also, the DEXA evaluation is simply a benchmark in time, without indicating how quickly bone is being lost. It is recommended there be up to a two year interval between screenings, which could allow significant deterioration during that time. Perhaps the strongest criticism of the DEXA is that the value of the test lies in its ability to forecast the future probability of fractures. However, as mentioned earlier, fracture risk is at least to some extent independent of BMD.

In 1998 the U.S. Food and Drug Administration approved the use of a second device that evaluates the BMD levels. The portable ultrasound device, a sonometer, transmits sound waves through the heel of the foot. The heel ultrasound is accurate enough for screening, but currently lacks the sensitivity of the DEXA, which is still seen as the "gold standard" for diagnosis of osteoporosis. Again, these tools may be adequate indicators of BMD, but oftentimes not good predictors of bone fractures.

When bone loss overcomes new bone formation, i.e., when resorption overcomes replacement, indicators of this are found in the blood and subsequently excreted in the urine. One of the materials contributing to bone formation is *deoxypyridinoline*, or Dpd, an amino acid that cross-links with collagen in the bone (and other tissues). During resorption, Dpd is excreted unmetabolized in the urine and can be measured by the Pyrilinks®-D urine test. Urine collection can be taken at home or in a doctor's office, after which the sample is mailed to the laboratory. To learn more about the Pyrilinks®-D urine test, call North Bay Diagnostics at (888) 689-8378.

Yet another test helpful in evaluating osteoporosis-related bone loss may be the most accurate of all. The Osteomark® NTx urine test, similar to the Pyrilinks test, measures a marker released during bone resorption. The marker, *N-telopeptides*, or Ntx, is present *only* in Type I collagen which forms about 90% of the organic bone matrix, and is exclusively related to bone as opposed to Dpd which can come from tissues other than bone. A person can be reevaluated in three months using the Osteomark. In this way, the results of

therapy can be monitored accurately. To learn more about the Osteomark NTx urine test, visit www.ostex.com, or call Inverness Medical at (609)627-8000.

■ For additional information about Osteoporosis, visit the Member's Area of *The Encyclopedia's* website.

PARKINSON'S DISEASE

In 1817, London physician James Parkinson published a paper entitled "Essay on the Shaking Palsy." Although this was the first "modern" formal description of the disease, in 175 AD the noted Greek physician Galen referred to the condition as "Shaking Palsy." Thousands of years previous, its existence was discussed in the ancient medical writings of both the Indian (Ayurveda; the disease was called "kampavata" and "atmagupta") and Chinese medical literature as long as 2,500-5,000 years ago. Parkinson's (PD) is a progressive and to date incurable neurological disorder resulting from degeneration of dopamine-producing brain cells (neurons) in the *substantia nigra pars compacta* (SNpc) and *corpus stratia* portions of the midbrain.

When dopamine secretion from the SNpc becomes deficient, the classical symptoms of the disease begin to manifest—tremor (trembling or shaking) of a limb (often beginning in one hand), especially when the body is at rest (and less so with movement); rigidity of the limbs; poor balance; slow movement (bradykinesia) or an inability to move (akinesis); a shuffling gait; stooped posture; difficulty swallowing; difficulty speaking; and lack of facial expression ("mask face").

The most common symptom of PD is known as the "pill-rolling tremor," where there is an uncontrollable movement of the thumb resembling the rolling of a pill between the thumb and other fingers. The disease also may cause mental disturbances including depression, personality changes, loss of sleep, and sexual problems. One tragedy of PD is that by the time any symptoms are noticed, 80-90% of the dopamine-producing cells have been lost.

Parkinson's disease exists throughout the world with the disease being more prevalent in some countries than others, although it remains unclear why these variations occur. PD is infrequently seen in those under 40 years of age, with the average age at onset being about 60. The disease afflicts about one percent of both men and women over age 70, with men being slightly more affected than women. About 500,000 to one million people in the U.S. have PD, with roughly 50,000 additional new cases annually.[1] As the population ages, its prevalence is expected to rise. Several well-known personalities suffering from PD, including Muhammad Ali, Michael J. Fox and the late Pope John Paul II, have brought the disease more into the public eye.

There have been many theories regarding the cause of PD—including pathogenic infection, genetic predisposition, toxic environmental exposure, and poor nutritional habits—although no single causative factor has been proven definitively, and there are likely multiple causes. The literature contains references to PD symptoms being caused by ingestion of illegal drugs contaminated with the substance MPTP. Studies of family histories and of twins suggest some may have a genetic susceptibility to PD which is influenced by environmental factors.

Whatever the ultimate causative factor(s), researchers believe there is oxidative damage to cellular structures in the SNpc area of the brain. This causes a deficiency of one of the three most important neurotransmitters, dopamine. Neurotransmitters are those chemicals that help the billions of brain cells both send and receive nerve impulses, and thereby communicate with each other.

Currently there are no blood tests or imaging techniques that can conclusively diagnose Parkinson's, although these tests are useful in excluding other diseases and identifying structural, vascular and metabolic anomalies that may be at the root of the disease. Neurologists use several means to attempt to diagnose PD, including PET and other brain scans. While not pointing to a specific diagnosis, the P300 brainwave speed and voltage test and the quantitative encephalograph (QEEG) are useful in identifying early cognitive loss.

Autopsied brains of affected victims show microscopic structures called *Lewy bodies*, the presence of which are considered a hallmark of classical PD. Autopsies of older persons without diagnosed PD often uncover Lewy bodies, a fact that has led some researchers to believe that known PD sufferers are only the tip of a much larger neu-ro-decaying iceberg—with as many as 20 affected people for each diagnosed PD patient.[2]

Treatment. As there is no cure for Parkinson's, therapies can only reduce its progression, minimize symptoms, and maximize the quality of life. Because PD creates a deficiency of dopamine, one form of treatment focuses on replacing dopamine with precursor substances such as levodopa (L-dopa; Sinemet® and Larodopa®), which the body converts into dopamine. One of the difficulties associated with the use of L-dopa is that it loses its effectiveness over time. Also, after about five years 50% of its users have motor complications such as involuntary movements (dyskinesias).[3] Additional side-effects can include nausea and vomiting, which are often treated with the addition of the drug *carbidopa*. Difficulty with swallowing, breathing and balance also can occur.[4] Despite their many potential side-effects, these drugs are often helpful in controlling Parkinson's symptoms.

Alternatively, other drugs such as selegiline (Deprenyl® and Eldepryl®) attempt to prevent the breakdown of dopamine by inhibiting *monoamine oxidase* (MAO), the enzyme that breaks down dopamine in the brain. Such drugs are referred to as MAO inhibitors. A third approach is the use of drugs such as bromocriptine (Parlodel®) and pergolide (Permax®) to directly affect dopamine receptors. Combinations of these drugs are often prescribed.

Two surgical techniques can be used in the later stages of PD, when all other forms of treatment have failed. Ablative surgery severs areas in the brain that control muscle movement, thus relieving symptoms of tremor, rigidity, and slow movement. Surgical complications can include stroke, cognitive impairment, difficulty swallowing, and vision defects.[5] Deep brain stimulation, discussed below, is another surgical procedure typically reserved for late-stage PD.

■ ***Deep Brain Stimulation.*** A relatively new surgical technique, Deep Brain Stimulation (DBS) is a surgical option for persons with Parkinson's disease, Essential Tremor, dystonia, and tremor resulting from multiple sclerosis. It often provides relief from tremors, rigidity, stiffness, slowness of movement, and balance problems. DBS is a new-and-improved version of the old surgical technique involving the destruction of small portions of the brain within the thalamus or globus pallidus. As currently practiced, the goal of DBS is the stimulation, not destruction, of brain tissue.

During the surgery, a small lead containing several electrodes is positioned within the brain at the specific area to be stimulated. Success of the operation depends on the correct placement of the electrodes. The target area is defined prior to the operation by use of magnetic resonance imaging (MRI), and is further defined by sophisticated monitoring instruments as well as patient-doctor interactions during the operation. Even though the patient remains awake during the surgical placement of the electrodes, the operation is painless as the brain itself does not have pain receptors and therefore does not generate pain signals. Other pain-producing tissue damage caused by the operation is treated with a local anesthetic.

The lead containing the electrodes is connected by thin, insulated wires through a small opening in the skull to an apparatus consisting of a battery and a programmable regulator (impulse generator) implanted under the skin below the collar bone in the chest area. The impulse generator, or pacemaker-like device, transmits the proper electrical signals to the target area of the brain, blocking abnormal neural activity which is the cause of the symptoms to be treated.

On average, DBS patients experience about a 50% improvement in walking and balance, from 60-80% improvement in symptoms of tremor and slowness of movement, and over 80% reduction in involuntary movements caused by medication. Following DBS, most patients are able to significantly reduce their medication levels.

There is a 2-3% risk of brain hemorrhage that may either cause no problem, or may cause problems such as paralysis, stroke, or speech impairment. Stated another way, for each 100 patients receiving DBS, two or three will experience a severe complication or permanent damage. There is a reported 15% risk of a minor or temporary complication. DBS is an FDA-approved procedure for the treatment of Essential Tremor and Parkinson's disease, and is covered for these conditions in most states by Medicare. Most other insurance policies also cover DBS. More natural treatments offer additional hope to those suffering from Parkinson's.

■ *IV Glutathione.* Composed of the three amino acids cysteine, glycine and glutamic acid, *glutathione* is one of the body's master detoxifiers and antioxidants. As a detoxifier, it helps convert fat-soluble toxic chemicals (such as pesticides and solvents) and heavy metals (such as lead, mercury, and aluminum) into water-soluble forms that can then be excreted in the urine and bile. As one of the brain's most active antioxidants, glutathione neutralizes harmful free radicals that are highly implicated in the development of Parkinson's. Although there are several means of increasing glutathione levels using glutathione precursors such as the oral supplements vitamin C, lipoic acid, and N-acetylcysteine, PD patients require therapeutic doses of glutathione that can be obtained only through intravenous administration.

In a 1996 study[6] by Italian researchers, 600 mg of IV glatathione was administered to PD patients twice daily for 30 days. Patient progress was assessed once a month over the next six months. The researchers reported a striking improvement in all of the patients receiving glutathione, with a 42% decline in disability. Following the 30 day treatment regimen, the benefits lasted from two to four months without further treatment.

World-renowned alternative medical practitioner Dr. Julian Whitaker highly recommends the technique for treating PD, has had many successes in treating his PD patients, and believes it should be the treatment of choice for PD. Pioneer glutathione researcher Dr. David Perlmutter has produced a video giving an overview of IV glutathione treatment. The video demonstrates the protocol he uses for simple and successful glutathione administration, and also presents clinical case studies. The video can be ordered by calling (800) 530-1982 or by visiting www.inutritionals.com. To locate a practitioner in your area who administers this treatment, contact the American College for Advancement in Medicine at (800)530-1982, or visit their web site at www.acam.org.

■ *Enhanced External Counter Pulsation* (EECP). A technique effective in treating various aspects of cardiovascular disease has recently shown promise in treating the symptoms of PD. EECP is a non-surgical treatment that uses a unique set of mechanical equipment to inflate and deflate a series of pneumatic compressive cuffs around the calves and lower and upper thighs. The cuffs inflate and deflate in a particular sequence which is correlated to the heart beat. The overall effect is to increase the oxygen supply of the heart, while decreasing its oxygen demand. Many experts believe PD may be associated with vascular problems. EECP's success in treating PD supports this view.

Several years ago Arkansas cardiologist Dr. Charles Fitzgerald serendipitously discovered that EECP treatment, in addition to helping his cardiac patients, also provided significant improvements in the symptoms of his Parkinson's patients, including ease of walking, mood enhancement, and increased facial expression. Fitzgerald believes the beneficial effects are probably the result of increased blood flow to the portion of the brain that produces dopamine, the *substantia nigra pars compacta*.[7]

Medicare covers EECP treatments only for angina. As more research demonstrates its effectiveness in relieving PD symptoms, insurance coverage could be expanded. To learn more about the technique, see EECP under **Cardiovascular Disease** and visit the website of its manufacturer Vasomedical at www.vasomedical.com, or call them at (800)455-3327.

■ *Coenzyme Q10* (CoQ10). Also known as ubiquinone, CoQ10 has antioxidant properties similar to vitamin E, although unlike vitamin E it can be manufactured by the body. CoQ10 is a lipid which is present in the energy-producing mitochondria of every cell in the body, and is found most abundantly in areas of the body requiring the most energy, such as the heart. It is a powerful antioxidant that increases stamina, may slow the aging process, and is helpful to the body in myriad other ways.

One of those ways was recently documented by researchers at the University of California, San Diego. In a 2002 article published in the *Archives of Neurology*,[8] the UC researchers reported the results of a 16 month study involving 80 patients with early Parkinson's. The patients were randomly assigned to one of four groups: 300 mg, 600 mg, or 1,200 mg daily, or a placebo. Symptoms of the patients in each of the CoQ10 groups progressed much more slowly compared to the placebo group

taking no Q10. The most pronounced effect was in the 1,200 mg/day group which experienced a 44% reduction in symptom worsening.

A good CoQ10 product will contain either an oil (such as borage, flax, etc.) or an advanced delivery system to aid in absorption. Two such products are oil-based Vitaline CoQ10 and Q-Sorb® by Jarrow Formulas, which have proprietary liposomal delivery systems. Both are available in health food stores and on the internet. Perhaps the best CoQ10 product is known as Ubiquinol, a reduced and more bioavailable form of the substance, which is also available online and in health food stores.

■ *Vitamin E.* Vitamin E is a fat-soluble vitamin of critical importance in the treatment and prevention of a number of medical conditions. The generic term vitamin E includes at least eight forms of tocopherol produced from plants, of which d-alpha tocopherol is believed to have the highest potency. In a 2002 study published in *Archives of Neurology*,[9] the mental decline of 3,000 men and women aged 65-102 was followed over a seven year period. Those participants whose dietary or supplemental vitamin E consumption was in the highest quintile (one fifth) experienced a 36% reduction in worsening of symptoms compared to those in the lowest quintile.

Both the natural (d-alpha tocopherol, d-alpha tocopheryl acetate, and d-alpha tocopheryl succinate) and synthetic forms (dl-alpha tocopherol, dl-alpha todcopheryl acetate, and dl-alpha tocopheryl succinate) of vitamin E are commercially available as a pill-form supplement.

Natural vitamin E is isolated from vegetable oils, whereas synthetic vitamin E is produced from petrochemicals. Natural vitamin E is significantly more biologically active and more present in various organs, blood and muscle tissue compared to its synthetic counterpart. When supplementing with vitamin E, be sure to select the natural version— "d," not "dl."

■ *Mucuna Beans.* Previous to the advent of synthetic L-dopa—the typical form currently obtained by prescription—various cultures throughout the world, particularly in Africa and the Middle East, have treated PD with cooked fava beans *(Vicia faba)*. Although those who used the beans for this purpose had no knowledge of their chemical composition, they nevertheless noted the beans helped relieve PD symptoms.

In Brazil and India, traditional healers have used mucuna beans (*Mucuna pruriens*) to treat PD. Ancient Indian medical texts describe its use 4,500 years ago. In 1936, two Indian researchers isolated L-dopa from the mucuna bean, although its connection to Parkinson's wasn't made until the 1960s.

A leading producer of Ayurvedic medicines, Zandu Pharmaceutical Works of Bombay, India, currently markets a mucuna bean product for the treatment of PD called Zandopa (HP-200). One clinical trial of the herbal preparation, reported in the *Journal of Alternative & Complementary Medicine*[10] in 1995, was conducted at the Texas A&M Medical School in Temple, Texas. Sixty Stage 2.5 (Stage 5 is the worst) PD patients averaging 59 years of age were given daily doses of Zandopa containing 1,250-1,750 mg of natural L-dopa. Following three months of treatment all of the participants improved significantly, averaging almost one stage of improvement. The study concluded that Zandopa is highly beneficial in the treatment of PD. No toxicity was noted and side-effects were mild, mostly relating to stomach upset.

Animal studies have shown that, dose for dose, mucuna is 2-3 times more effective than equivalent amounts of synthetic L-dopa.[11] This has led researchers to postulate there are other active constituents in the mucuna bean that help account for its relative effectiveness in comparison to the same amount of synthetic L-dopa. In addition to being a possible substitute for its synthetic counterpart, scientists hope to isolate the other compounds that may be helping the mucuna bean product achieve its effectiveness.

Zandopa is marketed in India, but is currently undergoing clinical trials in the U.S. Although self treatment for Parkinson's is not recommended, there are mucuna powder products available as nutritional (anti-aging) supplements. The product L-dopa is a mucuna-based formulation marketed by International Supplements.com. It can be purchased by calling (800)476-1720 or (561)626-4787, or by visiting www.internationalsupplements.com.

■ *Transcranial Magnetic Stimulation.* A technique still in the research stages for Parkinson's

offers hope of reducing the amount of medication required by patients by making the brain more sensitive to the medication. *Transcranial magnetic stimulation* (TMS), a relatively new technique of modern medicine, employs an electronic apparatus which stores energy in a bank of condensers. As the stored energy discharges into a wound coil, a magnetic field is created around the surface of the coil. According to Dr. Mikhail Lomarev, M.D., Ph. D., a neurologist at the U.S. National Institutes of Health, when the apparatus is applied to the brain of a patient, an electromagnetic field is induced in different layers of the motor cortex and there is a change of electrical activity in the treated areas of the brain.[12] The goal of this approach is to improve the motor function of patients so that they are less stiff, and able to move more quickly.

Lomarev has measured the walking speeds of Parkinson's patients before and after a two week treatment period of up to eight TMS sessions. Maintaining the same level of medication, as the number of treatments increased, the walking speeds of the treated patients increased proportionally. There was no improvement in the placebo group of PD patients who received no treatment.

The next step for Lomarev and his colleagues is upcoming clinical trials in which he will test different versions of the TMS equipment, including direct current (DC) stimulation of the brain, and high frequency stimulation. Although Lomarev's work is still in its relative infancy, progress to date is robust enough to believe that TMS will prove to be a beneficial adjunct in PD treatment. To learn more about the technique, its historical background, and its use in treating other illnesses, do a key word search for "transcranial magnetic stimulation," or visit www.earthpulse.net/TMS.htm, www.biomag .hus.fi/tms/Thesis/dt.html or http://transmagnet .med.br/mostra_resumos.php?seq=44. To track the research progress of TMS and its treatment of Parkinson's, do a key word search for "parkinson's tms."

■ *Stem Cell Therapy.* One of the most promising areas of research focuses on the use of stem cells, a type of basic (undifferentiated/unspecialized) cell which, under certain conditions, has the ability to transform into specialized cells such as cells of the heart muscle, pancreas, or even specialized brain cells. In a 2002 study reported in the *Proceedings of the National Academy of Sciences*,[13] researchers announced that for the first time they have successively transplanted mouse embryonic stem cells into the brains of rats with brain damage resembling Parkinson's disease. The transplanted stem cells spontaneously acquired many of the features of normal dopamine-producing cells, and the animals experienced a gradual reduction in PD symptoms. Brain scans showed the transplanted cells integrated into the surrounding area and began dopamine production. Although the stem cells did not survive in 25% of the animals, and an additional 20% developed tumors near the transplant site within nine weeks, this nevertheless was a significant step in the important and rapidly developing area of stem cell research.

In 1999, a human Parkinson's patient received a transplant of neural stem cells derived from the patient's own brain. Some benefit was attained. In 2001, a small trial produced disastrous effects in humans who received fetal stem cell transplants. Following the successful transplants, the cells continued to multiply, producing an irreversible over-production of dopamine.

In 2002, U.S. researchers successfully transplanted adult stem cells cultured *in vitro* from the Parkinson's patient's own brain. When the cells showed signs of producing dopamine, they were re-injected into the patient's own brain. The patient experienced a reduction in trembling, muscle rigidity, and dopamine production increased 58% after a three month period. While the dopamine production stopped in subsequent months, the progress was maintained and the symptoms did not return.[14]

Recently, progress has been made and stem cell therapy is being offered to PD sufferers by various medical groups. For more information, visit www.xcell-center.com or www.cellmedicine.com. To monitor the progress of this area of research, do an online search for "stem cell parkinsons."

■ **_NADH_**. Nicotinamide Adenine Dinucleotide (Hydrogen), abbreviated NADH, is the coenzyme (reduced, active) form of vitamin B_3. Chemically, it is vitamin B_3 (niacinamide), combined with the 5-carbon sugar ribose, a phosphate group, and an adenine nucleotide (a DNA component). NADH is required for the oxidation (burning) of fats, sugars, and amino acids into ATP, the chemical manufactured in the cells' mitochondria that produces energy for the body's many metabolic reactions. NADH is, in fact, the first of five enzyme complexes of what's known as the *electron transport chain*, where much of the ATP is manufactured. Each unit of NADH is able to generate three units of ATP energy. Additionally, NADH aids in cell regulation, DNA repair, enhancement of the cellular immune system, and repair of oxidative damage.

The first person to develop a stable and absorbable oral tablet-form of NADH was Georg Birkmayer, M.D., Ph.D., Medical Director of the Birkmayer Institute for Parkinson's Therapy in Vienna, Austria. Dr. Birkmayer is also a Professor at the University of Graz, Austria, where he heads the Division of Neurochemistry at the Department of Medical Chemistry. In addition to many additional honors and achievements he is on the editorial board of several distinguished medical journals, including the *Journal of Experimental and Clinical Cancer Research* and the *Journal of Tumor Marker Oncology*. Dr. Birkmayer founded Menuco Corporation in 1995 to promote the sale and distribution of NADH, which is also known as Co-E1.

In the mid-1980s, Dr. Birkmayer theorized that NADH might increase the brain's production of dopamine which, as discussed, is deficient in Parkinson's patients. In a study reported in 1993,[15] 885 Parkinson's patients were divided into two groups: 415 were administered intravenous NADH and 470 received oral NADH tablets at the dosage of up to 25 mg daily. About 80% of both groups showed overall good responses, primarily in motor improvements, walking, pushing motion, posture, and speech. Emotional and cognitive improvements were also noted in some patients. Improvements in both the oral and IV groups were almost identical, with the maximum overall improvement noted in the oral users. Specifically, 19.3% of the patients showed 30-50% (very good) improvement; 58.8% showed 10-30% improvement (moderate); and 21.8 % showed no improvement.

The extent of progress is correlated with the degree of disability prior to treatment; the duration of the disease; and the age of the patient. Increased urinary excretion of dopamine was also found in the patients, indicating a NADH-induced increase in dopamine production.

To learn more about NADH, visit www.enadh.com. To view a remarkable video on the NADH treatment of a Parkinson's patient, visit www.enadh.com/movies_parkinson.html.

■ *Hyperbaric Oxygen Therapy* (HBO). Some have suggested an infective component is implicated in PD. If this is the case it would help explain the beneficial results of HBO, as it is known that oxygen is effective against most infectious pathogens. See *Hyperbaric Oxygen Therapy* under **General Treatment Methods**.

■ A device that's shown effectiveness in treating PD is the Magnetic Molecular Energizer (MME). The MME offers hope for many difficult-to-treat medical conditions, including PD. To learn more about this technology, see *Magnetic Molecular Energizer* under **General Treatment Methods**.

■ PD may have an infective component such as that caused by microbial infection from viruses, bacteria, fungi, or parasites. Sodium chlorite (NaClO_2) is a powerful anti-infective. See *Sodium Chlorite* under **General Treatment Methods**.

■ If toxic exposure is involved, various forms of chelation therapy may be capable of producing significant improvement. See Chelation under *Alzheimer's Disease* and *Autism*.

■ See *Lyme Disease*. Some researchers believe Lyme is implicated in many cases of PD.

■ See also Omental Transposition under *Spinal Cord Injury*, and Parkinson's Disease in the Member's Area of *The Encyclopedia's* website.

Prevention. There is a long list of factors associated with PD, including exposure to:

❏ Chemical toxins such as pesticides and herbicides; carbon monoxide and methanol
❏ Solvents such as those used in paints, printing inks, and many other industrial applications
❏ Excess levels of dietary iron
❏ Infections such as encephalitis, influenza, measles, and sexually transmitted diseases

On the other hand, a diet rich in certain nutrients has been shown to offer protection from developing PD. Researchers at Baylor University have found the antioxidant compounds *polyphenols* found in green tea protect the dopamine-producing brain cells of mice against damage from a neurotoxin known to cause PD.[16] Green tea can be consumed either as a liquid or as a pill-form supplement.

Several studies have shown that consuming high levels of dietary vitamin E may protect against the occurrence of Parkinson's. One of the most often quoted studies, known as The Rotterdam Study, found that consumption of high levels of dietary vitamin E but not vitamin C or beta-carotene offers such protection.[17] Foods rich in vitamin E include dark green leafy vegetables (such as chard, kohlrabi, and turnip greens); nuts; and wheat germ. Animal foods rich in vitamin E include chicken, liver, many types of fish, and turkey.

In animal studies, minocycline (Minocin®), an antibiotic in the tetracycline family, was shown to protect the brains of mice given a chemical that induces symptoms of PD. Researchers suggest minocycline or similar drugs may be able to prevent the progression of neurodegenerative diseases including PD. It is speculated that minocycline derives its neuroprotective effect by blocking the action of nitric oxide (NO) in the brain. NO released from *glial* brain cells may be associated with the death of neurons in areas of the brain responsible for Parkinson's symptoms.[18] On the other hand, some researchers suggest PD may have an infective component, such as mycoplasma or other stealth pathogens. If this is the case, it may help explain minocycline's effectiveness.

It was reported in a 2003 article published in *Archives of Neurology*[19] that researchers at the Harvard School of Public Health have found that people who regularly used Nonsteroidal Anti-inflammatory Drugs (NSAIDS) such as aspirin, indomethacin, ibuprofen, and naproxen experienced a 45% reduced risk of developing PD compared to those not taking the drugs. These results suggest that inflammation plays a significant role in the development and course of PD.

Because NSAIDS are accompanied by such significant side-effects, discussed in detail in the section on *Arthritis*, other anti-inflammatories such as Lyprinol (also under *Arthritis*) or curcumin, derived from the yellow-colored spice turmeric, would be a possible substitute. Curcumin has been used as a medicament by the ancient Egyptian pharaohs as well as traditional Ayurvedic medical practitioners of India dating back some 6,000 years. It has been shown to be up to 75% more effective than cortisone as an anti-inflammatory.[20] This product should be purchased as "curcuminoids," available in health food stores or on the internet. A suggested dosage is 300 mg three times per day.

POISON INGESTION

Ipecac syrup has long been used to induce vomiting in cases of poison ingestion. Oral administration of another substance recently has been shown to be more effective, safer, and easier to use than ipecac syrup.

■ *Activated Charcoal.* A 2001 study of 115 children in *Pediatrics*[1] online reported that home treatment with activated charcoal averaged 38 minutes compared to 73 minutes to receive emergency room treatment. Depending on the toxicity of the poison ingested, this time differential could mean the critical difference between life and death. Because activated charcoal absorbs the poison upon contact rather than allowing it to be absorbed by the body, it should be taken as soon as possible following the poison ingestion, and preferably within one hour of ingestion.

To administer the activated charcoal, mix several tablespoons in water and drink. Because time is of the essence, it has been suggested this be done prior to visiting a hospital emergency room, or while in transit. Activated charcoal is inexpensive, and is available in health food stores.

POST OPERATIVE

Two techniques, both done preoperatively, can significantly reduce the pain of surgery: the *Sphenopalatine Ganglion Block* and the spinal epidural (see *Back*). Otherwise, refer to **Pain Relievers** and **General Treatment Methods**.

POST TRAUMATIC STRESS DISORDER (PTSD).

See Eye-Movement Desensitization and Reprocessing (EMDR) under *Stress*.

PROSTATE

The prostate gland is a spongy, walnut-sized structure situated at the base of and surrounding the urethra in human males. The gland secrets a milky or white-colored slightly alkaline fluid which neutralizes the acidity of the vaginal tract, thus prolonging the lifespan of sperm. This is the only known function of the gland. The prostate fluid secretion is a major constituent of ejaculatory fluid, in which sperm are expelled from the penis.

The three prostate-associated difficulties many men will encounter during their lifetimes are: 1) *Benign prostatic hyperplasia*, 2) *Prostatitis*, and 3) prostate cancer. Men over age 40 are subject to enlargement of the prostate wherein benign (noncancerous) nodules increase the size of the gland. This is known as *benign prostatic hyperplasia*, or BPH. It is also called *benign prostatic hypertrophy* and *benign enlargement of the prostate* (BEP). At least a minimal amount of prostate enlargement is present in 50-75% of men over 40 and 75-95% of men over 80 years old. Prostate enlargement is thought to be a normal process of aging—at least in modern Western societies. Men leaving in rural areas, however, have a much lower incidence of BPH symptoms.

The exact mechanism which leads to BPH is uncertain. However, excessive levels of two chemical are significantly implicated: *dihydrotestosterone* (DHT) and *5-alpha reductase*. Starting at about age 40, quantities of the hormone *prolactin* begin to increase, which stimulate the production of 5-alpha reductase, an enzyme that converts testosterone into DHT. DHT is the chemical that can trigger growth of the prostate.

As the prostate enlarges and presses against the urethra, a clamping action is exerted. The bladder wall thickens and becomes irritated. Increased frequency of urination occurs as the bladder begins to contract even though it contains only a small amount of urine. As the disease progresses, the bladder weakens and loses its ability to fully empty itself, causing urine retention. Thus, the constricture of the urethra and weakened bladder cause many of the symptoms associated with BPH.

About 70% of all men with BPH either never manifest any symptoms of the condition or are relatively symptom free, especially earlier in life.[1] As men age, symptoms tend to increase. When symptoms do occur, they can take the form of urinary hesitancy (slow, weak or delayed urine stream), nocturia (needing to urinate two to three or more times per night), pain upon urination, increased urinary frequency, urinary urgency, incontinence, or blood in the urine.

Modern medicine offers many tests to diagnose BHP, including the digital rectal exam (DRE) (digits = fingers); urinary flow rare; post-void residual urine; pressure flow analysis; X-ray analysis; urinalysis; and urine culture. If symptoms are severe, traditional Western medicine makes its standard offers—pharmaceutical drugs and surgery. These drugs include alpha-1 blockers such as alfuzosin, doxazocin, tamsulosin and terazocin, which are also medications for high blood pressure. They relax the urinary muscles and allow easier urination. They'll lower your blood pressure too, at no additional charge. They also can produce symptoms such as dizziness, tachycardia (rapid heart rate), tiredness, weakness, nasal congestion, and retrograde ejaculation wherein the ejaculate enters the bladder rather than being expelled through the urethra.[2]

Another pharmaceutical drug offered in the treatment of BPH is finasteride (Proscar,® a 5-alpha reductase inhibitor), which lowers prostate hormone levels, thereby reducing the size of the gland. Although the drug has been shown to increase urinary flow rates and decrease BPH symptoms, it may take up to six months before any benefit is noticed. Additionally, users may be affected by incontinence, a decreased sex drive, as well as impotence,[3] which won't take six months to notice.

Yet an additional available drug is Lupron,® which through some slight of hand and questionable business practices has become a best-seller for its manufacturer TAP Pharmaceutical, Inc. On October 3, 2001 the U.S. Department of Justice reached out and tapped TAP for a cool USD $875 million in fines. The charges, to which TAP pleaded guilty on all counts, were for inflating prices and engaging in improper sales and marketing practices to induce (a diplomatic word for "bribe") doctors to prescribe Lupron. TAP agreed to plead guilty to "felony conspiracy to violate the Prescription Drug Marketing Act." The fines included a $290 million criminal fine, $560 million for fraud-

ulent claims filed with Medicare and Medicaid, and $25.5 million to settle civil liabilities with all 50 states and the District of Columbia.[4]

In cases of more advanced BPH, surgical techniques are offered. These include techniques such as the Transurethral Resection of the Prostate (TURP)—considered the "gold standard" for BPH surgical treatment. According to this procedure, a 12 inch long instrument called a *resectoscope* is inserted through the urethral canal of the penis. The resectoscope contains an electrified loop which the surgeon uses to remove the obstructing tissue piece by piece. The loop cuts the tissue and cauterizes (seals) the blood vessels simultaneously. The pieces of tissue are flushed out at the conclusion of the operation. Speaking of "flushing," this technique has been referred to as being the equivalent of "roto-rootering" the urethra and prostate. The risks of the TURP include dysuria (difficult and/or painful urination), incontinence, retrograde ejaculation, sexual dysfunction, urinary retention, and urinary tract infection.[5] Another procedure in your friendly urologist's bag of surgical procedures is the Transurethral Incision of the Prostate (TUIP), wherein the urethra is widened by making several small incisions in the bladder neck where the urethra joins the bladder, as well as the prostate itself. Neither the advantages, disadvantages, nor the long-term side-effects of this procedure are currently known.[6]

There are several other "minor" (so-called minimally-invasive, "non-surgical") procedures designed to treat BPH. One such procedure is the Transurethral Needle Ablation, or TUNA. Sounds yummy. Another is Transurethral Microwave Thermotherapy (TUMT). The goal of both therapies is to heat the prostate sufficiently so that substantial necrosis (cell death) of the prostate tissue occurs. Thereafter, the dead tissue is reabsorbed by the body causing the prostate to shrink in size. Our favorite procedure is the TURN, wherein the prospective surgical patient simply turns and quickly exits the surgeons office with no further ado. Needless to say—based on the complications of both necessary and unnecessary surgeries—this latter procedure is often appropriate.

The *coup de grâce* for the walnut-sized appendage is the Radical Prostatectomy, wherein the gland *en toto* is surgically removed along with some of the surrounding tissue, and possibly lymph nodes in the area. Although many men have been cajoled into having this operation, two recently-published studies appearing in the *New England Journal of Medicine* shed glaringly painful light on the inadvisability of submitting to this procedure—unless it is deemed of absolute necessity due to the presence of metastatic cancer. Two Swedish studies followed the progress of 695 men with large prostate tumors over an average period of 6.2 years. Half of the men underwent radical prostatectomies, while the other half followed what is called "watchful waiting"—careful monitoring of the disease with no intervention unless required. One of the studies examined the differences in the mortality rates between the two groups, and the other study evaluated the differences in their quality of life.

Overall, no difference was found in life expectancy between the two groups, i.e., on average the watchful waiters lived as long as the surgical group. The researchers concluded, "current evidence indicates that radical prostatectomy, as compared to watchful waiting, has little or no effect on overall survival."[7] Concerning quality of life issues, 80% of the surgical participants experienced erectile dysfunction compared to only 45% of the watchful waiters. Furthermore, nearly 50% of the surgical group experienced incontinence, compared to only 21% not receiving surgery. The only statistic favoring the surgical group—28% to 44%—was urinary obstruction, which was higher in the watchful waiters' group.[8]

Given the choice between erectile dysfunction and incontinence versus a slightly reduced incidence of urinary obstruction, the choice seems obvious on the face of it. This is not even taking into consideration the fact that participants in these studies suffered from *large* prostate tumors. Men with smaller tumors would logically fare even better on their own. Additional factors which need to be taken into account are the alternative therapies discussed below. For methods of preventing metastasis—the spreading of cancer from the site of origin to distant sites—see *Cancer*.

Prostate cancer is the most common type of cancer and the second leading cause of cancer death in men. In 2004, 32,000 American men died of prostate cancer and over 320,000 new cases were diagnosed. Fifteen to 20% of all men will have prostate cancer during their lifetime, and virtually all

will have the disease if they live long enough. Since 1988, the *Prostate-Specific Antigen* test (PSA) has been modern medicines' tool for the early detection of prostate cancer. The PSA blood test measures prostate-specific antigen, which is produced by the prostate under several circumstances whether or not there is cancerous involvement. For example, the larger the prostate size, the more PSA is released into the bloodstream, and the higher the PSA reading. Consequently, the PSA test is a measure of *prostate gland size*, and only an indirect measure of possible cancerous involvement.[9] Therefore, PSA can be elevated in the case of prostate enlargement (BPH) with no cancerous involvement. Further, inflammation also causes the increased production of prostate-specific antigen.

The PSA test is notorious for giving false indications of possible cancerous involvement. An elevated PSA score may simply be caused by benign enlargement, inflammation, or infection. Even though the PSA may have some usefulness in diagnosing cancerous involvement, due to the high number of false positives (testing elevated when there is no cancer) and false negatives (not testing elevated when there is cancer—up to 30% of prostate cancers occur with a PSA reading of 4.0 or less)—the test is not an accurate stand-alone test to screen for prostate cancer.

Further, the PSA is useless as a means of determining either the size or severity of a tumor. In other words, the test is ineffective in determining the risk posed by a cancerous tumor. In an article published in the *Journal of Urology* in 2002, researchers at Stanford University School of Medicine examined the removed prostates of 875 men. When comparing PSA scores with the size of the prostates, they found that only 14% of the tumors correlated with their PSA values. For example, a PSA score of 9 was no more predictive of a large and/or aggressive tumor than a score of 2. Lead researcher Dr. Thomas Stamey commented, "I could get 15% by flipping a coin."[10] Also, PSA scores in this range have limited value in predicting surgical cure rates. A patient with a PSA score of 2 was no more likely to survive following surgical intervention than a patient with a score of 9.[11]

Following the detection of an abnormality in the prostate—as might be indicated by a false positive PSA—a *needle biopsy* is typically performed, the evaluative technique which has been the gold standard method of differentiating malignant from benign (non-malignant) tumors. As discussed in the *Cancer* section, needle biopsies can provide a path for cancer cells to spread beyond the area of cancerous involvement, while without a biopsy the cancer would have been contained. One study showed a 10-20% risk of the biopsy needle tracking cancer cells along the biopsy path. Therefore, an elevated PSA often leads to a series of unnecessary and potentially dangerous needle biopsies.

A new diagnostic technique accurately differentiates malignant from non-malignant prostatic tumors without the need of a biopsy. Called the 3.0 Tesla MRI Spectroscopy Scanner [3-T MRI; also referred to as the Proton Magnetic Resonance Spectroscopy (^{1}H MRS)], the test provides biochemical information about the tissues being examined. It is able to detect specific ratios of choline, creatine, and citrate compounds which are present in cancerous but not benign tumors, thus differentiating malignant from benign tumors—with even greater specificity than the *transrectal ultrasound of the prostate* (TRUSP) which is also used to evaluate potential malignancy. The 3-T MRI is not widely available in the U.S., but is currently available at the Diagnostic Center for Disease in Sarasota, Florida and the Department of Radiology at the University of California at San Francisco. To learn more, visit www.mrisprostatecancercenter.com.

Prostatitis, infection and/or inflammation of the prostate gland, is sometimes accompanied by symptoms such as sexual dysfunction—penile burning, itching, and discharge; ejaculatory pain; pelvic pain; impotence; infertility; fatigue; or fever. Referred pain is sometimes experienced in the lower back, groin, penis, testicles, and circumferentially around the rectum. Urinary symptoms can be similar to those experienced with BPH. In other individuals, there is virtually no manifestation of symptoms. Leading urologists believe that all men will eventually develop prostatitis if they live long enough. It is associated with virtually all cases of prostate cancer and is found in nearly all prostate biopsies.[12] The disease is difficult for many practitioners to diagnose and even more difficult to treat. Although a wide variety of treatments are available, few are effective in more that a small percentage of cases. The prominent American urologist Dr. Ron Wheel-

er believes prostatitis is a "four-lane highway leading to prostate cancer."

In about 5% of cases,[13] the cause of prostatitis is either acute or chronic bacterial infection that may be difficult to detect. It is also often recalcitrant, sometimes requiring antibiotic treatment of both the man and his partner.[14] To determine whether such a component is present, a culture and sensitivity test of the either urine or an EPS (see below) specimen should be performed before beginning any course of indiscriminate antibiotic treatment. In the remaining 95% of prostatitis cases—which are not caused by bacterial infection—antibiotic treatment is ineffective, a needless expense, and may suppress immunity and aid in the development of super-resistant microbial species.

In addition to some of the drugs used to treat BPH, other drugs used to treat prostatitis include the alpha blockers Cardura,® Flomax,® Hytrin,® and Uroxatrol.® Finasteride (Proscar) and dutasteride (Avodar®) are also prescribed. Although these drugs tend to improve urinary flow, they don't resolve the underlying cause of prostatitis or prevent prostate growth. Further, they must be taken indefinitely and have significant side-effects similar to those used to treat BPH, as described above.

An *Expressed Prostatic Secretions* test (EPS) is able to detect prostatitis by looking for white blood cells in the specimen. This test is performed by expressing a sample of prostate fluid from the penis by gentle-to-moderate massage during the DRE, and immediately analyzing it under a microscope. More than 10 white blood cells per high-power microscopic field (400X) is considered a definitive diagnosis of prostatitis. Unfortunately, many family care practitioners and even a significant percentage of urologists are not proficient in collecting an EPS specimen. One should inquire of the physician whether he/she is proficient in this technique. Based upon the difficulty of performing the EPS test properly, some practitioners have relied on a post massage urine test (VB-3). However, this test has been shown to provide a high degree of false negatives, missing some two-thirds of prostatitis cases.[15] The VB-3 does have value if performed both pre- and post-massage when comparing the increased presence of white blood cells in the post-massage specimen, but is not the most reliable and definitive test available.[16]

Ultrasonic examination of the prostate indicates prostatitis if cysts (fluid-filled sacs) and calcium deposits are detected.[17] The most convenient method of detecting prostatitis is the Prostate-Specific Antigen test. The PSA—while not being an accurate screen for prostate cancer—is a highly accurate screen for prostatitis, which is the principal cause of a rising PSA. When the PSA is over 1.0 ng/mL (nanograms per milliliter), the test is virtually 100% accurate in diagnosing prostatitis, and can be used as an indicator of the degree of inflammation. An unexplained rise in the PSA level is much more likely the result of prostatitis rather than BPH or cancer.[18] Nevertheless, it has been shown that in men aged 40-60, a PSA score in excess of 0.6-0.7 ng/mL increases the risk of prostate cancer by 300-400%, while a PSA between 2.0-4.0 ng/mL is associated with a 500-900% risk of aggressive prostate cancer in the subsequent 10 year period. A PSA of 1.0-4.0 is associated with a 20-30% probability that cancer is present.[19]

Based on the above, it can be concluded the PSA test is an accurate barometer of prostate health. A healthy prostate is one in which the PSA is 1 or less with a complete absence of urinary symptoms, while a PSA of 1 or greater is indicative of an unhealthy prostate. The lower the PSA score, the lower the risk of eventually developing prostate cancer. Prostatitis—having a PSA of 1 or over—is a precursor event to prostate cancer and therefore should be treated in order to avoid escalation from prostatitis to prostate cancer.

Depending upon the severity of the problem, BPH, prostatitis, and prostate cancer are often treated effectively and safely with individual plant extracts, a combination thereof, or other non-invasive or non-surgical techniques described below.

■ **Saw Palmetto** (**Serenoa repens**). Saw palmetto extract is obtained from the seeds and pulp of a scrubby palm tree native to the Atlantic coast of the U.S. and also the West Indies. This extract has been the subject of European research for more than 20 years. Saw palmetto's active ingredient *beta-sitosterol* works on the same principle as the prescription drug Proscar, by preventing the conversion of testosterone to DHT.[20] In a 1984 study reported in the *British Journal of Clinical Pharmacology*,[21] 110 participants who were adminis-

tered saw palmetto experienced a 45% decrease in nighttime urination, a 50% increase in urinary flow rate, and a 42% reduction of urinary retention. In another study, the results of a head-to-head comparison showed saw palmetto to compare favorably with the drugs Hytrin and Proscar.[22]

■ *Pygeum africanum.* The beta-sitosterol-containing powdered bark of the large, tropical pygeum tree has been used for centuries to treat a broad array of urinary disorders. This product is thought to derive its effectiveness from its anti-inflammatory properties and its ability to reduce swelling and decrease the testosterone uptake of the prostate. In a German study[23] of 263 men reported in 1990, urinary symptoms improved in 66% of the participants taking pygeum compared with only 31% improvement in the placebo group.

■ *Stinging Nettle* (**Urtical dioica**). Although touted as having a powerful effect on the symptoms of BHP, less research has been performed on stinging nettle in comparison to saw palmetto and pygeum. Several animal studies have been done, with the results indicating inhibition of prostate growth in mice. The steroidal components of stinging nettle root seem to suppress prostate cell growth.[24]

■ *Beta-Sitosterol.* Phytosterols are found in all plant foods and are substances that are particularly beneficial to the prostate. Beta-sitosterol is the specific phytosterol contained in saw palmetto and pygeum, and is the principal contributor of the beneficial effects of these two plants. Two large clinical studies, reported in the *Lancet* and the *British Journal of Urology* in 1995 and 1997, respectively, showed beta-sitosterol to increase peak urine flow and decrease voiding time and urine retention.[25] Beta-sitosterol aids in reducing the conversion of testosterone to DHT. It also has been shown to inhibit the growth of prostate, breast and colon cancer, as well as reduce and normalize cholesterol and triglyceride levels.[26]

The product neoProstate B-400 is one of the premier prostate products currently on the market. Each tablet of neoProstate contains 400 mg of standardized beta-sitosterol complex, or the equivalent amount of sterol found in 4,000 dried saw palmetto berries. It also contains 100 mg of IP-6,

10 mg of OptiZinc,® 100 mg of lecithin, and 1 mg of copper. Users of this product have reported rapid results, some within a matter of only a few days. Beta-sitosterol is non-toxic and without adverse effects. To order, call (888)803-5333 or visit www.bcn4life.com. An alternative is Source Naturals' Beta-Sitosterol Mega Strength,® containing 375 mg of beta-sitosterol per tablet.

■ **Crinum Latifolium.** A humble Vietnamese herb shows promise in becoming one of the leading treatments for both BPH and ovarian conditions including *polycystic ovary syndrome*. The herb may also be effective in treating prostate cancer. Although used traditionally as an elixir for longevity, the herb was so revered in its native country of Vietnam that its use was reserved for royalty—referred to as "Medicine for the King's Palace" and the "Royal Female Herb."

Identified botanically as *Crinum latifolium*, much of the early research using crinum was reported by the Hoang family of Vietnamese medical doctors. Three generations of Hoang family physicians have worked together to improve the uses of Vietnamese and Chinese herbs in the field of modern alternative medicine.

Hundreds of successful case histories using crinum for BPH have been reported. Seven years of research by the International Hospital in Vietnam showed good results for 92.6% of BPH patients. These positive results were confirmed by measurements of prostate size and clinical evaluations by urologists.[27] In another Vietnamese study[28] of 158 BPH patients, a crinum-based herbal preparation was given orally twice daily. Following 64 days of treatment, patients were evaluated by clinical and ultrasound examinations. Researchers found that prostate size returned to normal in 154 of the patients—a 97% success rate. A three-year follow-up confirmed a high rate of long-term success.

In 2005,[29] the Institute of Traditional Medicine of Ho Chi Minh City and the Institute of Aging Disorders of Hanoi tested crinum on 627 patients with BPH. The results showed a 33-93% reduction in urinary symptoms and a 90% reduction in prostate size. A significant number of patients achieved a normalization of prostate size and urinary health after three months of therapy. No significant adverse reactions were reported.

To learn more about *Crinum latifolium*, visit www.allergyresearchgroup.com/April-2007-Focus-Crinum-Latifolium-sp-29-html. It is available in the combination herbal formula Healthy Prostate & Ovary from Allergy Research Group.

■ **Peenuts.**® Urologist Dr. Ron Wheeler, mentioned above, has formulated the natural prostate formula Peenuts, which stands for "**P**ower to **E**mpty **E**very **T**ime While **N**ever **U**rinating **T**oo **S**oon." The product consists of anti-inflammatories, antioxidants, beta-sitosterol, immune boosters, vitamins, and minerals. Unlike most other prostate products, in double-blind, placebo-controlled studies Peenuts not only improved voiding symptoms in all of the men studied, but 69% of the participants improved in six-to-seven out of seven of the prostate-related categories measured. Additionally, all participants significantly improved in the two definitive markers of prostatitis—by an average decrease of 49% in their PSA scores, and a 66% reduction in white blood cells as measured by the EPS.

■ **EDTA Chelation.** Prostate difficulties often result from the accumulation of calcium in the prostate, along with heavy metals including lead and cadmium which displace the important mineral zinc. Rectal administration of the heavy metal chelating agent EDTA by means of a suppository, as discussed under Chelation Therapy in the section on **Cardiovascular Disease**, has been shown effective in treating prostatitis, BPH, and even some cases of prostate cancer.

■ **Sodium Chlorite.** The universal antibiotic sodium chlorite, discussed under **General Treatment Methods**, may prove be an effective treatment for prostatitis caused by microbial infection.

■ **Rectal/Vaginal Heater.** In 1930, Charles Robert Elliot patented a device for increasing the local temperature of either the rectal or vaginal vault. Elliot's device consisted of a bag-type unit which was inserted into either the rectal or vaginal orifice, after which heated water (up to 130°F) was circulated through the bag via connecting tubes. The application of this device brought seemingly miraculous cures for a host of ailments, including chronic male prostatitis, pelvic infections in women, bladder problems, and hemorrhoids. Even locations distant from the pelvic area benefitted from this therapy in many instances—seemingly unexplained.

The results of this therapy were reported in several prestigious journals, including the *Journal of Urology* and the *American Journal of Obstetrics and Gynocology*.[30] This therapeutic technique and the simple device used to deliver the treatments represent yet another case of an effective, forgotten technology being supplanted by more modern and often less effective techniques. Following the advent of modern antibiotics and their wide-spread introduction during WWII, many effective therapeutic techniques including this device were shelved and soon forgotten amidst the fervor of the high-tech wonder pills.

A modern version of the Rectal/Vaginal Heater is manufactured in Switzerland. To learn more, visit www.cheeenergy.com. To place an order for the device, call Dr. Charles McGee at (800)442-8029.

■ ***Photoselective Vaporization of the Prostate.*** Also called GreenLight PVP® and formerly referred to as the Niagara Technique, this treatment is performed with the use of a KTP laser [Potassium Titanium Oxide Phosphate (KTiOPO4)] which emits a beam in the green portion of the spectrum at 532 nanometers (nm). The technique is minimally invasive and produces a dramatic reduction of BPH symptoms with long-lasting results.

While under anesthesia—either local, light IV or spinal, depending on the patient's preference—an endoscope is inserted into the urethra, and a hair-thin fiber-optic cable which carries the laser beam is guided to the prostate gland. The pulses of green light are directed at the obstructive prostate tissue, the source of the pressure and constriction that causes most BPH symptoms. Because of the high absorption rate of blood hemoglobin of the vascular prostate tissues at 532 nm, the powerful 30-80 watt laser vaporizes excess prostate tissue in about 10-30 minutes, depending on the size of the prostate. At the same time, the beam prevents bleeding by cauterizing the surrounding tissues to a depth of 1-2 millimeter. This minimal intrusion allows rapid and painless recovery with virtually no adverse side-effects, according to the manufacturer.[31]

Within a period of about one week, BPH symptoms begin to disappear. Nearly 100% of those re-ceiving this treatment experience dramatic results. Urine flow increases an average of about 200%, and pain, urgency, hesitancy, and nocturia disappear. Also, there is no risk of loss of sexual function using GreenLight PVP. Its beneficial effects are long-lasting, with some patients having been monitored for up to five years with no relapse of symptoms.[32] To learn more and to locate a doctor in your location, visit www.laserscope.com, or call (800)356-7600.

■ ***Radio Wave Hyperthermia.*** If BPH escalates to prostate cancer, in addition to radical removal of the gland, Western medicine offers techniques such as external beam radiation and seed implant radiation therapy, which are often ineffective. However, at least one treatment has shown quite good results. The technique is hyperthermia, which is the therapeutic application of directed heat to the problemed area, in this case the prostate gland. Full-body hyperthermia also is effective in cases where the cancer has metastasized (spread) to other areas.

The rationale of this treatment method is that tumor cells are denser than normal tissue, and heat is more readily absorbed by denser tissue. Overheating of the cellular structures leads to the cancer cells' demise in several ways. Cancer cells have a primitive blood supply system in comparison to normal cells. As they are heated, their metabolism increases, thus increasing all of their cellular functions. Because of the limited ability of their vascular systems to supply nutrients and remove heat and metabolic wastes, the cancer cells either starve from lack of nutrients, become damaged from overheating, or suffocate in their own waste byproducts. Normal cells, on the other hand, have sufficient networks of blood vessels to adequately manage the increased metabolism.[33]

The hyperthermia technique as practiced by some U.S. urologists uses microwaves to heat the targeted tissues. This method has the serious side-effect of painfully burning the urethral tissue, a result that has caused some physicians to abandon the technique altogether. European physicians, on the other hand, use radio frequency waves to heat the tissue. This technique achieves about a 90% remission rate in Stage I and Stage II prostate cancers, without burning the urethra.[34]

To learn more about radio wave hyperthermia, visit www.klinik-st-georg.de. This is the website of Dr. Friedrick Douwes, founder and Medical Director of the St. George Clinic in Bad Aibling, Germany, and an expert on the use of radio wave hyperthermia. In the **Cancer** section, hyperthermia is discussed in greater detail and contact information for other clinics is given.

Untreated prostate or any other cancer can metastasize to other locations of the body. To learn about substances useful in preventing cancer metastasis, as well as the prostate treatment method High-Intensity Focused Ultrasound (HIFU), see the **Cancer** section. See also Prostate in the Member's Area of *The Encyclopedia's* website.

PSORIASIS

A chronic disease of the skin characterized by scaling and inflammation, psoriasis affects about two percent of the U.S. population, or about six million people. It typically manifests as patches of thick, red skin covered by silver-colored scales, and can occur anywhere on the body. These areas, sometimes referred to as *plaques*, may itch or burn, and may crack at the joints. Researchers believe about two thirds of psoriasis cases are linked to immune disorders, while the remaining cases are inherited—although it is a poorly-understood medical disorder and thought by some to be incurable.

Modern allopathic medicine has its lotions and potions, including Anthralin,® Calcipotriene,® coal tar, corticosteroids, retenoid, and salycylic acid, to name a few. In certain cases these may offer some relief. Systemic treatment is attempted with an arsenal of pharmaceuticals drugs including cyclosporine (Neoral®), hydroxyurea (Hydrea®), methotrexate, and retinoids (such as Soriatane®). Phototherapy techniques using UVB and UVA light wavelengths (in combination with the compound psoralen; PUVA) are often effective, and can be administered by skin specialists.

■ *Oregon Grape.* An extract from the bark of the Oregon grape, known botanically as *Mahonia aquifolium*, offers new hope for psoriasis sufferers. Historically, *Mahonia aquifolium* has been used to treat a variety of skin disorders. Researchers have discovered that an extract of the tree's bark inhibits keratinocyte (abnormal skin cell) growth.[1] Scientists at the U.S. National Cancer Institute have found the extract inhibits 5-lipoxygenase and lipid hydroperoxide (lipid peroxidation). These actions are thought to be responsible for the beneficial effects produced in its treatment of psoriasis.[2]

In a multicenter trial with 89 medical practices participating, German dermatologists studied the effects of *Mahonia aquifolium* ointment on 443 patients with both acute and chronic psoriasis. After 12 weeks the doctors concluded that psoriasis symptoms improved or disappeared in 81% of the patients. Tolerability without side-effects was evaluated as good or very good by 82% of the participants. At the start of the study, 30.1% of the patients had significant or severe symptoms. After the 12 week treatment with *Mahonia aquifolium* ointment, that number dropped to 5.6%.[3]

A product based on *Mahonia aquifolium* is marketed as M-Folia® and can be ordered from NorthStar Nutritionals at (800)913-2592, or visit www.northstarnutritionals.com.

■ *Tamanu Oil.* The phrase "oldies but goodies" certainly holds true for this product. Tamanu (TAW-man-oo) oil has been used for centuries by the inhabitants of the South Pacific islands where the tree from which it is derived proliferates. According to ethnobotanist Chris Kilham, tamanu is one of the most effective agents known in aiding scar formation at the site of a healing wound—a process called *cicatrization*. The oil has antioxidant, anti-bacterial and anti-inflammatory properties contributing to its regenerative abilities.[4]

Tamanu oil is produced from the large, blond nut of the apricot-sized fruit of the tree. In the Pacific Islands where the tree grows by the sandy beaches, the islanders use the oil for everything having to do with the skin. The Fiji islanders call the oil "dolno," meaning "no pain." Traditionally, the oil has been used topically to treat abrasions; acne; anal fissures; blemishes and wrinkles; blisters; body and foot order; burns (including chemical and X-ray); diabetic sores; diaper rash; dry or scaly skin; eczema; herpes sores; insect bites and stings; neuritis and neuralgia; psoriasis; rheumatism; sciatica; shingles; and sunburn.[5]

The Western world was briefly introduced to the oil after a French nun during the 1920s used it to treat symptoms of leprosy including painful inflammation of nerves (leprous neuritis). Due to the logistical problems of transporting the product to Europe, its use outside of its native homeland was never established—although some research on the oil has been conducted in the Pacific Islands, Asia and Europe. Recently, some major breakthroughs have helped shed light on the science behind the success claimed by Pacific Islanders. Japanese researchers at Meijo University have isolated various constituent chemicals from the oil, and found these constituents inhibit skin tumor promotion.[6] Canadian researchers at the Université de Sherbrooke demonstrated tamanu contains two chemicals known as HIV reverse transcriptase inhibitors.[7]

Tamanu oil has only recently become available to those in the Western world. One brand is True Tamanu,® harvested on the small, pristine island of Vanuatu. The nuts from which the oil is derived are hand-gathered, sun dried, and cold-processed using only a simple mechanical screw press. The resulting oil is rich, dark-green, and readily absorbed by the skin.

To learn more about True Tamanu or to order the product, visit www.new-chapter.com, or call (800)543-7279. Tamanu is also available in health food stores and can be ordered at a discount on the internet at www.mountainroseherbs.com.

■ *Fumaric Acid*. Taken orally, fumaric acid has been used for over thirty years to effectively treat psoriasis. One good product is Fumeric Acid by Vitamin Research Products. To learn more and order, visit www.vrp.com. Enter "fumeric acid" in the search box. A series of helpful articles is found under the heading "Research Center."

■ *Flax Seed Oil*. Two to four tablespoons of organic, cold-pressed flax oil (Barlean's Organic Oils or Omega Nutrition are recommended) often produce noticeable results.

■ *Hyperbaric Oxygenation*. Discussed in detail under **General Treatment Methods**, Hyperbaric Oxygenation is a very effective treatment for all types of skin ailments, including psoriasis.

■ *Honey*. Discussed in the section on **Burns**, certain types of medicinal honeys have been shown effective in treating psoriasis.

■ *Chlorine*. Removing chlorine from both drinking and shower water often produces noticeable results.

SCIATICA

The sciatic nerves are a pair of the largest nerves in the body that begin in the area of the lower spine, passing through the buttocks and down the back of the thighs. Sciatica is pain along the course of either of these nerves typically caused by inflammation, compression or reflex mechanisms. For treatment methods, see **Back** and **Neuropathy**. See also Benfotiamine under **Diabetes**, **Pain Relievers**, and **General Treatment Methods**, particularly **Bowen Therapy** and **Prolotherapy**.

SCOLIOSIS

Scoliosis is the term used to describe an abnormal lateral (side-to-side) curvature of the spine. In persons with scoliosis, the spine is "S" or "C" shaped rather than being straight. The muscles and ligaments of the spine are affected, causing a lateral twisting and rotation of the spine, ribs, and pelvis. This condition affects about 2% of women and 0.5% of men in the general population, with roughly six million Americans being affected.

Scoliosis generally develops in mid to late childhood, with the primary age of onset being 10-15 years old—although it can affect infants, adolescents and adults alike. In about 85% of the cases there is no known cause (idiopathic), although there is a genetic involvement. If a family member has scoliosis, there is a 20% increased likelihood of a second member acquiring it.[1]

Each year in the U.S., about 30,000 children receive braces to halt the progression of the disorder, and 38,000 receive spinal fusion surgery. The symptoms of scoliosis included digestive problems; headaches; limited activity; menstrual problems; leg, hip and knee pain; reduced respiratory function; and loss of self esteem.

The typical course of treatment consists of 1) observation, 2) bracing, and 3) surgery. Each individual case is assessed to determine the proper course of action depending on the age of the patient, severity of the curvature, and other factors. Orthopedic braces are generally used if the spinal curvature is in the range of 25-45 degrees. The braces are intended to prevent further curvature, not to correct the existing problem. The majority of scoliosis cases never require surgery. However, in cases where the curvature exceeds 45 degrees and the patient doesn't respond to bracing, spinal fusion surgery is typically employed.

During spinal fusion surgery, a metal rod is attached to either side of the spine using hooks which attach to the spinal vertebrae. The spine is then "fused" (grafted) with a piece of bone taken from the patient's hip. The metal rods position the spine so that the bone grows properly between the vertebrae, holding the spine straight.

■ *The Pneumex Technique.* A new treatment for scoliosis may help avoid unpleasant treatment by braces and/or surgery. It may even correct spinal curvature significantly. The treatment uses a series of exercises and a harness-type device. Pneumex rehabilitates the small muscles along the spinal column, allowing them to pull the spine into a more normal position. The technique is painless, involves no surgery, and is covered by most insurance policies. Changes in the curvature attained by Pneumex are permanent, so long as a course of home exercises is maintained for about one year following the major Pneumex treatment.

For more information and to locate a practitioner in your area, visit www.pneumex.com. For more information about scoliosis, visit www. scoliosis.com or www.iscoliosis.com.

SHINGLES

Also called herpes zoster, shingles is an acute inflammation of the spinal and cranial nerve ganglia. It is caused by a reactivation of the herpes virus—the same virus causing chicken pox—and manifests as grayish-colored blisters on the skin's surface. Herpes zoster is a localized form of chicken pox. Shing-RELEEV® (formerly Shingle-EEZE®), is a topical spray that some have found to bring pain relief within 30 minutes. It also helps the outbreak from spreading and helps existing lesions to heal, sometimes within 48 hours. The formula combines the antimicrobial benzalkonium chloride with herbal extracts which include echinacea and dandelion. For more information and to place an order, visit www.netriceuticals.com/products.asp.

Intravenous vitamin C, discussed in more detail in the **Colds and Flu** section, is an extremely effective treatment for shingles and post herpetic neuralgia. Topically-applied geranium oil and tamanu oil (discussed under *Psoriasis*) may significantly reduce the pain of post-herpetic neuralgia. Procaine injections, discussed under **Neural Therapy**, may offer relief. Many of the techniques/products discussed under **Pain Relievers** and **General Treatment Methods** are applicable. See also *Herpes*, Benfotiamine under *Diabetes*, and the Member's Area of *The Encyclopedia's* website.

SLEEP APNEA

According to the National Institutes of Health, more than 12 million Americans suffer from sleep apnea. The major risk factors include being male, overweight, and over 40 years of age, although even children have been known to suffer from the ailment.[1] The Greek word apnea means "without breath." People who suffer from this condition repeatedly stop breathing during their sleep, sometimes hundreds of times each night for a minute or longer. Obstructive sleep apnea (OSA), the most common form of the ailment, is usually caused by a relaxing and collapse of the soft tissues (uvula, soft palate, and tongue) at the rear of the throat.

The other common form, central sleep apnea, doesn't involve an obstructive blockage, but rather a malfunctioning of the brain's normal signals to the muscles responsible for breathing. Although unrecognized by many practitioners, prescription drugs may contribute to the disorder, some of the worst offenders being anti-arrhythmia drugs.

Although snoring and high blood pressure are possible indicators of the ailment, the majority of those having sleep apnea go undiagnosed and untreated. Traditional Western medicine recognizes that if left untreated, serious medical consequences can result, including behavioral changes, depression, heart attack, headaches, high blood pressure, impotence, loss of energy, obesity, and stroke.[2]

Those with sleep apnea generally suffer from sleep deprivation, as they may be awakened tens to hundreds of time each night. Sleep may be extremely fragmented and of poor quality. Sufferers sometimes awaken during the night choking and gasping for air, but more commonly are unaware of their unconscious struggle to breathe. Job impairment and motor vehicle accidents are not uncommon in those afflicted with the disorder.

Mild cases of obstructive sleep apnea often can be treated with various means of preventing the sufferer from sleeping on his/her back. Sometimes nasal decongestants are useful. One common treatment involves the application of air pressure during the sleeping hours. Known as "nasal continuous positive airway pressure" (CPAP), this method uses a mask and pump to prevent the normal obstruction by supplying positive pressure to the airway. When anatomical defects are present, surgery is sometimes performed.

In addition to the consequences commonly associated with sleep apnea, a number of additional medical consequences can result which would not typically be associated with the specific diagnosis of sleep apnea, including symptoms of seemingly unrelated ailments such as chronic fatigue syndrome, fibromyalgia, and even multiple sclerosis. This is not as unusual as it might appear at first glance, as a significant toll is taken by the body when it is deprived of oxygen and sleep—two of the most critical components of our ability to maintain a healthy state.

It is known that during apnea episodes the blood oxygen saturation falls from its normal 95-98% levels to 70% or below.[3] In an effort to supply the necessary oxygen to the body, the heart will beat faster and faster. The effort of the abdomen and chest increase, trying to enable a breath to be taken. Eventually, the person is aroused to the point that breathing occurs, at least momentarily, until the process repeats itself.

■ *Robson Splint.* Tacoma, Washington dentist Farrand Robson, DDS, has developed and patented an oral appliance designed to eliminate the symptoms of sleep apnea. Robson fashions a customized splint designed to pull the lower jaw forward. With the jaw in a more forward position, the patient's oxygen supply immediately becomes normalized, and symptoms disappear rapidly, according to Robson. Although the device is simple, he has reported some amazing remissions of symptoms not only related to sleep apnea, but with other conditions that otherwise wouldn't be thought of as being caused by this disorder. Robson believes that oftentimes unexplained symptoms are the body's reaction to lack of oxygen, and its attempt to maintain an adequate oxygen supply.

Hypertension and snoring are two of the main symptoms associated with sleep apnea. If you are experiencing these symptoms, any of the symptom described above, or suspect that additional symptoms not typically associated with the disorder may be the result of a sleep apnea problem, contact Dr. Robson's office at (253)272-8651 for a referral to a dentist who uses the splint.

Spinal Cord Injury

The horseback-riding accident of actor Christopher Reeve focused the attention of the world on the devastating severity which can result from spinal cord injury. Although he played Superman on the silver screen, Reeve was powerless to heal himself in real life. In fact, for years he had to be strapped into his wheelchair just to sit upright. Even the life-giving act of breathing, which occurs automatically and without consideration for most of us, was far from routine for Mr. Reeve. Following the accident, each and every breath required the assistance of a mechanical device. Although he improved somewhat, Reeve was never able to walk or perform most of life's day-to-day activities that most of us take for granted.

■ *Omental Transposition.* In real life there are medical supermen who may have been able to help Mr. Reeve. During the 1960s, Dr. Harry S. Goldsmith of the University of Nevada School of Medicine developed a surgical technique known as *omental transposition.*

The omentum is a large, fatty membrane that is attached to the stomach and intestines in the lower abdomen. This apron-like structure is rich in nutrients and growth factors (angiogenic and neurotrophic factors) that promote vascular development (increase blood vessel growth and blood supply) and stimulate healing. Omental transposition consists of freeing the biochemically-rich omentum from the abdominal cavity and, with its blood supply remaining attached and intact, transposing it over the injured area(s) of the brain or spinal cord.[1]

Although the technique has been largely ignored in the U.S., surgeons in many other countries including Brazil, Cuba, Germany, India, Italy, Japan and Singapore have used omental transposition effectively to treat a range of either age-related or traumatically-induced neuropathic conditions including Alzheimer's, cerebral palsy, Parkinson's, spinal cord injury, and stroke. In China alone over 5,000 procedures have been performed.[2]

One success story is the case of a gymnast who sustained a fractured neck at the age of 17, leaving him a quadriplegic who had to be strapped into his wheelchair much the same as Chris Reeve. The gymnast underwent omental transposition a year-and-a-half following his injury, and today has regained almost total use of both his arms—including the ability to power his own wheelchair.[3] In another dramatic case, a nun regained her ability to read within several weeks after receiving omental trasposition. She underwent the operation two-and-a-half years after suffering a stroke.

Hundreds of journal articles have been published on omental transposition, including nearly 100 by Dr. Goldsmith himself. To learn more about the technique, do a key word search for "omental transposition." Dr. Goldsmith still performs the operation. Contacted him at P.O. Box 493, Glenbrook, NV 89413; fax (702)749-5861.

■ *Laser Light.* A group of researchers at the Uniformed Services University in Maryland have performed groundbreaking research using laser light. For the first time ever, the severed spinal cords of mammals have been fused together using the coherent, low-intensity light of a laser at the 810 nanometer (nm) wavelength. A group of 10 rats with severed spinal cords received laser treatment over a two week period for about 50 minutes per day. When tested nine weeks after the treatments began, all of the animals had regained their mobility. A control group of ten animals not receiving light treatment showed no signs of improvement.[4]

Although the researchers do not fully understand the mechanism(s) behind the remarkable spine-mending results, they believe the light alters the behavior of cells, allowing the neurons of the spinal cord to "regroup," which in turn allows the spinal cord to refuse.

Lead researcher Professor Juanita Anders stated that advances in light therapy are being made which are "almost too incredible to believe." Christopher Reeve, the researchers believe, might have recovered had he been lasered in the days following his injury. The researchers believe it also might

be possible to treat long-term, non-recent injuries. In addition to spinal cord injuries, they intend to focus their technology on stroke victims as well. To learn more about this technique, search online for "juanita anders."

■ See also *Light* under **Pain Relievers**.

■ *Dimethyl Sulfoxide* (DMSO). According to the co-discoverer of its therapeutic properties, Dr. Stanley Jacob of the University of Oregon Medical School believes the substance (solvent) DMSO operates on an entirely new therapeutic principle. According to the medical and pharmaceutical literature, DMSO "is declared to have the widest range and greatest number of therapeutic actions ever shown for any other single chemical."[5]

As such, it benefits a wide range of ailments and performs a variety of functions. It is an anti-inflammatory, bactericide, diuretic, free radical scavenger, fungicide, immune booster, pain blocker, vasodilator, and virocide. In addition, DMSO is able to transport a variety of pharmaceuticals across cell membranes; reduce the incidence of blood platelet thrombi (clots); act as a tranquilizer when rubbed into the skin; stimulate wound healing; and a host of other benefits.

One of the most striking areas of benefit of DMSO is in the treatment of brain and spinal cord injuries. When administered intravenously (IV) within 90 minutes of such an injury, the substance can produce near miraculous results, including prevention of paralysis.[6] The sooner a patient is given DMSO, the more pronounced the beneficial results are likely to be. Dramatic results have accompanied DMSO administration even when given several hours after the initial trauma. There appear to be at least three factors responsible for this benefit. DMSO is an anti-inflammatory, a free radical scavenger, and the substance reduces the cellular requirement for oxygen.

When the brain and spinal cord (central nervous system, CNS) are traumatized by injury, there is compression of the nerves and tissues which produces swelling. As the swelling takes place within the skull in head injuries and the spinal column in spinal cord injuries, blood vessels constrict and blood and oxygen are cut off from the damaged areas, causing the injury or death of cells and tissues. With the timely infusion of IV DMSO, the swelling is prevented and there is an increased amount of blood flow to the damaged area.[7]

During head injuries, water and blood accumulate within the cranium causing a buildup of pressure that eventually compresses vital brain centers, resulting in permanent injury or death. Immediate treatment with DMSO significantly reduces intercranial pressure, helping the victim to avoid lasting injury or possible death. DMSO binds to the excess water and blood, takes it to the surrounding blood vessels, and carries it away from the brain. In effect, it dries out the brain from potentially-damaging water and blood.[8]

The production of hydroxy free radicals accompanies head and spinal cord trauma, which extends the damage by killing surrounding cells. DMSO is such a powerful antioxidant that it interrupts the ensuing free radical cascade, thus protecting neuronal tissues. Although it is not known why, DMSO reduces the amount of oxygen required by the cells for healthy functioning. This is particularly important in brain and spinal cord injury where oxygen deprivation is a major contributing factor to cell damage and death.[9]

In animal CNS injuries, when the animal is brought to a point of near death—as indicated by a flat electroencephalogram (EEG)—the IV infusion of DMSO restores the normal EEG in about 10 minutes. A normal respiratory pattern is also restored, with breathing becoming deeper and faster, a desirable effect in CNS-injured victims. Also, the elevated blood pressure that accompanies CNS injury in animals and man is stabilized.[10]

In one dramatic study, the blood supply to the midsection of the spinal cord was blocked for 30 minutes in 24 mongrel dogs. The 12 animals in the control group received a saline injection, while the experimental group of 12 received an injection of DMSO. Eleven of the 12 animals receiving the saline solution experienced total paralysis of the lower extremities. Eleven of the 12 DMSO-injected animals, on the other hand, had a complete recovery and were able to walk and run normally. The twelfth animal in the DMSO group had only a slight weakness. Microscopic tissue studies of both groups showed ischemic (oxygen deficient) changes and cellular damage in the control group but none in the DMSO-treated group.[11]

Administering DMSO to humans has had similar dramatic results. In one quadriplegic patient who had no sensation or muscle activity from the neck down, immediate administration of DMSO led to the patient moving his toes within two hours, and an eventual total recovery with full function.[12]

DMSO's co-discoverer Dr. Jacob reported two cases at his Oregon medical school in which DMSO was given within one hour for CNS accidents which would have resulted in immediate, complete quadriplegia. In both instances the patients walked out of the hospital after having made a complete recovery.[13] Dr. Jacob reported three additional cases where DMSO was administered five, six and nine hours following CNS trauma, where the likelihood of paraplegia was near 100%. Even though the 90 minute window of opportunity had passed significantly, two of the three patients were able to walk after receiving intravenous administration.[14]

There have been other similar cases, yet the technique is virtually unknown within the halls of emergency medicine. Those who understand its therapeutic efficacy believe DMSO should be carried in ambulances for rapid use, and should be a standard emergency medical tool in all emergency rooms. When IV administration is not possible, rubbing several tablespoonfuls of 70% DMSO/30% water on virtually any area of the skin (except at the injury site) should help prevent tissue swelling and CNS trauma including brain damage.

To learn more about DMSO, see DMSO under **Pain Relievers** or read Dr. Morton Walker's book *DMSO: Nature's Healer.*

■ ***Rolipram.***®[15] Inhibition of nerve cell growth in the spinal cord is a major contributing factor in preventing recovery in spinal cord injuries. Various chemicals have been identified which inhibit the regrowth of damaged spinal cord neurons, including NOGO, *myelin-associated glycoprotein*, and *oligodendrocyte myelin glycoprotein*. In 2001 it was discovered all three inhibitory chemicals function by binding to the same receptor site on the surface of nerve cells, which raised the possibility that blocking this site could prevent growth inhibition.

Researchers at the City University of New York recently discovered a drug that overcomes the effect of the growth-inhibiting chemicals. It does this by raising the level of the common signaling molecule *cyclic AMP*, or cAMP. The drug, rolipram, was once licensed for use as an antidepressant, but was removed from the market for causing nausea and vomiting in the oral form—which shouldn't be a problem when used in an injectable form for treating spinal cord injuries.

In a study of 20 rats which had their spinal cords severed in the neck region, half were administered rolipram two weeks after injury for an additional two weeks. Following treatment, 70% of the treated group regained significant function compared to 20% of the placebo group. The use of rolipram may eventually offer one aspect of a multipronged approach to treatment.

■ *Fusion Technology.* Yet another technique offering hope to those with nerve injuries has been pioneered by researchers at the University of Texas at Austin. As reported in the *Journal of Neuroscience*,[16] researchers first apply a sticky solution of polyethylene glycol (PEG) to the cut, crushed, or otherwise damaged nerve axons for a period of only one or two minutes. Thereafter, the PEG solution is washed off and the nerve endings are then soaked in calcium salt solutions resembling natural body fluids. The PEG solution basically removes water from cell surface membranes, allowing the membranes to fuse together. Within seconds to minutes after the (central or peripheral) nerves are rejoined, the repaired cells once again begin to conduct electrical signals. Between 5-60% of the nerve impulse level has been restored.[17]

Purdue researchers demonstrated similar results with PEG administered by IV injection.[18] Nineteen dogs with severe spinal cord injuries impairing their neurological function were injected within 72 hours of injury. Following injection, to reduce inflammation they received standard treatment for spinal cord injury including steroids and removal of stray bone chips. Thereafter, they received a second injection of PEG. The control group received the standard treatment only. Two days following the initial injection, the PEG-treated dogs scored higher on tests measuring early recovery of function. After six weeks, 68% of the PEG-treated dogs were able to walk, compared to 24% of the control group. Nearly 75% of the PEG-treated dogs were able to resume a normal life. Some healed so completely they continued to live as though nothing had happened. According to Dr. Richard Borgens of Purdue's Center for Paralysis Research,

> the results of this pilot trial provide evidence consistent with the notion that the injection of inorganic polymers in acute neurotrauma may be a simple and useful intervention during the acute phase of the injury.[19]

■ See **Stem Cells,** and Constraint Induced Movement Therapy and Nanotechnology under **Cardiovascular Disease**. See also **Magnetic Molecular Energizer** under **General Treatment Methods**, and Spinal Cord Injury the Member's Area of *The Encyclopedia's* website.

STEM CELLS

Stem cell therapy is now offered by many companies, including Cell Medicine (www.cellmedicine.com) and Xcell-Center (www.xcellcenter.com). Conditions treated include ALS; Alzheimer's; autoimmune diseases; cardiovasular disease; cerebral palsy; diabetes; M.S.; osteo- and rheumatoid arthritis; Parkinson's disease; spinal cord injuries; and stroke. See also the **Index**, and Stem Cells in the Member's Area of *The Encyclopedia's* website.

STRESS

Whether it be money, relationships, sickness, war, or the plethora of other potential stress triggers, modern man is more stressed-out than ever before. In the U.S., over $300 billion annually, or about $7,500 per employee, is spent on stress-related compensation claims, reduced productivity, absenteeism, health insurance costs, direct medical expenses, and employee turnover. It is predicted that depression, one of the manifestations of stress, will be the leading occupational disease of the 21st Century—responsible for more work days lost than any other single factor.[1]

In 2003, the British newspaper *The Guardian* published a report indicating that nearly 25% of the adult population of France are taking either a tranquilizer, antidepressant, antipsychotic, or other mood-altering prescription drug. In persons over aged 70, 40% are taking these drugs, as are 4% of all French children under age nine.[2] Although psychiatriac drugs can be useful, various categories of these drugs have recently been linked to an increased risk of diabetes, blood clots and stroke.

Stress is the mental and physiological reaction to perceived demands of daily life that exceed one's ability to cope or respond to the situation(s) in a reasonable manner. The symptoms of stress include anxiety, depression, insomnia and fatigue, and may lead to physical ailments ranging from the minor to the catastrophic. Medical researchers are now able to measure the direct detrimental effects of stress on the cardiovascular, immune, endocrine, muscular, genitourinary, and gastrointestinal systems, and on mental health.[3]

Not to be surprised, the pharmaceutical companies offer many solutions aimed at making us more tranquil in the face of our daily challenges. If we're too tranquil, i.e., depressed, the many varieties of anti-depressants (energizers) will lift us up. One pill makes us taller, and one pill makes us small—just ask Alice.

Tranquilizers are divided into two groups: Major tranquilizers include Clozaril,® Haldol,® Thorazine,® and Risperdal.® Minor tranquilizers have more familiar-sounding names: Ativan,® Librium,® Serax,® Valium® and Xanax® (street names include: "libs," "tranks," "benzos" and "vees.")

Tranquilizers such as the Benzodiazepines can be addictive even at prescribed dosages if taken for extended periods. Withdrawal may include diarrhea, delusions, depression, flu-like symptoms, general pain, hallucinations, heart palpitations, paranoia, psychosis, and stomach cramps. Withdrawal from some Benzodiapines can be life threatening.

Minor tranquilizers are designed to induce feelings of calm and relaxation. On the other hand, if they don't function as designed, one might experience blurred vision, disorganized thinking, dry mouth, hallucinations, headaches, hostility, impaired motor functioning, irritability, lethargy, memory loss, nausea, sweating and vomiting.[4] These are the tranquilizers. War is peace.

Antidepressants, on the other hand, are "mood-brighteners." You may need them if you have an adverse reaction to a tranquilizer. Two main types of antidepressants are tricyclic antidepressants (TCAs) and selective serotonin reuptake inhibitors (SSRIs; and their next-generation offshoot, SNRIs, serotonin-norepinephrine uptake inhibitors). These drugs function by reducing the uptake of neuro-transmitting brain chemicals such as serotonin so that more of the chemical remains available.

Serotonin, denoted 5-hydroxytryptamine (5-HT), is the brain's master molecule. Adequate levels produce feelings of calmness and relaxation. Low levels produce anxiety, depression, insomnia, and other negative feelings and behaviors.

Pharmaceutical antidepressants are effective for many, but when they're bad, they're very, very bad. While this classification of psychoactive drug is intended to help people, sometimes it has the opposite effect—with catastrophic results. As an example, many of the highschool and other senseless shootings which have plagued the U.S. and other countries were perpetrated by individuals taking the SSRI group of antidepressants.

The list of casualties includes such household names as Eric Harris (Columbine High; total killed: 13, wounded: 23; Harris was taking prescription Luvox®); Mark Barton (Atlanta day trader; total killed or injured at two separate brokerage firms: 22; he also killed his wife and two children; Prozac® was found in his car); Brin Hartman, wife of deceased *Saturday Night Live* comedian John Hartman, was also taking a prescription SSRI drug when she killed her husband; Joseph Wesbecker, a Prozac taker, killed seven of his co-workers at a Kentucky printing company with a semiautomatic rifle.

Before sitting down quietly in a chair to wait for the arrival of the police, 42-year old software engineer Michael McDermott killed seven of his co-workers using an assault-type rifle, shotgun and a semiautomatic pistol. McDermott was a Prozac user;[5] and the list goes on. Heard that from your local (legal) drug vendor lately? (Other popular SSRI drugs include Effexor,® Paxil,® Seroxat,® and Zoloft.®) To view an informative index of hundreds of violent SSRI-related incidents, visit www.ssri stories.com/index.php.

In January 2008, Dr. Erick Turner, Professor of Psychiatry at the Oregon State Health and Sciences University shocked the medical world when the *New England Journal of Medicine* published his article entitled "Selective Publication of Antidepressant Trials and Its Influence on Apparent Efficacy." In the article, Dr. Turner disclosed he had discovered evidence that the pharmaceutical firms who manufacture antidepressants maintained an ongoing policy of hiding from public and private view the results of clinical trials whose results are not favorable to the drugs being evaluated. Rather, only the studies showing positive results are published. The hidden trials Dr. Turner discovered showed that in 49%—nearly half—of these trials, the antidepressants had either negative or mixed results. Because such negative test results can be withheld from public awareness—as if they never existed—the unsuspecting public has no idea that many/most people using these drugs experience no greater benefit than taking a sugar pill. This is particularly reprehensible given the advertising spin that surrounds this group of drugs via the direct-to-customer marketing methods now permitted.

Another unpleasant fact regarding SSRIs, as discovered by researchers at the Harvard School of Public Health, is that SSRIs depress levels of the neurotransmitter dopamine—the brain's "feel good" molecule. Brains of individuals with Parkinson's disease produce almost no dopamine, and it is the absence of this neurotransmitter which is related to many symptoms of the disease. The Harvard researchers reported that persons taking SSRI antidepressants were almost twice as likely to develop Parkinson's as those not taking the drugs.

Because of the harmful effects experienced by so many users of the SSRI category of antidepressants, it's best to avoid them in favor of more natural alternatives, several of which are discussed below. It's important to note, however, that the use of SSRIs should never be stopped immediately, and any SSRI should be allowed to clear from the body before other products are taken.

■ **_Dilantin_**. One pharmaceutical that many have used effectively for treating "emotional problems" is Dilantin,® (phenytoin sodium), a drug that was approved by the FDA in 1953 for the treatment of epileptic seizures. Because the drug calms the nervous system, it's effective as a mood stabilizer—reducing anger, anxiety, and phobias. Anti-anxiety effects are achieved at a dosage of 100 mg twice daily. After his life was "rescued" by Dilantin, Jack Dryfus—financier and founder of the Dryfus Fund—wrote the book *A Remarkable Medicine Has Been Overlooked*.

■ **_Gamma Amino Butyric Acid_** (GABA). Eugene Roberts, Ph. D., a researcher at Washington University, discovered GABA in 1950. Several years thereafter GABA was found to be involved in the transmission of nerve impulses. Within a decade, researchers established GABA as a key neurotransmitter located throughout both the brain and body.[6]

GABA, an amino acid, is the most widely-distributed neurotransmitter in the brain. It is contained in 40-50% of all brain synapses—the junctions at which nerve impulses pass from one nerve cell to another. Of the 50-plus known neurotransmitters, it is 200-1,000 times more concentrated than the other well-known neurotransmitters serotonin, acetylcholine and norepinephrine. Its highest concentrations, in descending order, occur in the basal ganglia, hypothalamus, hippocampus, cortex, amygdala, and thalamus.[7]

Neurotransmitters are classified as either excitatory or inhibitory. GABA is the brain's main inhibitory neurotransmitter. It functions within the brain to regulate and inhibit anxiety, fear, grief, depression, pain, and panic. It also functions to inhibit the urgency of addictive cravings for alcohol, cocaine, and other prescription and recreational drugs. GABA is also effective in treating post-traumatic stress disorder.[8]

The *amygdala* (uh-MIG-da-la) is the brain's storehouse of emotions such as anger, anxiety, depression, elation, fear, and grief. The hippocampus (hip-o-CAM-pus) is believed to be the gateway to emotional experiences. GABA slows down or blocks emotional messages coming from these areas of the brain as they make their way to the cerebral cortex, the brain's decision-making center.

Therefore, because these messages are quelled by the presence of GABA in these areas of the brain, the cortex is not overwhelmed with impulses which we experience as the negative emotions of anxiety, fear, depression, etc. When GABA receptor sites are empty, pain and anxiety-related messages are experienced more intensely, sometimes overwhelmingly. When sufficient GABA is present within the body, it mutes these messages.[9]

The benzodiazepine group of tranquilizers—including Dalmane,® Halcion,® Lexotan,® Librium,® Paxipam,® Rohypnol,® Tranxene,® Valium,® Ativan,® and Xanax®—function by attaching to GABA receptor sites, thus mimicking the actions of GABA. In their wishful thinking, pharmaceutical companies refer to these as "benzodiazapine receptor sites," when in actuality they are provided by Mother Nature to be filled with gobs of GABA.

In order to be metabolized properly, GABA should be taken along with vitamin B$_6$ and the mineral magnesium, especially magnesium chloride. Also, there are four general grades or purity of amino acids and nutritional supplements, ranging from the purest to the least pure: I.V. grade, pharmaceutical grade, cosmetic grade and food lot grade. Especially in the case of using this important amino acid, the pharmaceutical-grade product is recommended. One product meeting these specifications is the patented product Anxiety Control 24,® developed by anxiety and pain control expert Billie Jay Sahley, Ph.D. This product can be ordered by calling either (210)614-7246 (questions), or (800)669-2256 (orders only).

■ *L-theanine.* L-theanine (THEE-uh-neen) is another alternative that is an effective stress reducer. Theanine is a neurologically-active amino acid that has been shown to promote deep muscle relaxation and combat insomnia. It is L-theanine, in fact, that provides the relaxing effects that are attributed to drinking green tea.[10] Although their names are similar, theanine is a different substance from yet another amino acid threonine.

Although the mechanisms of action are not fully understood, it is known that L-theanine is able to cross the blood-brain barrier—the biological firewall (tight cell-to-cell junction) that prevents many substances from leaving the brain and also from crossing into the brain. Having this ability to cross into the brain, it supports the function of various neurotransmitter chemicals,[11] chemicals that assist in transmitting nerve impulses.

In a recent study published in *Trends in Food Science & Technology*,[12] it was shown that 30 minutes after the administration of 50-200 mg of L-theanine, there is an increase in the production of alpha brain waves—thought to be a prime indicator of relaxation. Theanine also has been shown to stimulate the production of GABA, the inhibitory neurochemical discussed above. It also significantly increases the level of tryptophan, an important building-block amino acid of serotonin[13]—a mood-altering brain neurotransmitter that helps promote the feelings of relaxation and well being. In lab animals, the administration of theanine was shown to significantly increase the levels of serotonin and dopamine.[14] Additionally, theanine affects the car-diovascular system as well as the nervous system, and has been shown to help regulate blood pressure by slightly lowering elevated levels.[15]

Because L-theanine has been consumed for centuries in green tea with only positive effects, its use is viewed as both safe and effective for reducing anxiety and promoting relaxation. Furthermore, it does not cause the daytime sleepiness and mental fog often associated with pharmaceutical drugs.

■ *Kava kava.* Another stress buster is the herb *Kava kava*, botanically classified *Piper methysticum*. The herb grows on islands in the South Pacific, and is used by the indigenous peoples for social and cultural purposes. In the West, it is used as a stress-relieving agent when taken in moderation and, when taken in larger dosages, has slight inebriating and sleep-inducing qualities. According to published studies, Kava is an excellent stress reducer.[16]

In 2002, Kava was taken off the market in some European countries in connection with being a possible cause of liver damage. In response to this, several supplement trade associations hired toxicologist Donald Waller, Ph. D. to examine the evidence. Dr. Waller is Professor of Pharmacology and Toxicology at the University of Illinois, and a Diplomat of the American Board of Toxicologists.

On February 19, 2002 Waller reported to the U.S. Food and Drug Administration that "there is no clear evidence that the liver damage reported in the U.S. and Europe was caused by the consumption of Kava." He further stated that cases with a possible association between Kava use and liver problems "appear to have been hypersensitivity or idiosyncratic base responses."[17] Waller stated that many of the liver-associated problems were probably due to use of the herb in conjunction with alcohol and/or drugs that are recognized as having the potential to cause liver damage,[18] such as acetaminophen, and the statin cholesterol drugs.

In contrast to Europe and Canada, U.S. citizens still can purchase Kava kava in health food stores. Teas, tinctures and capsules are available. Products standardized to contain 20-30% *kavalactones*, the active ingredient, are recommended by many who have experience with this herb.

■ *Rhodiola rosea.* Adaptogens are plant materials that normalize the physiological and psychological functions of the body and return it to a state of balance, or homeostasis. Adaptogens increase the body's ability to function normally. Characteristic of these substances is their ability to increase daytime energy, endurance, and mental alertness while at the same time promoting deep and restful sleep. The herb *Rhodiola rosea*, known also as Russian Rhodiola and "Golden Root," may be the world's premier adaptogen—the first botanical to legitimately be called a "second-generation" adaptogen.

Russian scientist Dr. Nikolai Lazarev discovered the properties of these substances in 1947, and coined the term "adaptogens." His protégée, the late Dr. Israel Brekhman—a well-known name to those familiar with this field of research—conducted extensive studies on adaptogens, and was considered the world's foremost expert on these substances. Hundreds of clinical studies have been conducted on adaptogens, mostly in Russia and Germany, that have shown their outstanding stress-relieving, anti-depressive and immune enhancing properties. Russian athletes and cosmonauts rely on rhodiola to provide enhanced mental and physical performance. Its actions are of such broad scope and benefit they are too numerous to explore in this writing.

Key among rhodiola's properties is its ability to significantly reduce both physical and emotional stress. As reported in the journal *Phytomedicine*,[19] in a double-blind cross-over study of 56 young physicians performing stressful night duties in a hospital setting, 170 mg of standardized rhodiola extract significantly improved associative thinking; calculation and ability of concentration; short-term memory; and speed of audio-visual perception.

Another study[20] evaluated the adaptogenic effect of rhodiola extract on the fatigue of students caused by stress during an examination period. Statistically significant improvements were seen in mental fatigue, physical fitness, and neuro-motor tests in comparison to the placebo group.

In a study[21] of 150 persons suffering from depression who took rhodiola extract for a period of one month, two thirds of the participants had full remission of symptoms at the end of the study period. As in the many other studies evaluating the beneficial effects of rhodiola, no adverse side-effects were noted.

Researchers at the Chungnam National University in Taejon, Korea have confirmed via liquid chromatography that the Russian extract of rhodiola has twice the potency of other extracts, including the Chinese and Tibetan versions.[22] Those familiar with the various products available in the marketplace suggest that purchasers of rhodiola products should look for certain minimal standardized concentrations of the two active ingredients: rosavins: 2.5% and salidroside: 1%. Many products do not meet this minimal requirement, and may be ineffective. Now Foods and Enzymatic Therapy market a product containing 3% rosavins and 1% salidroside. An internet search or a trip to your local health food store will provide many more sources.

■ *Cranial Electrotherapy Stimulation* (CES). Also known as Transcranial Electrotherapy, Neuroelectric Therapy, Electroanalgesia and by other names, Cranial Electrotherapy Stimulation is the medical application of weak microcurrents of electricity to the head. The Russian scientist Rabinovich is credited for making the first claim (1914) that CES is an effective treatment for insomnia. To date, hundreds of research studies have been done which have evaluated the efficacy of CES as a beneficial treatment for anxiety, depression, insomnia, drug addiction, and general physical pain control.

CES gained public notoriety following the publication of a 1983 article in *Omni Magazine*, "Black Box—Secret Treatment of Rock Superstars," in which several well-known rock 'n roll legends including Pete Townshend of *The Who* told their stories of painless withdrawal from serious drug addiction, including heroin, using CES technology.[23] In the early 1980s, University of Southern California physics professor Bob Beck re-engineered the original "black box" device, calling the new instrument the Bio-Tuner® (also known as the Brain-Tuner). To listen to Dr. Beck's most informative 1983 lecture on the brain-tuner technology, visit www.braintuner.com/Bob-Beck-Brain-Tuner/Index.html. See link at bottom of the page.

The application of microcurrents to the brain is believed to increase the production of endorphins such as *beta-endorphin* and *enkephalin*, the body's own opiate-type analgesic substances produced naturally in the brain. Also likely affected are the limbic system, hypothalamus and the reticular activating system.[24] CES seems to mobilize the body's own painkilling capacities.

CES devices are similar in size and appearance to the TENS units described in the section on **Electricity** under **Pain Relievers**, although they use different waveforms and intensities of microcurrents for this specialized application. Some units are only slightly larger than a pack of cigarettes, and attach to the head either via clipping to the earlobes, or by means of a stethoscope-type headset by which electrodes are placed in the hollows behind the ears near the mastoid process bones. A typical CES session lasts from 20-40 minutes, and is generally accompanied by a feeling of relaxation and a heightened sense of well being. A comprehensive review of the CES literature was published in the 1985 book *Neural Stimulation* by Ray B. Smith, Ph.D. According to Dr. Smith,

> ...CES is effective in alleviating the symptoms of anxiety, depression and insomnia...CES appears effective as a treatment for withdrawal in the chemically dependent person...CES appears to be safe, with no harm or negative side-effects having been reported to date...[25]

In a study published in the *American Journal of Pain Management*,[26] the outcome of CES patients' self reports were peer reviewed for efficacy in many different areas of pain control, including anxiety, depression and insomnia. Patients ranked the effectiveness as either slight (less than 24% improvement); fair (25-49% improvement); moderate (50-74% improvement); or marked (75-100% improvement). The results were as follows: *Overall Stress*—4.88% had slight improvement; 24.39% fair improvement; 31.71% moderate improvement; and 39.02% marked improvement. In patients treated with CES for overall stress, 95% experienced either fair, moderate or marked improvement.

The categories were further broken down into the three main symptoms of stress: anxiety, depression and insomnia. *Anxiety*—10.16% of the patients had slight improvement; 22.66% fair improvement; 32.81% moderate improvement; and 34.38% marked improvement. In the patients treated with CES for anxiety, 90% experienced either fair, moderate or marked improvement. *Depression*—13.21% of the patients had slight improvement; 20.75% fair improvement; 43.40% moderate improvement; and 22.64% had marked improvement. In the patients

treated for depression, 87% experienced either fair, moderate or marked improvement. *Insomnia*— 6.13% of the patients had slight improvement; 28.83% fair improvement; 28.83% moderate improvement; and 36.20% marked improvement. In the patients treated for insomnia, 94% experienced either fair, moderate or marked improvement.[27]

The same study evaluated the effectiveness of CES in treating many different types of pain, including arthritis, back, cervical, hip/leg/foot, migraine, myofacial, RSD, shoulder/arm/hand, and TMJ. The results for overall pain were: 6.98% of the patients had slight improvement; 32.97% fair improvement; 38.02% moderate improvement; and 23.04% marked improvement, as defined above. In the patients that were treated with CES for overall pain, 93% experienced either fair, moderate or marked improvement.[28]

A chapter on CES from the book *Bioelectric Medicine* can be viewed at www.chronicpain reliefnow.com/research/ces_pain_depression_ anxiety_insomnia/1.html. A variety of CES units are available, some of which require a prescription in the U.S. Preferred units include the Bio-Tuner,® marketed by Sota Instruments (www.sota instruments.com; 800-224-0242) and the Alpha-Stim® SCS (www.alphastim.com; 800-FOR-PAIN). The Bio-Tuner is a non-prescription device, while the Alpha-Stim can only be purchased with a prescription and is more costly.

Another type of electromagnetic therapy, Transcranial Magnetic Stimulation, was approved by the FDA in October 2008 for use in adults with major depression which is unresponsive to pharmaceutical medication. See Transcranial Magnetic Stimulation under **Parkinson's Disease**.

■ ***Emotional Freedom Technique*** (EFT). This is a very unusual technique that fits best in this section on stress, although it could be considered a topical treatment as well as a general treatment method. EFT has been referred to as being a form of psychological acupressure—because it caters to psychological issues and involves the manipulation of acupressure points. It is used to remove negative emotions, reduce food cravings, implement positive goals, and reduce or eliminate pain.

Of all the treatment methods covered in this document, EFT is one of the most esoteric. That is, it is based on the concept that the electromagnetic energy flowing through our bodies is the regulator of our health. This concept is foreign to the scientific, Western mind which tends to appreciate things only if they can be weighed and measured. Nevertheless, based on the very positive results it achieves, the technique warrants being included.

EFT uses the same energy meridians and nine of the specific acupuncture points on the head and chest traditionally used to treat emotional and physical ailments. Unlike acupuncture, however, the technique uses tapping of the fingertips on these points rather than the insertion of needles. While tapping these points, the person thinks about their problem—anxiety, depression, pain in the body, etc.—and voices positive affirmations. The combination of tapping (activating) the energy points while voicing the positive affirmations works to clear the energy block from the body's bioenergy system, thus restoring the energetic balance.

In practice, the technique is simple and quick to perform. All one needs to learn is the location of the points and the proper method of formulating the affirmations. The series of nine acupuncture points with affirmations can be "tapped out" in less than a minute. Each point is tapped five to seven times—about the time it takes for one full breath.

An example of an affirmation would go something like this: "I love and accept myself even though I have this fear of public speaking." Or, "Even though I have this migraine headache, I deeply and completely love myself." This is spoken aloud, with energy and enthusiasm, as the successive nine points are being tapped. It doesn't matter whether or not the tapper believes the affirmation in order for the technique to be effective.

Dr. Joseph Mercola, a well-known osteopathic physician, is one of the main U.S. proponents of EFT. Dr. Mercola has only high praise for the technique, and states that "more than any traditional or alternative method I have used or researched, EFT works." Dr. Mercola markets a set of DVD/VHS materials to help assist interested persons in mastering the technique. To learn more about EFT or to order Dr. Mercola's materials, visit www.mercola.com/forms/eftcourse.htm. To locate an EFT practitioner in your location, visit www.alternatives for healing.com/cgi_bin/practitioner-eft-tft.php.

■ *Eye-Movement Desensitization and Reprocessing* (EMDR).[29] Typical psychotherapeutic techniques generally take many weeks, months or years to achieve beneficial results. This has been one of the drawbacks of standard treatments. A little-known technique is changing the landscape of certain aspects of traditional psychotherapy, as this new method often is able to accomplish in one session what has taken years with other methods of therapy.

In the late 1980s, Dr. Francine Shapiro began developing a form of therapy that focuses on treating the emotional stress brought on by traumatic experiences such as grieving over the death of a loved one, divorce, battlefield experiences such as post traumatic stress disorder—in short, any negative or traumatic emotions associated with specific thoughts and memories. While walking in a park in 1987, Shapiro serendipitously noticed that a back-and-forth (lateral) movement of her eyes seemed to decrease the negative emotions associated with certain distressing memories she was experiencing. Many years of further investigation led to the therapeutic technique now known as Eye-Movement Desensitization and Reprocessing (EMDR).

According to the technique, the client is led by the therapist to move his/her eyes back and forth following the therapist's fingers across the client's field of vision for 20-30 seconds (or longer), while at the same time consciously thinking about the most vivid visual image (negative thought and body sensations) of the traumatic memory. The same procedure is repeated numerous times throughout the session, with the therapist customizing subsequent imaging depending upon the client's feedback. The client is instructed to let the mind go blank and notice whatever thoughts, emotions, images, etc., come to mind. In only one session many clients experience a significant desensitization of the "intrusive mental images and feelings" associated with a particular traumatic event. Because results are achieved so quickly, practitioners have called EMDR "nothing less than astonishing."

Although it is still a matter of some debate, the simple lateral shifting of the eyes is believed to greatly increase the brain's own ability to process information. Consequently, according to proponents of the technique, EMDR results in rapid cognitive restructuring of the traumatic event. The individual still remembers the event, but somehow the associated negative emotions are "reprocessed," and thereby lessened—and for all intents and purposes fundamentally changed for the long term.

Similar accelerated reprocessing/restructuring occurs during dreaming as the eyes move back-and-forth in what is called "rapid eye movement," or REM sleep. Neurologists believe the back-and-forth movement of the eyes results from the increased processing that occurs during REM sleep. With EMDR, it is the purposeful shifting of the eyes that causes the mental reprocessing, even though the client is fully awake and alert during the session.

Based on many controlled studies, EMDR is designated an effective treatment for post traumatic stress disorder by the International Society for Traumatic Stress Studies, the Northern Ireland Department of Health, and the Israeli National Council for Mental Health. Many EMDR clinicians describe it as being more effective than any other method in treating stress, anxiety and trauma.

Interestingly, researchers at Manchester University in England have found that moving the eyes horizontally from side to side for about 30 seconds increases short-term memory of lists of words. The eye movements seem to enable the two hemispheres of the brain to communicate more effectively.

To learn more about EMDR, read Dr. Shapiro's books *EMDR: The Breakthrough Therapy for Overcoming Anxiety, Stress, and Trauma* (1997) and *Eye-Movement Desensitization and Reprocessing: Basic Principles, Protocols, and Procedures* (2001), or visit www.emdr.com.

An interesting offshoot of EMDR was developed by psychologist Dr. Allan Botkin. A practicing clinician for over 20 years—with extensive experience in counseling combat veterans—Dr. Botkin noticed that during EMDR sessions, his clients frequently would have "encounters" with deceased persons who were significantly related to the client and his/her emotional trauma. These experiences were deep, spiritual experiences which seemed to help resolve the traumatic event(s) under treatment. Dr. Botkin has developed a technique to "artificially" induce this experience more-or-less at will. He calls this process Induced After Death Communications (IADC), and has trained many clinicians in the practice of the technique.

Following the EMDR eye movement activity, the IADC practitioner applies "a sequence of therapeutic actions" Botkin discovered that precipitate the communication experience with the deceased. According to practitioners, there is a remarkably consistent resolution of grief resulting from the client's perception of a reconnection with the deceased person, and *in all cases* the grief remains resolved.

After the technique is initiated, the client remains seated with eyes closed. In the client's private mental experience they claim to see and speak with the deceased—be it a friend, loved one, or others. In nearly all cases, those having this experience not only immediately achieve a significant level of acceptance of the loss of the deceased, but also achieve complete resolution of the loss including related symptoms such as anger, grief, guilt, and sadness, as well as any intrusive mental images that may be impinging upon the patient.

As unusual as it may seem—even to those who administer the technique—in almost all cases the "communication" event is so profound that clients believe they have been in contact with the deceased. The occurrence and benefits of the experience seem independent of the clients' beliefs prior to the experience; religious beliefs or disbeliefs; or recency of the death. IADC practitioners state the essential healing ingredient is the perception of reconnecting with the deceased, regardless of the "origin" of the experience (i.e., how did the experience happen?; did the experience *really* happen?, etc.)

Botkin suggests that 1) the trained IADC practitioner can rapidly and reliably induce an after death experience in virtually anyone interested in having the experience, 2) IADCs always resolve grief resulting from traumatic loss, 3) the experiences are similar to those who have had near death experiences (NDEs), and 4) in every case for which follow-up data is available, the results are maintained indefinitely and appear to be permanent.

To learn more about IADC, read Dr. Botkin's 2006 book, *Induced After Death Communication: a New Therapy for Healing Grief and Trauma*, or visit his website at www.induced-adc.com. On his website, you can also read about the experiences of a journalist who personally had an IADC.

A further technique of contacting the deceased is described by Raymond Moody, M.D., Ph.D. In his book *Reunions: Visionary Encounters with De-*

parted Loved Ones, Moody describes the use of the *psychomantium*, an ancient form of mirror gazing.

■ ***Baclofen***. The prescription drug *baclofen* (Kemstro® and Lioresal®) is a muscle relaxant typically used to treat muscle spasms resulting from various conditions. In 2002, French-American physician Dr. Olivier Ameisen began self-medicating to treat his own problem with alcohol addiction after learning the drug is known to alleviate alcohol and cocaine addiction in rats, and after reading a 2000 *New York Times* article about a cocaine user whose addiction was cured after being prescribed baclofen for a muscle problem. After some experimentation with dosage, Ameisen cured his alcoholism and subsequently published the book *The Last Glass* which attained best-seller status in France in the fall of 2008. The English version of the book, *The End of My Addiction*, is currently available in the U.S.

Dr. James Garbutt of the Bowles Center for Alcohol Studies at the University of North Carolina School of Medicine reports the drug has shown good results, although the dosage and degree of effectiveness for all patients is undetermined. In 2007, a double-blind study[30] conducted at the Institute of Internal Medicine of the Catholic University of Rome found that 70% of baclofen-treated alcohol-dependent patients achieved sobriety compared to 30% of the placebo group. Dr. Ameisen, currently a visiting Professor of Medicine at the State University of New York Downstate Medical Center, believes baclofen affects areas of the brain which leads to a suppression of cravings for addictive substances such as alcohol, cocaine, and heroin.

■ ***Ibogaine***. The root of the plant *Tabernanthe iboga* has long been used as a religious sacrament by the Bwiti culture of Gabon and Cameroon in West Africa. The powder made from the rootbark of the plant is at the heart of their religious rituals. Depending upon the dosage and the individual experiencer, mild hallucinogenic states are produced when the plant is ingested orally. Aside from being a staple of Bwiti religious experience, the plant has another important use.

In 1962, 19-year-old heroin addict Howard Lotsof first experimented with *ibogaine*, as the oral preparation is called. Although he was only seeking a "high" from the drug, after the effects wore off 30 hours later Lotsof noticed he'd lost all craving for heroin—without experiencing *any* withdrawal symptoms. He then gave ibogaine to seven other heroin addicts, five of whom gave up their habits immediately after having one ibogaine experience.[31] Thus began a decades-long journey into the preliminary investigation of ibogaine as a treatment for many types of addiction including alcohol, amphetamines, cocaine, nicotine, and opioids.

Over the ensuing years, many mainstream scientists have taken up the ibogaine cause. Among those who have researched ibogaine are Dr. Ken Alper, Assistant Professor of Psychiatry and Neurology at New York University School of Medicine; Dr. Charles Kaplan, Department of Psychiatry and Neurology at Maastricht University, The Netherlands; Dr. Deborah Mash, Professor of Neurology, University of Miami School of Medicine.[32]

Dr. Mash has been one of ibogaine's main proponents. She is credited with the discovery of *noribogaine*, an active metabolite of ibogaine which may offer anti-addictive properties without the hallucinogenic effects. In 1996, Dr. Mash established a clinic on the Caribbean island of St. Kitts, where ibogaine treatments continue to be given. Other treatment centers have sprung up in many other cities throughout the world including Amsterdam, Holland; Copenhagen, Denmark; Vancouver, British Columbia; Tijuana, Mexico; and other locations.

Many of those who have "kicked their habits" using ibogaine say it is a miracle treatment. Others say it provides a "window of opportunity" of diminished cravings for several months following treatment, during which time other types of aftercare may be required to prevent possible relapse. Whichever the case, hundreds of former addicts attest to the ability of ibogaine to quickly reverse years of addictive behavior. Although its mechanism of action remains uncertain, ibogaine's unique molecular structure may satisfy certain neurological receptor sites that block the dependency feedback loop. Dr. Carl Anderson of McLean Hospital in Virginia speculates that addiction is related to a disrupted communication between the brain's two hemispheres, and that ibogaine may restore hemispheric reintegration.[33]

Ibogaine is a Schedule I drug in the U.S., one of the most highly controlled of all pharmacologic substances. Furthermore, it is illegal in many other countries throughout the world. Nevertheless, a number of treatment facilities in several countries offer ibogaine therapy. To locate a facility in your location, visit www.ibogaine.co.uk/options.htm. To learn more about ibogaine, visit www.ibogaine.org.

■ *5-hydroxytryptophan* (**5-HTP; hi-Drox-e-TRIP-tuh-fan**). Even a novice at chemistry will notice that 5-HTP has a very close chemical formula to serotonin, the brain's master molecule 5-HT. Used medicinally, 5-HTP is not a synthetic drug, but rather an extract from the African plant *Griffonia simplicifolia*. (Perhaps even its name is trying to suggest that we follow the K.I.S.S. principle—Keep It Simple Stupid.) 5-HTP is a precursor of serotonin, i.e., it provides the building materials out of which the body makes serotonin.

By increasing 5-HTP—which has rapid access through the blood-brain barrier directly to the brain—serotonin levels are also increased. Levels of other neurotransmitters also are raised by 5-HTP including dopamine, melatonin and norepinephrine. 5-HTP has been approved in Europe for decades as a treatment for many medical complaints including anxiety, depression, insomnia and weight loss. Medical practitioner and author Dr. Michael Murray has used 5-HTP with hundreds of patients with tremendous results, including mood elevation, increased energy levels—a basic rediscovery of the joys of being alive.

To learn more about the benefits of 5-HTP, read Dr. Murray's 1998 book, *5-HTP: The Natural Way to Overcome Depression, Obesity, and Insomnia*. This product is available in health food stores or can be ordered on the internet.

■ *St. John's Wort.* Known botanically as *Hypericum perforatum*, the herb St. John's wort has been used for centuries to treat a variety of both physical and mental disorders. It was used during the Crusades as a battlefield antiseptic. Disorders of mood and temperament have been treated successfully by St. John's wort for centuries. Its antidepressant and mood-stabilizing qualities result from its principal active ingredient, the compound *hypericin*.

A study of more than 1,700 patients comparing St. John's wort to pharmaceutical antidepressants was reported in the *British Medical Journal*[34] in 1996. Hypericum extract was found to be at least as effective as pharmaceutical drugs in treating mild to moderate depression, while having about half the reported number of side-effects. Almost twice the number of participants taking standard antidepressants dropped out of the study due to side-effects in comparison to the Hypericum group. Many other studies have reported similar results.

In Germany, extracts of St. John's wort are approved for the treatment of anxiety, depression and sleep disorders. The herb is considered quite safe when taken as directed, although it may cause sun/skin sensitivity in some individuals. Also, St. John's wort interacts with Coumadin,® digoxin, theophylline, oral contraceptives, transplant (anti-rejection) drugs, and several AIDS medications. St. John's wort can be purchased in health food stores or on the internet.

■ *S-adenosyl-methionine* (**SAM-e**). Pronounced "Sammy," SAM-e is produced from two substances normally found within the body—methionine and adenosine triphosphate (ATP). Methionine is an amino acid; ATP is manufactured within the cells, and provides the energy to fuel the body's many processes. SAM-e works by elevating the brain's serotonin levels and helping to balance numerous other neurotransmitters.

Seventy percent of depressed persons taking SAM-e notice mood improvement within days, as opposed to pharmaceutical antidepressants that typically require from two to four weeks to take effect. Dr. Richard Brown, Associate Professor of Clinical Psychiatry at Columbia University and co-author of the 1999 book *Stop Depression Now*, describes SAM-e as the breakthrough supplement that works as well as prescription drugs, in half the time, with no side-effects. SAM-e can be purchased in health food stores or on the internet.

■ *Essential Fatty Acids.* Sixty percent of the weight of the human brain is fat, the most fat-rich organ of the body. Of that, 30% is composed of essential fatty acids (EFAs).[35] Hence, the term "fat head" is accurate if not politically correct. EFAs are not manufactured by the body, and are obtained only through the diet. Two of the most important EFAs are omega-3 and omega-6. In the brain, omega-3 and omega-6 EFAs occur in a ratio of about 1:1, and should be ingested at that ratio.

To maintain proper brain function, ingesting adequate amounts of EFAs is necessary—specifically the omega-3s EPA and DHA. When deficiencies occur, the brain becomes imbalanced and abnormal behavior can manifest including addiction, anxiety, and depression. Ingesting adequate amounts of EFAs either from the diet or by supplementation has been shown to lift depression, reduce anxiety, decrease addiction and ease withdrawal from alcohol, cigarettes and drugs.[36] It has been documented that societies having the lowest consumption of fish also have the highest rates of depression, suicide and violence.[37] Many scientists believe inadequate consumption of omega-3s may account for the increasing societal levels of attention deficit hyperactivity disorder (ADHD), autism, bipolar disorder, and depression.[38]

Good sources of EPA and DHA are cold water fish and fish oils. Nevertheless, Neptune Krill Oil (NKO) is less subject to toxic continuants, better absorbed, and almost 50 times as potent an antioxidant as fish oil. Flax seed oil and ground flax seeds are also good sources. A specially-formulated product developed by the well-known nutritional scientist Udo Erasmus, Ph.D., is Perfected Oil Blend. Chia, discussed under **General Treatment Methods**, is also one of the best sources of EFAs.

■ *Ketamine*. A group of physicians at the Mood Disorders Research Unit of the National Institute of Mental Health have found that ketamine, a common anesthetic drug, is capable of eliminating the symptoms of severe depression in under two hours. Dr. Carlos Zarate, Jr., Chief of the unit, stated that "We have broken the sound barrier in depression treatment...We are not replacing depression with a manic phase. The effect is simply the elimination of depression. The patients, essentially, return to normal."[39] Ketamine, technically deemed an *N*-methyl-D-aspartate antagonist, is FDA approved for human use as an anesthetic, but is most commonly used as an anesthetic in veterinary medicine. It is also a popular street drug sold under names including jet, super C, kit, and kat.

The results of a randomized, placebo-controlled, double-blind crossover study of 17 participants diagnosed with treatment-resistant major depression (*DSM-IV*) were reported in 2006 in the *Archives of General Psychiatry*.[40] Twelve women and five men ranging in age from 16 to 60 (mean age 47) were given a single IV injection of ketamine hydrochloride (0.5 mg/kg) or a placebo. At 110 minutes, 24-hours, and one week post-injection the participants were given the written 21-item Hamilton Depression Rating Scale. At 110 minutes, there was a statistically significant drop in the depression ratings, indicating the participants were feeling much less depressed. After 24-hours, the decrease in the depression ratings was highly significant. Of the 17 participants who received the ketamine injections, 71% were significantly relieved and 29% experienced total symptom elimination the day following the injection. Thirty-five percent maintained that response rate for at least one week.

Because the trial was limited to participants with treatment-resistant major depression, it's not clear whether ketamine will be as effective or show results so quickly in persons with less severe depression. This study provides the proof-of-principle that rapid treatment of depression is possible.

■ *Get A Pet*. Many years ago in the U.S. and other countries, retirement homes, nursing homes, hospices and hospitals began to bring in small animals—dogs, cats, rabbits, etc.—for visitations with the residents. In fact, the practice has a name—Animal Assisted Therapy (AAT). The interaction that happens between man and beast can cause amazingly positive results in peoples' conditions whether it be depression, physical illness, or simply boredom. Animals are good communicators even without saying a word. Friendly, domesticated animals are "living toys" waiting to be played with by adults and children alike.

According to epidemiologist Maryellen Elcock of the Delta Society, a national U.S. non-profit organization that trains therapy animals for health facilities, schools, and libraries, the animal-human connection has many benefits. Pet owners live longer and are less lonely than non-pet owners. Children in homes with pets have higher self-esteem. Heart patients with pets have lower mortality rates. Elcock says that "the connection between humans and animals is a physiological effect, a measurable effect" that results in a heightened sense of well-being and better overall health, both mental and physical. Petting or just being near a loved pet relieves stress, with the measurable effect of reduced heart rate and blood pressure.[41]

Eighty percent of the Delta Society's pets are dogs, but there are also therapeutic cats, one donkey, one camel, a rooster, llamas and rabbits. For more information about the Delta Society, visit www.deltasociety.org. On the less than warm-and-fuzzy side, in Japan—where there is a rapidly aging population—one high-tech nursing home near Osaka has been cheering up residents with robotic teddy bears since 2000.[42] So to take the edge off the stress, get-a-pet, or play with your neighbors' (pet, that is...Sadly, playing with the neighbors is a behavior reserved only for children.)

■ *Get A Job*. It has been said that an idle mind is the devil's playground. Therefore, if you find yourself sitting around with time on your hands, do something useful—even if it's not getting a job. Volunteer at your local hospital, hospice, kindergarten or some variation thereof. If all else fails and you can't find anything useful to do, do something useless. But don't just sit around and stew in your own cranial contortions. Do something!

■ *Row A Boat*. In the hubbub of everyday activities, it's not difficult to lose one's perspective on life—especially in the 21st Century work-a-day, rat race world where the almighty buck rules supreme. Take time to breathe deeply, look around you and gather some appreciation for the simpler things in life. Smell the flowers. Plant some flowers. Watch a sunset 'til it turns dark. Laugh uproariously at least once a day, even if you have to rent a Mr. Bean or Austin Powers movie. It'll stimulate your immune system. Have a long talk with a friend. It's cheaper than psychotherapy and probably more productive. Take a break from your routine. Get the perspective back into your life. Buy a boat and do some sailing. Row your boat gently down the stream. Remember, even if you win the rat race, you're still a rat. If all else fails, fire your boss.

■ *Learn Some Philosophy*. Around 100 A.D. lived a Greek philosopher named Epictetus (Ep-ick-TEE-tus). He was a teacher of the stoic philosophy. Happiness, he believed, comes by being in the flow of life's events which are caused by natural laws largely beyond the control of man. Man, he believed, has control only over himself. "One can never fail to be happy," he argued, "if one learns to wish that things should be only as they are." Stated another way, in the words of Lennon and McCartney, "Let it be." This is not a bad thing to understand, if you can. We are free to make our requests—even demands—on life and the world that surrounds us. Yet in the end, regardless of the result, we must be brave enough and have the depth of insight and understanding just to "let it go."

One of Epictetus' famous sayings is that "men are disturbed not by things, but by the views they take of them." (Women, on the other hand, are disturbed not by things, but by not having enough of them...) Meaning, it is not the events themselves but our personal perceptions and interpretations of the events that contribute to how we "feel" about the situations that transpire around us. "Easy for him to say," you may be thinking—but there's a lot to his statement.

Implicit in Epictetus' words is the notion that *we learn our views and opinions* about the things which surround us. That is, we are encultured by the events and circumstances of our lives. If we learn them, we surely can unlearn them or at least modify them if they serve us no good. This takes some serious time and introspection, to say the least. Nevertheless, at least to some extent we are our own captains and, as such, have the power to effect change in our own lives. It's not necessary that our psyches be constantly at the mercy and whim of society at large, our neighbors, our relatives, or even our own craziness that may happen from time to time. We can learn, and change, and understand many things. These are our prerogatives, if we so choose. If all else fails, take a pill.

■ For additional information on Stress and Depression, visit these topics in the Member's Area of *The Encyclopedia's* website.

STROKE. See *Cardiovascular Disease*.

STUTTERING

Most people are quite familiar with this type of speech impediment, which is an involuntary disruption of vocal communication characterized by repetition (s-s-stutter) or prolongation (sssss-stutter) of vocal sounds. Unusual facial or body movements may also accompany the effort to speak. The terms stuttering and stammering are typically used interchangeably.

More than 55 million people worldwide suffer from stuttering, including about three million people in the U.S., at the ratio of four males to every female. Stuttering usually begins between two and five years of age, but occasionally appears in school-age children and more rarely in adulthood.[1] Even though early intervention is recommended, between 50-80% of children who stutter outgrow the disorder as they age.[2]

One fascinating aspect of stuttering is that many who have the disorder speak normally when acting, singing, speaking in a group, talking to pets, or whispering.[3] This indicates that stutterers have the ability to speak fluently, but rather experience some type of interference with that ability.

Although much is known about the cause of the disorder, many unanswered questions remain. It was once believed that stuttering was caused by underlying psychological difficulties. Today it is recognized that even though traumatic life events, illness or other environmental factors may trigger the onset of the disorder, researchers now believe there is often an underlying genetic predisposition or biological prerequisite.

■ *SpeechEasy.*® Capitalizing on the fact that stutterers generally speak more fluently while speaking in a group—a phenomenon known as "choral speech"—researchers from the Stuttering Research Group of the Department of Communications Sciences & Disorders at East Carolina University have developed a tiny, programmable in-the-ear device that increases the fluency of stutterers. Following 10 years of peer-reviewed research, inventor Joseph Kalinowski, Ph.D. and his team of researchers have developed several versions of a programmable speech-correcting device called the SpeechEasy®—a device that quickly and dramatically reduces chronic stuttering.[4]

Worn like a hearing aid, the SpeechEasy uses digitally-programmable software to adjust a range of possible settings. The device uses Delayed Auditory Feedback (DAF) and Frequency Altered Feedback (FAF) of the stutterer's own voice. Altered auditory feedback in the form of slightly delaying the sound of the speaker's voice, and frequency shifts in terms of varying the pitch of the speaker's voice, produce the effect of another person speaking along with the stutterer in the stutterer's own ear—a simulation of choral speech. The SpeechEasy allows the user to adjust the delay of the "echoed" voice, the pitch either higher or lower, or a combination of the two modes.

Since the first prototypes of the SpeechEasy became available in April 2001, it has been tested on several hundred people with impressive results. It has demonstrated an 80-90% success rate in improving stutterer's fluency from 50-95%. It reduces stuttering irrespective of the rate of speech, and has been shown effective in a variety of speaking situations including lecturing, phone conversations, restaurant ordering, and social conversations, according to its manufacturer. Users of the SpeechEasy claim there is no adaptation effect, but rather their fluency levels increase with continued use. The beneficial effects of the device are present while the user is wearing it, but there is no data suggesting fluency persists when the device is not being worn.

Prices range from USD $4,100-$4,900, depending on the model, and there is also a monthly leasing program. The device is warrantied for one year, and 90% of the purchase price is refunded if returned within 30 days of purchase. To learn more, visit www.speecheasy.com or call Janus Development in Greenville, NC at (252)551-9042.

TEETH AND GUMS

Tooth pain is one of the most troublesome pains of the human body. Whether caused by a cavity, infection, a lose tooth or a combination thereof, tooth pain can be debilitating even to the most robust of individuals. Aside from extraction, a root canal, or topical pain-killing ointments available in the pharmacy, several technologies are often successful in reducing tooth pain.

When a tooth is so damaged that it can't be saved, extraction is the recourse of last resort. With the exception of children, once a tooth is extracted, it is gone forever. At least, this was the case until recently. Researchers at the Dental Institute of King's College London have successfully grown new teeth in mice using stem cells[1]—the body's unspecialized "master cells" that naturally transform into a multitude of other, more specialized cells. The researchers believe that if the procedure is successful in mice—because the principles are the same—there's no reason the technology cannot be transferred to humans. The newly established company Odontis intends to pursue that goal with their product the BioTooth.®

During the procedure—which requires only a local anesthetic—small balls of specially-prepared stem cells are implanted into the gap previously occupied by a tooth. Within a period of about two months, the stem cells grow into a new, full tooth. During the growth process, stem cells also produce bone which anchors the tooth into the jaw.

The cost of the procedure will be about USD $2,500-$3,500. Researchers hope the technology will be available within the next several years. To learn more, visit www.odontis.co.uk.

The oral cavity is a breeding ground for harmful bacteria—which produce inflammation. Chronic inflammation of the gums and bones supporting the teeth has been linked to a number of systemic diseases including heart disease, arthritis, and cancer. The following natural remedies help prevent and treat gum, bone, and tooth problems.

■ *Peri-Gum*.® One product that's effective in treating gum disease is Peri-Gum, an herbal mouthwash combining the seven herbs bayberry, bloodroot, cayenne, echinacea, peppermint oil, tea tree oil, and white oak bark. Many users have found this product so effetive they've been able to avoid gum surgery. Also, some have experienced a reversal of infection-induced bone loss. In a four-week pilot study conducted by a major northeastern university, Peri-Gum was found to significantly improve gum and oral health with a 20% reduction in gingival inflammation and a 16% reduction in plaque. Peri-Gum is marketed as a concentrate, with a one-ounce bottle making about 90-ounces of mouthwash. To place an order call Lesko Care, LLC at (908)272-3081, or visit www.peri-gum.com.

■ *Fizz & Clean*. When it's inconvenient to brush after a meal, Fizz & Clean tablets produce a bubbling action that dislodges food particles from around the teeth. It has been shown to whiten the teeth and reduce plaque, decay-causing bacteria,

cavities, and bad breath as well. Its manufacturer, OraHealth Laboratories, calls the product "a toothbrush in a tablet." For more information, visit www.fizzandclean.com or call (800)969-5227.

■ *Coenzyme Q10* (CoQ10). Periodontal (gum) disease is associated with low levels of CoQ10. Even in the most severe cases of periodontal disease, increasing its intake through oral supplementation can produce dramatic benefits. Topical application of CoQ10 has been found to be a very effective treatment of periodontal disease. Q-Sorb® by Jarrow Formulas provides a highly-absorbable form of Q10. Ubiquinol, the reduced and even more bioavailable form, is perhaps the most effective form of Q10. Other beneficial aspects of CoQ10 are discussed in more detail in the section on *Cardiovascular Disease*.

■ *Xylitol*. The unique sugar substitute Xylitol has been shown to increase bone density. It is also known to prevent tooth decay by preventing bacteria from adhering to tooth surfaces. Xylitol also helps reduce periodontal disease by preventing bacteria from adhering to skin surfaces within the mouth. Either of these benefits can cause a significant reduction in pain over time. See the **Index** for additional information on Xylitol.

■ Electromagnetic Pulsing, as described under *Herpes*; *Electricity* (TENS units); *Light* and *Magnet* therapies as described under **Pain Relievers**; and *Olive Leaf Extract*, *Sodium Chlorite* (especially if caused by infection), and *Acupuncture*, as described under **General Treatment Methods**, often reduce or eliminate tooth and gum pain. A solution of activated sodium chlorite is particularly effective in eliminating bacterial infection and stopping/reversing gum inflammation.

■ *The Gerald Judd Protocol*. In an effort to entirely avoid tooth and gum problems, Gerald Judd spent years researching this topic. Gerard F. Judd, Ph.D., is Professor Emeritus of Chemistry at Purdue University. In his storied career, he was an industry researcher for 18 years and a chemistry professor for 33 years. In addition, he is a speaker, writer, radio host, and author of several books including *Chemistry: Its Uses In Everyday Life*.

Having lived his entire adulthood observing the chemical nature of everyday life, Dr. Judd turned his attention to a subject which concerns every human being—the good health of our teeth and gums. In 1997, he penned the book *Good Teeth, Birth to Death: The Prescription for Perfect Teeth.*

According to the American Dental Association, there is an epidemic of tooth decay in America. Over 40% of American's over 65 years old and 25% over 44 years old have no natural teeth remaining. Forty-four-year-olds have had an average of 30 cavities, 17-year-olds an average of 13, blacks and poor whites have twice this incidence, and Native Americans have even higher rates.

In his book *Good Teeth, Birth to Death*, Dr. Judd describes the chemistry that is the basis of tooth decay and gum disease. He states that he has learned the real causes of dental cavities and gum infection, and that an overwhelming amount of dental research proves the following:[1]

Cavities/Decay

❏ Only acids—which are introduced into the mouth from food and drink—are capable of eroding tooth enamel (calcium hydroxy phosphate), and causing cavities. Protons of the acid quickly pull phosphate from the enamel. Food and drink not containing acids have no action on tooth enamel.

❏ Sugars are not capable of having any action on tooth enamel. Sugars (fructose, glucose, and sucrose) were found in Dr. Judd's laboratory studies to be unable to dissolve calcium phosphate to any extent, even in a hot water solution. The reason for this is that the chelation process of sugar toward teeth is slow due to the large size of the molecule and perhaps due to the particular shape of the chelate formed. Sugars are not the cause of tooth cavities to any great extent, but still it would do no harm to rinse them off the teeth after consuming candy, especially the sticky variety. The adhering barrier will prevent re-enamelization.

❏ Bacteria are not capable of having any action on tooth enamel. Both human and animal remains show teeth and bones are resistant to earth-bound organisms such as bacteria. Teeth cannot be affected by bacteria, because enamel contains no carbon or hydrogen upon which bacteria subsist. Study of *Streptococcus mutans* as a source of so-called "decay" is a waste of government funding which is donated to dental organizations.

❏ When acids are properly removed from the teeth, cavities do not occur. Removal of acids is easily accomplished by simply sipping water, milk, coffee, or other non-acidic liquids while eating. The acids quickly react chemically with the liquids to form hydronium ions, thereby saving the enamel.

❏ Harmful acids (with a pH <4.0) which attack the enamel include lemons, grapefruit, oranges, pineapple, kiwi, tomatoes, vinegar, cider, vitamin C (especially chewable) and stomach acid. The lower the pH, the more rapidly the acid's attack.

❏ Teeth are able to re-enamelize when clean. Teeth are best cleaned by brushing with any bar (not liquid) soap. Bar soap does an excellent job in cleaning tooth surfaces, enabling the enamel to thicken and causing the teeth to become less sensitive.

❏ Toothpastes containing glycerine—which most do—are very sticky, requiring over 20 rinses to remove it from tooth surfaces. Glycerine-containing toothpastes leave a residual film, preventing the teeth from proper re-enamelization. Soap, on the other hand, is removed with two rinses.

❏ Dietary or supplemental calcium and phosphate result in tooth re-enamelization, but only when the teeth are clean. Re-enamelization is necessary on a daily basis as enamel leaches slightly with water over decades, even in the absence of acid. Without re-enamelization, having healthy teeth is not possible.

❏ Abscesses can be offset by holding Cepacol® (14% alcohol) in the mouth for five minutes.

Gum Infection

❏ *Gingivitis* is an irritation of the gums. It is usually caused by plaque, a poorly-formed, bacteria-containing crystalline structure that adheres to the outside of tooth enamel. Bacteria contained in the plaque accumulate in the small gaps between the gums and teeth, producing toxins that cause inflammation of the gums around the teeth. Over time, inflammation can cause deep pockets between the teeth and gums and loss of bone that anchors the teeth—a condition known as *periodontitis*.

Although bacteria do not cause cavities/decay, they are a source of irritation and inflammation which may lead to infection, according to Dr. Judd.

Gums are disinfected and plaque is prevented and eventually removed by brushing with any bar soap. Procedures which remove plaque dig holes through the enamel, causing food to adhere in these areas, attracting bacteria and causing gum infection.

❏ Gum pockets are formed not only when plaque pushes the gums away from tooth surfaces, but also by using toothpastes containing fluoride (or when fluoride is introduced into the oral cavity by other means)—which severs the protein molecules that bind the gums to tooth surfaces.

❏ Gums can be reconnected to the teeth by taking vitamin C [ascorbic acid; 1 level teaspoon (four grams)] with Arm and Hammer® baking soda (one-half teaspoon) in one inch of water in a glass. Let it fizz and then dilute to one-half to one cup with water; then drink. The resulting sodium ascorbate is non-acid, very pure and 1,000 times more soluble than vitamin C. Sodium ascorbate is more reactive than ascorbic acid in building connective tissue and antibody structures and more effective in killing some viruses and bacteria. This will help knit the gums back to the teeth. Pressing against the gums with the fingers forces adhesive materials from the gums onto the teeth, which helps the process. Receding gums and plaque are ended when soap is used for brushing and vitamin C is taken daily in the form mentioned.

❏ Phosphate is also an important ingredient in gum repair. Monosodium phosphate is the best supplemental form of phosphate since it is very pure and highly soluble in water. Dissolve about one-fifth teaspoon (one gram) in one inch of water in a glass; then fill the glass and drink daily. This is helpful for all the bones, teeth, DNA, RNA and at least 30 phosphate-containing enzymes. Phosphate also regulates body pH. (A good source of food-grade monosodium phosphate is V.L. Clark Chemical Company, 888-852-2436; www.vlclark.com.)

❏ Receding gum surgery, which may involve transferring flesh from the roof of the mouth to the excised area, is a heinous and useless procedure which ought to pass into oblivion, according to Dr. Judd. Receding gums are nothing more than gum pockets caused by the use of toothpaste and fluoride.

Fluoride
❏ Removal of fluoride from drinking water, tooth-

pastes and gels saves the enzyme adenosine diphosphatase so it can deliver phosphate to calcium at the tooth surface, resulting in a beautiful enamel.

❏ If fluoridation were effective in preventing cavities, Native Americans would have the least cavities. They have had forced fluoridation for approximately 60 years.

❏ Fluoride in water at one part per million (ppm) increased tooth cavities in four large, reliable studies (7%, 22%, 45% and 10%—averaging 21%). The reason is that adenosine diphosphatase is destroyed by fluoride and calcium fluoride, which slips into the enamel, is alien to the tooth composite and makes the enamel weak, brittle and discolored.

❏ Methyl mercury formed from amalgams is deadly. It causes brain disease. Fillings made of quartzite and epoxy are a safe substitute.

❏ Fluoride is the smallest negative particle on Earth. Since the fluoride particles are so small and so intensely negative, they connect with the hydrogen enzyme molecules at very low concentrations—around 1-3 ppm. The mechanism for destruction of enzymes by fluoride has been proven by x-ray analysis. Hydrogen bonds have been shown to be broken by fluoride.

❏ Avoiding fluoride prevents more than 114 ailments listed with references in Dr. Judd's book. These 114 medical side-effects range from cancer to headaches, which are caused by levels as small as one ppm of fluoride in the water.

❏ Fluoride harms the economy by requiring people to purchase sources other than fluorinated water. It also harms the economy by making people dependent upon undependable professionals that know nothing about its effects. Lack of knowledge about fluoride's detrimental effects is worldwide.

❏ The lethal dosage of the fluoride compound (fluoroacetic acid) for a 110 pound person is 2.5 mg, compared with 400 mg for arsenic oxide. Toothpaste companies are now required to place a warning on tubes so children will not consume enough of the 1,000 ppm (.1%) material to make them sick or cause death. This requirement arises out of lawsuits in which children were poisoned by fluoride-containing toothpaste.

❏ The best available data indicates about 120,000 cancer patients are killed annually because of fluoride in their drinking water. These include patients with every type of cancer. Dentists share some responsibility due to their efforts in convincing city councils to put fluoride in the water for "the children's teeth." The unique character of fluoride ions in destroying enzymes deserves attention.

In summary, according to Dr. Judd the health of our teeth will increase to be very nearly perfect if the regimen of water rinsing, soap brushing and taking calcium, phosphate and vitamin C in the diet is implemented. Wet the brush, swipe the bar two or three times, then brush the teeth thoroughly and the gums gently. Rinse with water three or four times. All oils are thus washed off the teeth and the gums are disinfected. The bacteria are killed by the soap. The teeth are then ready for re-enamelization with calcium and phosphate in the diet.

A special soap for teeth cleaning is offered at www.inspiredliving.com. *Good Teeth, Birth to Death: The Prescription for Perfect Teeth* can be purchased online from several sources.

■ ***Emdogain.***® Mild to moderate periodontitis affects most adults at some point in life, while 5–20% of any population suffer from severe forms of the disease. Straumann Holding AG of Basel, Switzerland has developed a regenerative system that offers treatment options to support both tooth preservation and oral bone augmentation. Emdogain is a gel topically applied by the dentist to root surfaces exposed by routine flap surgery, where the gums are lifted away from the tooth, plaque is removed, and the gums are re-sewn snugly around the tooth. The innovative product helps stabilize teeth and improve the outcome of periodontal surgery by stimulating lost bone and regenerating tissue structures that anchor the tooth.[3] Since its introduction in 1996, Emdogain has been used on more than a million patients worldwide. Studies show Emdogain patients regain about 65% of lost gum tissue within 16 months of treatment.

■ ***BoneCeramic.***® One in five dental implants requires bone augmentation either prior to or concurrent with implant placement. The patient's own (autologous) bone, from the jaw or elsewhere, is the preferred material. However, limited quantities are available and the procedure can result in pain and complications at the donor site. Bovine bone and human cadavers are two additional common sources. BoneCeramic is a very attractive alternative as it is fully synthetic. It supports the regeneration of and is gradually substituted by the patient's own bone. In comparison to bovine-derived material, BoneCeramic achieves equivalent new mineralized bone and more vital tissue after six to eight months. A 2007 study[4] showed that BoneCeramic combined with autologous bone achieved significantly better outcomes than autologous bone alone.

■ Additional information on Teeth and Gums can be found in the Member's Area of *The Encyclopedia's* website.

TOE AND FINGERNAIL FUNGUS

About 25% of all adults over the age of 30 have a nail fungus infection, according to podiatrists' reports. Fungal infestation of the toenails and fingernails usually brings more mental than physical discomfort—especially for those living near a beach or for those who like to wear sandals.

Several prescription and oral medications include itraconazole (Sporonox®), fluconazole (Diflucan®), griseofluvin (Fluvicin®), and terfinabine (Lamisil®). Although these systemic medications have been effective for many, they are quite expensive and carry with them the potential of side-effects including headaches, upset stomach, and most significantly, liver damage. There are more natural solutions that work quite well.

■ ***Tea Tree Oil.*** The age old, natural remedy for toenail and fingernail fungal infections is tea tree oil, known botanically as *Melaleuca alternifolia*. The tea tree is an indigenous species of New South Wales, Australia, and has been used as a general anesthetic by the native peoples of Australia for thousands of years. Captain James Cook, who visited Australia in 1770, made tea from the leaves of the melaleuca tree—hence the name tea tree.

Tea tree oil is an effective fungicide and bactericide, and is useful in killing a broad range of stubborn infections. It is safe for topical use, and does not inhibit normal cell growth. Continued application of 100% strength tea tree oil is effective in resolving many toenail and fingernail fungal infections—although it doesn't smell very well.

■ *Grapefruit Seed Extract.* Extracted from the seeds, membrane and pulp of the ordinary grapefriut, *grapefruit seed extract* (GSE) is a broad spectrum antimicrobial similar in molecular structure to the well-known antimicrobial benzalkonium chloride. It has been shown effective in treating toe and fingernail fungal infection. GSE is available in health food stores in capsule or pill form or as a liquid for topical application. For more information, read *The Authoritative Guide to Grapefruit Seed Extract* by Dr. Allan Sachs.

■ *SSKI.* Saturated solution of potassium iodide (SSKI) (one part DMSO to nine parts SSKI) is a very effective fungus remedy. See SSKI under *Iodine* in the seciton on **General Treatment Methods**. DMSO also can be added to tea tree oil and GSE. See DMSO under **Pain Relievers**.

■ Other products useful in treating toe and fingernail fungus are Listerine,®—the mouthwash—and 3% (drugstore) hydrogen peroxide. Soaking the feet or hands with either has been effective for many. Also, Vicks VapoRub® has been used successfully.

■ See also *Olive Leaf Extract* and *Sodium Chlorite* under **General Treatment Methods**.

TRAUMA (psychological). See Eye Movement Desensitization and Reprocessing under *Stress.*

TUBERCULOSIS

The bacterium *Mycobacterium tuberculosis* (TB; *tubercle bacillus*) is the most common cause of tuberculosis, an infectious and often deadly disease. Skeletal remains show that humans have been infected since prehistoric times, as long ago as 7000 BC. In the past TB was called consumption, as it seemed to consume its victims from within.

TB is a serious problem in some developing countries, but less so in first-world countries. Nevertheless, because it is transmitted by aerosolized droplets of a cough or sneeze, or the saliva (speaking or singing) of an infected person, there is always a danger of increased prevalence.

TB is treated by antibiotics, most commonly rifampicin and isoniazid. Drug-resistant TB (DR-TB) is a growing problem in many developing countries. Multi-drug resistant TB (MDR-TB) is resistant to both rifampicin and isoniazid, the two most effective front-line treatments. Extensively-drug-resistant TB (XDR-TB) is resistant to both rifampicin and isoniazid as well as three or more of the six classes of second-line antibiotics. XDR-TB is associated with high rates of mortality and accounts for at least 7% of TB cases worldwide.

Although some experts have feared that XDR-TB is effectively untreatable, researchers at Harvard Medical School have shown XDR-TB can be treated effectively. In the Harvard study, greater than 60% of the XDR-TB patients were cured using a combination of five or more antibiotics selected from a group of 12 anti-TB drugs to which the specific strain showed susceptibility. To learn more, Google "harvard xdr-tb."

Prior to the introduction of antibiotics, vitamin D was used effectively to treat TB. High doses of vitamin D_3 are also an effective TB preventive. See Vitamin D under *Colds and Flu*.

■ For additional information on Tuberculosis, see the Member's Area of *The Encyclopedia's* website.

URINARY TRACT INFECTION (UTI). See *Iodine* under **General Treatment Methods**.

VAGINAL. See *Prostate* (Rectal/Vaginal Heater).

VARICOSE VEINS

Also called varicoceles, varicose veins are knotted, enlarged blood vessels close to the skin's surface. The word varicose is derived from the Latin word *varix*, meaning twisted. Any vein can become varicose, but the most commonly affected are in the legs and feet. When veins in and around the rectal area become varicose, they're called hemorrhoids. Small varicose veins are often called spider veins.

Unlike arteries which deliver blood to the body as it leaves the heart, blood's return trip to the heart is through veins containing one-way valves which prevent the blood from flowing backwards. Varicose veins form when these valves fail or improperly-function allowing blood to pool, causing the veins to swell and appear as twisted, dark-blue vessels just under the skin's surface.

For most people varicose veins are merely a cosmetic concern, and are medically insignificant. For others, they can cause pain and discomfort in the form of muscle cramps and aching; fluid accumulation; and possibly blood clots. Varicose veins may indicate a more serious circulatory disorder, but because of their commonness many doctors believe they are largely the result of man's erect posture and gravitational forces at work.

According to proctologists—doctor's specializing in the area "where the sun don't shine"— hemorrhoids are a common occurrence, affecting nearly 75% of the Western world at some point during their lives. They even caused Napoleon to ride side saddle, and sidelined George Brett during the 1980 World Series. Hemorrhoids can be exacerbated by straining during a bowel movement, heavy lifting, or vigorous exercise.

Eating foods with a high fiber content such as fruits and vegetables, and drinking plenty of liquids can help prevent hemorrhoids from forming by softening the stool and easing elimination. A healthful diet which excludes processed foods is also a significant preventive measure.

Traditional medical treatment for serious cases of hemorrhoids can involve many different invasive techniques, including electro-therapy, injections, rubber banding, and surgery (naturally).

■ *Horse Chestnut.* One non-invasive treatment that attempts to address a long-term solution rather than merely the symptom(s) is standardized *escin* (also *aescin*), a saponin extract of the seed of the horse chestnut tree, *Aesculus hippocastanum*. Escin has been shown to decrease capillary permeability, thereby preventing edema (swelling). Escin also decreases vascular fragility, i.e., it strengthens blood vessels, rendering them less subject to forming varicosities. It also helps prevent the backward flow of blood by helping constrict damaged vein valves.[1]

European clinical trials have shown the effectiveness of horse chestnut in treating varicose veins.[2] In a recent study published in the *Lancet*,[3] horse chestnut seed extract was found to be as effective as compression stockings (which do nothing to treat underlying causes of the ailment) in patients with chronic venous insufficiency.

One product that is readily available is Venastat,® which is sold in many supermarkets and health food stores in the U.S. Other horse chestnut products are available at www.iherb.com. A dosage of 300 mg twice daily is recommended.

■ *Collinsonia.* Another substance shown to be effective in the treatment of varicose veins is the herb *Collinsonia canadensis*, also known as stone root. The action of this herb on varicosities has been well known for more than 100 years. In the 1919 book *The American Materia Medica, Therapeutics and Phamacognosy*, Finley Ellingwood, M.D. writes,

> [Collinsonia] is a specific remedy for hemorrhoids. If they are of recent origin they can be cured in a comparatively short time...The most intractable cases will be relieved and permanently benefitted by its persistent use. There is no therapeutic influence more reliable than this. I have relied upon it for years.[4]

Some physicians believe collinsonia is even more effective than the escin extract from horse chestnut. To locate a collinsonia product, do a key word search for "varicose veins collinsonia." One excellent product is Collinsonia Root, from Standard Process. To purchase this product, visit www.totalhealthvitamins.net.

VISION DISORDERS

Farsightedness, or *hyperopia*, is a condition in which near vision is impaired while distant vision remains intact. Over 60% of Americans over age 40 are affected. The eye of a hyperopic person focuses light behind, instead of directly on, the retina at the back of the eye. This is caused either by the eyeball not being long enough (front-to-back), the cornea being too flat, a weakened ciliary muscle that controls the lens, or a combination of these factors.[1]

Glasses, contact lenses, and corneal-steepening surgery are options used to improve vision. (The cornea is the transparent coating over the front of the eyeball covering the pupil and iris.)

In nearsightedness, or *myopia*, on the other hand, there is an impairment of vision at a distance, while near vision remains normal. The cornea of a myopic eye is too steep, the eyeball is too long (front-to-back) compared to a normal eye, and light focuses in front of the retina. Myopia affects about one third of the U.S. population[2] and a significant portion of most other cultures. Visual corrections are made with glasses, contact lenses, or surgical procedures which include flattening the central cornea or by implanting an intraocular lens (IOL).[3]

Presbyopia, meaning "aging eye" in Greek, is an age-related impairment that develops when the lens loses flexibility, preventing the eye from properly focusing on near images. Because this symptom is similar to farsightedness, the two conditions are often confused, even though the condition affects distant vision as well.

Presbyopia affects most Westerners over the age of 40, and nearly everyone over 50. It is estimated that over 90 million American baby boomers have or will soon develop presbyopia.[4] Presbiopics are typically treated with glasses or contact lenses.

Glasses (including bifocals) and contacts are the most popular non-invasive means of correcting refractive eye disorders, those disorders related to the bending and focusing of light within the eye. Both of these means of correction have drawbacks, however. Glasses and contact lenses adjust the focal length of the lens of the eye so that the incoming light focuses more directly on the retina.

In so doing, however, corrective lenses contribute to the progression of both near and farsightedness by allowing insufficient movement and thereby loss of tone of various important eye muscles.[5] Use it or lose it. Also, long-term use of glasses and contact lenses can lead to sensitivity to artificial light and loss of depth perception.[6]

Contact lenses can attract microbial contaminants that cause infection and inflammation of the cornea.[7] A study reported in the *Lancet*[8] found a 65% higher incidence of corneal inflammation in contact wearers compared to those not wearing contacts. The highest risk of infection occurred with the use of extended-wear soft contact lenses.[9]

Three types of refractive eye surgeries are in common use. They all have at least two similarities: the cutting of the cornea and potentially serious side-effects.

❏ *Radial keratotomy* (RK) treats myopia through flattening the cornea by making a series of incisions in the cornea in a radial pattern that resembles the spokes of a wheel. This procedure requires the surgeon to cut through 90% of the thickness of the cornea.[10] Cases where the cornea is completely penetrated typically result in blindness.[11] Because the eye is weakened by scar tissue that forms following the surgical incision, it is more subject to damage that may result from possible subsequent injury.[12] Also, radial keratotomy can lead to visual distortion, fluctuation, and nighttime glare.[13]

❏ *LASIK* (laser *in situ* keratomileusis) is a relatively recent procedure used to treat myopia, hyperopia, and astigmatism. A flap is cut near the apex of the cornea that exposes the cornea's middle layer, called the stroma. A laser is then used to vaporize some of the stromal tissue, after which the flap is reattached.

❏ *Photorefractive keratectomy* (PRK) also uses a laser to reshape the cornea, but without cutting the corneal flap. In PRK, the top layer of the cornea is scraped away so that the stromal layer is exposed for laser vaporization. PRK is accompanied by more short-term discomfort and a longer time before visual improvements are noticed.

According to *The Eye Care Sourcebook*,[14] both LASIK and PRK share these potential side-effects:

❖ Laser-created free radicals destroy keratocytes that assist the cornea in maintaining its integrity. Thinning and other corneal damage can occur.

❖ Diminished tear secretion—Dry Eye Syndrome.

❖ Patterns such as halos and starbursts appear around lights.

❖ A decrease in visual acuity

❖ Retinal detachment and tears, and macular holes and pucker, especially in myopics

❖ Damage and destruction of optic nerve (presumably caused by the high intraocular pressure that occurs during surgery).

■ **_Conductive Keratoplasty_** (CK; also called NearVision CK).[15] A new technique that's FDA approved for vision correction in hyperopia and presbyopia is much less invasive than the above surgeries. The elective procedure *conductive keratoplasty*, or CK, is an alternative to eyeglasses, contact lenses, LASIK, and PRK.

CK uses low-level radio waves applied in a circular pattern on the outer cornea to reshape the cornea. A small probe is used to release radio frequency (RF) waves that slightly heat and shrink corneal tissue. The circular pattern in which the treatment is applied acts as a constrictive band around the cornea—similar to the tightening of a belt—increasing (steepening) the curvature (slope) of the cornea which causes a refocusing of light more directly on the retina.

Thin as a human hair, the probe used to apply the RF energy is inserted into the cornea to a depth of about 80% of its thickness. As few as eight or as many as 32 insertion sites can be treated in one session (must be in multiples of eight) with each site taking only three seconds to complete.

The entire procedure takes only a matter of three to four minutes per eye. Either one or both eyes can be corrected, depending upon the need. Anesthetizing eye drops are used to insure the procedure is painless. The most common sensation reported is pressure on the front of the eye.

FDA approval was based on clinical data collected at the 12 month follow-up visit of those having had CK. The results were as follows:

• 98% of all study participants were able to read magazine- and newspaper-sized print (J5).

• 87% of participants were able to read phonebook-sized print (J3) and also see 20/20 at a distance.

Because CK is minimally invasive compared to the above-discussed surgical procedures, its potential side-effects are correspondingly less. Nevertheless, as with any procedure that physically touches the eye, there is the possibility of complications. Because hyperopia and presbyopia are progressive conditions—eyes change with age—CK is not considered a permanent correction. To locate a doctor trained in CK, call Refractec at (800) 752-9544, or visit www.myclearvision.com.

■ *Bates and Cambridge Methods*. There are non-invasive procedures useful in helping to correct vision. Two of the most effective are the Bates Method and the corrective vision program offered by the Cambridge Institute for Better Vision.

To view the Bates Method in a nutshell, visit www.i-see.org/bates_nutshell.html. To learn more about the method, read Dr. William Bates' 1981 book *Better Eyesight Without Glasses*, or do a key word search for "the bates method." To learn more about the Cambridge Institute, call (800) 372-3937, (978)887-3883, or visit www.bettervision.com.

■ See also *Cataracts*, *Glaucoma*, and *Macular Degeneration*.

WARTS

Many orthodox and unorthodox wart treatments exist. On the unorthodox side, rubbing the wart with a banana peel is sometimes helpful. Traditional Western medicine employs cryotherapy, where liquid nitrogen is used to freeze the wart. Recently, a very low-tech method has been shown effective.

■ *Duct Tape Occlusion*. In a 2002 study,[1] 51 participants received two months of treatment with either cryotherapy or duct tape. Following treatment, 60% were wart free, compared to 85% of those treated with duct tape.

A small piece of duct tape is used to cover the wart continuously for a six day period. The tape should be replaced as necessary. On the seventh day, the wart should be soaked in water and thereafter rubbed with an emery board or pumice stone. On the eighth day, begin the process again, and continue for two months or until the wart disappears. It is believed that the process stimulates the immune system which then eliminates the wart. The adhesive tape portion of ordinary band-aids is also very effective and may adhere better than duct tape.

■ *Grapefruit Seed Extract* (GSE). The extract of the seeds and pulp of ordinary grapefruit is often effective. GSE is sold in health food stores generally as a liquid solution of glycerin and grapefruit seed extract. Grapefruit Seed Extract is discussed in more detail under *Toe and Fingernail Fungus*.

WEIGHT LOSS.

■ *Integra-Lean Irvingia*.® An extract from the African plant *Irvingia gabonensis* has produced successful weight loss for many. To learn more about Integra-Lean Irvingia, visit http://search.lef.org/search/fault.aspx?s=1&QUERY=irvingia%20gabonensis. See also Weight Loss in the **Index** and in the Member's Area of *The Encyclopedia's* website.

■ *University of Georgia Cocktail*. A group of researchers at the University of Georgia have found that combinations of various over-the-counter nutritional supplements are effective in causing weight loss in many people. One of the most effective combinations is soy isoflavones (100 mg daily), resveratrol (100 mg daily), and quercetin (500 mg daily). To learn more, visit www.naturalhealthreference.com/natural-weight-loss/burn-body-fat-lose-fat-cells.

PART THREE: PAIN RELIEVERS

DMSO (Dimethyl sulfoxide)

For a short time during the 1960s, following an article in *Barron's Financial Weekly* and a *60 Minutes* television program discussing its many medicinal virtues, DMSO became known as a medical "wonder product" before briefly falling out of favor with the U.S. Food and Drug Administration. Its biological properties were co-discovered by Dr. Stanley Jacob of the Oregon Health Sciences Institute, the Director of Organ Transplant Research, where he demonstrated DMSO's many remarkable medicinal properties.

A product of wood pulp, DMSO is a solvent with an uncanny ability to penetrate the skin. Dr. Jacob explains that DMSO is water's "alter ego." Its molecular bond with water is 1.3 times stronger than water's molecular bond with itself. Because of this, it substitutes for water as it moves through cell membranes, pulling substances through cells that ordinarily would not penetrate them.[1] DMSO hydrates the cells, causing changes in the liquid structure of cellular water. Some believe its basic therapeutic principle is its ability to alter and restore damaged cells by hydrating them, changing their water structure, and increasing cellular permeability—which allows cells to nourish themselves and dispose of wastes more easily.[2]

Because of its penetrating abilities, DMSO is able to bring its healing powers deep within the body's tissues where it beneficially affects conditions including arthritis, both rheumatoid and osteoarthritis; athletic injuries; back pain and disc disorders; bursitis; burns; cuts and scrapes; fractures; gouty arthritic protuberances; herpes outbreaks; musculo-skeletal injuries; tendinitis; sprains and strains; whiplash; and a multitude of other conditions. Another unusual property of DMSO—which is very different from most other substances including pharmaceuticals—is that it has a cumulative effect rather than requiring larger doses.[3]

In his book *DMSO: Nature's Healer*, Dr. Morton Walker states that people now have a new breakthrough for pain: DMSO. The New York *Daily News* reported that some researchers believe DMSO "...may be the aspirin of the 21st Century."[4] Although all of the mechanisms of the substance are not fully understood, it is believed one mode of action is that it blocks C fibers of peripheral nerves on which pain signals are conducted. Because it tends to increase the blood supply to affected areas, especially to the lower limbs, it is an excellent treatment for soft-tissue injuries.[5] It also appears to be an excellent antioxidant and anti-inflammatory.

In the research conducted on the use of DMSO as a topical treatment, a 5%-90% DMSO solution was used several times daily, depending on the condition. Application to sensitive areas of the body may cause redness, stinging or a burning sensation. Allergic reactions are rare. DMSO is contraindicated in pregnant women and breast-feeding mothers. Although all DMSO products carry a notice that it's not to be used on skin, this is merely an FDA labeling requirement. High-quality DMSO is available in most health food stores, or it can be purchased on the internet. For more information, including research studies, visit www.dmso.org. See also DMSO under **Spinal Cord Injury**.

ELECTRICITY

Stone carvings 2,500 years old—from the Egyptian Fifth Dynasty—depict humans using an electrified fish to treat pain. For those who are vegetarians, non-fishermen, or just wanting an easier method, there is a modern-day analogue which is effective for many. TENS (transcutaneous electrical nerve stimulation) devices are typically pocket-sized, battery-operated units with wire leads that attach to the skin near the painful area (or on acupuncture points) by means of two or more electrodes. Non-painful, patient-controlled electrical impulses are sent through the skin to the nerve fibers where they interrupt the nerve impulses which transmit pain signals to the brain. TENS therapy also encourages the body to produce higher levels of *endorphins* and *enkephalins*, two of the body's natural pain-killing chemicals.[1] For some, pain relief continues even after the device is turned off.

TENS devices have been used world wide to treat both acute and chronic pain. Physicians, physiotherapists, pain clinics and sports coaches have used these devices with great success in treating a multiplicity of painful ailments including arthritis/bursitis/tendinitis, back, cancer, dental, fractures, headache/migraine, joint, labor, menstrual, muscle, peripheral nerve injury (including diabetic neuropathy), phantom limb, post operative, sciatica, shingles, sports injuries, sprains/strains, TMJ, trigeminal neuralgia, whiplash/neck, plus many other ailments.[2]

TENS devices are FDA approved in the U.S., are reimbursable by most insurance providers, and generally require a doctor's prescription. TENS therapy may be contraindicated for people wearing pace makers, expectant mothers, and in certain other situations. For more information on Transcutaneous Electrical Nerve Stimulation, do a key word search for "tens pain."

A device similar to the TENS unit applies weak microcurrents directly to the head. This form of therapy often produces a general lessening of pain due to its stimulation of the body's own painkilling substances, including endorphins. This technology is called *Cranial Electrotherapy Stimulation* (CES). To learn more about CES, see Cranial Electrotherapy Stimulation under **Stress**.

FARABLOC®

Some people can forecast changes in the weather by the subtle changes they feel in their bodies—a throbbing knee, a stiff thumb, the pain of an old

sports injury, etc. It is assumed these people are perceiving subtle changes in their immediate environments, one possibility being a shift in the surrounding electromagnetic fields. An unprotected, unshielded human being on the surface of planet Earth is subject to electromagnetic radiation of various wavelengths which impinge upon the body. Some wavelengths are harmful, while some are healthful.

In 1969, German scientist and inventor Frieder Kempe was motivated through necessity to invent something for his father, a war veteran with a limb amputation who suffered from "phantom limb" pain—pain associated with a former limb (healed stump), even though the limb is no longer physically present. At times of changing weather, his father's surgery site became very painful. In an attempt to find a remedy, scientist Kempe created a *Faraday Cage*, a physical device capable of shielding (i.e., blocking the penetration of) electromagnetic radiation of various wavelengths. His first prototype was in the form of a blanket fashioned of fabric made from fine steel mesh spun onto nylon thread. Although cumbersome, itchy and uncomfortable, the device significantly reduced his father's limb pain. The fabric material was named *Farabloc*.

Following its initial success, a more comfortable, light-weight, user-friendly version of Farabloc was produced and patented. The present product consists of a series of ultra-thin stainless steel threads woven into a nylon fabric, after which it is fashioned into garments such as blankets; cummerbunds (back); elbow and knee wraps; gloves; short- or long-sleeved jackets; socks; and limb covers for amputated limbs.

The specific mechanisms by which Farabloc achieves its analgesic and other beneficial effects are not fully understood. Farabloc is believed to reduce pain by shielding the wearer from high-frequency electromagnetic fields which are known to cause cellular damage, while at the same time allowing the passage of low frequency waves which are known to stimulate blood circulation and promote healing.

Farabloc is an effective electromagnetic shield at frequencies above 1 MHz, and is most effective in the high- and ultrahigh-frequency ranges. It has a limited shielding capability in the low-frequency electromagnetic field (EMF), particularly the very low (> 10 KHz) and extremely low-frequencies, and also the super and extremely high-frequency ranges > 10,000 MHz.[1]

In a 1993 Canadian study of phantom limb pain, at least a double thickness of Farabloc fabric worn for a minimum of four hours brought significant pain reduction compared to the placebo group.[2] In 2000, a study published in the *Clinical Journal of Sports Medicine*[3] examined Farabloc's ability to effect delayed-onset muscle soreness (DOMS) following severe exercise of the human thigh muscle. The blood serum levels of five markers indicative of muscle damage, pain and inflammation were measured: creatine phosphokinase and myoglobin (indicative of muscle cell membrane disruption), malondialdehyde (an index of lipid peroxidation that increases with free radical damage), and leukocytes and neutrophils (known to increase with severely strenuous exercise and muscle damage). Double layers of Farabloc wrapped around the thigh muscle of participating subjects significantly reduced pain, loss of strength, and reduced all five of the above muscle damage markers.

Clinical trials in Europe and Canada have shown Farabloc to be effective in reducing or eliminating pain of various types and causes. Anecdotally, users have reported help with pain in the back, hip pain, migraines, nerve pain, stiff neck, sports-injury-related muscle pain, and even pain from conditions such as arthritis and fibromyalgia. One version of the product is Equi-bloc,® which is used on horses to help reduce muscle fatigue and recovery time following strenuous exercise. Prices range from USD $70-700, depending on the product and size. The lightweight material looks and feels like linen, can be washed, and lasts for years with proper care. To learn more about Farabloc, call ABC Health Solutions at (253)631-8270, or visit www.abchealthsolutions.biz.

FREQUENCY SPECIFIC MICROCURRENTS

Frequency Specific Microcurrent (FSM) is a system of treating specific medical conditions using microamperage current and the resonance effects of certain frequencies. An ampere is a unit of electrical current, or amount of electric charge per second. Microcurrents are measured in millionths of

an ampere—very small electrical charges too weak to stimulate the sensory nerves and therefore can't be perceived by the average person. Microamperage currents are the same level of electrical charges produced by the cells of the body.

In his book *Energy Medicine*, James Oschman, Ph.D., explains that each part of the body—including each of the body's cells—is a portion of the whole, which forms a continuously interconnected network that communicates via frequencies. When there is an injury on any level—physical, toxic, emotional, etc.—discordant vibrational patterns are created in the tissues. It is the specific frequencies and the resonance effects used in FSM that are responsible for the beneficial healing effects by correcting the discordant vibrational patterns.

FSM is currently enjoying a resurgence of popularity in the U.S., Canada, and Australia, although the practice of stimulating the body with microcurrents has been employed for at least 100 years. It was, in fact, a popular method of treatment in the U.S. prior to 1950 when the American Medical Association deemed FSM devices "unscientific," threatened to remove the licenses of doctors who continued to use them, and outright outlawed the technology. Thereafter followed the emergence of the repressive influence of the large pharmaceutical firms and the relentless marketing of their "patent" medicines, pharmaceutical drugs.

In the 1950s, American physician Dr. Harry Van Gelder purchased a medical practice in Vancouver, B.C. Along with the practice came a 1920s version of a microcurrent device that was used at that time. Accompanying the device was a manual which included specific frequencies used to treat various medical conditions. The discovery of this old device along with the list of frequencies would mark the beginning of the renewed use of this technique, although it would take an additional several decades to reinstate the technology. In the 1980s, a form of microcurrent therapy was used by physicians in Europe and the U.S. for stimulating acupuncture points, stimulating healing of sports-related injuries, and stimulating bone repair in non-union fractures. In the 1990s, other instruments began to emerge.

Although there are presently a number of devices on the market capable of delivering micro-amperage current, a particularly effective unit is manufactured by Precision Microcurrent, Inc. of Vancouver, Washington. The instrument has two independent channels that allow the practitioner to set both the frequency and the current independently for each channel. The unique circuitry allows for long battery life and frequencies that are precise to 0.1% accuracy. This is the device used by Dr. Carolyn McMakin, an American chiropractor at the forefront of FSM therapy. Although the story is virtually unknown to the sports news media, it was Dr. McMakin who treated superstar wide receiver Terrell Owens of the Philadelphia Eagles following his severe ankle injury just seven weeks prior to Super Bowl XXXIX. Surprisingly, FSM treatment allowed Owens to make a spectacular recovery, contributing nine receptions for 122 yards in his Super Bowl effort.

FSM is used successfully to treat a wide range of ailments including allergies, asthma, carpal tunnel syndrome, fibromyalgia, hyperthyroidism, imbalanced emotions, inflammation, irritable bowel syndrome, kidney stone pain, liver dysfunction, muscle pain, nerve pain, toxins—the list is practically endless. Those who practice the technique as well as those who have benefitted from its use describe the results as near miraculous. Dr. McMakin has trained several hundred practitioners in FSM treatment, and home units are also available. To learn more about FSM and to locate a practitioner in your area, visit www.frequencyspecific.com. [Microcurrent devices, including the Precision Microcurrent instrument, are approved by the FDA for use and sale in the category of TENS devices (see *Electricity* in this section), even though TENS devices deliiver milliamperage current as opposed to microampere currents used in FSM devices.]

LIGHT

It is a well-established fact that light has powerful effects on living organisms. Especially over the past decade, significant research has focused on applying specific wavelengths of light directly to the skin of individuals in an attempt to effect positive changes in a wide range of ailments, including pain reduction of various origins, and tissue healing. The results are often dramatic and long lasting.

Light Therapy, also referred to as Photon Therapy and Phototherapy, uses different wavelengths, intensities and durations of application, depending upon the ailment. Light is absorbed by certain components—cytochromes—in the cells of both tissues and blood, thereby stimulating the natural capabilities of the body by energizing and normalizing the functions of these cellular components which may have been disrupted by injury or disease.[1] This causes beneficial changes in nerve fibers, muscle, connective tissue and blood. Both chronic and acute pain caused by many ailments are often quickly and effectively controlled.

Laser light, mostly in the red area of the spectrum [~635 to 904 nanometers (nm)] has received considerable research attention. Laser light is monochromatic, i.e., it is a single, discrete wavelength. The therapy is referred to as Low-Level Laser Therapy (LLLT), and certain adaptations of the technology can perform near miracles in pain reduction and wound healing. LLLT devices operate at such a low power level they do not burn the skin, and are completely painless. One such device is the advanced, pulsed laser system by LazrPulsr Systems. To learn more about this therapy, visit www.lazrpulsr.com.

Because of the physical properties unique to laser light, LLLT often accomplishes results not obtainable by *light emitting diodes* (LEDs). However, because of its cost effectiveness, portability, safety, and broader range of wavelengths from a single light source, the use of LEDs is gaining popularity as an effective pain control technology. Similar to lasers, therapeutic LEDs offering pain relief and enhanced tissue growth and regeneration also operate in the red portion of the spectrum. Because of its limited skin penetration, the visible red wavelength (~635 nm) is most effective for treating problems close to the surface, such as acupuncture points, cuts, scars, and the like.

A more promising wavelength of LEDs is in the near-infrared portion of the spectrum, at about 890-904 nm. Light of this frequency penetrates to a depth of up to nine inches.[2] (A simple experiment demonstrating the depth of penetration can be done with an inexpensive visible-light red LED by shining it through the palm of the hand in a darkened room). Because of its ability to achieve deep skin penetration, near-infrared LEDs are more effective in treating bones, joints, and deep muscles.

A more technical explanation of the effectiveness of Phototherapy is as follows: When light is absorbed within a cell, singlet oxygen is produced, which in turn causes a change in proton gradients across cell membranes including the mitochondria—the energy storehouse within cells which produces adenosine triphosphate (ATP). Cell membrane permeability increases, leading to increased ATP levels, i.e., the cells become more energetic. Increases in DNA production, endothelial cell production and fibroblast proliferation occur.

Also, the application of near-infrared energy increases the nitric oxide content of the blood and blood plasma, resulting in enhanced tissue perfusion, neovascularization and successful wound healing. Even though not simple, this explanation is simplistic in that there are additional mechanisms of action involved in the healing process, both understood and not understood.

According to Dr. Harry Whelan, Professor of Pediatric Neurology and Director of Hyperbaric Medicine at the Medical College of Wisconsin, "The near-infrared light emitted by these LEDs seems to be perfect for increasing energy inside cells...the LEDs boost energy to the cells and accelerate healing."[4] Dr. Whelan's NASA-funded research has demonstrated remarkable results using LEDs to promote wound healing of mouth ulcers caused by chemotherapy and radiation cancer therapies.[5] Whelan and his research team have shown that near-infrared treatment of skin and muscle cells grown *in vitro* produces a 150-200% increase in cell growth. They also demonstrated a 40% improvement in musculoskeletal training injuries in military patients treated with LEDs.[6]

Doctors aboard the USS Salt Lake City submarine reported a 50% increase in healing of crew members' lacerations when treated with near-infrared LEDs.[7] Red LEDs also have been used successfully in the treatment of burns, including third degree burns,[8] and in treating neuropathies, including diabetic neuropathy. For more information about this technology, visit www.cheeenergy.com; www.anodynetherapy.com; www.painxequine.com/Studies.htm or do a key word search for "led pain." See also **Spinal Cord Injury** for the latest laser treatment for that ailment.

MAGNETS

Magnetic forces have long been prized by man for their restorative properties. Ancient Greeks including the Father of Medicine, Hippocrates, used natural loadstone for therapeutic purposes. Likewise, the ancient Egyptians extolled the medicinal benefits of natural magnets. Bio-magnetics (aka magnetic field therapy) is currently well established in Austria, China, Germany, India and Japan. Pain control by the use of small magnets taped to the skin is growing in popularity in the U.S. Each year, Americans spend more than $200 million on various types of medicinal magnets. The Japanese biomagnet company Nikken surpassed $1.5 billion in 2000, with sales expected to be up sharply in the coming years.[1]

Typically, suitable magnets for use in pain relief range in strength from about 500 gauss to 10,000+ gauss. The strongest magnets—in the 10,000-12,000 gauss range—are rare earth neodymium magnets mixed with iron and boron. The stronger the magnet, the deeper the penetration and broader the effect, according to the researchers familiar with the various forms of electromagnets. Magnets in the 10,000 gauss range are believed to penetrate tissues to a depth of up to six inches.

Scientists at Baylor College of Medicine in Houston, New York Medical College, and Vanderbilt University in Tennessee have conducted research into the positive effects of magnets in pain prevention of many types. To the surprise of some researchers, magnets actually relieved many types of pain in about 70-80% of the people tested. No one knows exactly *how* magnets work. Robert R. Holcomb, M.D., Ph.D., Assistant Professor of Pediatrics and Neurology at Vanderbilt University School of Medicine, believes magnets alter the chemical interactions within the nerve fibers that mediate pain impulses. "In essence, you cut off chemical pain messages before they can reach the brain,"[2] says Holcomb. Another popular theory is that magnets produce an increase in blood flow to the affected area, thus speeding healing.

Magnets of various strengths can be purchased on the internet, in some health food stores, and in many golf shops. For more information on magnet therapy, visit www.garynull.com/Documents/magnets.htm. Magnet therapy is contraindicated for people wearing pace makers and for expectant mothers.

Dr. Dean Bonlie, president of the Scientific Committee of the North American Academy of Magnetic Therapy and owner of the Canadian firm Magnetico, has developed a magnetic mattress pad that is unique in both design and effect. The Magnetico pad is of *unipolar* design, as opposed to other magnetic mattresses that are *bipolar*.

All magnets have both a north and south pole—i.e., they are bipolar. Researchers have suggested the best results of short term treatment by magnet therapy is by using the negative[-] pole (against the skin) in the northern hemisphere, and by using the positive[+] pole in the southern hemisphere. Even in this situation, a bipolar effect will be present, but this is seen as beneficial for short-term use. Dr. Bonlie explains that the Earth's natural, unipolar magnetic field nourishes the body by its negatively charged electrical field descending from above in the northern hemisphere and its positively charged field emanating through the Earth from below in the southern hemisphere.

While short-term treatment with bipolar magnets often achieves effective results, as discussed, Bonlie suggests that long-term (hours at a time—such as sleeping on a mattress) magnetic treatment with bipolar magnets may be harmful. In order to reap the benefits of using magnets for extended periods of time, only one electrical field—negative in the northern hemisphere and positive in the southern hemisphere—should be present.[3] Dr. Bonlie has discovered a means of achieving that state in his unipolar mattress pad.

Contrary to other magnetic mattress designs in which the magnets are spaced at a significant distance from one another, Bonlie achieves a unipolar effect by placing powerful magnets very close together, so that the negative electromagnetic field becomes more prominent in the vertical plane above which a (northern hemisphere) person sleeps, while the positive field is moved to the perimeter of the mattress. A further improvement of the Magnetico mattress pad is that it is placed under the regular mattress, and therefore minimizes any positive-field energy spikes that may be present. During sleep, the body rests in a pure negative electromagnetic field (for northern hemisphere customers, and vice-versa for the southern hemi-

sphere) of five gauss, the strength that some researchers believe was present on Earth many thousands of years in the past, but now has waned to only one tenth of that strength.[4]

The body responds positively to being bathed in an electromagnetic field of the appropriate polarity and strength, resulting in benefits such as increased immunity, increased oxygen saturation, and decreased blood pressure. According to private communications between Dr. Bonlie and Dr. Gumiel of the World Development Organization, Gumiel stated he was able to increase the life span an average of 500% in 23 different species of insects using enhanced magnetic fields, while increasing the life span of human tissue by 250%.[5] Bonlie has done controlled clinical testing of his mattress pad, and found it helpful in treating many serious ailments including cancer, cardiovascular disease, chronic fatigue syndrome, fibromyalgia, and osteoporosis.

In an observational study of more than 900 cancer patients over an average 3.5 year period, there was a 78% reduction in the development of new cancers in comparison to the expected incidence.[6] Eighty-eight volunteers exercising for six minutes in a five gauss negative field experienced a 5.93% increased oxygen saturation level and a 13.15% decrease in heart rate.[7] Canadian physician Dr. Carolyn DeMarco conducted a pilot study on six of her worst chronic fatigue patients. Following six months of using the unipolar mattress pad, all patients showed improvement and three of the six patients were able to return to work.[8] In a controlled, double-blind study of 111 fibromyalgia patients conducted at the University of Virginia, the Magnetico pad was compared to the popular Nikken pad as well as a non-active control pad over a six month period of use. The Magnetico pad significantly reduced patient pain levels (32.4%) in comparison to the Nikken pad (10%) and the control (7.5%).[9]

Although no formal clinical trials have been done in the treatment of osteoporotic patients, Bonlie has found the unipolar pad so effective in maintaining or increasing women's bone density that he offers a 90% refund of the purchase price if no improvement in bone density is seen from an initial DEXA scan to an after-use scan within one year of using the magnetic pad. For all other conditions, there is a 90% unconditional refund policy within six months of the purchase date.

To learn more, visit www.magneticosleep .com, or call (800)265-1119 from within the U.S. or (403)730-0883 from outside the U.S.

MANUAL SPINAL NERVE BLOCK™

Dr. Stephen Kaufman is a chiropractor with 30 years experience, currently practicing in Denver, Colorado. The Manual Spinal Nerve Block techniques are an advanced form of PNT (discussed below) using spinal nerves to turn off muscle trigger points and their associated pain, which is a different approach than that used by the PNT techniques. Spinal nerve blocking is a form of spinally or centrally mediated PNT, while PNT uses local muscular neurological reflexes. One technique doesn't replace, but compliments the other. The techniques can be used alone or in combination. According to those who have witnessed or experienced the results of manual spinal nerve blocking, the outcomes are equally as dramatic or even more so than those of the PNT. Dr. Kaufman also offers a set of instructional DVDs for this technique. To inquire, call (800)774-5078.

NATURAL RELIEF 1222™

H. Edward Troy, Ph.D., a research pharmacologist for a major international pharmaceutical company, spent 14 years developing the formulation that eventually became Natural Relief 1222. The number "1222" indicates the total number of separate attempted formulations before success was achieved, "1222" being the final, perfected product. Natural Relief 1222 is an odorless, fast-acting topically-applied cream formulation that some users say is in a class of its own. It's a proprietary, all-natural formulation combining more than 18 separate compounds, and is useful in bringing pain relief to ailments caused by both muscles and joints, including sports injuries; muscle sprains; tendinitis and bursitis; osteo- and rheumatoid arthritis; and fibromyalgia. The all-natural formulation is currently used by members of the U.S. Olympic track and field team, as well as players from all 32 National Football League (NFL) franchises. For more information and to order, visit www.natural-relief .com/natrelief.html or call (979)422-1177.

PAIN NEUTRALIZATION TECHNIQUE™

Dr. Kaufman, the originator of the Manual Spinal Nerve Block discussed above, has added another powerful pain-relieving technique to his armormentarium—which is now available to the public. Kaufman always wondered if there weren't something like a "magic switch" that could turn pain off instantaneously—like a light switch. In 1989, he began a research project to find this "Holy Grail" of pain relief, his goal being to discover some way to easily and instantly turn off pain using only light pressure on neurological reflexes. After more than a decade, he has developed numerous procedures that seem to do just that, in many cases. One of these procedures is called the Pain Neutralization Technique™ (PNT).

Kaufman discovered a method of combining several simple, standard neurological reflexes to immediately change the tone in a painful muscle, eliminating many chronic painful areas and symptoms. The doctors and practitioners (D.C.s, L.Acs, M.D.s, D.O.s, P.T.s, N.D.s and body workers) who have taken his PNT course acclaim this as a major breakthrough in the treatment of pain.

Much of the pain people experience is located in the muscles and tendons. This is where PNT focuses. All of the body's muscles have opposing muscles. As one muscle contracts, the opposition muscle relaxes. In daily life, the nervous system reflexively relaxes the muscle opposing the contracting muscle. At times, a muscle may unnecessarily remain in a state of contraction, causing discomfort or pain.

Although there are a number of techniques employed by Dr. Kaufman, the following is a simple explanation one of the most important. PNT treats the muscle opposing the contracted muscle. The practitioner manually stimulates the neurological receptors in the tendons of the opposing muscle while applying a slight pressure to the painful area. The nervous system senses the opposing muscle is contracting and reflexively relaxes the painful, contracted muscle. The formerly painful, contracted muscle now has a new muscular and neurological "set point" and, once reset, the pain is eliminated.

Dr. Kaufman demonstrates PNT at medical meetings throughout the U.S. The following are several commentaries from physicians who have themselves received PNT treatments:[1]

> Here's a miracle I wouldn't have believed if I wasn't there to witness it. A previously unknown chiropractor delivered a talk about... instantly relieving the pain of trigger points. He claimed to immediately restore motion and eliminate pain...I listened with curiosity and healthy skepticism. Then he performed his technique on many of my esteemed colleagues including some very famous ones. The majority got immediate relief, even with very long term chronic problems. It was absolutely incredible!   —Robert Rowan, M.D.
> Editor-in-Chief, *Second Opinion* newsletter

> For 9 months, I have suffered with left sacroiliac/lower lumbar pain. With just 1 session of less than 5 minutes (of PNT), my low back pain is 80% better. The next day, it's 90% better. WOW! I gotta learn how to do this stuff!
> —John Parks Trowbridge, M.D.
> Best selling author of *The Yeast Syndrome*

> Thank you Dr. Kaufman for the immediate relief you provided me yesterday. I have had continuous back pain since fracturing the transverse process of L1-2-3-4 in 1974. You found the painful point and with P.N.T. the pain was completely gone in a few seconds. It is still gone. Follow up 18 months later: the pain never came back after that one treatment!
> —Ted Rozema, M.D.
> Former President, American College for Advancement in Medicine and the International College of Integrative Medicine

A set of instructional DVDs is available to health practitioners. Dr. Kaufman has trained many practitioners around the U.S. in the technique of PNT. For more information and to locate a PNT practitioner in your area, visit www.kaufmantechnique.com/index.html or call (800)774-5078.

PENETRAN+PLUS®

Healthy cells maintain a balance (equilibrium) between particles inside and outside of cell membranes. Electrically-charged ions within the extra-cellular fluid help maintain this balance. Damaged cells have difficulty maintaining this equilibrium, as both the cells' internal environment as well as the composition of the extracellular fluid undergo change. Adjacent cells are negatively affected by this altered environment, causing a domino or cascading effect which is perceived as pain.

Penetran+Plus contains ammonium-based compounds (quaternary amines) which supply nitrogen ions to the damaged cells. The presence of nitrogen helps reestablish the normal electrical balance within and around the cells, thereby effectively and dramatically reducing pain.

A 1998 study evaluated the effectiveness of Penetran+Plus in the treatment of arthritis, bursitis and tendinitis. Seventy percent of the study participants experienced significant pain reduction compared to only 4% in the placebo control group. The effects began about 20 minutes following application, and lasted an average of four hours.[1] Penetran+Plus is effective for pain caused by bruises, burns, cuts, insect bites, muscle strains, sprains, and also may be effective for pain caused by diabetic neuopathy. Purchase Penetran+Plus from some health food stores and pharmacies, or on the internet by searching for "penetran plus."

PROLOTHERAPY. See *Prolotherapy* under **General Treatment Methods**.

SOOTHANOL X2®

This liquid product is intended to treat sprains, strains, joint injuries—in fact, any minor aches and pains of muscles or joints. Soothanol X2 contains 12 ingredients, including arnica oil, calendula oil, cayenne pepper, DMSO, emu oil, ginger, limmonene oil, methanol, MSM, olive oil, St. John's wort oil, and wintergreen. According to the manufacturer, pain relief occurs within several minutes of application. For more information and to place an order, Google "soothanol," or call the manufacturer NorthStar Nutritionals at (800)913-2592.

SPHENOPALATINE GANGLION BLOCK

Along the back surface of the inner nasal cavity lies a small triangular cluster of nerve fibers comprising the largest number of neurons (nervous tissue cells capable of transmitting electrical impulses) outside of the brain itself. Called the *sphenopalatine ganglion*, or SPG (also referred to as the pterygopalatine, nasal or Meckl's ganglion), this bundle of fibers is a major junction point of nerve fibers through which pain impulses must pass before reaching the brain. Nerve impulses of headache pain, facial pain, neck pain, back pain, musculoskeletal pain, and even a pain in the butt all must pass through this "switch box" en route to the brain. The SPG seems to play a pivotal role as an important major relay center of the autonomic nervous system.[1]

By inserting an applicator into the nasal cavity and topically applying an appropriate anesthetic solution onto this small bundle of nerve fibers, the ganglion becomes anesthetized. Pain messages originating in many locations throughout the body often can be effectively blocked before reaching the brain and being perceived as pain. In this case it would be appropriate to say, "no brain, no pain."

The technique was pioneered during the early 1900s using topical anesthetics such as cocaine which, among other uses, is a powerful topical anesthetic. A series of five daily treatments typically brings pain relief lasting weeks or months, possibly even years. Because cocaine in the U.S. is currently in such political disfavor—although its medicinal use has not been outlawed—even for medical applications such as the SPG block, U.S. doctors may be hesitant to use this effective topical anesthetic for fear of repercussions by their Medical Boards or the DEA. As the technique is most often practiced today in the U.S., lidocaine (Xylocain®) or a mixture of lidocaine and diazepam (Valium®) are used, which are not likely to be as effective. Some South and Central American countries use the more effective cocaine treatment, as do practitioners in most European countries.

Although a Q-Tip can be inserted into the nasal cavity to apply the topical anesthetic solution to the SPG, this technique is bothersome to many patients. (On the other hand, many patients have been taught to self administer the anesthetic.) The preferred method seems to be the use of an intratracheal cannula which is preloaded with the anesthetic solution.[2] Prior to insertion of the cannula into the nasal cavity, the patient can be made more comfortable by anesthetizing the nasal cavity itself using a lidocaine aerosol spray. Depending upon the severity of the medical condition and the amount of pain experienced, the sphenopalatine block could be an answer to many chronic pain conditions. To learn more about this procedure, visit www.painphysicianjournal.com/2004/april/2004;7;283-286.pdf.

TAMANU OIL. See *Psoriasis.*

THE MVT RELIEF™

Microvibration therapy is a unique and patented technology that synergistically combines four separate therapy technologies into one device: The MVT Relief. The unit, not much larger than a penlight, combines the sciences of massage therapy, light therapy, sound therapy and magnetic therapy for the relief of physical pain. No electrical stimulation or TENS is used.

From sensation to perception, pain is the perception of discomfort at one for several points in the body. Sensory information or "pain signals" are transmitted by *pain transmission neurons* (PTNs). PTNs, in turn, relay the pain messages to the brain. Scientists believe that it is at the first nerve connection, or synapse, where the peripheral nerve meets the central nervous system, that both pain (hyperalgia) and pain relief (analgesia) are processed. It is through the blockage of this pathway that acupuncture is theorized to relieve pain, via a mechanism that has not yet been clearly established. The MVT Relief device may or may not achieve its beneficial results due to this same principle.

The device is believed to function by stimulating the cells and tissues, causing them to rapidly and dramatically improve circulation as well as other vital activities within the cells. According to the inventors Robert Milne, M.D. and Walter Spawr, the device seems to "wake up" sluggish cellular activity, revitalizing cells into healthy function, at least in part by stimulating the harmonic vibration of atoms within cells and improving intercellular communication. This allows the body's own healing processes to take place, thereby increasing muscle relaxation, relieving discomfort, improving energy, and increasing well being. Additional studies will be needed to more precisely elucidate the device's mechanism(s) of action.

For those who may appreciate a more technical explanation, the present paragraph is offered. A prerequisite for life is the ability to maintain electrochemical imbalances across biomembranes. It is known that the plasma membrane potential of a human cell is maintained at approximately -70 mv. Milne and Spawr theorize that when the body is injured (or the biomembrane is less bioactive), the proton pump within the cellular membranes becomes stagnant. The membrane potential of affected cells, therefore, becomes less electronegative (e.g., -45 mv). When "healthy" cells come into close proximity to "sick" cells having decreased electronegativity, an intercellular voltage disparity exists, and cell to cell communication is impaired. This impairment produces a signal carried by nerves to the brain that humans may interpret as "pain." When the painful area is treated with the MVT device, it is theorized that the area is flooded with multi-resonant frequencies, and cybernetic cellular energy induction is produced which may temporarily increase cellular electro-negativity. Once local cellular communication is re-established, the pain signal rapidly disappears. Most likely the MVT inductively and resonantly stimulates the cells to increase the proton pump and enhance cell-to-cell communication.

The MVT Relief device is initially placed on three key acupuncture points that have direct access to the central nervous system. It is thereafter placed on any point of the body that has discomfort. Relief is felt in a matter of minutes and lasts an average of from 45 minutes to several days, depending upon the individual and the nature of the discomfort. Most individuals find that consecutive, daily treatments produce longer-lasting results with each use, according to Milne and Spawr.

Mechanical vibration, the first of the four technologies employed by the device, uses very fine physical oscillations to produce therapeutic benefits. Over the past 40 years, studies have shown that vibration therapy causes many physiological changes in various organ systems, including the musculoskeletal, endocrine, and nervous systems. Vibration therapy has been shown to decrease back pain and increase bone strength in patients with osteoporosis and osteopenia. Vibration therapy has also resulted in endocrinologic changes within the body, including as high as a 460% increase in growth hormone production, up to a 7% increase in testosterone production, and a 30 fold decrease in cortisol levels. It can also affect the nervous system, with one study illustrating reduced tremor in conditions such as Parkinson's disease, according to research compiled by the inventors. The MVT Relief uses micro-fine vibrations with an amplitude of 0.01 mm.

The second technology used by The MVT Relief is light microvibration. Every living cell absorbs and emits light energy in the form of biophotons. It may be for this reason that therapies utilizing light energy have been shown to affect cells by providing an external source of photons for cellular function. Light energy harmonically vibrates atoms within cells. The MVT Relief uses light emitting diodes (LEDs). The beneficial effects of low level light therapy include increasing the body's production of ATP and endorphins to reduce pain; decreasing inflammation, swelling, and improving lymphatic drainage; increasing blood circulation (particularly to the areas of trauma); increasing the proliferation of fibroblasts and osteoblasts to increase bone strength; and causing up to a 75% increase in enzymatic activity.

Acoustic sound vibration is the third technology used by the device. For many years, medical practitioners have utilized sound vibration, in the form of ultrasound, both diagnostically and therapeutically. Basic science has shown that direct stimulation of living cellular tissue using sound frequency vibration can cause a marked cellular organelle response, a corresponding measurable increase of cellular metabolism and, therefore, a possible mobilization of the cellular healing response. This increase in cellular vibration may improve, and thus theoretically restore cellular communication. The sound waves also stimulate motion of fluids through the body and brain, bringing oxygen and other nutrients to tissues, which in turn increases serotonin, dopamine, and other neuropeptides, helping to alter one's perceptions.

Also, it is believed that each of the body's organs has its own specific frequency at which it resonates in a healthy state. Some believe that exposing unhealthy organs to such frequencies will assist them in returning to their normal state of resonance and health.

By delivering specific frequencies through the body directly, an entirely different system of the body—the brainstem and spinal cord—are brought into play, offering the possibility of direct cellular stimulation.

Magnetic Vibration is the final technology employed by The MVT Relief. There is growing evidence that living organisms are affected by magnetic and electric fields. Even the simplest life forms make use of electric and magnetic field effects, illustrated in the process of signal transduction through the gated transport of sodium, potassium, calcium, and chloride ions in neurons. An important aspect of magnetic fields is that they permeate all body tissues without interference. Various cell structures, including mitochondria, are stimulated by magnetic fields and relatively small magnetic energies are required to affect chemical reactions in cells. These effects are widespread and include increases in intracellular calcium through changes in the calcium channel, changes in the sodium-potassium pump, increases in RNA/DNA production, increased conversion of ATP to ADP, and stimulation of cyclic AMP. Additionally, free radical production can be significantly decreased by magnetic fields at magnetic field strengths of as little as 10-100 gauss. There is evidence that magnetic fields decrease vascular resistance, thus increasing tissue oxygen perfusion. This effect reduces swelling and decreases clotting and platelet adhesiveness. Human and animal studies have shown decreased nerve cell firing after exposure to magnetic fields, which may effect pain perception. Magnets produce very rapid specific and direct actions on acupuncture points and meridians.

The MVT Relief has been found useful in treating the following disabilities: allergies, chronic arthritis, dental pain, diabetic neuropathy, fibromyalgia, gastrointestinal discomfort, migraine headaches, muscle & tendon injuries, and neck and back pain. To learn more about this device, visit www.mvtrelief.com.

TENNANT BIOMODULATOR® *PLUS*

The precursor device to the Biomodulator, known as the SCENAR, was originally developed by a team of over 40 Russian scientists and doctors. The device was created for their cosmonauts who make long-duration space flights. The Russian therapy, known as Cybernetic Biofeedback therapy, was developed as a means for promoting the body's own healing process. Although the device has been widely used in Russian hospitals since the early 1980s, it remained a military secret until *perestroika*. At that time, the inventors were issued a patent for the device, and the Russians thereafter began to make the technology available to the West.

In early 2005, Jerry Tennant, M.D. introduced the long-awaited replacement of the original Russian SCENAR device. The Tennant Biomodulator®

PLUS is a device with advanced circuitry, frequency set, and a digital circuit board. It is the next generation of SCENAR technology. After years of working with similar devices, Dr. Tennant was able to create an entirely new set of therapy frequencies unlike any previously available. These new treatment modes allow the practitioner to operate the device more efficiently and effectively.

Every cell and every organ in the body is controlled by and communicates with other cells and organs via electrical signals. The skin, the brain and the nervous system are closely related since they all are derived from the same embryonic origin. The Biomodulator sends low energy electrical signals to the brain by way of the nervous system—including the C-fibers—to stimulate the brain into activating the body's own self-healing resources. A series of signals is sent through the skin and the feedback response is measured. Each signal is only sent out when a change in response to the previous signal is recorded in the electrical properties of the skin.

Visible responses to the device include reddening of the skin, numbness, stickiness (the device will have the feeling of being magnetically dragged), a change in the numerical readout, and an increase in the electronic chattering of the device. People treated with the device usually report a pleasant, relaxed feeling of well being—and usually report they experience an immediate reduction in pain and feel "energized" after a therapy session. Patients with various types of pain have reported remarkable pain reduction using the device.

The Tennant Biomodulator® *PLUS* is a biofeedback-controlled electrostimulator. It's regulated by the U.S. Food and Drug Administration under 21 CFR 882.5890: transcutaneous electrical nerve stimulator for pain relief, Product Code GZJ, Class II medical device. The device is best used for symptomatic relief and management of chronic, intractable pain, and adjunctive treatment in the management of post-surgical and post-traumatic pain. The FDA requires the Biomodulator to be used by or upon the recommendation of a licensed health practitioner, and its use requires a written prescription.

The Biomodulator offers an effective and non-invasive, drug-free alternative, integrative or adjunctive medical treatment for pain relief. Treatment is painless and is conducted by placing the device directly on the skin or by using accessory electrodes that are available for purchase. The Biomodulator is not intended for use with persons using a pace maker or other electronic implants. For more information on the Tennant Biomodulator® *PLUS*, visit www.senergy.us/tennantbiomod.htm, or contact the Senergy Medial Group at (972)580-0545.

TRAUMEEL®

Used as a natural pain-reliever and anti-inflammatory in European hospitals and private clinics for the past 30 years, Traumeel is a homeopathic product made from a combination of 12 botanical and two natural mineral ingredients. Available as either a sublingual tablet, oral liquid, or topical ointment, the product is an anti-inflammatory and analgesic which is effective in treating acute trauma, arthritis, and repetitive use injuries. It quickly relieves pain and speeds up healing in instances of nerve pain, physical trauma, pulled muscles, post-surgical pain, sprains and strains, swelling, and wound healing.

Ingredients: 50 grams of ointment contain: 0.75 grams each of *Arnica montana* 3X, *Calendula officinalis* 1X, *Hamamelis virginiana* 1X; 0.50 grams each of *Aconitum napellus* 3X, *Belladonna* 3X; 0.25 grams each of *Bellis perennis* 1X, *Chamomilla* 1X, *Echinacea angustifolia* 1X, *Echinacea purpurea* 1X; *Millefolium* 1X 0.15 gram; *Hepar sulphuris calcareum* 8X 0.125 gram; *Mercurius solubilis* 8X 0.06 gram; *Symphytum officinale* 4X 0.05 gram and *Hypericum perforatum* 6X 0.045 gram in a hydrophilic base. Traumeel can be purchased in health food stores or online.

URINE

An effective remedy for pain control is only as far away as...your bladder. Many cultures around the world have recognized the effectiveness of the topical application of fresh urine on painful areas of the body, including arthritic joints. This method of pain control is a Russian folk remedy for treating arthritis, a Bedouin nomad technique for treating burns, and a Carribean islander's remedy for jellyfish stings.[1] The scientific rational behind the treatment's efficacy is that urine supplies nitrogen-rich ammonium which helps restore the electrical balance of the affected cells, as discussed in the section on Penetran+Plus above. You don't have to go to the internet to obtain this product.

PART FOUR:
GENERAL TREATMENT METHODS

ACUPUNCTURE

Acupuncture is one component in the system of medicine called Traditional Chinese Medicine (TCM). In addition to acupuncture, TCM incorporates the use of herbs, diet and massage. The origin of acupuncture can be traced back at least 3,000 years to the Shang Dynasty, where hieroglyphs showed the use of acupuncture needles—although the needles were much different than those in use today. The true origin of the technique is based in Taoist tradition dating back over 8,000 years, which predates recorded history.

TCM and Western medicine view the human body quite differently. According to TCM, the body has 12 major channels (meridians) of flowing energy. The energy, which can't be measured or perceived by the present techniques of Western medicine, is called *chi* (Chee) or *qi* (Key). Chi, according to this tradition, is the life force of existence. Along these 12 channels lie 365 specifically-mapped acupuncture points which lie close to the surface of the skin. In addition to these points, there are over 1,000 additional points located on the ear, hand and scalp.

TCM first diagnoses the patient's ailment in a much different manner than is done in Western medicine. Observations of the tongue, physical monitoring of the pulse in several locations of the body, and a patient interview are the principal means of diagnosis. The diagnosis attempts to evaluate patterns of deficiency or excess which may lead to disease, as well as the state of health of the body's internal organs and energy channels. Disruptions or blockages in the chi, it is believed, are responsible for illness and disease.

Following the diagnosis, and in accordance with its outcome, a series of very thin stainless steel needles are inserted along the energy meridians in order to promote the flow of chi and restore balance to the body. Following insertion, the needles can be manipulated in various ways to assist the flow of chi.

Acupuncture uses several other techniques in addition to needles. *Cupping*, the use of suction cups, draws heat from the body. *Guasha* describes the use of spoons to apply friction to the skin. Burning mugwort is used to heat the needles in a technique called *moxibustion*. *Tuina* is the technique of Chinese massage.

Electroacupuncture uses an external source of small microvoltages of electricity which is attached to the acupuncture needles. This creates an electrical potential across two or more acupuncture points. There are now small, self-contained electroacupuncture units available which are used to stimulate the acupoints. The electrical current is so small that the patient hardly notices the application of these small microcurrents to the skin.

When first introduced to the West within the last 50 years, Western physicians laughed at the techniques of acupuncture. Now, following decades of experimental research in the U.S., Europe, and other Western countries—as well as many hundreds of research papers published in prestigious Western journals—many previously-biased doctors are changing their opinions of the technique.

Acupuncture has been found to be a most efficacious treatment for a host of ailments and diseases including addiction, allergies, angina, anxiety, asthma, depression, dysmenorrhea, erectile dysfunction, fibromyalgia, headaches (including migraines), high blood pressure, infertility (male and female), menopausal symptoms, osteoarthritis, psoriasis, shingles, stroke rehabilitation, tinnitus (ringing in the ears), and urinary tract infections. Many types of pain seem to be amenable to acupuncture treatment in addition to the above-named, including dental, low back, myofacial and post operative. This may be due at least in part to the demonstrated release of opiod peptides that accompanies the administration of the technique.[1]

To learn more about acupuncture, do a key word search for "acupuncture." To find more information about acupuncture treatment for a specific ailment, e.g., headaches, do a key word search for "acupuncture headaches."

BOWEN THERAPY

The inventor and developer of this technique was the Australian osteopath Tom Bowen (1903-1982). Bowen referred to his work as "soft tissue therapy," and it later took on the name of its originator. His philosophy was that the body is a self-regulating bioenergetic and biomechanical entity that tends toward self regulation. As long as the proper neurological and neuromuscular context exists, the body has the innate ability to self regulate and return to balance. Neuromuscular imbalances can develop throughout the body, according to Bowen, causing the manifestation of illness. If these imbalances could be resolved, the body would once again regulate itself.

Bowen was an astute observer of his patients' illnesses. He came to realize that when the body is stimulated in a certain specific way, its innate intelligence begins the process of normalizing the neuromuscular imbalances. Part of the brilliance of his contribution to the healing arts is his development of the system of techniques that allow the body to automatically and systemically reintegrate via stimulation of the central, peripheral and autonomic nervous systems. The result is the removal of pain and imbalanced physiological conditions that manifest as a host of ailments. As the techniques are applied, there is an orchestrated response involving alpha and gamma motor neurons, spinal reflex arcs, the motor cortex of the cerebrum, the cerebellum and the basal ganglia.

Depending on the extent of the imbalance, treatment takes from one to several 30-45 minute sessions to achieve a desirable and long-lasting result. The sessions are very gentle and non-invasive, with no forceful manipulation. The treatment consists of a sequence of specialized "moves," as they are called, which are directed in a specific and systematic manner. The moves are a cross-fiber gentle manipulation of muscles, tendons, ligaments and nerves, using varying pressures, spaced by resting periods that allow the body to reintegrate.

Treatments can be done either through the patients clothing, or directly on the skin. This therapy allows the body an opportunity to comprehensively reorganize itself by the activation of various neural reflexes. Despite its simple appearance, practitioners of Bowen Therapy continue to report its amazing results in treating a multiplicity of ailments.

The following disorders generally respond favorably to Bowen therapy:

Angina, asthma, attention deficit disorder (ADD), autism, back pain, Bell's palsy, bursitis, chronic fatigue syndrome, colitis, constipation, deafness, depression, digestive disorders, dyslexia, dysmenorrhea, fibromyalgia, gallbladder pain, headaches (including migraines), herniated disks, infertility, liver pain, Mennier's disease, multiple sclerosis, pain (of many types), Parkinson's disease, prostate, sciatica, scoliosis, seizures, shin splints, sinusitis, tennis elbow, TMJ, urinary disorders, vision problems, and others.[1]

To learn more about Bowen Therapy, visit www.bowenworkacademyusa.com or www.bowtech.com. To locate a practitioner in your location, call the United States Bowen Registry at (866)862-6936.

Throughout his long career, Tom Bowen shared the intricacies of his techniques with only five other people. After he died in 1982, various offshoots of his system came into being as the result of these other practitioners taking Bowen's message to a larger audience. One of the variations is called Neurostructural Therapy (NST). A major proponent of NST is Joseph Mercola, D.O., a well-known osteopathic physician who has a strong internet presence. Dr. Mercola describes this therapy as "the most consistent form of a miracle treatment that I have ever learned." To learn more about NST, visit Dr. Mercola's web sites: www. mercola.com/nst/explain.htm, and www.mercola .com/nst/therapist.htm. From these sites you can locate a practitioner in your area.

DEL-IMMUNE V®[1]

John Sichel, R.Ph., P.D., is a retired pharmacist with 50 years experience in the world of pharmaceuticals and medications of all sorts. Several years ago, when his daughter became ill with an influenza virus, Sichel seized the moment to evaluate some samples he had on hand of a unique immune-boosting product manufactured in Russia. Upon trying the product, he was pleased to find the results exceeded his expectations. Not only did the product work, it worked spectacularly. In just eight hours, his daughter was free of all symptom of the flu virus.

Based on this success, Sichel's daughter continued taking the product with the hope of defeating her hepatitis C infection, which had increasingly worsened to a viral load of 200,000+, compared to the normal value of "0" for a healthy person. Because the product had worked so spectacularly in combating influenza—and since hepatitis is caused by a viral infection as is the flu—they hoped the Russian product would once again rise to the occasion. They were not disappointed. True to form, within several months of taking the product, all symptoms of hepatitis had vanished, and Sichel's daughter's viral load normalized to "0" where it has remained for over five years.

Thus began the medical adventure that brought John Sichel from the ranks of the retired to being the president and owner of his own company—which now retains the exclusive world-wide manufacturing and marketing rights to this marvelously-effective immune enhancing product developed in the Soviet Union decades previously. The impetus behind the initial development of this product, now called Del-Immune V® (and previously Preparate and Extrabiolat), is a fascinating story in its own right.

So impressed was Sichel with the performance of the product, that he traveled to Russia to investigate it further. During informal discussions with key Russian officials, Sichel was told that during the Cold War in the early 1980s, the Soviet government realized the need for a safe, inexpensive, easy-to-use, and effective antidote for biological warfare weapons which might possibly be used against their troops. He was told of the team of esteemed M.D.s and Ph.D.s that studied the problem with the hope of developing a solution to defend against bioweapons—including anthrax and smallpox. The classified research was performed at the State Scientific Center Research Institute of Highly Pure Biopreparations—the top Soviet bioweapons research and manufacturing facility.

During the ensuing years of research, the Soviet scientists evaluated many potential approaches to solving the problem, including the use of vaccinations and antibiotics. None of the normal, logical approaches seemed to fulfill their requirements, as antibiotics were too expensive and also ineffective against certain pathogens such as viruses, and vaccines would become ineffective upon mutation of the pathogenic strain. The scientists decided to look "outside the box" for a solution. They reasoned that the immune system itself held the greatest hope of defeating such a broad array of challenges, but *only* if it was functioning optimally. In the end, the research led to the discovery of a "probiotic" preparation that would boost immunity so powerfully as to provide a potent and practical means of protection against 1) an array of biological warfare agents, 2) the radiation sickness that occurs in the aftermath of a nuclear event, and 3) a diversity of ailments and diseases—although interestingly, during the development phase, civilian use was not a consideration.

On April 25, 1986, the world's worst nuclear disaster occurred at a nuclear facility in Chernobyl, in the former Soviet Union, currently Ukraine. Although only several dozen plant workers died in the explosion, radioactive fallout became a serious problem. During the years following the accident, Russian medical authorities noticed a substantial increase in the incidence of various forms of cancer in those who lived in the path of the fallout—an occurrence which came to be known as "the Chernobyl effect." This provided an opportunity to test Del-Immune on cancer patients. At the State Research Institute for Transfusiology and Hematology (The State Cancer Hospital) in St. Petersburg,

Russia, the product was and currently is used to treat cancers of many types, and has been shown to greatly benefit patients with depressed immune systems resulting from chemotherapy and radiation treatments. Following supplementation, chemo and radiation patients often experience a reduction or cessation of the side-effects that so typically accompany these procedures. As a logical offshoot, the use of Del-Immune could have important health ramifications in current combat and non-combat environments where depleted uranium (DU) munitions cause radiation sickness in both soldiers, local citizens, and others as the DU is carried to distant locations on the wind—often as components of giant dust clouds.

The product itself is manufactured from a unique strain of the lactobacillus bacterium, one of the many bacteria which are naturally occurring in the intestines, nose, mouth and throat. While lactobacillus is present in milk, cheese and yogurt as well, the strain used by the researchers was *Lactobacillus delbrueckii* ssp. *bulgaricus* (which was later more accurately identified by American researchers as *Lactobacillus rhamnosus*), an unusual strain that would prove to have powerful immune-boosting capabilities. The Russians discovered that by rupturing (lysing/fractionating) the bacteria's cell walls, their contents become available to help stimulate and produce important weapons used by the immune system, the body's ultimate arbiter of good health. Without this physical breaking of the bacteria's cell wall—creating immune-potentiating "cell wall fragments"—these key ingredients remain locked within the cell, totally unnoticed by the immune system, and therefore unavailable for its use.

The idea of fractionating the bacteria's cell walls came from research conducted in Bulgaria during the mid-1970s. However, it is the lysing of this special strain of *Lactobacillus rhamnosus* (D-V strain), and not other bacteria or other strains of lactobacillus such as acidophilus or casei, that provides the dramatic immune-enhancing capabilities. During the research phase, over 600 strains of lactobacillus were evaluated before determining the rhamnosus strain to be the most potent. Originally taken from a sample of unpasturized milk from a farm near St. Petersburg, Russia, there are unique properties of this strain that enable it to provide such dramatic immune-boosting capabilities.

When the cell walls of the bacteria are broken, certain proteins, peptides, complex sugars, organic acids, balanced microelements, activated nutritional fibers, vitamins of bacterial origin (including B_1, B_2, C and E), and other cell constituents activate switches in the immune system. As part of this immune activation process, the production of interleukins is also stimulated, helping to protect the tissues of the nose, throat, lungs, and kidneys (interleukin I) and reducing inflammation (interleukin VI). This in turn activates and stimulates the immune system's T-cells, B-cells, NK (natural killer) cells, and phagocytes, as well as other components and processes which remain activated for about 36 hours. It's also important to note that immunity is activated only on an "on-demand" basis, thereby not exacerbating an overactive immune system that may result from a condition such as autoimmunity.

Most of the original research on Del-Immune was conducted in the former Soviet Union during the Cold War, and was strictly classified. Much of the work was compartmentalized, and researchers were kept informed of various aspects of the project only on a need-to-know basis. For example, those scientists working on product development weren't always informed of the results of the animal and human testing. Although some of the research was eventually published in the open literature, translating it into other languages has remained a problem.

We do know, however, that the product was developed as the primary means of combating biological warfare agents—including anthrax, smallpox, botulism, plague, tularemia (Rabbit fever), and typhus—as well as fighting the symptoms that accompany exposure to ionizing radiation which follow a nuclear event. Scientists who worked in product development have stated that, with reference to the above-named biowarfare agents, mortality of the untreated experimantal animals was 30 times higher than those treated with Del-Immune. The only caveat to these results is that Western scientists have not yet attempted to replicate this research.

Del-Immune can be used prophylactically, to elevate immunity in advance of a pathogenic infection; interventionally, in response to pathogenic infection; and adjunctively, post-exposure, along with antibiotics or other medications. Del-Immune has the following pharmacological actions, as determined by the Russian researchers and translated from their scientific literature:

- Stimulates humoral and cell immunity
- Stimulates non-specific resistance factors
- Exhibits adjuvant action
- Augments blood-making processes
- Performs cancer-protective action
- Stimulates protective mechanisms against infective bacterial and viral agents
- Shows anti-allergenic action
- Increases cholesterol dissociation, and decreases cholesterol levels in blood serum
- Prevents dysbacteriosis development during antibiotic and chemotherapy
- Forms a natural shield against growth of pathogenic microflora
- Enhances reproduction of normal microflora
- Stimulates mucous membrane regeneration in the stomach and intestine
- Stimulates protein metabolism
- Normalizes enteric pH
- Stimulates pancreas secretatory activity
- Increases motor-evacuative function of intestine
- Diminishes risk of osteoporosis development by supporting calcium metabolism
- Strengthens detoxification function of liver
- Prevents synthesis of carcinogenic substances by pathogenic bacteria

Del-Immune is a powerful anti-infective agent by means of providing immediate immune system support. As such, it has been shown effective in the treatment of:

- ❖ Allergies
- ❖ Cancer
- ❖ *Candida albicans* and athlete's foot
- ❖ Chronic inflammation
- ❖ Colds and cough
- ❖ Dermatitis
- ❖ Fatigue
- ❖ Gastro-intestinal upset
- ❖ General immune suppression
- ❖ Hepatitis and other liver disorders
- ❖ Hospital-acquired infection
- ❖ Non-healing bone fractures
- ❖ Radiation sickness
- ❖ Respiratory infections including influenza, bronchitis, tuberculosis, and pneumonia
- ❖ Surgical (post-operative) complications resulting from infection

The current Del-Immune V formulation has been shown to be some 10-30 times more potent than the original Russian product. It is manufactured in the U.S. by a freeze-drying process, followed by encapsulation of the powdered product. Each vegetarian capsule contains 25 mg of (lysed cell wall) *Lactobacillus rhamnosus* powder (approximately two billion cell wall fragments per capsule), and is available in 30 and 100 count bottles.

The recommended preventive/maintenance dosage is from one to three capsules daily, or as directed by your healthcare professional. The treatment dosage is two capsules two to three times daily, beginning at the first sign of infection. Immune system enhancement begins quickly, and peaks approximately six to eight hours following administration. Dosages as high as 12 capsules per day have been shown safe, with virtually no accompanying side-effects. Because the product contains no live bacteria, refrigeration is unnecessary. Lactose-intolerant persons should not experience side-effects, as the special lactobacillus strain is not cultured in milk. Del-Immune is also safe for use with pets. To learn more about Del-Immune V and its many dramatic product testimonials, visit www.delimmune.com. To order, call (888)IMMUNE5 (466-8635), or visit the Del-Immune website.

Several years ago, American television's *20/20* produced a documentary on this wonder product. However, the show was "scrubbed" before production was completed, and the segment never aired. In an effort to gain notoriety for his product, John Sichel has himself contacted members of the U.S. military, U.S. Senators and Representatives, and other politicians—to no avail. Is this a case of, "We're not interested because it's NIH?" (Not Invented Here) Or, perhaps the government representatives are holding out for a fix by the pharmaceutical firms in the form of very lucrative vaccination contracts—one of the approaches which the Russians rejected outright? Whatever the case, you and your loved ones now have access to this potent immune system booster—a product that could literally save your life.

ELECTROMAGNETIC THERAPY

See Magnetic-Field Therapy under **Cancer**; 3.0 Tesla MRI Spectroscopy under **Cancer** and **Prostate**; The Rebuilder® under **Diabetes**; Blood Electrification and Magnetic Pulsing under **Herpes**; Electromagnetic Therapy under **Multiple Sclerosis**; **Electricity, Farabloc,® Frequency Specific Microcurrents, Light, Magnets, Tennant Biomodulator® PLUS, The MVT Relief®** under **Pain Relievers**; and **Magnetic Molecular Energizer** under **General Treatment Methods**. To view a multiplicity of electromagnetic therapy devices, visit www.braintuner.com.

EXERCISE WITH OXYGEN THERAPY (EWOT)

About 20% of the air we breathe is oxygen, which provides much of the body's biological energy. Oxygen is transported from the lungs/heart to the tissues of the body via red blood cells. Specifically, the iron-containing pigment *hemoglobin* present within red blood cells carries oxygen throughout the body via the blood.

At sea level on Earth, the atmospheric pressure is roughly 15 pounds per square inch (psi). This is known as "one atmosphere" of pressure (one atmosphere absolute, or 1ATA). In healthy individuals, hemoglobin saturates with oxygen to the level of about 97% at sea level elevation. As the blood travels away from the heart through the arteries, smaller capillary vessels supply the oxygen that nourishes the body's trillions of cells.

Beyond the membranes of the capillaries through which the oxygen diffuses, the cells are nourished by oxygen which is dissolved within the watery environments of the body such as blood plasma—the watery liquid in which the red and white blood cells are suspended. Because the solubility of oxygen—i.e., the ability of oxygen to dissolve—is dependent upon the pressure which surrounds it, a lower-than-optimal arterial pressure will not adequately provide all of the cellular oxygen requirements. In youth, the pressure of oxygen in the arteries closely matches the pressure in the lungs. This is the optimal pressure necessary to provide all of the cells with life-giving oxygen, which maintains them at an optimal level of vitality.

As a person ages, the pressure driving the oxygen drops significantly. The volume of oxygen within the blood does not change unless there is a medical condition that affects the oxygen-absorbing capacity of hemoglobin. It is still maintained at the level of about 97% saturation. However, due to the reduction of pressure and the reduced efficiency of the capillary membranes to pass oxygen and other nutrients as a result of hormonal imbalances, free radical pathology, and other degrading factors that accompany aging, optimal cellular oxygenation does not occur. Consequently, if a person has an arterial blood-oxygen saturation level of 97%, this is no guarantee the cells furthest from the heart are receiving an adequate/optimal supply of oxygen. The key factor is how much oxygen is being *transferred* from the blood to the cells—*not* how much oxygen is *contained* within the blood.

Because every cell in the body requires an adequate level of oxygenation, the transfer of oxygen from the capillaries to the cells critically affects our level of health and well-being in every aspect. This process is perhaps the most important factor in whether a person lives a healthy life, or one plagued with illness and disease. Especially in aging individuals or those with disease, injury, or microbial contamination, by increasing oxygenation of the cells to their previously youthful levels, significant health and anti-aging benefits are gained.

Exercise With Oxygen Therapy (EWOT), also called Multi-Step Therapy, involves breathing pure oxygen while exercising. By practicing EWOT, additional oxygen is absorbed not by the red blood cells—which are already at their maximum absorption capacity of about 97%—but by the body's watery components including the blood plasma and tissue fluids. This allows additional oxygen to be absorbed by the cells and deep tissues.

The EWOT process restores to proper functioning the oxygen transfer mechanism that becomes damaged with age. Capillary endothelial cells—which over time have become swollen with salt and water due to low oxygen pressure—become rejuvenated, normalized, and regain their thin, flattened shape which allows increased passage of oxygen and other nutrients contained within the blood. The pressure driving the oxygen is also raised to its previously youthful level which makes available additional oxygen. Consequently, oxygenation of the cells is restored to youthful levels, the aging process reverses, the body begins to repair itself cell-by-cell—and the benefits last for years.

There are two principal variations of the basic EWOT technique—the long form and the short (so-called "quick") form. In both variations, a drug-nutrient combination which assists in oxygen uptake and utilization is taken 30 minutes before the EWOT session begins. The combination consists of 30 mg of thiamin (vitamin B$_1$), 100 mg of magnesium orotate, and 75 mg of the prescription drug Dipyridamol (Persatine®). While exercising, oxygen is delivered via an oxygen mask.

When practicing the long form, one exercises two hours each day over a course of 18 days while breathing oxygen at the level of 4-6 liters per minute. Every 20 minutes, the individual exerts a maximal but comfortable level of effort, thereby enhancing cardiac output and oxygen delivery to the cells. In the quick form, the individual performs aerobic exercises at a moderate level for 15 minutes while breathing 10 liters of pure oxygen per minute. A combination of the two forms is also practiced. Oxygen is supplied either from a bottled oxygen source, which requires a prescription, or from an oxygen concentrator, a device which concentrates oxygen from the room atmosphere.

In addition to the above-described benefits, EWOT is useful in treating a diversity of specific medical conditions including amyotrophic lateral sclerosis; autism; cancer; dementia; infection; ocular conditions such as cataracts; respiratory conditions such as emphysema; and a host of additional ailments. Although EWOT has been practiced in Germany for decades, it is relatively unknown to the rest of the medical world. Of all the medical techniques useful in addressing a multiplicity of diseases and medical conditions, EWOT is at the top of the list. To learn more, read Dr. William C. Douglass' book *Stop Aging or Slow the Process: Exercise with Oxygen Therapy (EWOT) Can Help*. To locate an EWOT practitioner in your area, call the American College for Advancement in Medicine at (800)532-3688 or visit www.acam.com.

HYPERBARIC OXYGEN THERAPY (HBOT)

Hyperbaric oxygen therapy delivers oxygen to the body within an enclosed chamber at pressures greater than occur at sea level. Two basic types of chambers are used. Mild hyperbaric uses a pressure of about 1.3 atmospheres within a thin-walled chamber, while high-pressure hyperbaric uses pressures in the range of 2-3 atmospheres within a metal chamber. Both types of units have shown significant beneficial results for a diversity of medical conditions.

Because the solubility of oxygen is largely dependent upon the pressure which surrounds it, as described in the preceding section on EWOT, under the increased pressure of hyperbaric oxygenation, oxygen easily dissolves in the watery environments of the body including blood plasma, tissue fluids, and synovial and cerebral fluids. Irrespective of the circulatory system, hyperbaric oxygenation super saturates the body's cells. Therefore, even if the oxygen supply is cut off from a body part or area due to blood vessel damage as the result of injuries including physical trauma such as a sports or automobile injury where brain or spinal damage is involved—or any other damage such as crush wounds, burns or the like—hyperbaric oxygenation is able to continue to supply the damaged area(s) with life-giving oxygen. HBO can increase the oxygen tissue levels at least 12 times that of normal sea level oxygenation.[1]

Currently, there are only 15 FDA-approved uses for HBOT, including decompression sickness ("the bends"); osteomyelitis (bone infection); and carbon monoxide poisoning. However, many additional conditions known as "off-label" uses are also effectively treated. Because oxygen is so vital to the body, virtually every bodily activity is increased in efficiency by increasing oxygenation. HBOT is effective in treating a long list of ailments including ALS, autism, Alzheimer's, cerebral palsy, Crohn's disease, hepatitis, infection, MS, postoperative surgery, and psoriasis. It is also an effective treatment for any vascular event where circulation is compromised, and for invasion of microbes such as bacteria—including the flesh-eating variety. It is well known that most pathogens thrive in a low-oxygen environment and cannot survive under conditions of high oxygenation.

High oxygen levels cause the immune system, including the T-3 defender cells, to become supercharged.[2] These cells use oxygen to kill infective pathogens with an "oxidative burst" of weaponry. British and German HBOT practitioners have successfully treated chronic fatigue syndrome, fibromyalgia, and any ailment involving circulatory impairment such as stroke.[3] Also, HBOT improves health, fitness, stamina, endurance, and helps reverse the physiological and psychological effects of low oxygen levels caused by air and water pollution, and aging.

A 2006 study published in the *American Journal of Physiology*[4] reported that a single two-hour HBO exposure at two atmospheres of pressure doubles the number of circulating stem cells in humans, while 20 two-hour sessions increase stem cell production by 800%. This elucidates one of the principal mechanisms by which HBOT exerts such profoundly beneficial effects across a wide range of medical conditions.

To learn more about HBOT, visit www.hbo treatment.com. With a prescription, portable HBOT units are now marketed to the public. These units range in price starting at about USD $10,000. To learn more about portable units, visit www. hyperoxy.com or www.hyperbaric-oxygen-cham ber.com. To view a list of medical conditions treated by HBOT which are covered by Medicare (i.e., those conditions approved by the FDA), visit www.hbotofaz.org/conditions/index.html. To view a list of "off-label" conditions which have benefitted from HBOT, visit www.hbotreatment.com/ conditions.htm. To locate a practitioner in your area, call the American College for Advancement in Medicine at (800)532-3688.

INSULIN POTENTIATION THERAPY

As explained in the section on **Diabetes**, insulin is a hormone secreted by the *islets of Langerhans*— small clusters of cells within the pancreas of mammals. It is named after the German pathologist Paul Langerhans (1847-1888) who discovered the "islets" or "islands." The term "islands" is translated into Latin as "insula," the root derivation of the word insulin. Insulin itself was discovered in 1921 by a team of researchers at the University of Toronto, headed by an unsuccessful orthopedic surgeon named Dr. Frederick Banting. Success comes late for some. Banting and his colleague J.J.R. Macleod were awarded the Nobel Prize in Medicine/Physiology in 1923 for the discovery of insulin.[1]

In the pages that follow, Insulin Potentiation Therapy will be examined in conjunction with traditional chemotherapy agents for the treatment of cancers. It will also be evaluated as a potential treatment method for non-malignant diseases.

The Physiology of Insulin. The human body is composed of many tens of trillions of cells—the basic building blocks of our bodies. Each cell functions as a tiny biological factory contributing to the overall functioning of the body.

The food we eat provides the energy that powers our vast array of cells. What we consume as food is converted into the form of food that nourishes our cells—*glucose*, the typical form of sugar in which dietary proteins and carbohydrates are assimilated in man and animals. Glucose molecules are transported throughout the body via our "freeway to the cells," the blood supply. Insulin (a large, polypeptide molecule with a molecular weight of 5808) is secreted into the blood stream by the pancreatic beta cells in direct response to an increase in blood glucose concentration. It is one of the primary functions of insulin to maintain the proper blood-glucose level. It does this by allowing glucose to leave the blood stream and enter the cells.

On the surface (and much less so on the interior) of most all mammalian cells are *insulin receptors*—chemical groups or molecules that have an affinity (attraction) for insulin. Each cell in the body has between 100 to 100,000 insulin receptors.[2] It is rare that cells have no receptors at all. As insulin molecules circulate throughout the body via the blood stream, they are attracted and attach to the vast quantities of receptor structures largely on the surfaces of cells.

It is this attachment of the insulin molecules to the cells via the receptors that allows the glucose within the blood to pass into the cells, and thus provide cellular nourishment. In a very real way, insulin is the "gatekeeper" of the cells, as it facilitates the diffusion (transport) of glucose across the cell membranes of the body's different types of cells. In addition to the receptor-specific transfer of glucose, it is believed that insulin has a general tendency to "permeablize" the cell membranes to glucose.

[A few words about the insulin-diabetes connection: As explained in the section on **Diabetes**, in Type I diabetes the pancreas produces too little insulin to effectively regulate the blood-glucose levels. Even though there is "food" within the blood, the cells starve due to the lack of insulin which would otherwise allow the glucose to permeate the cell membranes. Type I diabetics require an external source of insulin, such as that received from daily hypodermic injections. Type II diabetes, in which the body inefficiently produces and/or utilizes insulin, is related to obesity, high cholesterol, high blood pressure, and insulin resistance—the inability of the insulin molecules to attach properly to the receptors, thus preventing or decreasing the glucose transfer into the cells. This produces an excess of sugar within the blood, a condition known as *hyper*glycemia. Low blood sugar is referred to as *hypo*glycemia.]

Traditional Chemotherapy. Chemotherapy is a scary word for most people familiar with the method. Administered either orally or by IV injection, high-dose "chemo" is the primary treatment for recurrent cancers, and metastatic cancers of the liver and lung.[3] Chemotherapeutic agents are powerful drugs designed to kill cells, which they do reasonably well. The difficulty is that because chemotherapeutic agents circulate systemically throughout the entire body, they kill cells indiscriminately—without differentiating healthy cells from diseased or unhealthy cells. Chemotherapy's unstated goal is to attempt to kill the disease before the treatment kills the patient. This represents the first strike against high-dose use of chemotherapy drugs.

Because these toxic chemicals must be administered in high doses—doses that are high enough to force the toxic chemical across the membranes of cancer cells—there is toxicity to both normal cells as well as significant side-effects relating to the chemo treatment in addition to the initial goal of killing some cancer cells. Also, cancer cells actively resist the chemo agents, further requiring large doses to breach their cell membranes.[4] For example, a common tumor-treating drug is cyclophosphamide. If 20 mg of this drug needs to be delivered to a tumor site, it would require the administration of 100 times that amount, 2,000 mg of cyclophosphamide, to achieve the desired result. A little math shows that 1,980 mg of the toxic drug is free to poison other cells in virtually any location where it may circulate.[5] Even though the frequency of administration of high-dose chemotherapy is low, e.g., one treatment every three to four weeks, the dose is so massive that the damage is difficult to avoid. Strike two.

Many chemotherapeutic agents are designed to aggressively attack cells that are in a rapid state of growth, as are many cancer cells. The difficulty is that there are other, healthy cell systems within the body which grow rapidly as well, including cells of the gastrointestinal tract such as the mouth and throat, hair follicles, and bone marrow cells.[6] Knowing this, it is understandable why many recipients of chemotherapy experience sores of the mouth and throat; nausea and vomiting; hair loss; weight loss; loss of appetite; general immune suppression, as well as a host of other symptoms. Strike three, you're out—sometimes literally!

After all is said and done about traditional, high-dose chemotherapy for use with many cancers, including recurring and metastatic cancers, the results are abysmal. Take, for example, a 1993 study conducted by the Clinical Oncology Unit at Guy's Hospital in London. In this study, 758 patients were treated for recurrent or metastatic breast cancer. The median time to the progression of the disease was 3.7 months. The median survivability was 7.9 months. Death was the ultimate result for over 99% of the women.[7] (The lack of success of high-dose chemotherapy is discussed in more detail in the section on **Cancer,** under Chemotherapy.

Recent research on a technique called "low dose" chemotherapy is a modification of the high-dose method discussed above. According to this new method, both Canadian and U.S. researchers have found that, in animal studies, smaller but more frequent doses of chemotherapy drugs are able to eradicate tumors permanently.[8] Two of the top researchers in this area of exploration are Dr. Robert Kerbel of the University of Toronto, and Dr. Judah Folkman of Harvard. They believe the low-dose, higher-frequency technique does not directly target tumor cells, but rather the blood vessels that nourish them.[9] Human clinical trials are currently ongoing, and the results are encouraging. Patients are reporting few if any side- effects—no hair loss, bone marrow loss, nausea or vomiting.

Researchers have theorized that the typical three week interval between high-dose chemotherapy treatments allows time for the tumor-nourishing blood vessels to (re-) grow, whereas the low-dose technique given more frequently prevents this from occurring. A further interesting observation about the low-dose technique (using the agents adriamycin, methotrexate, arabinoside and cytosine) is that some researchers believe this method may stimulate the immune system to produce an array of "defensive" immune system chemicals such as interferons, interlukins, and tumor necrosis factor.[10]

Insulin Meets Chemotherapy. In the same way insulin makes cell membranes permeable, allowing the transmembrane transport of glucose into the cells, *insulin also opens the door for the passage of other substances into the cells as well*, including chemotherapy agents. The first person to make this observation was Donato Peréz García, Sr., M.D. (1896-1971), a surgeon lieutenant in the Mexican military. The year was 1926, only five years after Banting's discovery of insulin. García's discovery seems to be yet another case of the right person being in the right place at the right time. A serendipitous event—a confluence of optimizing circumstances, if you will. Dr. García had himself suffered for years from a chronic and unresolvable gastrointestinal condition, including malnutrition. Upon reading about the use of insulin for the treatment of non-diabetic malnutrition, he effectively treated himself. After a short time he was symptom free and regained the weight he had lost.

Theorizing about insulin's mechanisms of action which brought about his seemingly-miraculous recovery, Dr. García reasoned the insulin had helped his body assimilate food. Stated another way, the insulin had assisted the glucose within the blood to enter into and thereby nourish his cells. To Dr. García, it was logical to assume that insulin may assist other substances, such as medications, to enter the cells. Thus sprouted the seed of discovery which has led to the therapeutic technique called *Insulin Potentiation Therapy* (IPT; also called Insulin Potentiation Therapy Low Dose) (IPTLD)—"potentiation" meaning to increase the effectiveness of.

Although the foundation for Insulin Potentiation Therapy was laid by the senior Dr. García, IPT has been pioneered by two subsequent generations of García physicians: Dr. García Sr.'s son, Dr. Donato Peréz García y Bellón (referred to as Donato II), and then García y Bellón's son, Dr. Donato Peréz García (Donato III), the surviving García currently practicing in Tijuana, Mexico.

The combined efforts of three generations of the García family of physicians represent nearly eighty years of experience in treating a multiplicity of illnesses with IPT, including many types of cancers. Over the years, the Garcías have made great efforts to interest the general medical community in their technique, with little success as we shall see. Currently IPT is experiencing a mini-renaissance with over 300 physicians worldwide either practicing or having been trained in the technique.

Insulin Potentiation Therapy: How It Works. Insulin Potentiation Therapy represents a new rationale in the approach to treating cancer that does not involve new chemotherapy drugs. Rather, the therapy uses insulin as a *potentiator* to increase the pharmacological effects of traditional chemotherapeutic agents by working as a "biological response modifier" in several ways. This enables the use of greatly reduced quantities of the toxic chemo agents, thereby reducing the customary side-effects of traditional chemotherapy treatment.

Although there have been no formal clinical trials demonstrating the effectiveness of IPT in treating *any* ailment or disease, the long history of its use by a significant number of physicians has revealed a most interesting and significant body of information. The basic rationale behind the technique, for example, is immanently simple. It is well known that cancer cells are nourished almost exclusively by the uptake of glucose, as opposed to normal cells which can also burn fats. For this reason, cancer cells produce a significantly larger number of insulin receptors on their cell membranes—in search of the competitive advantage of attracting more nourishment. It has been discovered that cancer cells have as many as six to 15 times the number of insulin receptors in comparison to normal cells.[11] Because of this, they are able to uptake (digest) up to 15 times more glucose than normal cells.

After eating a meal and the blood-glucose levels are high, the pancreas secretes insulin which assists with glucose assimilation into the cells. The insulin molecules bind to the receptors on the cells, signaling the cells that "their meal has arrived." When high insulin levels in the blood are *artificially induced* during the administration of the Insulin Potentiation Therapy protocol, the cells are fooled into believing it's time to dine.

When chemotherapy drugs are given along with the insulin, significantly greater amounts of the toxic drugs are able to pass across the membranes of the cancerous cells, potentiating their toxic effects. This means that cancer cells can be more *selectively targeted* using IPT. That is, for the same amount (quantity) of chemotherapy chemical used, the cancer cells ingest much more than their fair share.

An example of this dramatic potentiating effect was reported by researchers at George Washington University, and the Laboratory of Pathophysiology at the National Cancer Institute, part of the U.S. National Institutes of Health. The researchers reported that in the presence of insulin, the killing effectiveness of the chemotherapy drug methotrexate can be increased up to 10,000 fold. According to the research, at every level of concentration of methotrexate, insulin increased its cancer-killing effectiveness. The researchers concluded the following:

> ...it is possible that the 10,000-fold increase in methotrexate cytotoxicity produced by insulin may establish not only a new way to increase the therapeutic effect of methotrexate but also the principal that metabolic modifiers should be examined as a means to increase the tumoricidal effects of chemotherapeutic agents.[12]

The toxic chemotherapy drugs enter normal cells as well, but because insulin increases the "access" of the chemo drugs so significantly, greatly reduced quantities of the drugs are required for effective treatment. Only 10-25% of the typical dosage of a chemotherapeutic agent need be given using IPT. Because the dosages can be reduced so significantly, the typical side-effects associated with traditional chemotherapy are *all but eliminated*. At times, up to three or four chemotherapy agents can be given during a single session, each agent aiming to deliver its lethal blow via a different mode of action.

In addition to the large number of insulin receptors present on the surfaces of cancer cells in comparison to normal cells, many cancer cells also have an equally increased number of receptors for Insulin-Like Growth Factors (IGFs).[13] IGFs are structural homologues (similar structure) of insulin, with IGF-1 sharing 43% of its main genetic sequence and IGF-2 sharing 41%.[14] Because these substances are so structurally similar to insulin, their receptors cross-react with each other, enabling insulin molecules to attach to IGF receptor

sites, and vice versa, thereby potentiating the therapeutic effects as the cell membranes become increasingly accessible.

Another key factor that contributes to the apparent effectiveness of Insulin Potentiation Therapy is that insulin is known to encourage cancer cells to enter a growth phase of their development.[15] Because many modern chemotherapeutic agents are specifically designed to target rapidly-growing cells, as mentioned earlier, the effect of IPT is significantly potentiated. This growth-stimulating effect is significant, as it's often the case that as much as 90% of the cells in a tumor mass are not actively growing at any given time, leaving only 10% of the cells susceptible to the chemotherapy drug.[16] By boosting the number of cells into a growth phase, more cancerous cells are able to be targeted. Also, because insulin and IGF receptors cross-react, as insulin molecules bind to IGF receptors, growth-stimulating messages are communicated to the cancer cells.[17]

Cellular structures are known to have regular phases of growth, referred to as the *cell cycle*. Cancer cells also typically follow these phases:[18]

G_0 *Phase*: Cancer cells are not actively replicating, and are therefore resistant to chemotherapy medications. Cells in this phase can function as a reserve pool of cells, reactivate, and become part of the proliferative pool even as the total number of cancer cells decreases.

G_1 *Phase*: (Growth) Cancer cells are proliferating, synthesizing RNA, enzymes, structural proteins and cell organelles. The G_1 Phase is sometimes referred to as the "first gap," or first growth period.

S Phase: (Synthesis) After sufficient quantities of RNA, enzymes and proteins are produced in G_1, cells progress to the S Phase where DNA is synthesized.

G_2 *Phase*: (Growth) After DNA synthesis concludes, RNA and protein synthesis resume.

M Phase: (Mitotic) This is the final phase of the cell cycle, during which the cell undergoes mitosis (cell division), and two offspring cells are formed.

Chemotherapy drugs are designed to be either cell-cycle-specific, or not. As the name implies, cell-cycle-specific drugs attack cancer cells at a specific phase in the cells' cycle. For example, the common chemo agent Taxol (Paclitaxel®) works between the G_0 and G_1 phases. Other common chemotherapy agents such as Platinol (Cisplatin®) and adriamycin (Doxorubicin®) function in a more general way, and are non-cell-cycle-specific. Interestingly, as is the case with many pharmaceutical drugs, many chemotherapy agents are based on plant extracts, including Aminocamptothecin,® Bleomycin,® Docetaxel,® Doxorubicin,® Mitomycin,® Paclitaxel,® Vinblastine,® Vincristine® and many others.[19]

The following are some of the more common chemotherapy drugs, denoting the phase of the cell cycle in which they function:[20]

Phase of Cell Cycle	Chemotherapy Drug	Trade Name
Go . . . G_1	Taxol	Paclitaxel®
G1	None	—
G1 . . . S Transition	Hycamtin, Camptosar	Topotecan,® CPT-11®
S	Cytosar, Cladribine	Ara-C, 2-Chlorodeoxyadenosine
S . . . G_2 Transition	Etoposide	VP-16®
G_2	Blenoxane	Bleomycin®
M	Oncovin, Taxol	Vincristine,® Paclitaxel®
Nonspecific	Platinol	Cisplatin®
Nonspecific	Adriamycin	Doxorubicin®
Nonspecific	Cytoxan	Cyclophosphamide®

Many modes of action have been proposed to explain the effectiveness of Insulin Potentiation Therapy. The following is a reasonably comprehensive list of what is known, as well as what has been proposed (theorized) to explain why IPT is often so effective:[21]

1) *Insulin Receptors.* It is known that virtually every cell in the human body has receptor structures to which insulin has an affinity. These receptor sites occur mostly on the outsides of cell membranes, but also have been found in cell nuclei. It is also known that cells have receptors for the growth factors IGF-1 and IGF-2, which cross-react with insulin receptors. That is, either molecule will cause the same basic effect(s) when attaching to either of the receptor sites. Cancer cells have from six to 15 times more insulin as well as an equally greater amount of IGF receptors in comparison to normal cells. Therefore, for a given amount of insulin—or chemotherapy drug—within the blood, diseased cells will "absorb" up to 15 times the amount of treatment agent, allowing a selective targeting of diseased cells.

2) *Cell Permeability.* It is assumed that insulin increases the permeability of cells due to an alteration of lipid (fat) synthesis, making the cells more fluid, and therefore more permeable.

3) *Tissue Permeability.* It has been observed that IPT increases the penetration of medications into various tissue structures around the body that are otherwise difficult or impossible to penetrate. These areas include the central nervous system (CNS), including the brain; solid tumors; joints; and perhaps even the eyes.

4) *Cell Growth Stimulation.* It's known that both insulin and IGFs encourage cells into a growth phase, where they can be targeted by chemotherapy agents that specifically attack rapidly-growing cells.

5) *Metabolic Changes.* Insulin may alter the metabolism of some cancer cells such that they become more susceptible to chemotherapeutic agents. The previously-cited George Washington University/NIH study (where the toxicity of methotrexate was increased by 10,000 fold) may be demonstrative of this process.

6) *Changes in Blood Chemistry.* As one of the most basic metabolic and control hormones, insulin produces profound changes in blood chemistry. The first two generations of García physicians studied these effects. They believed a major factor contributing to IPT's effectiveness could be the result of an improvement in the "biological terrain," rendering it less nurturing to disease states and more supportive of a healthy condition. These effects are long lasting, and could be permanent.

7) *Immune System Potentiation.* Insulin promotes rapid healing of infections and wounds, and reduc-

es symptoms in immune over-reactive diseases such as arthritis and allergies. It's likely the immune system is being potentiated in a number of ways, one of which is that the insulin and IGF receptors on immune cells are stimulated.

8) *Detoxification.* If cell membranes are made more permeable by insulin, toxins within the cells would likely be removed more easily. IPT's effectiveness in treating alcoholism, drug addiction and smoking lend support to insulin's ability to detoxify the cells. Liver-detoxifying drugs are often used when detoxification is the goal of therapy.

9) *Angiogenesis.* It has been shown *in vitro* (in the lab) that insulin stimulates the growth of new blood vessels. Perhaps this aids healthy tissues by bypassing blocked or injured blood vessels.

10) *The Worm Theory.* This theory was proposed by Chris Duffield, Ph.D., who since 1998 has been a Visiting Scholar with the Center for Latin American Studies at Stanford University. Dr. Duffield is the creator of the web site iptq.com, which he originated and maintains without monetary reward, solely for the purpose of educating people about this potentially life-saving treatment.

Dr. Duffield suggests that, in terms of the evolutionary process, insulin-like molecules are quite likely an ancient vestige that has accompanied us all the way to the 21st Century. Even in nematodes (a small worm), Duffield points out, insulin-like molecules play key roles in the basic functions of reproduction, metabolism and longevity. He believes insulin may trigger one or a series of "ancient biological mechanisms" that were crucial to the life processes/cycles of our earliest ancestors, as they may be today. These mechanisms may be initiated, Duffield suggests, through the expression of some otherwise normally-inactive gene(s).

The Effectiveness of Insulin Potentiation Therapy. Three generations of the Peréz García family of physicians, as well as numerous other highly-credentialed doctors, believe that cancer is one of the most successful applications of IPT. The worst case scenario is that it will have no positive effect— unlike the effects of typical high-dose chemotherapy where treatment is often accompanied by a diverse range of highly unpleasant symptoms.

Again, even though there have been no formal clinical trials to evaluate the effectiveness of IPT in treating cancer or any other disease or malady, these doctors' experiences have shown the technique regularly produces spectacular results in treating a wide range of cancers. If there is a chemotherapy agent known to attack cancer cells of the variety for which treatment is sought, complete remission is commonplace with IPT, depending upon the state of disease progression. If complete remission is not achieved, relief of pain and other symptoms is likely, with an improved quality of life, say the IPT doctors.

Cancers in the following areas of the body have been treated successfully using IPT:[22]

Biliary • Blood • Bone • Brain • Breast • Cervix • Colon • Esophagus • Lip • Liver • Lung • Lymph • Mouth • Neck • Nose • Ovaries • Pancreas • Prostate • Rectum • Skin • Small Intestine • Stomach • Testicles • Throat • Thyroid • Uterus • Vagina

Cancer is typically treated with one to five treatments per week for the first week or two, and then weekly. None of the physicians who have ever practiced IPT have claimed the technique to be a panacea. As with any treatment for a disease such as cancer, not everyone is a success story. Diabetic patients require special care by experienced practitioners to achieve good results. Patients whose livers and/or immune systems have been compromised by high-dose chemo (or for other reasons) do less well than those without these limitations.

Cancers for which no chemo drug treatment is available are less responsive. Although patients who are moribund (approaching death) may no longer have the physical resources necessary to recover, IPT can reduce suffering and increase the quality of life.

The third generation Dr. Peréz García who currently practices in Tijuana, Mexico, is the most experienced IPT physician living today, having begun practicing the technique with his father in 1983. Dr. García has made some general statements about IPT's effectiveness in treating various cancers:[23]

❏ For patients recently diagnosed (either by needle biopsy or direct removal of tissue) with a tumor smaller than 4 centimeters (cm), who have not previously received chemo, surgery or radiation, the response rate for a full remission is 95%, when properly administered by an experienced IPT physician.

❏ For patients recently diagnosed (either by needle biopsy or direct removal of tissue) with a tumor larger than 4 cm, who have not previously received chemo, surgery or radiation, the response rate for a full remission is 80%, when properly administered by an experienced IPT physician.

❏ For patients with recurrence/metastasis who were previously treated by chemo, surgery or radiation, the response rate for a full remission is 25%, when properly administered by an experienced IPT physician.

❏ For patients with recurrence/metastasis who were previously treated by chemo, surgery or radiation, the response rate for a partial remission is 70%, when properly administered by an experienced IPT physician.

❏ For patients with recurrence/metastasis who were previously treated by chemo, surgery or radiation, the response rate for quality of life improvement is 98%, when properly administered by an experienced IPT physician.

❏ For terminally ill patients, if no liver impairment, the response rate for quality of life improvement is 40%, when properly administered by an experienced IPT physician

❏ For patients with a brain tumor, either primary, recurrent or metastatic, the response rate is 65% for tumors smaller than 2 cm when IPT is administered as the primary treatment form.

A Typical IPT Session. The administration of Insulin Potentiation Therapy is a simple and painless procedure requiring a minimal amount of time. The subjective art to the practice of the technique lies in the *selection and dosage levels of the therapeutic medications to be given.* Over many years a compendium of information has been amassed regarding the use of various medications to treat many different illnesses, including cancers. This information is made available to doctors who receive formal training in IPT.

A typical session may use from five to 25 different medications, which are selected to cover three levels of treatment, as follows:

Primary Medications. These are the medications used to treat the primary medical condition for which the patient is being seen. Typically, these are the same medications ordinarily used to treat the condition, but in greatly reduced quantities—10-25% of the usual dosage. Multiple drugs usually can be given simultaneously with full effect or better, but with reduced chance of interaction due to the low levels administered.

Secondary Medications. Any secondary medical conditions are simultaneously treated.

Tertiary Medications. Medications that are intended to improve the general over-all health of the patient are also administered, such as immune stimulants and detoxifiers. In addition, vitamins such as C and B complex are often given.

Insulin Potentiation Therapy in General Medical Practice. As discussed, when chemotherapy drugs are given along with the insulin, significantly greater amounts of the drugs are able to pass across the membranes of the cancerous cells, potentiating the drug's toxic effects. In the same way, when *virtually any medication* is given along with insulin, the effect of that medication is significantly enhanced. This is the interesting little trick played by insulin when it is administered during a session of IPT. In the case of the chemotherapy agent methotrexate, the drug's effectiveness against certain cancer cells increased up to 10,000-fold.

When other medications are given at this time—regardless of their intended purposes or modes of action—significantly greater quantities are able to pass across the membranes of all the cells in the body, both diseased and healthy. Insulin serves as a Trojan Horse in that it allows these other molecules, including therapeutic ones, to sneak into the cells along with the expected glucose, whether it's present or not. In the case of IPT, glucose isn't present, but whatever medications your doctor prescribes could be, IF you know about Insulin Potentiation Therapy!

By taking advantage of an inherent biological mechanism to bring about a desired result, a knowledgeable physician can apply already-existing, known medications in order to treat more effectively a wide range of illnesses and diseases. If there is a known substance (e.g., a pharmaceutical drug, natural preparation, etc.) with a demonstrated effectiveness against a specific ailment, IPT is likely to increase its effectiveness significantly. Oftentimes more effective treatment is achieved using a reduced dosage, thereby reducing or eliminating harmful and/or unpleasant side effects. Sometimes IPT turns good medicines into super drugs.

The United States, if not the world, is plagued by ailments ranging from the annoying and debilitating—to the deadly. Particularly in modern times, debilitating and death-causing diseases are at an all-time high. The following prevalence statistics show how serious the problem is in the U.S.:[24]

Systemic Lupus Erythematosus: *500,000* people
AIDS: *1 million* people
Colitis and Ileitis: *2 million* people
Diabetes: *20 million* people
Arthritis: *38 million* people
Asthma or other allergies: *43 million* people
Genital Herpes: *68 million* people
Chronic Respiratory Problems: *73 million* people
Each year *1.2 million* people are diagnosed with cancer, now the number two killer in the U.S.

Insulin Potentiation practitioners believe IPT to be the cancer therapy for the new millennium. Many also think IPT may be the general medical treatment for the new millennium as well, since it's been used successfully to treat such a broad spectrum of ailments including allergies, auto-immune disorders, cancer, a host of infections, and neurological conditions.[25] Other advantages include the relatively modest cost in comparison to more traditional treatments, and the absence of both harmful and/or bothersome side-effects.

Furthermore, many of the conditions successfully treated by IPT are conditions for which traditional allopathic medicines and treatments are ineffective, such as the following. Researchers are discovering that some of these maladies may have an infection at their origin:[26]

Auto-immune Disorders • Chronic Body Pain • Central Nervous System Diseases • Multiple Sclerosis • Chronic Fatigue Syndrome

The following list includes many of the medical conditions for which IPT has been found successful:[27]

❖ Allergies—Chemicals, food, medicines, metals, respiratory, the sun
❖ Cancers—Breast, bone, cervix, intestine, liver, lung, prostate, skin, + more

❖ Circulatory—Angina, headaches, hemorrhoids, hypertension, migraine
❖ Dermatological Acne—Contact dermatitis, eczema, psoriasis, shingles
❖ Digestive—Biliary, dyskinesia, colitis, hypoglycemia, viral hepatitis
❖ Genito-Urinary—Cystitis, neoplasia of the prostate and cervix, prostatitis, pyelonephritis
❖ Infections—Bronchitis, cervicitis, herpes, viral hepatitis, osteomyelitis, + more
❖ Intoxications—Alcohol, drugs, tobacco
❖ Nervous/Neurological—Facial paralysis, hemiplegia, migraine, multiple sclerosis, sciatica, herniated disk, thoracic shingles
❖ Respiratory—Asthma, allergic bronchitis, respiratory allergies, chronic sinusitis, emphysema, vasomotor rhinitis
❖ Rheumatic/Rheumatoid—Arthritis, arthrosis, gout, polyarthritis, osteoarthritis, osteomyelitis

IPT Treatment of Auto-Immune Diseases. The human immune system is the body's first line of defense against all forms of illness. The lymphatic system, liver, spleen, thymus and bone marrow interrelate in the immune systems normal defense strategies. The tonsils, appendix and Peyer's patches (lymphoid tissues within the small intestine) are also related to immune function.

The structures and functions of the human immune system are intricate and complex. Much has been learned about the immune system—even since the discovery of AIDS—but no doubt there are a great number of other nuances that remain unknown.

A healthy immune system is able to ward off most challenges by infective microbes such as viruses, bacteria, fungi, yeast, parasites, and a host of toxic substances. However, those with a suppressed immune function such as the infirm, elderly and the very young are at higher risk.

Modern times have seen not only the rise of illness and disease, but also the rise in what has come to be known as "auto-immune diseases." The term "auto" refers to "self." In the case of auto-immune diseases, one's own body (self) is mistakenly identified by the immune system as a foreign substance ("not self"), and one's own immune system attacks mistakenly-identified, (formerly) healthy body structures.

The cause of auto-immunity is speculative, but believed by some to occur as the result of a similarity (resemblance) between foreign molecules and molecules of "self."[28] Other researchers believe the immune system is not actually attacking the self, but possibly attacking some heretofore unobserved infective agent such as *mycoplasma* or *nanobacteria*.

The following are some of the more prominent auto-immune diseases, and the areas of the body they affect:[29] IPT is often effective against many of these diseases, depending upon the degree of progression of the illness:

☞ *Addison's Disease*—Adrenal glands
☞ *Auto-immune Hemolytic Anemia*—Red blood cells
☞ *Crohn's Disease*—Intestines
☞ *Graves' Disease*—Thyroid
☞ *Insulin-dependent Diabetes Mellitus*—Pancreatic beta cells
☞ *Multiple Sclerosis CNS*—Brain and spinal cord
☞ *Myasthenia Gravis*—Nerves and muscle synapses
☞ *Pernicious Anemia*—Gastric parietal cells
☞ *Psoriasis*—Skin
☞ *Rheumatoid Arthritis*—Connective tissues
☞ *Scleroderm*—Heart, lungs, intestines, kidneys
☞ *Systemic Lupus Erythematosis*—DNA, blood platelets

Auto-immune diseases are so wide-spread within Western countries that many people suffer from their symptoms without ever knowing they have such a disease. Common symptoms include depression, dry skin, fatigue, joint pains, malaise, skin rashes, stiffness, stomach upset and weakness.[30] It's not surprising that an effective treatment for these conditions would be welcomed by the afflicted.

When an auto-immune disease is present, protein structures called *auto-antibodies* are produced by the immune system. The auto-antibodies seek out and combine with the foreign antigens that initially triggered their production. In the case of auto-immune diseases, the antigens are not foreign at all, but only mistakenly recognized by the body as such. Blood tests are currently available which are able to detect auto-immune diseases by identifying various auto-antibodies. To locate a medical prac-titioner who is knowledgeable about these blood tests, contact the American College for Advancement in Medicine, (800)532-3688, www.acam.org.

If auto-antibodies are detected, a Polymerase Chain Reaction test (PCR) can be done which will identify a microbial component to the disease if one is present. PCR tests are able to detect a wide range of infective organisms, some of which include:[31]

○ Candida albicans
○ Chlamydia pneumoniae
○ Chlamydia species
○ Chlamydia trachomatis
○ Cytomegalovirus
○ Epstein-Barr
○ Hepatitis A, B and C
○ Herpes Types 1,2 and 6
○ Lyme Disease
○ Mycoplasma fermentans
○ Mycoplasma genitalium
○ Mycoplasma hominis
○ Mycoplasma orale
○ Mycoplasma pneumoniae
○ Mycoplasma species
○ Ureaplasma urealyticum

[An interesting aside: The Polymerase Chain Reaction test had an unusual beginning, and the conditions under which it was "invented" are worth a quick review. Much to the dismay and exasperation of many conservative researchers, the handsome young surfer-scientist Kerry Mullis, Ph. D., conceived of the PCR while on...vacation. That is to say, he was taking a little trip—on LSD-25! For this he was awarded the 1993 Nobel Prize in Chemistry "for contributions to the developments of methods within DNA-based chemistry," and "for his invention of the polymerase chain reaction (PCR) method."[32]]

IPT in the Treatment of Infectious Diseases. Never before in the history of man has there been such a prevalence of diseases—infectious and otherwise. As mentioned, even many auto-immune diseases are thought to be of microbial (infectious) origin.[33] The list of diseases is growing, and effective treatments are sorely needed.

Many of the infections with which humans are plagued are difficult to treat with standard pharmaceutical medications because the organisms that cause these diseases live intra-cellularly, i.e., within the cells. The standard array of antibiotics (anti-microbials) used to treat these diseases—including anti-viral, anti-bacterial, and anti-fungal drugs—are most often unable to gain sufficient access to the cells to accumulate the amount of medication necessary to effect the desired result. That is to say, the medications can't penetrate the cells in sufficient quantities to kill the infective microbes.

IPT opens cells up to a wide range of standard but otherwise relatively ineffective, already-existing drugs. Because of this, IPT holds great hope for the future in the treatment of diseases that are currently either ineffectively treated or untreatable.

IPT practitioners are reporting improvements in conditions previously thought untreatable, and in some cases there is complete recovery in a variety of these previously untreatable and difficult-to-treat diseases. In part, this is due to insulin's ability to carry other medicinals into the cells of the central nervous system.

A primary reason that many disorders of infectious origin are untreatable or poorly treated is that the prescribed medications are not able to traverse the *blood-brain barrier*, the "biological fire-wall" that prevents or restricts most substances from entering the brain, including chemotherapy agents as well as many other compounds that would be useful in treating brain or spinal cord diseases.

The following several paragraphs are rather technical, but are presented as an explanation of the *physiological basis of the potential effectiveness* of IPT in treating diseases of the brain. Technical material is not included simply to fill pages. There are important points behind the subjects discussed, and the more that is understood about how all of the elements fit together, the more leverage you'll have in taking care of yourself, your family, and your friends. Here we go...

The blood-brain barrier consists of both anatomical structures and transport mechanisms that oversee the passage into the brain of various classes of substances. Anatomically, the blood-brain barrier is a "high-resistance tight junction" that joins 99% of the brain's capillary endothelial cells.[34] In other parts of the body such as the kidneys and intestines, capillaries are made porous by tiny openings in the capillary walls called *fenestrations*. The capillaries of the blood-brain barrier have no fenestrations, markedly restricting the free flow of substances from the blood to the brain's interstitial fluid.[35]

Once a substance penetrates into the interstitial areas of the brain, molecules have free access to brain cells. Therefore, molecules circulating within the blood—all of which are potentially suspect of being toxic—are allowed to pass the blood-brain barrier and into the brain only if they have access to one or more of a variety of transport systems located in the capillary's endothelial cells of the blood-brain barrier.

Specific transport systems within the blood-brain barrier have been identified that govern the uptake of various nutrients into the brain (e.g., the known transport substances include adenine, adenosine, arginine, choline, glutamate, lactate and phenylalanine.) The transport mechanisms for insulin are insulin, IGF-1 and IGF-2 receptors that reside along the internal bore (luminal aspect) of brain capillaries of the blood-brain barrier.[36]

This receptor-mediated transport of insulin across the blood-brain barrier explains the presence of relatively high levels of insulin within the brain itself. Insulin thereby moves from the blood to the insulin receptors within the blood-brain barrier, into the brain. And where there is insulin, there could likely be whatever molecules of therapeutic treatment that your holistic physician prescribes, IF you know about Insulin Potentiation Therapy.

[Of interest is that insulin receptors have been found on glial structures within the substance of the brain, but generally not on other brain cells. One of the most outstanding differences between a normal brain and that of Albert Einstein is that Einstein's brain had a larger-than-normal number of glial cells, which serve very important functions in the brain. Not to feel intimidated. While at Princeton University—where he had been teaching for some time—Professor Einstein is alleged to have inquired, on more than one occasion, as to the whereabouts of his own residence...]

An additional factor regarding IPT's potential as a treatment of nervous system diseases is that both insulin and its receptors are prominent throughout the entire central nervous system. Also, IGF-1 and IGF-2 receptors, with insulin cross-reacting capabilities, are widely distributed throughout the CNS as well. This has the effect of influencing developing brain cells including the regulation of brain cell maturation. It is believed that insulin influences the growth and development of the nervous system.[37]

The fact that insulin has such a powerful regenerative effect on the CNS helps to explain the many beneficial effects that IPT practitioners have experienced in treating CNS-related diseases. There is hopeful exuberance that more research will confirm the beneficial experiences reported by the IPT doctors in treating such diseases as the following:[38]

Cytomegalovirus • Epstein-Barr Virus • Herpes Virus • HIV • Lou Gehrig Disease • Lyme Disease • Multiple Sclerosis • Mycoplasma • Polio

Why Hasn't IPT Been Accepted by Mainstream Medicine? One would think that with such a promising medical treatment as Insulin Potentiation Therapy the medical world would be beating a path to its door. On the contrary, until only recently it is as if the treatment method fell into a medical black hole. Have any "mainstream" scientists taken a look at IPT and, if so, what were their conclusions? Did anybody tell the U.S. National Cancer Institute about IPT and, if so, what was their response? Have any health authorities told the citizens about IPT? Have three generations of physicians deliberately hidden the technology away so that their family could be seen as the family of "miracle makers?"

As you recall, Banting and Macleod's discovery of insulin occurred in 1921. Shortly thereafter in 1924, Dr. Donato Peréz García Sr. received his medical diploma at the age of 27. Two years later, in July of 1926, Dr. García first injected himself with insulin. In 1928, at the age of 32, he treated his first patient with IPT, at the time called Insulin Cellular Therapy.

From the time of his initial discovery of the technique in the mid-1920s, Dr. García Sr. made every attempt to publicize the information widely. He was well known within the Mexican military establishment, with aspirations of becoming the Mexican Secretary of Health. Although he didn't achieve that position due to a change in government, his retiring rank of Brigadier General is indicative of the prominence he enjoyed within Mexico's military elite.

The following is a chronology of the attempts made by Dr. Peréz García Sr. to bring Insulin Potentiation Therapy to the world:[39]

☐ 1935 Dr. García Sr. is invited by Harvard University to make a presentation on Insulin Potentiation Therapy. He is 38 years old.

☐ 1935 Mexican government sends Dr. García to San Antonio, Texas for a one year period to demonstrate IPT. At the Austin State Hospital, IPT causes rapid and complete recovery of seven patients with late-stage syphilis.

☐ 1938 Dr. García invited by U.S. Secretary of War Harry H. Woodring to demonstrate IPT at Saint Elizabeth Hospital in Washington, D.C.

☐ 1939 Dr. Alberto P. Leon, Mexican Secretary General of the Department of Health, signs a declaration acknowledging the effectiveness of IPT.

☐ 1939 U.S. Patent 2,145,869 is granted to Dr. García for treating syphilis.

☐ 1940 J. Agustin Castro, Mexican Secretary of Defense, signs an official document recognizing the effectiveness of IPT.

☐ 1941 Dr. García establishes a clinic which successfully tests IPT on the Mexican military.

☐ 1943-44 Dr. García is invited to demonstrate IPT at the U.S. Naval Hospital in San Diego, California.

☐ 1944 *Time* magazine publishes an article about Dr. García and IPT entitled "Insulin for Everything," reporting on successes in the treatment of syphilis, typhoid fever, malaria, peritonitis and rheumatic fever. García is now age 47.

☐ 1947 Dr. García makes other presentations in the United States.

☐ 1948-50 Dr. García cures ulcers using antibiotics and IPT 49 years before antibiotic treatment of ulcers became standard practice (for the treatment of the *Helicobacter pylori* bacterium, the principal infective cause of ulcers). García presents ulcer treatment before the 9th Congress of Surgeons in Mexico City.

☐ 1953 Dr. García publishes his book *Cellular Therapy (Terapia Celular)*, which is a detailed treatise of his work. García is now 56 years old.

The 1940 document signed by the Mexican Secretary of Defense referred to above was particularly complimentary to Dr. García Sr. and his newly-discovered, broad-ranged treatment called

Insulin Potentiation Therapy. Following the establishment of an experimental clinic to evaluate the effectiveness of IPT, the following statements were made part of a document signed by J. Agustin Castro, Mexico's Secretary of Defense and Juan Felipe Rico Islas, Brigadier General of the National Army:[40]

• That the results obtained...greatly exceeded expectations in each case treated, without a single accident.

• That said therapy was 100 percent effective.

• That its application proved innocuous even in many cases where accepted methods were dangerous.

• That it was applied without danger to patients of all ages.

• That it did not require special equipment or locale.

• That this therapy obtains positive permanent results in an amazingly short time.

• That from an economic standpoint there is absolutely no comparison between this therapy and those to this day accepted since its cost is insignificant.

• That this method proved not only applicable to neurosyphilis but also to many other diseases of a bacterial nature, as was proven in treating members of the family of military personnel at this clinic for different ailments.

• That because of its economy, ease of application, safety, rapidity and effectiveness, it is my opinion that this therapy should be officially adopted by all branches of the Armed Forces of the Republic, and its use extended to other Federal and State agencies. Specifically in view of the ease with which the technique is administered, for example, the operators at this hospital were often only skilled nurses.

Dr. Peréz García Sr. achieved some remarkable successes in his practice of Insulin Cellular Therapy, now called Insulin Potentiation Therapy. In 1955, Dr. García and his son Dr. Peréz García II reversed children's paralysis of polio with IPT. Other great successes are documented in *Cellular Therapy*, his *magnum opus*. Dr. Donato Peréz García Sr. died in December 1971 at the age of 75.

As Dr. Peréz García II, and then Dr. García III took up the cause in their familial predecessor's footsteps, many other attempts were made to bring IPT technology forward. Due to the limitation of space, only several will be mentioned.

❐ In 1986 Dr. Steven G. Ayre, a transplanted Canadian now practicing IPT in Burr Ridge, IL, along with Drs. García II and III publish an article in the well-respected, peer-reviewed journal *Medical Hypothesis*: "Insulin Potentiation Therapy: A New Concept for Management of Chronic Degenerative Diseases."

❐ In 1989 Drs. Ayre and Garcías II and III make a presentation to the 42nd Annual Symposium on Fundamental Cancer Research: Cellular and Molecular Targets of Cancer Therapy. Case studies are reported on the remarkable results obtained in treating breast cancer. This was at the M.D. Anderson Cancer Center at the University of Texas in Houston.

❐ In 1991 Drs. Ayre and Garcías II and III make a presentation at the Third Int'l. Congress on Neo-Adjuvant Chemotherapy in Paris, France entitled "Insulin Plus Low-Dose CMF as Neo-Adjuvant Chemo-hormonal Therapy for Breast Carcinoma."

❐ Because of the above presentation, the journal *Oncology News* featured IPT in their lead article of the July/Aug 1991 issue.

The remainder of this intriguing story must remain until another time. Suffice it to say that between the years 1991 and 1993, a flurry of interaction took place between a core of IPT physicians including Dr. Ayre and the Drs. García II and III, and the U.S. National Cancer Institute's (NCI) Cancer Therapy Evaluation Program (CTEP). After much discussion, etc., NCI made the decision to fund testing of IPT, but then they changed their minds...but then they decided to fund...but then not. And in the end, they didn't. There's much more to the story, but with space as a limiting factor enough has been said to help one understand why IPT is not a household term.

Other dialogue occurred including contacts with some hospitals and other government agencies, all the way up to the present time, seemingly all to little or no avail. There continues to be a slowly-growing group of dedicated physicians who form the core of the IPT doctors, currently numbering about 110 in 19 countries.

The upshot seems to be that many have come to listen, but few have heard the message. Why would this be so? For one reason, IPT doctors practice a little-known technique. Approved? Yes. Legal? Yes. Acknowledged? Yes. But well known, popular? It is not. There must be something to the notion that, just as average citizens grapple with issues of "political correctness," so too must physicians struggle over issues of what could be called "medical correctness," which would be something like political correctness within the medical community.

These strong influences likely result in a type of "self-policing," on both a personal mental level, professional, and social level. There is also legal policing as well. Doctors face more and more scrutiny over their specific medical practices. These pressures influence everything from the choice and quantities of drugs a doctor prescribes, to any type of medical procedure they may *or may not* perform for their patients. IPT may be more easily accepted by a doctor who is personally courageous, and imbued with a sense of vision about IPT's potentially bright future.

One small additional detail could be involved in helping keep IPT in relative obscurity. That detail has to do with how the financial story would play out if IPT were accepted into mainstream medical practice. The math looks fairly simple: More insulin would be sold, and the sales of many other types of medications would fall precipitously. Because remember, if doctors use only 10% of the typical dose of whatever type of medication they select for treatment, it necessarily follows they will use 90% less medications overall.

This would obviously benefit the patient, which should please the doctor. But to the corporations who market the pharmaceuticals, as is the case in the business world in general, more is better. In this case, more drug sales are better. "Please don't tell me about some newfangled technique that'll cut our sales by 90%. That just won't do. If granny or mom, or heaven forbid junior, contracts some life-threatening disease, we'll keep the list of IPT doctors for such emergencies. Just don't cut my pay check (or the company revenues) by 90%. Again, that just won't do." Nothing like this could be happening behind the scenes in both subtle and not-so-subtle ways, could it? Furthermore, the less

illness and disease present within society as the result of an effective super-treatment such as IPT, the less revenue for both the medical and pharmaceutical communities.

So why hasn't Insulin Potentiation Therapy been accepted into the flow of mainstream medicine? Whatever the reason(s) may be, it certainly hasn't been for lack of trying on the part of a small core group of IPT practitioners. Dr. Chris Duffield describes his experiences in trying to bring IPT to the fore, and offers a couple of explanations about what has kept IPT from enjoying greater popularity:

> In my efforts to seek interest, involvement, support, and even just acknowledgment of IPT, I have been ignored or turned down by many rich and powerful people and organizations, by millionaires and billionaires, by famous actors, by some of the biggest names in medical research, by drug companies, by some of the best known foundations. I have been sneered at in person by the head of the National Institutes of Health (NIH), and given bureaucratic redirection (or no answer at all) by administrators and their regional, national, and international health organizations. This has been a source of continuous amazement for me, for years. Again and again I have gotten excited about a new contact, only to find that yet another famous, powerful, high-level person or organization that states publicly their desire to help patients and humanity, and to advance science and medicine, will simply ignore or politely reject the IPT information...it is clear that IPT, not being a patentable new drug, and reducing the dose of existing drugs, does not fit their business models. Probably for similar reasons, venture capitalists and other financial people quickly lose their smiles or move away when they hear the details of the IPT innovation. News reporters have not yet been interested because IPT clinical trials have not yet been done, and it has not appeared in mainstream journals.[41]

Emergency Use. It may have occurred to some readers that the IPT procedure may lend itself to home administration in certain circumstances such as in exceptionally rural areas, or in a time of dire emergency such as a bioterror attack or a large-scale biological accident. In the latter two situations, depending on the size of the spread of contamination, hospitals could be full to capacity, leaving the average person to fend for him/herself and their family.

Many people don't like to think about such possible future events, understandably. It's painful to contemplate such possibilities. On the other hand, even the Boy Scout motto suggests it's often prudent to be prepared and to plan ahead.

If one were to plan for such a possible future event, the type of medication to administer, the dosage of medication, and the proper "recovery" system would be critical. Consultation with an "understanding" physician could resolve these issues. Dr. Chris Duffield has some interesting thoughts on this topic at www.iptq.com/low-tech_ipt.htm.

Conclusion. Is the technique safe? Dr. Peréz García III explains that in his 20 years of experience using IPT, "my father's 44 years of practice, and my grandfather's 41 years of experience with IPT, no patient has died as a result of the procedure, during the procedure, or after the procedure."

After nearly eighty years of use by three generations of the García family of physicians, as well as dozens of additional, highly-credentialed physicians—most of whom are in current practice—the preliminary results are in. Insulin Potentiation Therapy holds great promise as being a true breakthrough in the treatment of many forms of cancer, as well as many other maladies both major and minor.

As one of the basic controlling hormones of the body, insulin alters the dynamics of biological systems at a very basic level. One of the effects this has, as the molecules interplay within the body at the tiniest levels, is to increase the effectiveness of chemotherapy drugs—the same drugs being used today at toxic levels that produce unpleasant and damaging side-effects.

By reducing the medications to safer levels while still delivering more of them into the cancer cells, side-effects are reduced; the treatment is more effective because more toxic drug reaches the diseased cells; and the introduction of insulin into the body in and of itself seems to favorably change the biological terrain so that the body is less hospitable to disease processes and more supportive of good health.

Dr. Chris Duffield calls IPT "the second discovery of insulin." He suggests that any physician may use the IPT protocol currently, as it requires chemotherapy drugs that are already FDA approved and in use, and common insulin. (IPT is an approved, "off-label" use of the drugs.) In cases of cancer types with a history of successful treatment by IPT, a month-long "safe trial" period could be employed initially, and closely monitored for progress. If ineffective, the patient could undergo normal treatment.

Although no clinical trials have been performed using IPT, even the casual reader can see the great potential it holds for humanity. Whatever the politicians, bureaucrats, and misguided money moguls may do about IPT, now *you* know about the treatment method that may one day save your life, or that of a loved one. Congratulations—you have hereby added one more important tool to your inventory of medical knowledge. A comprehensive list of doctors who practice IPT can be found at http://iptforcancer.com/index.php?md=13.

IODINE

Discovered in 1811, the chemical element iodine is generally known for its use as a disinfectant (antiseptic), water sanitizer, and for its ability to protect the thyroid gland against radiation poisoning. It is well known in medicine as being critical for the proper functioning of the thyroid gland and the prevention of goiter (enlarged thyroid) and cretinism (congenital hypothyroidism). The U.S. Food and Drug Administration currently recommends 150 micrograms (mcg) as the daily adult dosage of iodine. For the past four to five decades it has been the accepted view of modern Western medicine that amounts significantly in excess of this dosage are toxic.

Prior to the 1940s, physicians used iodine in quantities several orders of magnitude higher than those commonly used today—without toxicity and to the benefit of general health and several medical ailments including both hyperthyroidism (overactive thyroid) and hypothyroidism (underactive thyroid). The current daily intake of 13.8 mg by 60 million Japanese—one of the healthiest Western societies—supports the safety, indeed the benefit, of higher levels of iodine than those currently suggested by the FDA.

Over 100 years ago, doctors had an understanding of iodine that would surprise modern Western physicians. It was referred to as "The

Universal Medicine," and used to treat several medical conditions in amounts far in excess of today's standard. Illustrative of its recognized importance in times past is the statement of Dr. Albert Szent-Györgyi, the famed Hungarian physician and winner of the Nobel Prize in Physiology/Medicine in 1937 for his discovery of vitamin C. Györgyi commented,

> When I was a medical student, iodine in the form of KI [potassium iodide] was the universal medicine. Nobody knew what it did, but it did something and did something good. We students used to sum up the situation in this little rhyme: *If ye don't know where, what, and why, prescribe ye then K and I.* Our medical predecessors...were keen observers and the universal application of iodide might have been not without foundation."[1]

Several contemporary, pioneer physicians are opening the door to a new understanding of both the importance of iodine in many aspects of the body's functioning as well as the body's requirement for larger amounts of the substance than are currently recognized. One of the physicians at the forefront of iodine use and research is the well-known integrative/alternative physician Jonathan Wright, M.D., director of the Tahoma Clinic in Kent, Washington. Dr. Wright has written extensively on the uses of potassium iodide, which is iodine in a form that's chemically referred to as a salt of iodine. Specifically, Dr. Wright uses and recommends SSKI, or Saturated Solution of Potassium Iodide—a concentrated liquid form of the substance. Many of the suggestions in this writing regarding medical treatments with iodine are adapted from his writings on the subject.[2]

Baby boomers know from childhood that tincture of iodine is a good disinfectant for cuts and scrapes. When teenagers "pop a zit," rubbing SSKI on the site will eliminate the zit in 24-48 hours. Airline travelers can protect themselves from microbes causing unwanted respiratory illness and other conditions by ingesting 10 drops of SSKI in water. Rural travelers or hikers can sanitize "questionable" water by adding a few drops two to three minutes prior to drinking.

Dr. Wright reports in his book *The Patient's Book of Natural Healing* that the SSKI form of iodine is able to cure even the most severe cases of fibrocystic breast disease. In less serious cases—"medium" to "minor"—six to eight drops of SSKI taken daily for three to six months in a few ounces of water will often reduce fibrocystic breast disease to an insignificant concern. Iodine helps eliminate fibrocystic breast disease and ovarian cysts at least in part through helping the body metabolize two potentially-harmful forms of estrogen (estrone and 16-alpha-hydroxyestrone) into the non-harmful estriol.

Other fibrotic conditions helped by iodine are Dupuytren's contracture and Peyronie's disease. Dupuytren's contracture is the abnormal thickening of fibrous tissues beneath the skin of the fingers and palms, curling the related finger(s) toward the palm. In Peyronie's disease, a similar tissue thickening and contracture occur along the shaft of the penis, making erections curved and painful. In both of these conditions, rubbing SSKI into the thickened tissues at least twice daily will soften the fibrotc tissue over a period of several months and help restore normal function. Dr. Wright suggests that in addition to iodine, sufferers of these conditions also take two grams of para-aminobenzoic acid (PABA) three times daily, and rub a mixture of vitamin E and DMSO into the affected area. Unusually thick scars known as *keloids* can also be treated by rubbing SSKI into the affected area at least twice daily.

Two common types of *fistulas*—abnormal tunnels through the tissue—are peri-anal and recto-vaginal. Frequent swabbings with an SSKI-soaked Q-tip both outside and within the affected orifice can often heal this type of ailment, although it can take several months for complete healing. Adding DMSO to the iodine often speeds the process. Hemorrhoids can sometimes be cleared literally overnight by applying a mixture of 20 drops of SSKI and one ounce of flaxseed oil.

Bladder infections, formally referred to as urinary tract infections (UTIs), can usually be cured by taking 10-15 drops of SSKI in water or juice every three to four hours until the infection clears. It's also known that the naturally-occurring simple sugar D-mannose is 90% effective in curing UTI. The D-mannose coats the sticky bacteria such as *E. Coli* and prevents them from attaching to the walls of the bladder. Thereafter, they're simply washed away during normal urination. Both cran-berry and pineapple juices have significant levels of D-mannose, but are usually ineffective in curing serious infections.

Atherosclerotic plaque—the deposit of fat and other substances along the inner walls of the artery—can be reduced by the combined use of iodine and niacin. This was observed over 30 years ago by ophthalmologists who found that several month's use of the tablet Iodo-niacin (120 mg iodine and 15 mg niacin) reverses atherosclerotic clogging of the arteries. This was confirmed by taking before and after retinal photomicrograph pictures of clogged arteries of the eyes. Following treatment, the photographs showed a significant reduction of athersclerotic plaque.

Afflictions of the lungs such as chronic bronchitis, emphysema, and other COPD-related ailments can be helped greatly by iodine use. Iodine permeates all bodily secretions, including thick and often difficult-to-expel bronchial secretions. Oral iodine use loosens these secretions, making them easier to clear, as well as reducing the growth of microorganisms.

Iodine combined with DMSO (see Dimethyl Sulfoxide under **Spinal Cord Injury**) is effective in combating toe and fingernail fungus. Twenty to thirty drops of SSKI in water is effective in clearing vaginal infections when used as a douche. And last but not least, if beans are soaked for about an hour in water containing one to two drops of SSKI (add fresh water before cooking), intestinal gas will be significantly reduced.

Although Dr. Wright uses the SSKI form of iodine, other effective iodine preparations include the liquid products Lugol's solution and Iosol.™ Dr. Wright is very adamant that persons supplementing daily with iodine have their thyroid function monitored regularly so that iodine overdose doesn't occur.

A physician with a more radical view of iodine supplementation—at least compared to the "current medical understanding"—is Guy Abraham, M.D., former Professor of Gynecology, Obstetrics, and Endocrinology at the UCLA School of Medicine. Dr. Abraham's research is set to turn modern medicine's view of the necessary/optimal level of iodine supplementation on its ear. After completing an extensive literature search on the medical uses of iodine, Dr. Abraham conducted his own

clinical research—which led to the development of a tableted form of Lugol's solution named Iorodal.™ In addition, his research led to several interesting and "surprising" conclusions about iodine use.[3-11]

❒ The nutrient iodine is essential for every cell of the human body.

❒ In non-obese persons without a defective cellular transport system for iodine, optimal concentrations can be achieved with daily intake of 12.5 mg to 50 mg of elemental iodine. (Note this is from almost 100 to almost 350 times greater than the current FDA daily recommended value.) The adult body retains approximately 1.5 gm of iodine at sufficiency. At such time, the ingested iodine is excreted in the urine as iodide.

❒ Goiter and cretinism are evidence of extremely severe iodine deficiency, because the smallest intake of iodine that would prevent these conditions, 0.05 mg per day, is 1,000 times less than the optimal intake of 50 mg of elemental iodine.

❒ The thyroid gland has a protective mechanism which limits the uptake of peripheral iodide to a maximum of 0.6 mg per day when 50 mg or more of elemental iodine are ingested. This amount therefore would serve as a preventive measure against radioactive fallout.

❒ An intake of 50 mg of elemental iodine per day achieves a peripheral concentration of iodide at a level which would protect the body against oxidative damage to DNA, providing an anticarcinogenic effect.

❒ Preliminary data suggest that iodine supplementation results in detoxification of the body from the toxic metals aluminum, cadmium, lead, and mercury.

❒ Most persons on a daily intake ranging from 12.5 mg to 50 mg of elemental iodine report higher energy levels and greater mental clarity, particularly with 50 mg daily (4 tablets of Iodoral). Patients with fibrocystic breast disease respond faster and more completely when ingesting 50 mg per day.

❒ For best results, supplementation should be part of a complete nutritional program, emphasizing magnesium instead of calcium.

❒ A beneficial effect of supplementation was observed in the following clinical conditions: autoimmune thyroiditis; cardiac arrhythmias; diabetes types I & II; fibrocystic breast disease and breast cancer; Grave's disease; hormone resistance syndromes; hypertension; obesity; polycystic ovary syndrome; recurrent and chronic infections; subclinical hypothyroidism; and thyroid nodules.

❐ Iodine supplementation may be the safest, simplest, most effective and least expensive way to solve the healthcare crisis crippling our nation.

The side-effects reported with the use of iodine include acne-like skin lesions in certain areas of the body, headache in the frontal sinus, an unpleasant brassy taste, and increased salivation and sneezing. Based on the experience of clinicians with several thousand patients using Iodoral, with daily amounts ranging from 6.25 to 50 mg for up to three years, the incidence of the above side-effects has been estimated at one percent.

Two tests are useful in assessing the body's need for iodine, the first being less accurate than the second. With a Q-Tip, paint a two inch by two inch diameter circle of 2% iodine tincture (use *only* this form of iodine) on your stomach (near the navel) or inner thigh. If the iodine stain can be seen 24-hours later, your body is less likely to be iodine deficient. If your body is deficient in iodine, the skin will uptake the iodine and the stain will disappear in under 24-hours.

The second, more accurate and comprehensive test was developed by Dr. Abraham. The iodine/iodide loading test is based on the concept that the normally functioning human body has a mechanism to retain ingested iodine until whole body sufficiency for iodine is achieved.

After taking 50 mg of an iodine/iodide combination (Iodoral), 24-hours of urine is collected at various time intervals. The amount of iodine excreted is measured. When there is an iodine deficiency present, little iodine will be excreted during the testing. When there is a sufficient body iodine level present, larger amounts of iodine will be excreted.

After determining an iodine deficiency is present, according to Dr. Abraham, supplementation should begin gradually because iodine mobilizes toxic metals and other toxic substances from their storage sites which may cause symptoms. Testing should be repeated every three to four months to monitor proper iodine levels. The test is performed by using a Test Kit: Iodine Sufficiency Test, which is available from Vitamin Research Products. To learn more about iodine supplementation and to order the Test Kit, visit www.vrp.com (enter"iodine" in search box. See articles on right side of screen.) or call (800)877-2447.

Four beneficial forms of iodine are readily available: Three liquids—SSKI, Lugol's solution, and Iosol™—and the tableted Iodoral.™ Labeling instructions on each product will explain the quantity of elemental iodine per drop/tablet. For example, Iosol and SSKI contain 1.83 mg and 19 mg of elemental iodine per drop, respectively. Lugol's and Iosol are available on the internet. To order SSKI, visit www.tahomadispensary.com. Enter "sski" in the search box. Persons with iodine sensitivity should not use these products.

MAGNETIC MOLECULAR ENERGIZER

Science has revealed that the Earth was formerly surrounded by a much stronger magnetic field than is present today. The U.S. Geological Survey has been recording Earth's magnetic fields for almost 160 years, and has shown the strength of the field continues to decline at the rate of about five percent each hundred years. The present average strength is only 0.4 gauss (unit of measurement of magnetic strength). Four thousand years ago it was 4 gauss, which has been confirmed by several evaluation techniques. It is believed that at the time the dinosaurs roamed the Earth, the geomagnetic field could have been as high as 200 gauss. Therefore, life on present-day Earth exists in a drastically reduced electromagnetic environment in comparison to thousands or even hundreds of years ago.

It's known that all living cells have an electromagnetic component. There are only two natural sources of magnetism that affect humans: the brain and the Earth. The energy generating capacity of the brain is derived from the *astrocyte cells*, which comprise about 80% of the total number of brain cells. The Earth provides a supportive steady-state field from which the body draws energy to enhance molecular action, while the astrocyte cells produce a pulsed, living magnetic field. These two magnetic fields work together to produce a magnetic resonance occurring primarily during restorative hours of sleep. This resonance dramatically enhances the chemical reactions of the body. When a magnetic field of the correct orientation passes through the atoms which comprise the molecular structures including the cells of the body, it increases the cells' energy state which in turn enhances the sharing of electrons between cells. This increased action is a catalyst to all of the body's myriad chemical reactions.

The critical importance of the strength of Earth's magnetic field is not generally realized. The fact that the geomagnetic field is so drastically depleted is even less well known. This depletion undoubtedly explains why people respond so well to an artificially-induced magnetic state such as that created by MME. Evidence of the importance of magnetism to human life was shown by Dr. E. N. Gumiel, chief consultant in biological research to the World Development Organization and Director of the Genesis Project. Gumiel reported that insects live five times longer in substantially enhanced magnetic fields, and human tissue cells live up to two-and-one-half times longer.

The initial 20th Century finding of the necessity of Earth's geomagnetic field was made clear when early Russian cosmonauts were found to have up to 80% mineral loss in their bones as a result of their extended space flights. Artificially generated magnetic fields are now used in space capsules to prevent these losses and assist in maintaining health during space voyages. Dr. Valerie Hunt, a former researcher at U.C.L.A., was able to create a geomagnetic-free cubicle in which human subjects were placed. Appropriate monitoring devices indicated mental and physical activity and physiological responses. Soon after being subjected to this environment, the subjects lost emotional control and began to weep. Thereafter, they began to lose muscular co-ordination, and shortly thereafter began to show effects on the heart muscle—at which time they were removed from the magnetic-free environment. As Dr. Hunt demonstrated, humans could exist only a few hours without the influence of Earth's magnetic field.

Magnetic Molecular Energizer (MME) technology takes advantage of both the biochemical and electromagnetic aspects, and positively affects the body's healing capability in a multiplicity of physical ailments. The MME is closely related to the familiar medical device Magnetic Resonance Imaging (MRI), although the MRI focuses on diagnosis while the MME is a treatment tool. When the MME is applied, there's a temporary increase in the magnetic field affecting every atom in every cell. Some of the electrons on these atoms begin to increase in speed, leading to an acceleration of normal chemical reactions, including oxygen carrying capacity, nutrient assimilation, metabolic waste removal, enzyme synthesis, reduction of free radicals, tissue regeneration, and healing.

More technically, the theory behind the MME device is derived from the application of physics, specifically the Lamar Frequency Formula—which states that by increasing the magnetic field in which an atom exists, the velocity of electrons and protons will increase proportionally. With the MME, theoretically the speed of some electrons can be increased 10,000 to 20,000 times faster than normal. At this dramatically increased velocity, magnetic resonance occurs much more readily. Magnetic resonance is a phenomenon that occurs when the pulsed electromagnetic current coming from the brain is at a harmonic of the frequency of the targeted tissue. This is described by Robert O. Becker, MD—a noted researcher, author, teacher, inventor and expert in biomagnetism—in his famous books *The Body Electric* and *Cross Currents*. The net result of the enhancement in magnetic resonance is increased efficiency of chemical reactions and increased available energy to the specific area affected.

MME technology was invented by the Canadian researcher Dr. Dear Bonlie, inventor of the Magnetico mattress discussed under **Magnets** in the **Pain Relievers** section. The MME consists of two electromagnets which apply a strong, direct current (DC) electromagnetic field to the body. The magnetic field ranges in strength from 3,000 to 5,000 gauss. MRI scanners, on the other hand, operate at up to 20,000 gauss. MME treatment is safe, painless, non-invasive, and its physical layout does not cause claustrophobic reactions as are sometimes experienced with MRI treatment. MME offers the hope of successfully treating many diseases previously considered untreatable by conventional methods. Thus far it has been successful in treating a wide variety of ailments including the following conditions listed along with the average number of hours required to accomplish the beneficial results. Treatment costs are USD $50 per hour.

Patients Experiencing Substantial Improvement. Osteoarthritis in the hip (88-112 hours); Spinal nerve injury and chronic pain from radiation (200); Chronic obstructive pulmonary disease (COPD) (100); Pain in the spine and joints (60); Femoral nerve pain, surgical injury (160); Cervical disc disease pain (200); Parkinson's disease and stroke (353); Fractured wrist (40); Degenerative disc, back pain (428); Trauma and lower back pain; osteoarthritis in both hips (215); Herniated disc pain (144); Paralysis (460); Fibromyalgia, low back pain, neuropathy in both feet (456); Feet, ankle neuropathy (110); Neck, upper back pain (100); Lower back pain with left leg nerve impingement, surgical injury (106); Torn right rotator cuff, bulging disks in neck (100).

Patients Showing Some Improvement. Osteoarthritis in the right knee (66); Osteomalacia (pain from osteoporosis) in the right wrist (10); Osteoarthritis in both knees (234); Parkinson's disease (350); Spinal cord injury, neck pain (228); Postherpetic neuralgia (520); Spinal stenosis (281); Alzheimer's disease (480); Cartilage tear in the right knee (100); Intractable hiccups; involuntary aspiration (146); Stroke (336).

Patients Having No Improvement. Dementia (156); Parkinson's disease (239-298); Diabetic neuropathy (142); Brain trauma (severe) (1011); Macular degeneration (dry) (100); Extreme overall muscular pain (20).

As of the spring of 2009, the unique MME treatment is currently being actively researched, so the full extent and limitations of this treatment method are not fully known. Research is being conducted under the auspices of an Institutional Review Board (IRB) as outlined in FDA regulations. The IRB consists of five or more physicians or health professionals who determine specific protocols and review the records of all cases treated. Because extensive toxicity studies have already been conducted, MME research currently focuses on responses or benefits to an array of diagnosed conditions. When significant numbers of cases in a given category of treatment have been accumulated, the collective information will be submitted to the FDA for approval of the MME as an effective treatment for that particular condition. At that time

treatment will become available on a broader basis. Presently, MME treatment is available in the following U.S. cities: Seattle, Washington; Sterling Heights, Michigan; Mocksville, North Carolina; Toledo, Ohio; Tucson, Arizona; Virginia Beach, Virginia. Specific treatment site information is available at www.amri-intl.com/clinics.html. AMRI International, manufacturer of the device, is based in Calgary, Canada. To learn more about the MME, visit AMRI's website at www.amri-intl.com, or Google "magnetic molecular energizer." (Another interesting magnetic technology is magnetic-field therapy, a therapy used in many German cancer clinics. In addition to cancer, magnetic-field therapy has application for a multiplicity of health challenges, as does MME. To learn more about magnetic-field therapy, see Magnetic-field Therapy under **Cancer**.)

NEURAL THERAPY

Every function of the body is under the control of the autonomic nervous system, which consists of the sympathetic and parasympathetic nervous systems. Together, these systems control heart beat, hearing, pain perception, smell—virtually all bodily functions. They also control blood pressure and blood circulation to all of the body's glands and organs.

Neural therapists believe that *interference fields* may develop within the body that cause dysfunction of the autonomic nervous system. An interference field is defined as any pathologically damaged tissue which acts to stimulate the autonomic nervous system in an abnormal way. Tissues can be damaged as the result of physical trauma (slight or severe), surgery, an infected tooth or root canal, even scars—no matter how large or small, recent or old.

Neural Therapy works by stopping the interference field from producing a stimulus which adversely affects the autonomic nervous system. Once this occurs there is more optimal functioning of the organs, glands and tissues, and the body is in a more advantageous position to eliminate abnormalities and disease conditions.

Interference fields are eliminated by injecting a local anesthetic such as procaine (Novocain®) or lidocaine (Xylocaine®) directly into the interference field(s) in areas such as acupuncture points, autonomic ganglia, glands, peripheral nerves, scars, skin, trigger points, and other tissues. Because the interference fields produce abnormal bio-electrical states within the nervous system, these injections normalize and stabilize the bio-electrical signals. According to the Physician's Desk Reference (PDR), local anesthetics such as procaine and lidocaine function by "stabilizing the membrane's bio-electrical potential, thus returning the organ to its original state."[1]

The administration of anesthetics is often able to restore and normalize the physiological structure that has been compromised, with a corresponding restoration and normalization of function. The result is rapid and long-lasting pain relief and the correction of chronic and previously untreatable ailments, with no side-effects.[2]

Neural Therapy was originally developed in Germany, and much of the scientific literature is from that country. According to that literature, interference fields can cause many types of illnesses and diseases including asthma, allergies, confusion, eczema, headaches (including migraines), chronic fatigue, chronic infections, chronic pain, gallbladder disease, liver disease, lupus, menstrual irregularity (and pain), rheumatoid arthritis, sinusitis, tonsilitis, vertigo, and other chronic degenerative conditions.[3]

According to Neural Therapy practitioners, this therapy offers many positive benefits, including:[4]

♦ Restoration of natural body functions; often produces quick results, called a *segunden*, or lightning reaction.
♦ Effective in a broad range of nerve and injury-related cases; often used in cases where surgery has failed.
♦ Can improve or resolve so-called "incurable" cases.
♦ Results are permanent.
♦ Compared to many other therapeutic approaches, Neural Therapy is a very conservative, non-invasive approach.
♦ There are no significant side-effects.

To learn more about Neural Therapy, visit www.neuraltherapy.com. To locate a practitioner in your location, call the American Academy of Neural Therapy at (425)637-9339.

Nutrition: Detoxification & Deficiencies

Our Potential for Good Health

Research has shown that chronic disease is caused chiefly by environmental factors (~75%) with some contribution from genetics (~25%). Our genes interact with the environment and give rise to expression. The expression of our genes is polymorphic—having the potential for more than one expression—and significantly influenced by the environmental factors to which they are subjected.

Every cell contains the genetic information of the whole body, yet depending upon the environmental stimuli to which precursor cells are exposed, some will differentiate into muscle cells, others nervous tissue, and so forth. Of the various environmental factors that influence our health, diet is the most influential factor. Former U.S. Surgeon General Dr. David Satcher stated that 80% of the leading causes of death in the United States are related to diet and alcohol consumption.

Medical science and the popular media sometimes suggest we are victims of our genes. Genetic predisposition is only one of many factors that contributes to disease. By taking an active role, the power of natural foods and properly tailored nutritional supplements help us to be personally accountable for our health. Nature's arsenal wields powerful weapons capable of battling against even the most serious diseases. This has been the message of ancient healing systems for thousands of years.

Many chemicals found in fruits and vegetables contain disease-fighting substances called *phyto* (plant) *nutrients*. These substances have been shown effective in preventing and treating a host of debilitating diseases and ailments. Dietary changes, appropriate nutritional supplementation and exercise are mainstays in the foundation of the holistic approach to chronic disease and the maintenance of health. All of these modalities will be discussed in detail within this section.

The Other Face of Progress

Notwithstanding our potential to live a healthy life, a host of environmental influences deter us from this goal. Our modern world has been the subject of many revolutionary forces. While the human being once foraged for his daily bread, the Domestication Revolution slowly ushered in the first dramatic transformation of human societies. Once a hunter and gatherer spending most of a typical day in search of the next meal, man's control over plants and animals for use as a food source forever changed the landscape of human civilization, both figuratively and literally.

Over the past several hundred years, many other revolutionary forces helped shape our modern world. The Scientific Revolution in all its many aspects transformed man from a campfire-building, spear-making animal into a space traveling being—all within a short number of years, all in the name of "progress."

In the Western world, the word "science" is inexorably connected to our notion of progress. Over a few short decades, man has transformed Earth by means of putting scientific principles into practice. Science has been the tool whereby people have gained increasing control over their lives—which is viewed by most as being coincidental with "improvement" and "progress." Indeed, in many ways science has transformed our planet into what our ancestors would surely think of as a "Fantasyland" of imagination—the embodiment of cleaver invention and creation manifesting as automobiles, skyscrapers, jet planes, and a plethora of additional high-tech wonders.

Few would argue that science has ushered in changes which as a whole have benefitted man greatly. On the other hand, tagging along with the benefits have come many negative consequences, some of which are only recently becoming known. One of the most formidable of these challenges is the degree to which our environment has become poisoned by substances which themselves are the very products of science. This poisoned, toxic environment is where man lives, and we're finding it increasingly difficult to escape these toxic surroundings.

Xenobiotics (zee-no-by-AWE-tics) is the term used to describe chemical compounds that are foreign to living organisms. These toxins are referred to as being *exogenous*, or coming from outside the body, as opposed to *endogenous* toxins which originate from within. Each year more than 1,000 such new chemicals are synthesized,[1] adding to the current total of more than 100,000 xenobiotic substances. These toxic substances include such familiar classifications of chemicals as food additives, industrial chemicals, pesticides, and pharmaceutical and other drugs.[2]

Industrial Chemicals

According to the U.S. Environmental Protection Agency (EPA), each year the following number of chemicals is pumped into the environment:[3]

❖ More than 500 million pounds of industrial chemicals are dumped into the public sewage system.
❖ More than 1 billion pounds of chemicals are released into the ground, threatening to contaminate the ground water that is held in underground aquifers. This ground water is the source of roughly half of our drinkable water supply.
❖ The other half of our usable water supply is sourced from rivers, streams and reservoirs. Nearly 200 million pounds of chemicals are discharged into surface waters annually.
❖ Nearly 2.5 billion pounds of toxic emissions are pumped into our atmosphere.
❖ More than 5.5 trillion total pounds of chemicals are released into the environment.

Household Chemicals

Once thought to be safe, there is mounting evidence that human exposure to chemicals even at low levels can be harmful. Exposures are linked to adverse biological effects including endocrine disruption, chemical sensitivity, and cancer. Aside from industrial chemicals, scientists are beginning to understand that household chemicals also pose a threat.

It is becoming increasingly clear that chemical substances used in combination are potentially many times more toxic than when isolated chemicals are used by themselves. For example, a single chemical by itself may cause no bodily harm; however, when another chemical or group of chemicals is introduced in combination with the first, the results can be deadly toxic.

As long ago as 1969, Dr. Irving Selikoff, Professor of Environmental Medicine at Mount Sinai School of Medicine, stated that,

> We may eventually see diseases that we don't begin to understand at this time. Also, the sum total of these various low-level contaminants—each in itself not very important—may be to generally shorten life [due to the] total body burden of environmental contaminants.[4]

What Dr. Selikoff foresaw more than four decades ago has now come to pass. Dr. Michael Dufresne, Adjunct and Research Professor at the University of Windsor in Ontario, Canada has recently published data suggesting that thousands of household items previously believed safe are now thought to pose significant health hazards, including carcinogenicity.[5] "People are blindly being led in the use of these products. They assume they are tested and safe, and they're not,"[6] says Dufresne. He continues to point out that scientists are discovering exposure to a variety of trace chemicals over the span of many years (or a lifetime) poses a significant threat to good health, and that his greatest worry is the lack of information available to the public about potentially-harmful products used on an everyday basis.

Dr. Dufresne's research points out that many home cleaning products used on a daily basis in millions of households contain dangerous chemicals. Such products, according to Dufresne, include Ajax;® Arm & Hammer® heavy duty laundry detergent; Joy;® liquid Spray 'N Wash;® Lysol;® Murphy's Oil Soap;® Palmolive;® Pledge;® Sunlight;® Tilex;® and many others.[7] Today's home contains more chemicals than a well-stocked laboratory at the turn of the 20th Century. As early as the mid-1990s, the American Association of Poison Control reported nearly 1.5 million toxic exposures in persons under 19 years of age, and over 1 million poisonings in children less than six years old.[8]

One of the biggest culprits is the cosmetics industry. According to Dufresne, the following is a partial list of products that may pose a health threat: blush, concealer, deodorant, eye shadow/mascara, facial powder, hairstyling products, nail polish, shampoo/conditioner, soap, tampons, and toothpaste.[9] Although cancer-linked chemicals are found in such products, there are virtually no FDA regulations overseeing their production or use.

Agricultural Contamination

The agricultural industry is one of the most significant polluters, with more than 50,000 different pesticide formulations currently in use.[10] The *Lancet* recently reported there are more than three million severe pesticide poisonings each year world wide, with 220,000 deaths.[11] In the U.S., pesticide-related illnesses occur at the rate of 150,000-

300,000 per year.[12] The EPA has ranked pesticide contamination as the number three cancer risk, behind cigarette smoke and radon gas.[13]

Fertilizer contamination is also a problem. According to a recent article in *The Seattle Times*,[14] industrial chemical waste from industries such as cement, metal, paper and wood product companies is recycled as an ingredient of fertilizer, the same fertilizer used in both commercial farming and family gardens. This waste is laden with heavy metals such as aluminum, arsenic, beryllium, cadmium, dioxins, lead, mercury, and titanium.

Pharmaceutical Drugs

As discussed earlier, in 2002 physicians wrote Americans over three billion prescriptions for drugs.[15] This is prescription writing at the rate of one each month for every living human being residing in the United States. With Americans spending over $200 billion per year on prescription drugs, we can see there's a very powerful potential for toxic reactions among the populous.

In the July 2000 issue of the *Journal of the American Medical Association*,[16] Dr. Barbara Starfield of the Johns Hopkins School of Hygiene and Public Health confirmed that each year in the United States more than 100,000 hospital deaths occur as the result of adverse reactions to prescription pharmaceutical drugs which are prescribed by physicians in accordance with the directions given by the pharmaceutical companies who manufacture them. These figures do not include data from other medical settings such as doctors' offices or outpatient deaths. Additionally, these totals are only for deaths and do not reflect negative effects associated with adverse reactions which do not cause death, but are nevertheless associated with disability and/or pain and discomfort. In addition to the 100,000 annual deaths caused by correctly-prescribed pharmaceutical drugs, an additional 125,000 deaths occur in the U.S. each year as the result of incorrectly-prescribed prescribed drugs.[17]

Food Additives

Substances present in the food other than the basic foods themselves are a further source of contamination. The food industry intentionally adds many such substances for a variety of purposes, including extending the shelf-life with preservatives; enhancing or masking flavors to make foods more palatable; and modifying the texture and/or color to make foods more attractive. In 1955, 419 million pounds of chemical additives were used in the U.S. food supply. Today, over one billion pounds of more than 10,000 different chemicals are used, with the average American consuming more than 50 pounds of food-additive chemicals per year.

Other Exogenous Toxifiers

Additional sources of toxification include alcohol consumption, cigarette smoke, dietary deficiencies, ionizing radiation, iron overload, microbial (viral and bacterial) infection, strenuous exercise, and tissue injury.

Endogenous Toxicity

In addition to the external (exogenous) sources of pollutants, internal (endogenous) pollutants also contribute to toxicity. Normal systemic metabolism can produce lactic acid, pyruvic acid, urea and other intermediary metabolites that add to the overall toxic burden within the body. Even the body's own detoxification processes can produce free radicals that are toxic to cellular structures.

Toxic Consequences

The three most vital necessities of man are air, water and food. It's clear from the above statistics that all of these necessities are being severely compromised—poisoned. Because our bodies live within this polluted ecosystem, just as fish exist within contaminated waters, there is no escaping the consequences of the toxic pollution that surrounds us. It should therefore not be surprising to learn that the average adult Westerner carries within his/her body at least 500 xenobiotic chemicals, according to the World Wildlife Fund. Several other agencies have confirmed these numbers.

In the month preceding a baby's birth, the umbilical cord—the lifeline between mother and baby—pulses over 300 quarts of blood each day back and forth between the nutrient- and oxygen-rich placenta and the rapidly growing baby. While scientists previously believed the placenta shielded the umbilical cord blood from the developing baby, they now realize the mothers' contaminated blood carries not only the building blocks of life, but also a steady stream of industrial chemicals and pollut-

ants directly to the developing human life nestled within the mothers' womb.

In July of 2005, the Environmental Working Group published the study *Body Burden: The Pollution in Newborns*.[18] Two hundred and eighty seven xenobiotic chemicals were detected within the umbilical cord blood of American newborns, with an average of 200 chemicals per baby—each baby ranging from 154 to 231 chemicals. Of these 287 chemicals, 108 have been shown to cause cancer in humans and animals; 217 are toxic to the brain and nervous system; and 208 cause birth defects or abnormal development in animal tests. The potential dangers of this toxic brew of carcinogens, neurotoxins, and developmental toxins have never been evaluated.

Included in the 287 xenobiotic chemicals detected are: polyaromatic hydrocarbons (PAHs)—18 tested for, nine detected; polybrominated dibenzodioxins and furans (PBDD/Fs)—12 tested for, seven detected; perfluorinated chemicals (PFCs)—12 tested for, nine detected; polychlorinated dibenzodioxins and furans (PBCD/Fs)—17 tested for, 11 detected; organochlorine pesticides (OCs)—28 tested for, 21 detected; polybrominated diphenyl ethers (PBDEs)—46 tested for, 32 detected; polychlorinated naphthalenes (PCNs)—70 tested for, 50 detected; polychlorinated biphenyls (PCBs)—209 tested for, 147 detected; and a range of heavy metals including aluminum, arsenic, cadmium, cesium, mercury, nickel, and strontium.[19]

Although many of these substances have unfamiliar-sounding names to most of us, the following list of sources of these toxic chemicals brings the picture more clearly into focus: stain and grease-resistant coatings used in food wrap, carpets, furniture—Teflon,® Scotchgard,® and Stainmaster® (PFCs); fire retardants—TVs, computers, furniture (PBDEs, PCNs); electrical insulators (PCBs, PCNs); pesticides (OCs, PCNs); garbage incineration and plastic production wastes (PCDD/Fs, PDBB/Fs); automobile emissions and other fossil fuel combustion (PAHs); and power plants, e.g., coal burning (methyl mercury).[20]

The radical changes in our society over the span of the last 100 years have not come without their significant, detrimental consequences. If it weren't for these consequences, the endless variety of our modern, high-tech wonders would be a joy, as most currently believe them to be. Little do we realize the toxicity associated with most of our high-tech accoutrements are killing us—and making us crazy—even if slowly. For many in the Western world, the connection between our toxic environment and disease, both physical and mental, is not readily apparent. Even those who understand this insidious connection cannot escape their polluted fish bowl Earth.

Over the last 50 years or so, many health conditions of relatively non-obvious origins have skyrocketed, including allergies; asthma; attention deficit and hyperactivity disorder (ADD & ADHD); autism (one in 166 American newborns have some form of the disease); birth defects (3-5% of U.S. babies are born with birth defects); chronic fatigue syndrome; fibromyalgia; infertility (5-10% of American couples are infertile); insomnia; migraines; neuropathies; and miscarriage (up to 50% of all pregnancies in the U.S. end in miscarriage).

Equally disconcerting is the rise in the more serious conditions of heart disease and cancer, America's number one and number two killers of humans, respectively. In 1900, heart disease accounted for 8% of all deaths in the U.S., and cancer about 3.5%. Since 1900, the number of cases of heart disease has increased some 400%, and the number of cases of cancer by over 700%. Childhood brain cancer and acute lymphocytic leukemia have increased dramatically over the past 30 years. Mathematically speaking, for a person living in the U.S. *there is a 75% probability for men and more than a 50% probability for women of being afflicted either with heart disease, cancer or both.* These are unacceptable odds, even for a confirmed gambler.

Animal Research

Western scientists base much of their evaluation of potentially-toxic substances on laboratory animal testing. It is assumed that if a chemical tests negative (non-toxic) in a rat, mouse, or rabbit model, for example, it will likewise be non-toxic to humans. Although this is sometimes the case, often it is not. Some researchers believe animal research is an unscientific methodology for assessing chemical toxicity. According to this view, animal toxicity studies produce staggering amounts of contradictory and invalid data that allow researchers to draw their (sometimes invalid) "scientific" conclusions.

An example of this is illustrative. Dr. Bruce Ames, Director of the National Institute of Environmental Health Sciences at the University of California at Berkeley, reported that,

> Of 392 chemicals in our database tested in both rats and mice, 226 were carcinogens in at least one test, but 96 were positive in the mouse and negative in the rat, or vice versa. Conversely, important human carcinogens may not be detected in standard tests involving rodents; this was true for a long time for both tobacco smoke and alcohol, the two largest identified causes of neoplastic [cancerous] death in the United States.[21]

What this means is that if there is a low correlation between the toxicity of many substances even in the rat versus mouse model, the extrapolation of such data from animals to humans is not as accurate as it may appear on the surface.

Detoxification

The term detoxification refers to the elimination of toxins (poisons) from the body. Throughout the ages the body has evolved complex systems which enable the excretion of a wide range of toxins the body has never previously encountered. These processes involve the biotransformation of non-water soluble (lipophilic) compounds into water soluble compounds which are then excreted via the urine.

Even though the body has a powerful capability to detoxify itself, the extent of the pollution present in today's world often exceeds the body's ability to detoxify. To a considerable extent this is dependent upon one's health and the strength of the immune system, as well as the proper functioning of the kidneys, liver, lungs, and gastrointestinal tract. Researchers recognize that every individual has a specific detoxification profile characterized by his/her own unique detoxification capacity. One's capacity to detoxify is a function of both environmental and genetic factors. This explains why, when presented with the same toxic stimuli, some persons become ill while others do not.

When overly polluted by toxic build-up or an inability to detoxify, the body reacts by producing states of illness and disease. Effects can range from bothersome symptoms such as allergic reactions; cardiovascular and gastrointestinal tract irregularities; cold-like symptoms; depression; fatigue; flu-like symptoms; headache; irritability; and muscle and joint pain[22] on the one hand, to more serious maladies such as being a contributing factor to other serious diseases including Alzheimer's and Parkinson's disease.[23]

Exposure to metals may well underlie persistent, chronic symptoms of allergic hypersensitivity, chronic fatigue, depression, musculoskeletal pain, neurological disorders, and poor cognitive function/memory.[24] Especially with exposure to toxic metals, overt symptoms may not manifest until later in life. Warning signs indicative of general toxicity include:[25]

• Increase in sensitivity to exogenous exposures such as odors, household chemicals, and medications
• Musculoskeletal disorders such as fibromyalgia
• Cognitive dysfunction
• Unilateral paresthesia
• Autonomic dysfunction
• Recurrent patterns of edema
• Worsening of symptoms following anesthesia or pregnancy
• Unusual reactions to medications or supplements

In addition to the above observational signs of toxicity, several clinical tools are used to access a toxic state:[26]

☞ *Challenge Testing.* These tests assess a person's ability to detoxify in the presence of certain "probe substances" such as acetaminophen, aspirin and caffeine. In addition to measuring metabolites of these substances in the blood, saliva and urine, they have well-known detoxification pathways which also can be monitored.

☞ *Organic Compounds.* Assessment of exposure to organic compounds can be done either via responses to detailed questionnaires or by laboratory tests that evaluate exposure to specific compounds.

☞ *Heavy Metals.* Exposure to heavy metals is typically evaluated by hair, blood or urine analysis.

☞ *Microbial Imbalances.* Several lab tests are used to evaluate the presence of potentially-pathological organisms such as bacteria, fungus, viruses and yeast. For example, the urine indican (Obermeyer) test evaluates the bacterial activity in the small and large intestines. Immunological tests are used to quantify bacterial and yeast antibodies.

If the body is unable to detoxify naturally, a course of detoxification can be initiated. In order to be most effective, a thorough detoxification program must target the 1) blood, 2) lymph, 3) colon, and 4) liver.

While the liver and colon are the primary targets of typical detoxification regimens, not detoxifying the blood and lymph continues to expose the organs, tissues and cells to harmful contaminants. It has been suggested that detoxifying the liver and/or colon without cleansing the blood and lymph is analogous to changing the oil filter on an automobile without changing the oil.

Blood. To animals, blood is liquid life. As it courses throughout the body, blood brings vital substances to the organs, tissues, and cells. Oxygen is transported from the lungs; nutrients are transported from the small intestines; hormones are transported from the glands; toxins are transported to the liver for filtration and disposal; waste is transported to the kidneys for excretion; and immune cells are transported to all parts of the body to fight infection and inflammation.[27] Perhaps the best-known blood cleanser is the root of the plant *burdock*, known botanically as *Arctium lappa.*[28] Red clover, yellow dock, cayenne, echinacea, garlic, pau d' arco and Oregon grape root are other natural blood cleansers.[29] One interesting product is Blood Detox® by Crystal Star. Order at (800)736-6015 or visit www.healthyhealing.com.

Lymph. Also referred to as a secondary circulatory system, the lymphatic system is composed of a network of vessels (tubes) having one-way valves that carry the waste-containing lymph fluid from tissues and cells to the final elimination organs (liver, kidneys, lungs); to nodes which filter the lymph fluid as it flows through the nodes; and to the thymus gland, tonsils, and spleen. Unlike the circulatory system (blood) which is powered by the heart, the lymph system relies on breathing and movement (exercise) alone to circulate the lymphatic fluid. Red clover extract, astragalus extract, and echinacea extract are powerful single herb lymph cleansers.[30] A lymph detox kit is available from www.healthyhealing.com, or by calling (800) 736-6015.

Colon. Although the largest amount of detoxification activity occurs in the liver, a significant portion of the remainder occurs in the intestinal walls. In fact, the highest concentration of detoxification enzymes are present in the tips of the intestinal villi.[31] Detoxifying the colon includes freeing stored toxins from intestinal walls and binding them to certain substances for elimination from the body.

Many popular bowel detox programs center around the herbs senna (*Cassia agustifolia*) and cascara sagrada (*Rhamnus purshiana*). The drawback to these herbs is that they can deplete vitamins, minerals and enzymes while leaving the user fatigued.[32] Enemas and colonics also are used to cleanse the bowel. Magnesium hydroxide is a gentle laxative that causes bowel contents to swell and soften by drawing water into the intestines. Once softened, toxic substances become loosened and cleansed from intestinal walls.[33] Slippery Elm bark, marshmallow root, and peppermint leaf extract also are used to detoxify the intestines.[34] Once the intestinal lining has been scrubbed, natural fibers are used to bind the toxic substances which assist in their removal through the intestines. Such fibers include oat bran, citrus pectin, psyllium husk and guar gum, or combinations thereof.[35] Probiotics, discussed below, also help restore healthy intestinal functioning.

Liver. It has been estimated that up to 75% of detoxification activity takes place in the liver,[36] the human body's second-largest organ—the skin being the largest. Within the liver, the conversion of toxic substances into forms able to be eliminated entails complex chemical processes. The detoxification process consists of two distinct phases, each involving a battery of enzymes.[37] During Phase I, a family of enzymes commonly referred to as the *cytochrome P450 system*, reduces, oxidizes, and hydrolyzes toxins, a process known as *functionalization.* The intermediate metabolites so produced are then further transformed during Phase II by other specialized enzymes in the liver. Following Phase II, the biotransformed substances are then able to be eliminated in the urine and feces.

In order for detoxification to be effective, the proper functioning of both Phase I and II is critical. Because the intermediate metabolites produced by Phase I can be more toxic than the initial toxins (e.g., harmful free radicals are often produced), Phase II must be functioning efficiently so that the intermediate-stage toxins can be rendered harm-

less, whereupon they are excreted from the body and the detoxification process is complete.[38] Persons undergoing a course of detoxification sometimes feel worse shortly after the procedure is begun. This could be explained by the increase (upregulation) of Phase I enzymes, with a corresponding lack of antioxidants and/or a corresponding lack of Phase II enzymes.

Proper detoxification is dependent upon adequate levels of supporting nutrients, including protein, carbohydrates, fat, antioxidants, and other factors. These dietary factors alter the efficiency of liver detoxification as well as the manifestation of secondary symptoms resulting from the detoxification process.

Cytochrome P450 enzymes require adequate dietary protein in order to actively detoxify xenobiotic chemicals. Restriction of dietary protein in laboratory animals has been shown to increase the toxicity of certain pesticides and other carcinogens.[39] High carbohydrate intake may reduce the efficiency of the cytochrome P450 enzymes.[40] This effect is particularly prominent with the use of common table sugar, as opposed to other polyglucose sources. A diet higher in protein and lower in carbohydrates seems to provide optimal activation of the cytochrome P450 family of enzymes.[41] Proper sources of both mono and polyunsaturated fatty acids also optimize the activity of the cytochrome P450 enzymes.[42] Free radicals produced during Phase I can be quenched by antioxidants such as vitamins C and E, as well as flavonoids and the mineral selenium. A high intake of pure (not tap) water also enhances the elimination of toxins along the detoxification pathways.

(Note: Fasting has been used both historically and in contemporary times as a means of detoxification. Both water and juice fasts, but particularly water fasts, may create more harm than benefit because of the lack of adequate levels of nutrients that support the detoxification process. Because of the absence of protein and/or excessive levels of carbohydrates that can accompany a juice fast, the production of pro-inflammatory and immune-inhibiting chemicals (prostaglandins and leukotrienes) is often increased.[43] Fasting with water alone allows the production of Phase I-produced free radicals to go unchecked.[44] Generally, because of the lack of antioxidants, carbohydrates, fat, protein, and other micronutrients, fasting can have significant adverse effects upon the safety and effectiveness of the detoxification process.)[45]

In addition to the above-named nutrients necessary for efficient and effective detoxification, other substances (cofactors) are required.[46] These include the amino acids methionine, cysteine and N-acetylcysteine; vitamins such as carotenoids, vitamins C and E; and the minerals copper, iron, magnesium, selenium and zinc. The following is a more comprehensive list of nutrients required for effective detoxification:[47]

Nutrients Supporting Phase I P450 Enzymes: Ascorbic Acid (vitamin C) • Coumarins • Flavonoids • Folic Acid • Indoles (cruciferous vegetables) • Methylxanthines • Minerals • Niacin (vitamin B_3) • Phospholipids • Riboflavin (vitamin B_2) • Thiamine (vitamin B_1)

Antioxidants and Nutrients Supporting Intermediate Phase:

Ascorbic Acid (vitamin C) • Beta-carotene (vitamin A) • Coenzyme Q_{10} • Flavonoids • Minerals • Tocopherols (vitamin E)

Nutrients Supporting Phase II Enzymes:

Carnosic Acid (rosemary) • Curcumin (turmeric) • Diallyl Sulfides (garlic) • Ellagic Acid • (red grape skin, raspberries) • Indole-3-Carbinols (cruciferous vegetables) • Isoflavones (soy) • Monoterpenoids (mormilin and limonene from citrus)

One comprehensive detoxification product is Detoxitech by Natural Factors. More information on blood, lymph, colon, and liver detoxification is found in Linda Page, Ph.D.'s book *Healthy Healing*. To order, visit www.healthyhealing.com or call (800)736-6015.

■ *Glutathione.* One of the most important protective substances synthesized by the body is *glutathione*, also referred to as GSH. Consisting of the three amino acids cysteine, glycine, and glutamate (glutamic acid), glutathione is a waterphase molecule present in all human cells. The presence of this substance is a sensitive indicator of a cell's overall state of health and may ultimately prove to be the single most accurate indicator of cellular health.[48] Conversely, its intracellular depletion ultimately results in cellular death.[49]

Glutathione plays a role in many diverse biological processes including cell maturation, enzyme catalysis, intermediary metabolism, protein synthesis, receptor action, and transmembrane transport.[50] It is most abundant in the liver, and is also significantly present in the spleen, red blood cells, lens of the eye, kidneys and leukocytes.[51] One of the major functions of glutathione is as a master antioxidant, fighting damaging substances called *free radicals*. As such, it exerts a direct and powerful effect as an immune system enhancer, radioprotective agent, and detoxifier.

Antioxidant. Molecules are composed of groups of atoms having even pairs of electrons that orbit the centers of the atoms (nuclei) similar to the manner in which planets orbit the sun. A free radical is an atom, molecule, or fragment of a molecule in which one electron has been knocked off, leaving at least one single, unpaired electron orbiting a nucleus. An atom or molecule in such an unbalanced electron arrangement becomes unstable and is aggressively reactive with other substances. In order to restore its own stability, the free radical indiscriminately "steals" an electron from another molecule, thus imbalancing that molecule and making it a free radical as well. This process of electron theft is called *oxidation*, and typically involves the formation of a chain reaction of many billions of free radicals that can occur within the span of a mere fraction of a second.

This cascading chain reaction of free radicals attacks any cell membrane or structure it contacts, causing cellular damage in many locations throughout the body. Approximately every 10 seconds, each of the body's trillions of cells is attacked by a free radical, amounting to over 600 quadrillion (600 followed by 15 zeros) damaging attacks per day. To help you imagine how large this number is, if you begin counting only to one trillion (a much smaller number in comparison to one quadrillion) and count a new number every second—1, 2, 3, etc.—it would take you 32,000 years to finish your count, give or take a few days.

Free radicals including superoxide, peroxide, the hydroxyl radical, and others threaten the integrity of cells, tissues and organs including critical bodily constituents such as DNA, RNA, enzymes, and other proteins.[52] The body's trillions of cells face the continual challenge of neutralizing free radical reactions before they lead to cell impairment and destruction. An impressive body of evidence indicates that free radical damage is a principal contributor to progressive loss of organ function (aging), as well as to maladies such as allergies, Alzheimer's disease, arteriosclerosis, asthma, cancer, cataracts, coronary artery disease, diabetes, immune dysfunction, Parkinson's disease, and stroke.

Antioxidants, as the name implies, are substances that operate against (anti) oxidants. They comprise a group of substances including vitamins, minerals, and enzymes that help neutralize the damaging effects of oxidation within the body. Antioxidants include any substance that delays, inhibits or destroys free radicals. They protect the cells and tissues by scavenging harmful free radicals throughout the body and by breaking the cascading chain reactions of electron thefts.

Glutathione is one of the body's master antioxidants, effective against free radical oxidation that can occur as the result of burns; cigarette smoke; dietary deficiencies of GSH precursors and enzyme cofactors; environmental toxins; heavy metals; household and industrial chemicals; inflammation; pesticides; pharmaceutical drugs; septic shock; strenuous exercise; surgery; ultraviolet (sun) and X-radiation (sun and medical); and viral and bacterial infection.[53]

In addition to its significant antioxidant capability, glutathione also assists in the restoration of other antioxidants that have been oxidized.[54] The many forms of free radicals against which glutathione has been shown effective include 1) hydroxyl radical quenching, 2) secondary radical quenching, 3) quenching of radical centers on DNA, 4) quenching of DNA peroxyl radicals, and 5) reduction of lipid peroxidases.[55]

Immune System Enhancer. The immune system is the body's front-line defense against all forms of illness. A healthy immune system is able to ward off most challenges by infective microbes including bacteria, viruses, fungi, yeasts, and parasites. The immune cells, as is the case with other cells as well, depend upon glutathione to grow and proliferate. Adequate levels of glutathione are required by both T and B lymphocytes to differentiate. Intracellular glutathione is also necessary for T-cell proliferation and other T-cell functions, activation

of T "killer cells," and metabolism of interleukin-2.[56]

Experimental depletion of glutathione has been shown to inhibit immune cell functions, and its intracellular levels in lymphocytes have been shown to be the determining factor of the magnitude of the immune system's capacity.[57] The ability of lymphocytes to combat oxidative damage is a function of their capacity to regenerate intracellular levels of glutathione.[58] Treatment methods which replenish cellular glutathione are therefore expected to optimize the immune system's capability.

Radioprotective Agent. Free-radical-producing radiation is potentially harmful to the human body. Various types of radiation are present in the environment, and there are several main sources. Radiation from cosmic rays and radioactive minerals does not typically endanger the body. Ultraviolet and other forms of radiation from the sun, through the mechanism of free radical production, can cause damage to DNA, the eyes and skin, and play a role in the development of some types of cancers. X-radiation from medical procedures such as X-rays, mammograms, CT-scans, and radiographs are other significant sources of harmful radiation. Yet other sources include waste from nuclear power plants, certain building materials, and residue from the use of military weapons. Studies have shown glutathione acts as a natural protector from potentially-harmful radiation. The supplement beta glucan, as well as Del Immune V (discussed under **General Treatment Methods**), also offer radiation protection.

[Note: Clouds of depleted uranium (DU), a product of U.S. military weapons used in Bosnia, Afghanistan, and Iraq, have been carried by the wind to many countries throughout the world. Japanese physicist Dr. Katsuma Yagasaki of the University of Ryukyusin, has estimated that the atomicity equivalent of at least 400,000 Nagasaki bombs has been released into the global atmosphere since 1991 as the result of the use of DU munitions. The toxic DU brew was found in glaciers and ice sheets globally one year after Gulf War I].

Detoxifier. As discussed above, detoxification is the process whereby the body rids itself of poisonous substances such as xenobiotic chemicals present within the body. It is estimated that up to 75% of detoxification activity takes place in the liver, and glutathione is the cornerstone of the detoxification process. About 70% of the total dietary intake of glutathione is used in the liver where it is stored and exported to other organs.[59] There is also a high concentration of glutathione in the lower regions of the lungs where it aids in neutralizing inhaled toxins such as cigarette smoke and also free radicals produced by activated immune cells within the lungs.[60] The kidneys and intestines, where significant detoxification takes place, also have high levels of glutathione. Its free radical scavenging ability is the key to its systemic detoxification activity at the molecular, cellular and tissue levels.[61]

A vast number of individual ailments are related to glutathione deficiencies:

Arthritis. As is the case in many other illnesses and diseases, free radical production plays a significant role in the inflammatory process which is a component of rheumatoid arthritis. Studies of patients with high persistent disease activity show depleted levels of glutathione in serum, red blood cells, and white blood cells.[62] Increasing glutathione by supplementation would be assumed to beneficially modify the course of the disease.

Cancer. The development of cancer has been associated with a drop in glutathione levels.[63] In both humans and animals, the incidence of cancer increases progressively with age. Two theories attempt to explain this phenomenon. The free radical theory of aging suggests that oxidative stress may account for carcinogenesis due to nonrepairable tissue damage over time. Another explanation is the accumulation of toxic burden that accompanies increased toxic exposure over time. Substantiating this later notion is the fact that many known carcinogens are detoxified by glutathione, including aflatoxin B_1, benzidine, dimethylhydrazine, dimethylnitrosamine, N-methyl-4- aminoazobenzene, and many others.[64] These two theories suggest glutathione to be a cancer-protective agent due to its dual function as both an antioxidant and a detoxifying agent.

Cardiovascular. Researchers have observed that heart attack patients and males with a family history of coronary artery disease have lowered levels of glutathione.[65] Atherosclerosis, deposits in the inner layer of arteries, has been linked to oxidative damage of arterial walls.[66] Oxidative stress within diseased arteries depletes glutathione, other anti-oxidants, and shifts the body's balance from anti-inflammatory to pro-inflammatory.[67] Intravenous administration of glutathione prior to heart bypass surgery favorably influenced postoperative kidney function and systemic arterial function.[68] Administration of glutathione and/or combinations of antioxidants can raise the threshold of platelet aggregation, thereby protecting the sensitive endothelial layer from further damage.[69]

Chronic Fatigue Syndrome. Chronic Fatigue Syndrome (CFS; also called Chronic Fatigue and Immune Deficiency Syndrome, CFIDS) is a group of symptoms of unknown cause including fatigue, cognitive dysfunction, and sometimes fever and abnormal enlargement of the lymph nodes. As the name CFIDS suggests, chronic fatigue seems intimately related to a deficient immune system. Also, studies have shown it to be related to toxic exposure with impaired detoxification. With both of these causative factors, glutathione is a major player, and shortages are common in CFS patients. Studies have shown glutathione supplementation increases immune function as well as improving symptoms of CFS by aiding in detoxification.[70]

Diabetes. Subjects with reduced insulin sensitivity, a common symptom of diabetes or prediabetes, show reduced blood levels of glutathione. Both red blood cells and platelets can experience low glutathione levels.[71] It has been shown that mild to moderate exercise helps normalize glutathione levels in diabetics,[72] but strenuous exercise tends to cause depletion.[73]

Exercise. Movement of the body is accomplished through muscles. The more strenuous the movement (exercise), the more oxygen the muscles require. Physical exercise increases by 300% the difference between arterial and venous oxygen levels, and increases blood flow through tissue by 3,000%.[74] It is this use of oxygen which produces free radicals. The more strenuous the exercise, the more oxygen consumed, and the more free radicals are generated in the process. As free radicals are generated, antioxidant defenses are depleted, particularly glutathione in both the muscles and total body glutathione pools.[75] Studies have shown that low glutathione levels decrease exercise endurance by up to 50%, while causing far more oxidative damage to the muscles.[76] Raising glutathione levels increases performance in all of the cells of the body, including muscle cells. This is one cornerstone of building a stronger, more muscular body. One recent study[77] found that when glutathione was raised by supplementation, both peak power and work capacity increased by 13%.

Infection. As discussed above, a properly-functioning immune system requires adequate levels of glutathione. In HIV infection, for example, there is systemic glutathione depletion.[78] Glutathione levels are lowered in blood plasma; red blood cells; T-cells and other lymphocytes; and monocytes.[79] Depleted levels of lung epithelial lining fluid (ELF) may predispose those with HIV to opportunistic lung infection. Symptoms of AIDS wasting may be helped by glutathione replenishment, and ELF may be replenished using aerosolized glutathione.[80] At all stages of HIV infection, oxidative stress is elevated and can benefit from glutathione replenishment.

Liver. Because glutathione stores are highest in the liver, it stands to reason that its deficiency is implicated in liver disease. In a study[81] of 48 patients with liver cirrhosis, a 400-800% decrease in plasma glutathione was found compared to healthy patients. Plasma and liver glutathione decreases have been found in patients with acute viral hepatitis, chronic hepatitis, alcoholic liver disease, and non-alcoholic cirrhosis.[82] Acetaminophen, other pharmaceutical drugs, as well as other xenobiotics can deplete liver glutathione levels.

Lungs. There is a high concentration of glutathione in the lungs of healthy persons, and its deficiency is linked to many pulmonary diseases including chronic obstructive pulmonary disease (COPD), acute respiratory distress syndrome (ARDS), neonatal lung damage, and asthma.[83] This is not surprising as the lungs are especially vulnerable to oxidative attack from several inhaled sources including airborne toxins, oxygen, and oxygen free radicals released by active white blood cells within the lungs. Glutathione replenishment has been shown to speed ARDS patients' release from intensive care.[84] The administration of nebulized (aerosolized) glutathione has been used successfully in the treatment of emphysema.[85]

Neurological. The pathological hallmark of Parkinson's disease is loss of dopamine-producing neurons in a portion of the midbrain called *sub-stantia nigra pars compacta*, or SNpc. When dopamine secretion from SNpc becomes deficient, the classical symptoms of the disease begin to manifest. Research has shown that free radical-induced oxidative stress is an important causative factor in Parkinson's.[86] Of the various biological alterations that occur in clinically-detectable Parkinson's disease, only loss of total glutathione is detectable in presymptomatic Parkinson's. This appears to be an early event in the causation of the disease.[87]

Although alterations in glutathione levels appear secondary in the pathogenesis of Alzheimer's, oral vitamin E intake has been shown to delay its progression in patients with moderately severe impairment. This supports the notion that oxidative stress plays a role in the pathogenesis of the disease.[88]

Because only trace amounts of glutathione precursors are found in food, other sources are required to boost the body's stores. This can take the form of glutathione itself, or various orthomolecular glutathione precursors, discussed below.

Oral Glutathione. Traditionally, it has been believed that oral glutathione supplementation does not increase systemic bioavailability.[89] However, studies have shown it is efficiently absorbed across the intestinal epithelium, reaches the blood intact, but is broken down prior to its accessing the liver.[90] Therefore, oral glutathione supplementation would be more advantageous for certain diseases, e.g., diseases of the gastrointestinal tract such as Crohn's disease.[91] Various case studies of neurodegenerative diseases such as Parkinson's disease have shown benefit from intravenous glutathione.[92] It appears glutathione levels in healthy subjects is so well buffered that it is difficult to increase its levels in this population.

Other Methods of Administering Glutathione. The intact glutathione molecule can be effectively delivered directly into the lungs via aerosolized particles where it is absorbed by pulmonary alveolar cells.[93] The enterocyte cells lining the intestinal tract absorb it by diffusion, and export it to the blood.[94] Blood vessel endothelial cells, retinal pigmented epithelial cells, and cells of the kidney's proximal tubule also absorb intact glutathione. The molecule is also able to cross the blood-brain barrier[95]—the brain's biological firewall which prevents toxins from entering the brain.

Glutathione is now available in a liposomal form for oral supplementation. Liposomes are tiny spheres (100-500 nanometers) made from essential phospholipids—the same material as cell membranes. The glutathione is contained within these tiny spheres and when taken orally, have an absorption rate of about 90%. Two liposomal glutathione products are Lipoceutical® Glutathione, available at www.autismcoach.com, and ReadiSorb® Liposomal Glutathione, available at www.readisorb.com.

■ *N-Acetyl Cysteine* (NAC). The amino acid cysteine is one of glutathione's most important precursors, and is the precursor which most significantly limits the body's synthesis of glutathione. Although supplementation with cysteine can replenish glutathione levels, it may be unsafe for high-dose oral administration as it degrades into potentially-toxic byproducts and is a neural excitotoxin.[96] The potent antioxidant NAC, however, is a bioavailable source of cysteine that safely and effectively replenishes glutathione levels in depleted individuals.[97]

Intravenous administration can improve lung function in patients with septic shock.[98] Dosages of 600 mg/day have been shown beneficial and innocuous, while one researcher found 1,200-1,800 mg/day caused side-effects.[99] Other studies have used significantly higher dosages in the treatment of HIV patients, with negligible side-effects.[100] According to a study reported in the *European Journal of Clinical Investigation*[101] in 2000, 31 HIV-infected patients supplementing with oral NAC had near normal levels of glutathione at the termination of the two month trial. The study authors concluded that NAC increases protection against oxidative stress, improves immune function, and detoxifies acetaminophen and other drugs.

■ *S-Adenosyl Methionine* (SAM-e). The amino acid L-methionine is another precursor of glutathione, and is another means of GSH replenishment. Methionine is an essential amino acid, and must be obtained from food. However, methionine occurs "metabolically upstream," and must first be converted to cysteine before it is available for synthesis into glutathione. Many cofactors are involved in this process, and these complex metabolic pathways may be inactive in certain adults,

children, and patients with liver disease.[102] SAM-e is an activated methionine metabolite that is effective in raising red blood cell and liver glutathione levels when taken orally at 1,600 mg per day.[103] It has been shown effective in treating liver cirrhosis and cholestasis (a problem with the flow of bile).[104]

■ *Alpha-lipoic Acid* (ALA). Alpha lipoic acid is a broad-spectrum antioxidant that functions in both lipid (fatty) and aqueous (watery) environments. ALA is a powerful antioxidant with potent electron-donating capacity. Supplementing with alpha-lipoic acid has been shown to be an effective means of glutathione replenishment. When taken orally, it has been shown to raise GSH levels in HIV patients, while being extremely safe and well tolerated. As a Krebs cycle cofactor and metal chelator, ALA has added biochemical versatility.[105] Further, it is able to cross the blood brain barrier, the tight junction of tissues which prevents most substances from gaining entrance to the brain. R-lipoic acid is a potent new form of lipoic acid which is likely to substantially increase its benefits in every aspect of its use. To learn more, visit www.r-lipoic.com.

■ *Infrared Sauna*. Saunas are another means of detoxification. The word "sauna" is Scandanavian, and refers to a method of heating the body that results in many positive effects. Generally, heating within an enclosed space is supplied either by wood, gas, rocks, or electricity. The rationale is to raise body temperature by several degrees after which, in an attempt to reduce its temperature, the body generates copious amounts of sweat. Saunas have been used for centuries by cultures around the globe for their health-promoting benefits. The Native American tradition of the sweat lodge exemplifies this practice. While saunas of times past used hot air, modern technology provides a more healthful alternative in the form of the infrared (IR) sauna.

One of the most efficient and effective means of detoxifying the body is through the use of the IR sauna. As the name implies, this technology supplies heat by producing energy in the form of infrared rays. This type of energy (heat) is also known as radiant heat, which heats objects directly through the process of "conversion" rather than by heating the surrounding air. IR energy produces temperatures in the range of 110-130° Fahrenheit, penetrating the body 1.5-3 inches. IR saunas produce a very uniform warming effect, with the skin absorbing more than 90% of the infrared rays.[106] Conventional saunas produce temperatures in the range of 180-235° F.

Although IR saunas have been shown to provide many health benefits including general pain relief, normalizing blood pressure, improving digestive disorders, and weight loss,[107] they are unsurpassed as a means of bodily detoxification. When our total toxic burden exceeds the body's ability to eliminate these environmental poisons, they begin to accumulate—compromising good health by causing chronic disease states. If detoxification is not initiated, the internalized poisons continue to negatively influence our health.

The body eliminates toxins via several routes, including the feces, urine, respiration, and perspiration. IR saunas remove toxins via the perspiration, and are effective in removing both chemical and heavy metal toxins.[108] Especially if the kidneys and/or liver have been damaged by toxins, the body's ability to detoxify through excretion of feces and urine becomes severely compromised.

IR saunas are effective in removing both lipid- (fat) stored and aqueous- (water) stored toxins. Toxic substances such as mercury, lead, and chlorine—or toxic gasses such as sulphur or carbon dioxide—contact water molecules and are encapsulated by clusters of these molecules. As the infrared waves contact these large water molecules they begin to vibrate, reducing the ion bonds that hold the molecules together. As they are gradually broken down, encapsulated substances are released such as toxic gasses and heavy metals.[109] Many toxins are stored in fatty tissues, which are broken down in a similar manner. Just below the surface of the skin lies a layer of fat and oil. As the skin temperature increases, these fatty substances "melt" and ooze from the skin's oil glands. By showering following the sauna, the toxins are washed away, reducing the body's toxic burden.

In one recent study,[110] conventional saunas were compared to infrared saunas. The sweat produced by a conventional "hot air" sauna was 95-97% water, while the sweat produced by the IR sauna was 80-85% water, the remainder of the non-water portion being cholesterol, fat-soluble toxins, heavy metals (such as aluminum and mercury),

ammonia, sodium, sulfuric acid, and uric acid. This concentration of fat-soluble toxins and heavy metals isn't found in sweat from normal exercise.

According to a 1992 article in the *Townsend Letter for Doctors and Patients*,[111] IR saunas are 7-10 times more effective in releasing toxins than conventional saunas, and produce 2-3 times the sweat volume while operating at an air temperature 70-100° cooler. The study authors conclude that IR saunas accomplish the following:[112]

• Detoxification of heavy metals, including aluminum, cadmium, lead, and mercury
• Detoxification of Agent Orange, arsenic, formaldehyde, industrial chemicals, and pesticides
• Detoxification of alcohol, nicotine and drugs
• Purification of the body on a cellular level

Most commercially-available infrared saunas use zirconium ceramic elements as their heat source. These elements produce wavelengths in the *far* infrared portion of the electromagnetic spectrum. Some health practitioners have suggested that incandescent, electric light infrared (infrared heat lamp)—which emit full-spectrum infrared—provide more health benefits compared to the more narrow emissions of ceramic elements. (250 watt incandescent IR bulbs are available in hardware stores. Halogen infrared lamps are believed by some to output a less healthful spectra compared to the incandescent bulbs.) To learn more about IR saunas and their ability to detoxify, visit www.gaia saunas.com or www.sunlightsaunas.com.

[Here's an interesting aside regarding detoxification, although a slightly different meaning of the word. While the above discussion focuses on detoxification of living organisms, there is a new technology for detoxifying (decontaminating) deceased organisms. More precisely, the technology focuses on decontamination of decaying biomass such as the large number of potentially-disease-producing human remains resulting from either natural or man-made disasters (hurricanes, tsunamis, war, etc.). It is also used to decontaminate water, and also structures, from organisms that can produce infection, odor, etc. Used since 1982, Effective Microorganisms® (EM Technology) consists of three types of microorganisms: phototropic bacteria, lactic acid bacteria, and yeast. The Thai Army used EM following the Asian tsunami disaster to spray decomposing bodies with the ecologically harmless microbial culture. The German government used EM to decontaminate standing toxic waters following the flooding of the Elbe River in 2002. EM-America, the U.S. company that markets EM, can be contacted at (866)369-3678, www.emamerica.com.]

Nutritional deficiencies exacerbate the body's inability to detoxify. The remainder of this section disusses what specific nutritional factors are of most importance not only for detoxification but for general health as well.

Superfoods

Americans spend about 90% of their food budgets on processed food, with roughly 10,000 new processed-food products being made available to American households each year. These types of foods contain lower levels of fiber, minerals, phytonutrients, vitamins, and other valuable food components in comparison to natural, unprocessed foods such as fruits, vegetables, seeds, nuts, and whole grains. Processed, low-nutrient-dense foods are unquestionably linked to poor health and decreased vitality, and studies have demonstrated a relationship between the modern, Western diet and the increase of chronic diseases over the past century.[113]

Superfoods represent a practical solution to our severely-deficient food supply by supplying high-quality food substances such as amino acids, carbohydrates, enzymes, essential fatty acids, fiber, minerals, phytonutrients, protein and vitamins.

Algae. The microalgaes such as *aphanizomenon flos aquae*, *chlorella*, *dunaliella*, and *spirulina* qualify as "superfoods," having a superabundance of compact nutrients that provide numerous documented health benefits. It is known that seaweeds and microalgae have been used as a food source since time immemorial, and are still used by various native tribes throughout the world. Microalgae is a rich source of essential amino acids, essential fatty acids, minerals, protein, and vitamins.[114] In today's polluted world, it's difficult to locate sources of "clean" trace and ultra-trace minerals. Microalgaes are one such source, relatively free of contamination, depending upon the location of harvest. Because they have been a staple of man for centuries, they are known to be safe and effective.

Stabilized Rice Bran (SRB). Another powerful superfood is *Stabilized Rice Bran* (SRB), a product derived from rice. This superfood is not only quite delicious, it is one of Earth's most nutrient-dense substances. Rice bran is comprised of a coating that surrounds the white rice kernel. This coating is stripped off during the milling process known as "polishing," leaving only the familiar white rice. In the past, the rice bran polishes were removed and discarded, largely because an enzyme component of the bran causes it to turn rancid within hours of milling. Ironically, this wasted resource has been found to contain a gold mine of concentrated nutrients. Until recently, however, these nutrients could not be cultivated as there was no means of preventing the bran from becoming rancid. Now, a stabilization technique involving dry heat extrusion allows the bran to retain its inherent nutrients in a biologically-active form. Stabilized Rice Bran is this form of rice bran—one of the most nutrient-dense foods in the world.

Stabilized Rice Bran is a significant source nutritional fiber, hypoallergenic protein and myriad phytonutrients and natural antioxidants. Antioxidants 100 times more potent than vitamin E have been identified in SRB, and it is a source of more than 100 different antioxidants, the significance of which is that most antioxidants act synergistically rather than separately. Stabilized Rice Bran is also a good source of essential fatty acids (EFAs)—otherwise known as "good fats"—fats that promote good health. If that weren't enough, SRB contains a storehouse of minerals, trace minerals, and other vital substances including:[115]

❏ B-complex vitamins, including a natural source of IP_6, which is important to immune function.

❏ Vitamin A compounds, including beta-carotene (pro-vitamin A) and mixed carotenoids (which are vitamin A compounds, of which there are over 800 types), including alpha-carotene, beta-carotene, lycopene, lutein, and zeaxanthin. The presence of the many carotenoids in SRB has important health implications.

❏ Vitamin E family. SRB is a rich source of the *entire* vitamin E complex. It contains the highest natural source of mixed *tocopherols* and mixed *tocotrienols* in nature, the two main categories that comprise the eight different types of vitamin E.

(Evidence has shown the various forms of vitamin E are best taken together.)

❏ High quality omega-6 and omega-3 EFAs

❏ Fiber—both soluble and insoluble

❏ Gamma-Oryzanol—the only sizeable source of Gamma-Oryzanol in nature. All other Gamma-Oryzanol is synthesized in a laboratory.

❏ Phytosterols, including beta-sitosterol, beta-sitosterolin and nearly a dozen others which have important beneficial effects in the human body. These substances, derived from the non-nutritive portion of plants, help lower cholesterol, act as anti-inflammatories, and support immunity. By inhibiting abnormal cell growth, they also help prevent cancer.

❏ Dimethylglycine (DMG) and Trimethylglycine (TMG). Because the human body produces only small amounts of DMG, the diet is the main source of its availability. Present in the cells of plants and animals, DMG's consumption in the diet may improve the health by improving the utilization of oxygen at the cellular level. TMG and DMG function in the biochemical processes related to neurotransmitter production, cardiovascular health and DNA repair. They also are thought to improve mood, well-being, and concentration, and to decrease the risk of cancer and cardiovascular disease.

❏ Fructooligosaccharides (FOS), which help support intestinal ecology, bowel regularity and health. As such, FOS is useful in the treatment of irritable bowel syndrome. It has been shown to significantly reduce fasting blood glucose levels, thus helping to control Type 2 diabetes.

❏ Lecithin, which contains substances such as phosphatidylcholine and phosphatidylserine that help the brain learn and remember.

❏ Ferulic acid, which helps block the harmful effects of sunlight's UV radiation, protects the arteries and reduces the tendency of blood to clot.

❏ Para-coumaric acid, which may protect against stomach cancers through the blocking of pro-carcinogenic compounds.

❏ Proanthocyandins—very powerful flavonoid antioxidants—protect against capillary fragility by strengthening blood vessels and connective tissues.

❏ Co-enzyme Q10 (CoQ10), which is cardio-protective and necessary for proper heart function.

❏ Squalene, which is chemically similar to beta-carotene (provitamin A). It has documented cholesterol-lowering effects and anecdotally has been touted as an anti-cancer agent (which has not been substantiated).

❏ Alpha-Lipoic-Acid (ALA), which helps replenish glutathione levels and may help retard aging.

Clinical trials demonstrate that Stabilized Rice Bran helps maintain normal blood sugar levels, and lowers cholesterol and triglycerides as well. Patents have been issued in these areas attesting to its effectiveness.

Chia. A relative newcomer on the superfood scene in the Western world is really one of man's oldest superfoods. Known as *salba*, or more commonly as *chia* (both terms are used interchangeably)—and botanically as *Salvia hispanica*—this super seed has been used by man since 2500 B.C. If the name "chia" sounds familiar, it's probably due to a 1980's TV commercial in which sprouted chia seed was used to grow "hair" on a variety of small terre-cotta pet figures. The catchy tune accompanying the words "Ch-ch-ch-chia" may ring a bell for baby boomers.

Chia was used by both the ancient Mayan and Aztec cultures. It was an integral part of the Aztec diet as well as a survival ration of their warriors who claimed to be sustained for an entire day on the equivalent of one tablespoon of seed. Chia was also used as endurance food by Aztec runners, and was nicknamed "running food." It was sometimes used as currency, and was also a component of Aztec religious ceremonies—thought to impart mystical and supernatural powers. When the Spanish conquistadors invaded Mexico in 1519, they all but destroyed the chia crops in favor of planting foods familiar to the Spaniards.

The modern resurgence of this nutrient-dense seed is due in large part to the efforts of Dr. Wayne Coats, a retired research professor at the University of Arizona. In 1991, Dr. Coates took seed from Mexican crops and replanted in Argentina, thus beginning the general availability of the seed to modern man. Coates' book *Chia: Rediscovering a Forgotten Crop of the Aztecs*, is the definitive treatise on the subject of chia.

At 16% by weight, chia has more protein than soy—and of a higher quality. Unlike soy, chia's protein contains all of the essential amino acids needed by the body. With 38% of its weight as fiber, it has more fiber than flaxseed. It has 31% fat and is the highest plant source of omega-3 fatty acids, most of which is in the form of alpha-linolenic acid (ALA) which is converted by the body into DHA and EPA. Because the seed has a natural resistance to insects, it's grown without the use of pesticides and is therefore contaminant free—unlike many varieties of fish (and their oils) which are increasingly plagued by contaminants such as mercury, PCBs, and other potentially dangerous chemicals.

Chia has six times more calcium than whole milk, 15 times more magnesium than broccoli, and three times the antioxidant power of fresh blueberries. It's lower in carbohydrates than other grains, low in sodium, and is an excellent source of both soluble and insoluble fiber. The fact that the grain is non-allergenic, non-GMO, and doesn't contain gluten are additional benefits.

Studies have shown that chia is equally as effective as fish oil in lowering triglyceride and LDL cholesterol levels, while raising the HDL. Daily use of the seed has been shown to significantly decrease blood pressure, C-reactive protein, and fibrogenic factors, as well as improving the omega-3 to omega-6 ratio. It also has been shown to help stabilize blood sugar levels and aid in weight loss by slowing the conversion of carbohydrates into sugar. The chia seed is very hydrophilic (water absorbing), and can hold up to 12 times its weight in water, thus prolonging hydration.

There are three urban legends, or myths, surrounding chia—all of which have been debunked by Dr. Coates, the Sage of Salba, if you will. The first is that it's best to consume chia after it has been soaked in water. According to Coates, soaking the seed releases the soluble fiber, which is of no significant benefit. Traditional use involves soaking the seed into a gelatinous form and adding sugar and other ingredients. Unlike flax, the chia seed is easily digestible without grinding or otherwise altering its natural from—although it can be ground and soaked.

The second myth is that there is a difference between more expensive white (sometimes denoted "salba") and more reasonably priced black "chia" seed. Dr. Coats explains it is only a marketing ploy which attempts to differentiate between the two colors of seed. Their compositional characteristics are virtually identical. (See www.arizonachia.com/blackwhite.html to view Dr. Coates' comparison chart of the protein, oil, and fatty acid profile of white versus black seed.)

The third point of contention is that some companies market "certified, organically grown" seed. Because no pesticides are needed to grow chia, and there is no use of solvents, irradiation, or the like, all chia seed is relatively comparable in purity and can't legitimately be claimed "certified organic."

Unlike fruits and vegetables which are largely air and water, chia offers densely-packed nutrition. Accordingly, the daily recommended serving is only two to three tablespoons for adults and one tablespoon for children. Because of its neutral taste in any form—whole seed, soaked, or ground—it can be sprinkled on a variety of foods, including cereal; blended in a smoothie or shake; mixed with flour and baked in breads, cakes, and cookies; or otherwise consumed in most any fashion. Unlike flax, chia seed can be stored without refrigeration for long periods of time without spoiling—so long as it's kept dry. A variety of companies market chia at significantly different prices. Two good companies are Hidalgo Foods (www.hidalgofoods.com) and Good Cause Wellness (www.goodcausewellness.com).

The shift from natural, whole, nutrient-dense foods to their perverted, nutrient-deficient, lifeless counterparts is linked to virtually every degenerative disease known to afflict mankind, including the four major chronic diseases: cardiovascular disease, cancer, diabetes and neurological illness. Superfoods offer an opportunity to prevent and even reverse a significant amount of our modern ailments by providing a nutrient-packed source of nourishment. They are nature's answer to the misguided oversight of mankind that fails to recognize the relationship of food to health. Superfoods are nature's champion in the battle against disability and death, empowering those who consume them to deliver a decisive blow to poor health and chronic disease.

Enzymes

Enzymes are so essential they have been termed "the fountain of life." Biological enzymes are the basis of the chemical life of man. They initiate, catalyze (accelerate) and regulate all chemical reactions in the body in an orchestration of intelligence and control. Up to 40% of the body's daily protein synthesis is used in the production of upward of 50,000 enzymes the body requires.

Dr. Edward Howell, author of several books on enzymes and the man considered the Father of Enzyme Therapy, is a true pioneer in the field. Howell has suggested that "the length of life is inversely proportional to the rate of exhaustion of the enzyme potential of an organism."[116] They are the life force, the *élan vital*, present in every biological system. The principal difference between healthy and unhealthy food, according to Howell, is related to its enzyme content. Enzymes are, as it were, the true yardstick of biological vitality. "Life is an enzyme process." They power our very existence—breathing, our mental functions, and even reproductive functions. They also aid in assimilating nutrients from food, destroy harmful microorganisms, and modulate chemical processes such as detoxification.

There are three categories of enzymes: food, digestive, and metabolic. Food enzymes are present within the foods we eat, especially in raw, natural, unprocessed foods. Even in raw foods, however, they are destroyed by prolonged heating over 118° F, as happens when foods are cooked. Food enzymes, when present, begin digestion in the stomach so that the contents reaching the duodenum continues to be easily broken down and assimilated. It is nature's plan for food enzymes to aid in digestion so that the body's endogenous digestive enzymes aren't called upon to carry the entire burden.[117]

There are two basic sources of enzymes. Either they are synthesized by the body from proteins or supplied by ingesting enzyme-rich foods through the diet. When food enzymes are present to assist in the workload, less digestive enzymes are required to be produced, enabling the body to devote more of its resources to the synthesis of the metabolic enzymes that power the entire body's myriad chemical reactions. When enzymeless, processed foods are consumed, a significant drain is placed upon the body's pool of enzyme machinery needed to manufacture metabolic enzymes. Over a lifetime, the body suffers in both health and longevity when metabolic enzyme production is not aided by the presence of dietary enzymes. The key

to preserving life-giving enzyme activity is to remove the burden from the digestive enzyme-making machinery.

Enzymes are so crucial to the body's healthy functioning that without adequate enzyme production, a "deficiency-like" state occurs that has been linked to chronic disease, accelerated aging and premature death by various well-known researchers including Dr. Edward Howell, Dr. William Kelley, Dr. Francis Pottenger, Dr. Royal Lee, Dr. Weston Price and Dr. Nicholas Gonzales. Animal studies have shown that organisms consuming smaller amounts of food routinely live longer than those which consume larger quantities. It is believed this effect is significantly related to the sparing of the need to produce digestive enzymes, thereby enabling maximal enzyme activity throughout the remainder of the body.[118]

There is a familiar adage which states that, "You Are What You Eat." In reality, a more correct rendition would be "You Are What You Eat, Digest and Assimilate (Absorb)," or, "You Are What You Don't Excrete." Digestive enzymes help break down and liberate protein, carbohydrates, fats, herbs, and vitamins within food. Therefore, they are essential for the maximum absorption and proper utilization of nutrients.

The consumption of foods with low enzyme content contributes to weight gain and obesity. Raw foods are usually nutrient dense, low in saturated fats, high in enzyme content, high in fiber and low in calories. According to Dr. Howell, "raw foods are relatively non-stimulating to glands and tend to stabilize weight."[119] Processed (cooked and otherwise manipulated) foods, on the other hand, are usually nutrient deficient, high in saturated fats, low in enzyme content, low in fiber and high in calories. Calories derived from cooked foods excite glands and tend to cause weight gain. As a general rule, cooked foods are much more fattening than raw foods, as raw foods are naturally endowed with enzymes that help the body properly utilize fat. Fat is not fattening, especially when present in its raw state, as fatty foods in their raw state are naturally endowed with copious amounts of lipase, an enzyme which helps break down and metabolize fat.

Consuming certain foods has been associated with significant health benefits including disease prevention. Foods such as aged cheeses and meats (preferably organic), sprouted grains, and raw fruits and vegetables—largely lacking in Western societies—provide a diet rich in enzymes. Fermented foods such as Kim Chee, pickles, miso, tofu, natto, and certain soybean products such as soy sauce, are replete with enzymes. It must be acknowledged that enzymes are a necessary part of our diet, and recognized that they have always been a constituent of *all* natural foods. Because enzymes fulfill an essential biological function, they should be considered an essential nutrient.

Research has shown that enzyme deficiency leads to a variety of chronic health conditions. There is a confirmed link between the intestines/digestion and rheumatic, auto-immune, allergic, and mental conditions. All of these ailments are interconnected to the enzyme content of our diet. The general degeneration of health likely involves a deficiency of enzymes. Enzyme therapy has been shown to benefit many health conditions, including acute and chronic bronchitis, aging, arthritis, autism, blood clotting, cancer, colitis, Crohn's disease, eczema, edema, fibrocystic breast disease, food allergies, gum disease (Gingivitis), headache, hives, inflammation, lymphedema, malabsorption/malnutrition, multiple sclerosis, pancreatitis, pancreatic indigestion, pelvic inflammatory disease, sinusitis, soft-tissue injuries, stroke, tissue healing, ulcerative colitis, venous and arterial disease, and vomiting. Other conditions known to respond to enzyme therapy are asthma, eczema, hay fever, loose bowels, psoriasis, and weight loss. The increase in the incidence of these illnesses corresponds to the reduction of enzyme content in the Western diet.

Various forms of cancer are often helped by enzyme therapy. The high death rate of this disease is associated with changes in enzyme chemistry. Because enzyme supplementation reduces the body's burden of making digestive enzymes, it allows the body to channel more metabolic enzymes to the site of the malignancy. The works of Drs. Max Wolfe, William Kelley and Nicholas Gonzales have proved this approach valuable. Dr. Wolfe was one of the first to demonstrate that supplementation of enzymes by individuals afflicted with cancer helps re-establish the ability to destroy tumor cells.[120] Dr. Gonzales has had excellent success in treating pancreatic cancer patients with enzymes. In addition to the above conditions, en-

zymes are indicated for anyone who wishes to practice preventive healthcare and to build a strong foundation of health.

The most healthful diet would consist of at least 50% raw food, preferably 75%. This allows one to absorb up to 90% of nutrients such as vitamins and minerals, while those who eat cooked, enzymeless foods may absorb nutrients in the range of 15-20%.[121] However, consuming high levels of raw foods is a practical impossibility for many. Therefore, supplementing with enzymes would be prudent for these people. How enzymes should be consumed and what enzyme forms are the best, however, are items of some debate.

The historical record shows that sprouted seeds have been consumed by man for millenia. Used both medicinally and nutritionally, ancient Chinese physicians reported over 5,000 years ago the disease-treating and health-benefitting role of the humble sprout. Although accounts of sprouting are reported in manuscripts including the Old Testament book of Daniel, it is only recently that the nutritional and medicinal merits of sprouting have been recognized.[122]

Enzymes from sprouted grains may have advantages over animal or fungal-derived enzymes. Fungal enzymes are made by a fermentation method using cultured fungi such as the Aspergillus species, and may cause allergies in people sensitive to molds or fungi. Nevertheless, they are a source of potent enzyme potential that can function in a variety of acid or base levels. Digestive enzyme supplements derived from fungi begin their work in the upper stomach, unlike animal-derived enzymes which don't function until reaching the lower stomach and intestines.[123]

Animal enzymes such as *pancreatin* and *pepsin* assist in the digestion of food in the intestinal tract and lower stomach. Stomach acid is needed for the activation of this type of enzyme. Low levels of stomach acid may fail to activate animal enzymes, thereby blocking their ability to perform digestive functions. (The condition of non-optimal levels of stomach acid, termed *hypochlorhydria* or *achlorhydria*, is very common in the elderly and may further contribute to deficiencies of vitamins B_2, B_6, B_{12}, and zinc as well as improper digestion and poor absorption). Furthermore, animal enzymes carry concerns of BSE (Mad Cow Disease).

However, there is ample documentation on the use of certain animal enzymes—namely trypsin and chymotrypsin—in modulating inflammation, and they are not without merit.

Sprouted grains, on the other hand, are a tremendous source of enzymes without the risk inherent in animal-based enzymes. They contain *amylases* (carbohydrate-digesting enzymes), *proteases* (protein-digesting enzymes) and *lipases* (fat-digesting enzymes), as well as roughly 1,000 additional classified and unclassified enzymes.

Sprouting involves germinating seeds over a three-to-four day span. During this time enzyme activity reaches it maximum level. To insure maximal enzyme potential, therefore, it's best to eat sprouts before the fifth day, as their enzyme potential decreases dramatically thereafter.

Sprouting multiplies the level of enzymes, vitamins and minerals contained in the cereal germ, liberating many varied types of enzymes. Sprouted grains are also a rich source of vitamins A, B-complex, C, D, E, and minerals such as calcium, magnesium, phosphorous, manganese, iron, zinc, potassium, selenium, silicon, chloride, chromium, and iodine, to name just a few. Certain grains such as spelt, Kamut® and rye are virtually superfoods in their own rights as well as being enzyme and nutritional storehouses.[124]

While enzymes are abundant in raw vegetables and fruits, their concentration in these foods is minuscule compared to sprouted seeds. Amazingly, there are 10 to 100 times more enzymes in sprouted seeds than in vegetables or fruits, and there is no food source higher in enzymes than sprouted seeds.[125] (Enzymes produced from sprouted grains are derived from seeds, not from the plant. Accordingly, they are gluten free.) Spelt, Kamut and rye are three of the most enzyme-rich and nutrient-dense sprouted grains.

The consequences of food-enzyme deficiency constitutes a serious oversight to optimal nutrition. Degenerative diseases such as cancer, heart disease, and premature aging are intimately connected to a compromised metabolism resulting in large part from the lack of enzymes in our modern foods. Enzymes are catalysts that lower the energy required to drive every chemical reaction in our bodies, without which these thousands of processes could not occur. Dr. Howell remarks,

Constituents of unprocessed natural foods have had countless eons of time to mold and shape the form and function of living organisms and have created a dependence to fill a need. Therefore, to remove any part of natural food from the normal diet could not be sanctioned because of the possibility of harm to the health and well-being. By eating food with their enzymes intact and by supplementing cooked foods with enzymes, we can stop abnormal and pathological aging processes... if we postpone the degradation of metabolic enzyme activity, what we now call old age could become the glorious prime of life. Enzymes, thus, may be the "fountain of life" so earnestly sought and so mysteriously illusive.[126]

Minerals and Trace Elements

Minerals are naturally-occurring, inorganic chemical elements found in the Earth and sea. As rocks and stones are broken down over millennia by the processes of environmental erosion, the remaining dust and sand particles form the basis of our soil. Other soil ingredients consist of varying amounts of organic matter originating from plant and animal debris, as well as microorganisms such as algae, bacteria and fungi. Mineral elements are assimilated by plants as part of their life processes, and in turn provide nourishment as the plants are consumed by both man and animal. Animals also provide mineral nourishment as they are consumed by both man and other animals.

Minerals are classified as either major minerals or trace elements, and together they compose about 4% of the body's total weight. Major (macro) minerals are the familiar elements calcium, chloride, magnesium, phosphorus, potassium, sodium and sulfur, and each element makes up no less than 0.01% of the body's total weight. These minerals make up all but a very small amount of the body's total mineral content. Humans require a daily intake of major minerals of at least 350-2,000 *milligrams* (mg; thousandths of a gram), depending upon the specific mineral.

Trace elements, or micro minerals as they are sometimes called, are those elements present in the Earth's soil in amounts less than 0.1% by weight, and each makes up less than 0.01% body weight. Although several trace elements are required in larger amounts, most are required in *microgram* quantities (mcg; millionths of a gram).

Examples of some of the more well-known trace elements include arsenic, barium, chromium, cobalt, copper, fluoride, iodine, iron, lithium, nickel, selenium, tin, zinc and zirconium. Some trace elements are present in the body in such small quantities they are difficult even to measure. Nevertheless, the presence of such minute quantities or the small requirement levels of these elements do not represent an accurate measure of their importance to the health and proper functioning of the body. For example, the absence of slightly more than one millionth of an ounce of iodine causes thyroid gland enlargement.

Although iodine was recognized as being related to thyroid function as early as 1850, the importance of many trace elements has only recently been discovered. It was only during the 1980s, for example, that boron and vanadium were recognized as playing important roles in several specific bodily functions.

As many as 80 chemical elements have been detected in the blood, brain, muscle and organs of human and animal tissue. Research over many decades has demonstrated either a proven or suggested beneficial role for nearly 50% of these minerals. The remaining mineral elements have gone largely uninvestigated, and their biological role will likely be identified at some future date.

In the same way an automobile engine requires the proper fuel and other fluids to function efficiently and produce energy, our body's tiny cellular engines require a proper fuel source as well. In the case of the human body, the fuel source is a supply of certain specific nutrients. Over 60 of these nutrients are essential for the body's basic functioning, health and longevity. At least 30 mineral elements (some experts believe as many as 60), 16 vitamins, 12 essential amino acids, and three essential fatty acids must be consumed in order for the body to maintain itself in a healthful state. Of these 60 plus essential nutrients, it is often the minerals that are the most difficult for many people to obtain.

Minerals are required as co-factors for the proper functioning of vitamins, DNA, RNA as well as the body's enzyme and hormone systems. That is, they operate in conjunction with other factors to allow the proper functioning of these vital systems and processes. Magnesium, for example, is the activator mineral for over 75% of all enzyme systems. Adequate levels of a full spectrum of minerals are essential for the proper functioning of the endocrine system, a group of glands consisting of the thyroid, parathyroid, pineal, adrenal and pituitary glands as well as the testes, ovaries, and pancreas. These structures produce and regulate the activities of hormones such as estrogen, testosterone, progesterone, adrenaline, and thyroxine.

Hormones are responsible for activities including body growth and development, homeostasis, and metabolic and immune system functioning. Improper functioning of any aspect of the endocrine system can lead to serious medical difficulties including debilitating diseases. The mineral iodine, for example, is required for the production of the hormone thyroxine; chromium and zinc are involved in the production of insulin; and so forth.

The body simply cannot perform the basic functions of life without the utilization of minerals either as major factors or as co-factors. Amino acids (proteins), enzymes, hormones, and vitamins are dependent upon minerals as co-factors. Vital roles are played by minerals in building and maintaining the structure of the body, and in maintaining proper brain function, intestinal function, and blood sugar balance. These substances are involved in virtually every aspect of bodily activity. Vitamin A, for example, cannot be assimilated without the presence of proper levels of the mineral zinc; the absorption of vitamin B_{12} is dependent upon the presence of calcium; iron is a component of hemoglobin; and so forth.

An ancient Chinese proverb states that "the strength of a nation depends on the strength of her topsoil." The famous doctors Bernard Jensen and Royal Lee also championed this truth. Unfortunately, throughout most of the Western world the topsoil which grows our food crops is severely nutrient deficient. The vital nutrients that fuel man's bodies—especially the minerals—are no longer present in sufficient quantities in the soil which grows the crops we eat and depend on for our good health and prosperity. The fruits, vegetables, and grains we consume today provide only a shadow of their nutritional content in comparison to several hundred years ago, even 100 years. Because of this, supplementation with bioavailable forms of minerals is recommended. Several sources of minerals are available, including 1) chelated, 2) sea vegetation, 3) liquid colloidal, and 4) ionic.

The process of chelation (key-LAY-shun) binds an easily-absorbable organic amino acid, peptide or enzyme to a mineral molecule, thereby allowing the mineral to "hitchhike" a ride through the intestinal wall into the bloodstream. Although some conflicting data have been published, a wealth of research shows that chelation significantly increases the bioavailability of minerals, depending upon the specific mineral and the chelating agent being used.[127] Products using chelates often label the ingredient with a suffix such as aspartate, picolinate, EAP, or gluconate (a weak chelate)—e.g., selenium aspartate, chromium picolinate or copper gluconate.

There are many varieties of sea vegetation, also referred to as sea vegetables, seaweeds, or algae. Sea plants contain most of the mineral elements found in sea water, with some of the elements being highly concentrated.[128] Unlike plants grown in nutrient-depleted soil, sea plants thrive in the same mineral-rich environment that existed hundreds of years ago. The landlocked croplands may become depleted through overuse, but the rivers flowing into the sea provide a continual source of remineralization. (Organically-grown crops, on the other hand, have been shown to contain significantly higher levels of nutrients in comparison to foods produced by non-organic farming practices.) Various mineral-rich sea vegetables include *Aphanizomenon flos aquae*, chlorella, Irish moss, kelp, and spirulina. Kelp, for example, contains more vitamins and minerals than virtually any other food substance.[129]

Although colloidal minerals have been commercially available since the 1930s, they have recently experienced a resurgence in popularity. Colloids are simply particles of one medium suspended within another medium. Within a colloidal system, the particles are more-or-less discrete, and insoluble. The particles are said to be in a suspension or dispersion throughout the host medium, as opposed to being dissolved. The term colloid also is used to define particles in the size ranging from .01-.001 microns (one ten-thousandth to one hundred-thousandth of an inch). In the case of colloidal minerals, tiny mineral particles are suspended in the liquid medium of water. When supplementing with colloidal minerals, consumers should select varieties which originate from a plant source. Organic, liquid colloidal mineral supplements are in a form that can be used efficiently by the cells of animals and man, and are a form that the human body is able to store, transport, and utilize.

In the case of ionic minerals, the term "ionic" refers not to the electrical charge (valence) of the particles, as is often a common usage, but to particle size. When minerals are totally dissolved (dissociated) into solution, they are referred to as being in an ionic or ionized form. One of the best sources of ionic minerals is sea salt. The health benefits of salt harvested from the active oceans have long been recognized by man. Sea salt contains all of the broad spectrum of major minerals and trace elements found in sea water, many of which have been stripped from the soil and therefore our food supply. Even though over 50 of these minerals occur only in parts per billion (ppb) or less, the minute quantities of many of these substances are vital for proper functioning of the body and the prevention of illness and disease.[130] Natural, unrefined sea salt—not refined salt which is falsely represented as sea salt—is light grey in color, not white. In its natural state, before being ground, it is moist to the touch and retains its moisture even when kept in cool storage for long periods. One true sea salt is Celtic (KEL-tic) sea salt which is manually harvested from the coast of France, sun dried, and without additives. It is available in better health food stores, or from the Grain & Salt Society of Arden, N.C.: (800) TOP SALT.

When supplementing, it is prudent to take balanced proportions of recommended levels of minerals rather than a significantly higher dosage of any one mineral. A high-quality multi-vitamin and mineral or multi-mineral supplement using chelates should provide major mineral requirements, as well as some trace mineral requirements. Supplementation with chelated minerals, on the other hand, will not supply a broad spectrum of trace minerals which are required on a regular basis. This can be accomplished by using a high-quality, organically-bound supplement such as algae, colloidal minerals, or ionic minerals. (Sea salt should not be relied upon as one's *only* source of minerals.)

Simply put, minerals are necessary for upward of 95% of the body's daily functioning, although their importance as part of the daily diet has not been widely recognized. One of the best assurances against disease and d egeneration is to obtain an adequate supply of bioavailable minerals on a regular basis.

Essential Fatty Acids (EFAs)

Essential fatty acids are labeled "essential" because they cannot be manufactured within the body and therefore must be derived from the diet. Unlike unhealthy fats, essential fatty acids are absolutely necessary for good health and do not increase the risk of heart disease or contribute to obesity. EFAs are a structural component of each of the body's trillions of cells. As such, they seem to confer protection on every cell, tissue, organ, and organ system of the body. EFAs help keep the cell receptors configured so that they properly respond to chemical messengers such as glucose, neurotransmitters, hormones and immune-hormones (cytokines).

Dutch, Italian, Japanese, and U.S. studies have shown that deaths from vascular diseases can be reduced more than 50% by consuming one to two weekly meals of fish high in EFAs.[131] The consumption of essential fatty acids from fish is inversely associated with heart disease risk. Researchers believe this to be the result of EFA's influence on arrhythmia, blood viscosity, blood clotting, cholesterol metabolism, blood pressure, inflammation, and through other unknown mechanisms. EFAs also offer benefits to persons with hypertension, often helping to lower blood pressure 10-20%.[132]

Another area of the body heavily influenced by EFAs is the neurological system. The brain and other neurological tissues are dependent on EFAs for their proper maintenance, repair and function. The brain, for example, is 60% fat by dry weight and requires the appropriate types of fat for its proper structure and function. Illustrating the importance of EFAs to the brain are studies which show their capacity to decrease neurological disease and dementia. Eating fish high in EFAs on a regular basis, for example, may decrease Alzheimer's risk by 50%. EFAs also reduce ADHD, autistic symptoms, developmental disorders, depression, learning disabilities, mania, mental illness, schizophrenia, as well as improve behavior. Not only are they protective against lowered IQ and learning disabilities, consuming EFAs actually improves learning.[133]

EFAs also have powerful anti-inflammatory and pain-blocking properties. Tissues that get bumped or bruised (or those that bear structural stress such as joints and bones) benefit greatly from EFAs. Many studies confirm their effectiveness in reducing arthritis pain and stiffness, increasing bone density, and in other rheumatologic disorders such as Raynaud's and Sjögren syndromes. In a study of arthritis sufferers, supplementation with EFAs decreased up to 40% the production of Tumor Necrosis Factor Alpha (TNF-alpha), resulting in relief from arthritis.[134] In another study, supplementation with EFAs for 18 months increased lumbar spine density 3.1% and femoral (thigh bone) density 4.7%.[135] They also have been shown to reduce menstrual pain and discomfort and mastalgia (breast pain), and to decrease the frequency and severity of migraine headaches.[136] Further, EFAs have been shown to improve symptoms of intestinal disorders such as ulcerative colitis and Crohn's disease.[137] The following are additional beneficial effects of EFAs:[138]

❖ Significantly decrease cancer risk and improve outcomes in cancer

❖ Improve hormone balance

❖ Improve blood sugar regulation and insulin sensitivity in diabetics and help the body maintain a healthy weight.

❖ Are necessary for proper retina and vision development and may help prevent Age Related Macular Degeneration (ARMD)

❖ May help protect the kidneys, treat nephropathy and prevent renal failure in End Stage Renal Disease (ESRD)

❖ Support skin health and improve skin conditions such as atopy and eczema

❖ Support respiratory function and health

❖ May be protective against stomach or intestinal ulcers and may support the integrity of the intestinal wall lining

❖ Help to protect against as well as treat cardiac arrhythmias such as ventricular tachycardia and fibrillation

Essential fatty acids are found in such foods as avocados, borage, evening primrose, flax, nuts, and cold water fish (EPA and DHA) such as salmon, herring, sardines, and mackerel. However, when supplementing the diet one should consider that studies show those who seem to benefit most from supplementation respond best to the types of essential fatty acids in fish (DHA and EPA), especially EPA. Furthermore, there is evidence suggesting some people may have an impairment in the enzyme *delta-6 desaturase* which prevents them from being able to efficiently utilize the types of fatty acids from non-fish sources. Compared to fish oil, on the other hand, Neptune Krill Oil (NKO) has the advantages of being less subject to toxic contamination; being better absorbed, thereby requiring a lesser daily amount; and being about 30 times as potent an antioxidant. (Note for vegetarians: There is a marine source of EPA from algae that is "vegetarian safe," marketed under the brand name Neuromins.®)

Essential fatty acids function by turning on health-promoting genes and interacting with receptors that only can be stimulated by these types of fat. The wrong types either can't turn on the right genes, turn on the wrong genes, or cause the signaling of wrong messages. EFAs are one of the most versatile and powerful health-promoting substances, and are an essential component of anyone's diet who wishes to maintain good health. Chia, discussed above, is one of the riches sources of EFAs.

Phytonutrients

Also called phytochemicals ("phyto" means "plant" in Greek), *phytonutrients* are biologically-active plant substances whose classification encompasses many compounds not traditionally considered essential. They are *vitamin-like* compounds that function to actively prevent disease, regulate bodily functions, and fine-tune metabolic processes. These substances are completely natural, safe, beneficial to the body, and are not synthesized in a laboratory but created by the master chemist, nature. They work on many levels and perform myriad health-promoting biological functions.

Alkaloids, isoflavones, terpenes, indoles, and phenolic acids are only several of the classifications of phytochemicals which are found in plants, fruits, vegetables, and grains. Phytochemicals have been associated with the prevention and/or treatment of at least four of the leading causes of death in the Western world—cancer, cardiovascular disease, di-

abetes, and hypertension. They are also associated with the prevention and/or treatment of other ailments including abnormal bowel function, arthritis, neural tube defects, and osteoporosis.[139]

Flavonoids are phytochemicals that supply the water-soluble colors to fruits, vegetables, leaves, grains, seeds, and bark. Once referred to as vitamin P (referring to protecting the "permeability" of blood vessels), they are a chemically-diverse group of phytochemicals comprising over 4,000 different compounds. Nobel laureate Dr. Albert Szent-Györgyi reported in the early 1900s that flavonoids reduce blood-vessel wall fragility and capillary permeability, whereas simple vitamin C does not confer these benefits. Although they are chemically unrelated, flavonoids work synergistically in performing many of vitamin C's well-known functions.

Free radicals, as discussed above, pose a significant threat to our health and longevity. Excessive free radical production is associated with many disease processes. By damaging cell membranes, DNA and protein bonds, highly-reactive free radical molecules are implicated in arthritis, auto-immunity, cardiovascular disease, cataracts, chronic fatigue, HIV, macular degeneration, neurological illness, unhealthy or accelerated aging, and other degenerative conditions.[140] Phytonutrients fight excessive free radicals and assist the body in replenishing its antioxidant stores. For example, supplementing with whole food phytonutrients has been shown to increase antioxidant levels by an average of 239%.[141] By consuming whole foods that contain a broad spectrum of antioxidants, the body is able to quench free radicals before they cause excessive damage.

By acting as natural antioxidants, phytonutrients are protective of the cardiovascular system. The medical establishment is now acknowledging the importance of antioxidant protection in cardiovascular health as illustrated by the fact that more doctors take antioxidant supplements than aspirin as a means of preventing heart attacks. Raising antioxidant levels reduces cardiovascular disease by up to 47%.[142] In addition to reducing the risk of cardiovascular disease, they have been shown to reverse high cholesterol, triglycerides, free radical damage, platelet stickiness, high homocysteine (a toxic metabolite in the blood that damages blood vessels and is strongly linked to cardiovascular disease) and degeneration of blood vessel walls. *Each single serving increase in daily fruit and vegetable intake achieves a 4% lower risk of coronary heart disease.*[143]

A recent study showed a 35% lower risk of atherosclerotic cardiovascular disease in women who consumed 3-10 servings of fruits and vegetables per day compared to those whose consumed 2.5 daily servings.[144] Lycopene is the phytonutrient antioxidant that gives tomatoes their red color. Other studies show that women with the highest amounts of lycopene in their blood have half the risk of cardiovascular disease. Lycopene also is known to reduce prostate cancer risk.[145]

Phytonutrients also protect against stroke. Studies show that by consuming approximately three servings of either whole grains or fruits and vegetables per day, a 50% reduction in stroke can be achieved.[146] Surprisingly, simply adding a few servings of whole grains to the diet reduces chances of stroke by almost 20%.[147]

Dr. Caldwell Esselstyn, head of Thyroid and Parathyroid Surgery at the Cleveland Clinic, questions the value of procedures such as coronary artery bypass surgery, angioplasty and stents in treating the "symptoms" of heart disease. He found that a plant-based diet is more effective in treating such ailments, stating that:

> ... mechanical interventions treat only the symptoms and not the disease. It is therefore not surprising that patients who receive these interventions often experience progressive disease, graft shutdown, restenosis, more procedures, progressive disability, and death from disease. Thus, the leading killer of men and women in Western civilization is being left untreated...in contrast, a five-year experience has shown excellent results in patients with severe coronary artery disease who followed a plant-based diet...[148]

A plant-based diet would help patients suffering from myriad diseases and ailments, including cancer, diabetes, hypertension and obesity. In addition to promoting cardiovascular health, by activating the body's detoxification systems and neutralizing the action of carcinogens, phytonutrients are one of nature's strongest weapons for defeating and preventing cancer. The American Institute for Cancer Research and the World Cancer Research Fund estimate that overall cancer rates could be decreased by as much as 20-40% if people consumed the recommended daily five or more servings of fruits and vegetables.[149] An additional 15-60% reduction in cancer might be achieved for some cancers such as breast, colon and lung.

As a way to maintain proper antioxidant reserves, The National Research Council and numerous other agencies have recommended consuming five servings per day of fruits and vegetables. However, less than 10% of the U.S. population consumes this daily amount. Considering that on a randomly-selected day 45% of the population consumes no fruits and vegetables, the impact of adding fruits, vegetables and whole food supplements to the diet would be substantial.

Several mechanisms are responsible for the cancer-protective effects of phytonutrients, including antioxidant protection, nutrient deficiency protection, detoxification stimulation, and in ways still largely unknown. A diet high in fruits and vegetables is associated with a reduced risk of developing cancers of the lung, colon, breast, cervix, esophagus, oral cavity, stomach, bladder, pancreas, and ovary as reported in a recent, comprehensive epidemiological study.[150] Studies suggest that up to 80% of colon cancers can be prevented by dietary changes alone. This further confirms that a low daily fruit and vegetable intake results in about twice the risk of cancer.

Other benefits of phytonutrients include:[151]

❑ Possible prevention of age-related mental decline and dementia

❑ Support of healthy hormone levels and proper hormone metabolism

❑ Support of respiratory health and help in the prevention, or improvement, of asthma, bronchitis and Chronic Obstructive Pulmonary Disease.

❑ Influence metabolic enzymes in benefit of the entire body

❑ Boost immune response by activating different classes of immune system components

❑ Inhibition of destructive enzymes and bacterial, viral, fungal and parasitic attack

❑ Protect connective tissues comprising joints, muscle, tendon, ligaments and blood vessels

❑ Reduction by one third the number of cancer deaths each year due to poor dietary practices

❑ Protection against mental decline/dementia

❑ Possible reduction of pain

❑ Promotion of healthy bowel function and possible protection against intestinal maladies

Amounts of phytochemicals needed to achieve optimal health or reverse disease may be difficult to consume from dietary sources alone. This is partially due to erosion of our top-soil and the associated depletion of its mineral and nutrient content, and more recently from genetic engineering of the food supply. Therefore, supplementing the diet is now more crucial than ever. It is important, whenever possible, to choose supplements derived from "whole foods" as opposed to fractional components.

The benefits of a diet high in fruits and vegetables often are not seen when consuming individual nutrients in supplement form, emphasizing the importance of supplementing with whole foods. Although it is important to supplement with whole food phytonutrients, this should be done *along with* a diet already rich in a variety of plant foods.

(Interestingly, people who consume a meat-laden diet have a significantly increased risk of cancer, heart disease, and other serious health challenges. In countries whose populations consume much less meat, there is a lower incidence of most of the debilitating diseases found in many Western countries. T. Colin Campbell, Ph.D., a researcher who has studied the health patterns of the Chinese, comments about meat consumption:

> ... People who eat more meat have higher blood cholesterol levels and higher blood albumin levels, which is a function of protein intake [which increases systemic acidity]. As blood levels of albumin and cholesterol go up, the diseases we get in the West—cancer, heart disease and diabetes—also start going up. It's quite remarkable.[152])

When considering supplementation, the free-radical-quenching (antioxidant) strength of supplements should most resemble that of whole foods. Several measures to quantify the activity of free-radical-quenching compounds have emerged. For many years, the scientific gold standard for testing free radical (antioxidant) potency has been the ORAC (oxygen radical absorbance capacity) test —considered by most experts to be the most accurate and reliable. By looking for products that are ORAC rated, one can be more assured of the activity level of antioxidants.

For example, a supplement with 2,700 ORAC units would be the equivalent of eating five mixed servings of fruits and vegetables per day. Only about 10% of the American population consumes five servings of fruits and vegetables per day, with most averaging less than 2,700 daily ORAC units. ORAC unit intakes as high as 6,000-7,000 can be achieved through dietary intake alone if fruits and vegetables with a high antioxidant capacity are consumed. For example, 100 grams of blueberries deliver about 2,400 ORAC units. Combinations of antioxidants from a variety of whole foods, combining many phytochemicals, provide the best ORAC potential to effectively combat free radicals. The latest medical understanding is that the body needs a minimum of 5,000 ORAC units daily which, as mentioned, is difficult for many Westerners to achieve by diet alone.

While the ORAC assay measures the level of antioxidants present in the sample being evaluated, the CAP-e assay (Cell-based Antioxidant Protection in Erythrocytes) measures the degree to which the antioxidants actually enter and protect living cells. Foods having high ORAC values sometimes rate much lower on the CAP-e evaluation, and vice versa—indicating the antioxidant *potential* of an ORAC measurement doesn't necessarily accurately reflect the food's ability to confer or not confer antioxidant protection to living cells.

The simple addition of whole, unrefined foods such as fruits and vegetables has tremendous benefit to overall wellness. In a study reported in *The New York Times*,[153] women who avoided refined foods and added only 1-2 servings of fruits and vegetables experienced a 13% reduction in cholesterol, a 16% reduction in LDL cholesterol, an increase in glutathione levels, and improved bowel function in 82% of the participants.

Most Americans are exposed to increased risk of heart disease, cancer and other diet-related disease from eating too much animal fat and too few fruits, vegetables, whole grains, beans, seeds and nuts. Since the many phytonutrients are what give color to plants, "eat a lot of color" through the arsenal of plants nature provides to protect against unnecessary aging, sickness, disability and death.

Probiotics

In the late 1800s, microbiologists identified forms of bacteria (microflora) in the intestinal tracts of healthy individuals that are beneficial to the health of their hosts. These beneficial microbes are called *probiotics*, which literally means "for life." The term "friendly bacteria" is often used interchangeably with probiotics.

Probiotics are intricately linked to the health of the intestine. One proponent of the link between the intestines and health was Dr. Bernard Jensen, who found that gastrointestinal tracts of healthy individuals differ from those of the unhealthy. Probiotics are an essential part of our evolutionary intestinal health. They play a role in detoxification; support liver function; protect and nourish intestinal cells; help digest food by producing enzymes; help form the gut-immune barrier; protect against infections (viral and bacterial), such as antibiotic-induced and traveler's diarrhea; and they help promote the secretion of natural antibiotics. In addition, probiotics aid in the secretion of nourishing substances which are used by the intestines to repair and grow themselves.

These and other mechanisms help them protect against and improve inflammatory bowel diseases such as necrotizing enterocolitis, non-specific colitis, Crohn's disease and ulcerative colitis. The power of probiotics is demonstrated by one study which showed they reduced the symptoms of Crohn's disease by almost 75%.[154]

Imbalance (dysbiosis) of the delicate balance of friendly bacteria in the intestinal tract is linked to a variety of disorders. The following is a partial list of symptoms often accompanying such an imbalance:[155]

❍ IBS (Irritable Bowel Syndrome)
❍ Diarrhea and/or constipation
❍ Skin problems such as acne, eczema and psoriasis
❍ Bad breath and foul body odor
❍ Delayed development in children
❍ Yeast infections/candida overgrowth
❍ High cholesterol
❍ Chronic fatigue
❍ Muscle pain, such as fibromyalgia
❍ Joint pain and arthritis syndromes
❍ Frequent colds and flu

Humans have over 100 trillion bacteria in our intestinal tracts, comparable to the total number of cells in the human body. The ideal ratio of beneficial to harmful bacteria is about 5 to 1. Most Westerners, however, have a reverse ratio of good to bad bacteria, largely due to the overuse of antibiotics and the underconsumption of fermented and raw foods. This can seriously compromise the immune and digestive systems, leading to a number of chronic diseases.

Probiotics promote healthy bowel regularity and transit time. Not only are they supportive of intestinal health and balance, they have a variety of systemic benefits as well. For example, they support vitamin synthesis and assimilation of nutrients, thus promoting intestinal and overall health. In addition, they modulate local and systemic inflammatory responses; local and systemic immune responses; and antagonize "bad" bacteria, yeast and infection.[156] They also protect against and help treat food allergies.

Furthermore, probiotics have the following effects:[157]

❒ Support healthy cholesterol metabolism. In one study, administration of *L. sporogenes* caused a significant inhibition of cholesterol. Furthermore, probiotics have been shown to lower blood cholesterol levels up to 30% when taken in therapeutic doses over a three month period.

❒ Protect against bladder and colon cancer, and stimulate the immune system.

❒ Help prevent urinary tract, vaginal and intestinal candida (yeast) infections. Help degrade toxins such as viruses, bacteria, fungi, molds and yeast.

❒ Increase digestive enzyme activity up to 85%.

❒ May help promote mental well-being.

❒ Essential in combating the negative effects of antibiotics (which means "against life"). Through what is called *microbial interference therapy*, they also play a vital role in combating antibiotic-resistant organisms. As such, the World Health Organization has deemed probiotics to be an important immune defense against virulent infection.

❒ Help to quench inflammation of the gastrointestinal (GI) tract. Arthritis, allergies and eczema are conditions that can be exacerbated by such inflammation. Treatment of these disorders with probiotics is often beneficial as modulation or down-regulation of the immune-inflammatory system can be achieved.

A decrease in the consumption of fermented foods, a natural source of probiotics, has caused a substantial increase in the immune-related and intestinal-linked health problems faced by Western society. Also, changes in our soil health, farming methods and a decrease in fruit and vegetable consumption have decreased the amount of probiotics in our diet. Furthermore, the rampart overuse of antibiotics in medicine and agribusiness has impacted the availability and viability of probiotics. Historically, methods of food preparation and preservation involved either the natural fermentation or drying of foods which provided the human diet with many times the amount of probiotics in comparison to today's diet. These changes have come at an astronomical cost.

A highly recommended probiotic product is Essential Formulas' Probiotic 12-Plus® probiotic formula, the creation of Okayama University's esteemed microbiologist Iichiroh Ohhira, Ph.D.—recipient of Japan's coveted "Scientist of the Year" award in 1991. Probiotic 12-Plus is itself the winner of Japan's 1991 "Best Product" award. This product is a non-dairy, vegetarian formualtion consisting of a blend of 12 strains of live bacteria, 4 types of organic acids, 10 vitamins, 8 minerals, 18 amino acids, fructooligosaccharides, hydrogen peroxide, natural antibiotics (bacteriocins), and 92 varieties of organic crops including plants, vegetables, fruits, leaves and seaweeds. Probiotic 12-Plus is manufactured using a 3-5 year natural-temperature fermentation process, and has been shown *in vitro* to be effective against Methicillin-Resistant Staphylococcus Aureus (MRSA), *E-coli O157:H7*, and possibly even intestinal anthrax. Probiotic 12-Plus is available in health food stores or on the internet. To learn more about this potent natural supplement, do a key word search for "omx 12 plus," or visit www.crohns.net/page/C/ROD/PROD/OMX 1030.

Fiber

The material that gives plants bulk and texture, fiber is an essential, health-promoting substance lacking in most Westerner's diets. It is found in many plant foods including fruits, vegetables, legumes, seeds, nuts, and whole grains. Although it has important health benefits—unlike many of the other nutrients such as fats, carbohydrates, and proteins—fiber is indigestible. Foods with higher fiber content tend to be healthier, more nutrient dense, have a high enzyme content, and have fewer calories. Fiber also helps satisfy the appetite by increasing the sense of fullness and stabilizing blood sugar levels. It also helps the body eliminate toxins; provides a food source for healthy intestinal flora; promotes healthy bowel ecology; promotes healthy cholesterol levels; promotes bowel regularity; and provides cancer protection. According to Dr. Betty Kaman, author of *New Facts About Fiber*, "fiber is the most important element in digestive tract health."[158]

Although fiber has a broad range of health-promoting effects, it is probably best known for its role in digestive health. Cultural taboos regarding digestion (biological functions) have hindered the progress of digestive health issues. This is at a time when the rate of digestive ailments has reached epidemic proportions. According to the American Gastroenterological Association (AGA), half of the U.S population is affected by some variety of digestive disorder.[159] Over 25 million Americans will suffer from an ulcer during their lifetimes.

Colon/rectal cancer is now the second leading cause of cancer-related deaths in the U.S., according to the American Cancer Society (148,300 new cases were diagnosed in 2002). This epidemic of digestive disorders is responsible for nearly 200,000 deaths per year, 10 million hospitalizations, 6 million procedures (14% of all procedures), 50 million physician office visits, almost 1.5 million cases of disability, and costs American society over $200 billion annually.[160]

There are two types of fiber—insoluble and soluble. Insoluble fiber does not dissolve in water. It provides weight and bulk to the diet, softens the stool, and passes quickly through the digestive system facilitating regular elimination. Soluble fiber dissolves in water and generally passes through the intestinal tract more slowly, thus slowing digestion and the rate of nutrient absorption. Soluble fiber adds some bulk and softness to the stool through its property of water absorption and, therefore, also normalizes stool regularity and proper elimination. This type of fiber is associated with its ability to decrease cholesterol absorption and control blood sugar levels by slowing the absorption of consumed foods. Soluble fiber also increases satiety, the feeling of fullness.

Similar to many vitamins and minerals, dietary fiber also has a daily recommend value (DRV). The current DRV for dietary fiber is 25 grams per day. The National Cancer Institute recommends consuming 25-30 grams of fiber daily. However, this is only about 20% of the intake level of one hundred years ago, and many believe this is too low a level to maintain optimal health. Forty, 50 or even 60 grams per day more accurately reflects a healthful diet.[161]

The American Dietetic Association believes that consuming more fiber-rich foods will have a significant impact on the prevention and treatment of cardiovascular disease, obesity, and Type-2 diabetes. In addition, fiber has been demonstrated to:[162]

• Decrease polyps (a precancerous condition) and cancer. This cancer protection is especially evident in hormone-dependent cancers (e.g., breast cancer) and colon cancer.

• Promote a healthy weight. A recent study found that young adults who ate at least 21 grams of fiber per day, on average, weighed eight pounds less over a 10-year period than those who ate less fiber.

• Promote bowel regularity and healthy bacterial ecology. A recent study showed those with chronic constipation ingested 20-30% less fiber.

• Promote the binding of heavy metals in the intestine (which is a main route of heavy metal elimination by the body); thus fiber helps promote toxin removal.

• Bind bile acids in the intestines, which can act as pro-carcinogens

• Help regulate and modulate blood sugar and significantly reduce the chance of becoming diabetic. One study showed that seven grams of fruit fiber given to diabetics before meals reduced by 35% their need for insulin. Through the incorporation of a high-fiber diet, many insulin-dependent and non-insulin-dependent diabetics no longer need supplemental insulin.

• Help prevent stroke and other cardiovascular diseases by up to 30%

• Decrease cholesterol and LDL levels

• Decrease hemorrhoids

Fiber powerfully supports the structure and function of the intestines. For example, appendicitis is primarily associated with a decrease in fiber intake.[163] Diverticulitis (blown-out or inflamed pockets in the intestinal wall) is directly related to low fiber intake. A high-fiber diet, on the other hand, is an effective treatment for the condition.[164] Furthermore, there is an association between diverticular disease, varicose veins, hernias, hemorrhoids and lack of fiber. In addition to playing a role in all of these conditions, it decreases gallstones and improves certain liver pathologies.

Our modern techniques of food processing, including the bleaching of flour and grains, have led to a decline in the fiber content of our typical diets. This has more impact than merely negatively affecting regularity and colon health. Fiber is known to be a "messenger" that communicates with genes to promote a healthy intestinal environment, including proper immune function; bowel tone; promoting an intact gut barrier; and the cultivation of healthy intestinal flora.

The consumption of whole grains and other fiber-rich foods is one health habit that has been shown to increase life-span and health-span. Epidemiological studies have shown fiber consumption to be inversely related to the risk of cancer, cardiovascular disease, diabetes, neurological illness, obesity, stroke, and other degenerative diseases.[165]

Increasing fiber consumption is an effective and simple step to improve overall health. One finding illustrating the importance of fiber was reported by British surgeon Dr. Densi Burkitt, who studied the amount of fiber consumed by various cultures and compared this information to the size of the cultures' respective hospitals. Dr. Burkitt found that the smaller the stools, the larger the hospitals, and the larger the stools, the smaller the hospitals.[166]

Exercise

A new disease is becoming epidemic. It's called *"Couch Potato Disease"*—more commonly it is known as *inactivity*. Couch Potato Disease is linked to over a dozen chronic diseases and many lesser health conditions. In the U.S. it is responsible for over a quarter million deaths each year.[167] Only smoking, which kills nearly one-half million people yearly, causes more preventable deaths. In addition to lost lives, inactivity-related illnesses cost close to $1 trillion per year.[168]

The lack of physical activity is wide-spread throughout all age groups. Roughly 22% of adults engage in some type of physical activity on a daily basis. Only 15% routinely exercise vigorously. Nearly 50% of all youth are not active on a daily basis. Enrollment in physical education classes has dropped by almost 50%. More than 60% of adults do not achieve the recommended amount of regular physical activity, and 25 % of all adults are totally inactive. Regular exercise is uncommon in the elderly. Less than 10% of this age group engage in physical exercise. About two thirds of elderly persons are either inactive or completely sedentary.[169]

The above statistics are alarming in light of the fact that exercise is likely as powerful as any "drug" ever created. If medicine could put all of the benefits of exercise into one-pill, it would be one of the greatest scientific achievements of all time. The following are just a few benefits of the "wonder-drug" exercise:

☞ Could help prevent at least 300,000 deaths each year in the U S.[170]

☞ Decreases physiological age, partially reverses aging and increases life-span. Persons who routinely exercise vigorously live up to seven years longer than those who do not. Furthermore, exercise has been shown to slow and even reverse several components of aging.[171]

☞ Protects against all major chronic diseases, including coronary artery disease, diabetes, hypertension, obesity, arthritis (all types), and osteoporosis. Exercise increases cardiac output, increases blood flow to muscles and can improve vascular disorders such as blood clots and intermittent claudication (vascular type).

☞ Significantly decreases risk of stroke.[172]

☞ Prevents and treats high blood pressure. A meta-analysis of over a dozen controlled studies on exercise shows that on average systolic blood pressure can be lowered by 11.3 points and diastolic blood pressure by 7.5 points. Exercise also reduces LDL cholesterol (the "bad" cholesterol) and increases HDL cholesterol (the "good" cholesterol).[173]

☞ Improves the body's sensitivity to insulin, allowing it to utilize blood sugar more efficiently. Can reduce insulin resistance by 40%. In addition to being an effective treatment, exercise reduces by 50% the risk of getting diabetes, and may be more effective than medication in treating Type 2 Diabetes.[174] Diabetes is the principal cause of kidney failure, limb amputations, and blindness in adults. The development of heart disease and stroke are also significantly related to diabetes. In a study of over 21,000 physicians, it was found that even infrequent exercise decreased the risk of developing Type 2 Diabetes by 24-39%. The study authors conclude that at least 25% of Type 2 diabetes is attributable to a sedentary lifestyle.[175]

☞ Improves muscle mass, flexibility, enhances balance and improves joint health.

☞ Helps prevent bone loss and increases bone strength.

☞ Can reduce anxiety and distress and elevate mood. Also improves sleep quality, mental functioning and has been shown to be *at least as effective as antidepressants* in ameliorating mild to moderate depression.[176]

☞ Decreases body weight and distribution of body fat. More pronounced effects are seen in those who are most overweight.

☞ Reduces the incidence of cancer. For example, at least 10% of all breast cancer cases are directly caused by a lack of exercise. By exercising 30 minutes or more daily, 15% of new colon cancer cases could be prevented.[177]

☞ Lowers gallbladder disease and decreases tendency towards gallstones.[178]

☞ Reduces pain. Exercise increases circulation and hence the blood supply to the uterine muscle, thus improving gynecological pain. It also helps the body produce endorphins, opium-like substances within the body that decrease all types of pain.

☞ Improves respiratory function, even in those with asthma or COPD. The authors of one study stated, "A six-month endurance-training program reverses the equivalent of thirty years of aerobic decline."[179]

☞ Improves brain function by 11% or more, as shown with Magnetic Resonance Imaging.[180]

☞ Improves immunity: The Appalachian State University exercise physiology department has shown that exercise improves immune function, as those who exercise moderately show double the resistance to viral illness.[181]

Over the last 100 years we have witnessed a tremendous increase in chronic disease, affecting over 90 million Americans and occupying 65% of each healthcare dollar spent. Chronic disease accounts for over one trillion dollars annually in lost productivity. Heart disease, diabetes and obesity are the three principal causes of non-accidental deaths in the U.S., each of them being directly related to a lack of exercise. These diseases can be modified, and their incidence reduced by 65%, by the simple addition of moderate physical exercise. Exercise is a powerful messenger that turns on health-promoting regions of genes and turns off health-negating ones.

Simple, moderate exercise has more health benefits than any known substance. Exercise is, therefore, an essential component of health. Anyone wishing to be healthy or stay healthy must include a rational exercise program. Our ancestors walked the equivalent of 10 miles a day *more* than we do today.[182] The decline in physical activity ushered in by the industrial and information revolutions is linked to every major chronic disease known today. Exercise is the movement of life, essential to health and an expression of vitality. Indeed, when combined with diet modification, it is likely the most promising single intervention in reducing the risk of virtually all chronic diseases simultaneously. Exercise holds an important answer to the chronic disease crisis.

The *quality* of one's life-span, not the *quantity*, is termed the "health-span"—which simply means the number of years one lives a healthy life, not necessarily the number of years one lives. A healthy lifestyle, incorporating all of the above-discussed items, not only increases life-span, but increases health-span by decreasing the period of "sick years," and can partially reverse aging. This phenomenon is called "compression of morbidity," which basically means that incorporating a healthy life-style decreases the duration, frequency and severity of chronic disease over one's life-time and compresses it at the very end. A healthy lifestyle can significantly increase one's health-span and compress sick years, thus significantly contributing to an enjoyable and fulfilled life.

OLIVE LEAF EXTRACT

An old cure has recently been rediscovered—from the leaves of the common olive tree, botanically classified as *Olea europaea L.* Documentation of the effective medicinal uses of the olive tree dates back some 6,000 years. In the *Bible*, the olive tree is called "the tree of life." Over this long span of time, various parts of the tree have been used medicinally. Olive oil, for example, was used by Hippocrates as a cure for cholera, muscular pains and ulcers. The leaves of the tree have been used as a medicinal tea for centuries, although this remedy has been practically unknown to modern, Western medicine—until only recently.

During the years 1827-1855, there were reports in the medical literature of olive leaves being used to brew a tea that was viewed as a potential cure for malaria. Later that century, biochemical analyses were performed on powdered olive leaves, and an active ingredient was isolated and given the Latin name *oleuropein* ($C_{25}H_{32}O_{13}$). By 1969, researchers at the pharmaceutical giant The Upjohn Company had done further analyses of oleuropein and found the principal ingredient to be a calcium salt of elenolic acid, which is chemically identified as *calcium elenolate*, a chemical byproduct of oleuropein.

The studies performed by Upjohn found that olive leaf extract—calcium elenolate—inhibited the growth of every virus, bacterium, fungus, yeast and parasitic protozoan it was tested against.[1] The pharmaceutical firm intended to patent the extract and market it as a drug. They abandoned their efforts, however, after finding that calcium elenolate binds to proteins in blood serum, rendering it ineffective as a treatment. By the mid-1990s, other researchers discovered a remedy to this obstacle, thus opening the door for the extract's use as an antimicrobial nutritional supplement.

In his book *Olive Leaf Extract*, Morton Walker, D.P.M. reports many seemingly miraculous benefits of this substance including:[2]

❖ the generalized degradation of pathological microorganisms of all types—viruses, retroviruses, bacteria, spirochetes, rickettsiae, chlamydiae, fungi, yeasts, molds, protozoa, helminths, and other parasites

❖ the relief of arthritic inflammations, especially osteoarthritis and rheumatoid arthritis

❖ the reduction of insulin dosage for better control over the risks of symptomatic diabetes

❖ the elimination of chronic fatigue and the symptoms associated with its syndrome

❖ the creation or restoration of abundant energy with prolonged stamina

❖ the normalization of heart beat irregularities (arrhythmias)

❖ the improvement of blood flow in cardiovascular and/or peripheral vascular disorders

❖ the lessening of pain from hemorrhoids

❖ the attenuation of toothaches

❖ the antioxidant quenching of free radicals

❖ the obliteration of fungal infections such as mycotic nails, athlete's foot, and jock itch

❖ the permanent relief of malaria (from a protozoa), dengue fever (from a virus), and other exotic and deadly tropical diseases which produce fever as a primary symptom

❖ the prevention and effective treatment of all types of viral diseases, including the Epstein-Barr virus, cytomegalovirus, the herpes viruses, human herpes virus-6, the retroviruses, the influenza viruses, viruses of the common cold, and the human immunodeficiency virus (HIV)

❖ the reversal of almost all symptomology connected with *Candida albicans* and other organisms causing the yeast syndrome

❖ the death and excretion of a variety of parasites, including microscopic protozoa and macroscopic helminth worms

Dr. Walker describes the above as a *partial* list of the benefits provided by the oral administration of olive leaf extract! This powerful germ fighter is not only effective, but safe. In 1969, The Upjohn Company conducted a battery of tests to determine the exact toxicity of calcium elenolate. The tests were performed on a variety of laboratory animals, and showed the substance to be "exceedingly safe and non-toxic."[3]

Dr. Walker's book cites a list of more than 125 infectious diseases for which olive leaf extract acts as an antimicrobial agent—as determined by Upjohn and others. The list is impressive, and its veracity is documented by over 25 published studies spanning more than four decades. Ranging from AIDS to Yellow fever, some of the list entrants include athlete's foot, bladder (urinary tract) infection, candidiasis, chicken pox, chlamydia, cholera, chronic fatigue syndrom (CFS), colds, cold sores, crabs, cytomegalovirus (CMV), diarrhea, diphtheria, ear infections (otitis media), ebola Sudan, ebola Zaire, *E. coli* O157:H7, Epstein-Barr, food poisoning, fibromyalgia (FM), genital herpes, genital warts, German measles, giardia, gonorrhea, head lice, heart arrhythmias, hepatitis A/B/C, influenza (all known strains), Legionnaire's disease, leprosy, lockjaw, Lyme disease, malaria, Marburg virus, measles, mycoplasma pneumonia, mumps, plague, pneumonia, polio, psoriasis, rabies, retroviruses, rheumatoid arthritis (microbially induced), ringworm, Rocky Mountain spotted fever, salmonella, scarlet fever, shingles (herpes zoster), smallpox, sexually transmitted diseases (STDs), syphilis, thrush, tuberculosis, typhoid fever, warts, whooping cough, and almost 100 others.[4]

Your local health food store carries a selection of olive leaf extract products in a variety of strengths, in either tablets or capsules. Dr. Walker recommends an oleuropein concentration of greater than 6%. Some products contain 15% or higher. Olive leaf extract is best taken on an empty stomach, according to the manufacturers.

Photoluminescence

Photoluminescence is the term used to describe the medical procedure of withdrawing a small amount of blood from a vein in the arm or hand—usually between 10-300 cubic centimeters (cc)—and irradiating it (shining a light on it) for a short period of time with selected wavelengths of light before returning the blood to the donor, generally at the same site from which it was taken. Before this technique was lost in the publicity that accompanied the introduction of pharmaceutical antibiotics during the 1930s and 40s, it was used effectively and extensively in the U.S. and elsewhere to defeat a broad array of both serious and minor diseases and illnesses. Treated diseases range from arthritis, asthma and insect bites, to polio, tuberculosis, and cancer. Photoluminescence holds the promise of offering a simple, inexpensive and effective treatment for many of medicine's modern challenges, including HIV/AIDS, SARS, Bird Flu, and bio-warfare agents.

Introduction. It does not make a great deal of sense that irradiating a small amount of someone's blood with a certain wavelength of light would have a particularly beneficial effect on the recipient of such a procedure. The fact is that it *does* have a very curative effect on a long list of ailments from the most minor to the most serious. What would be the proposed theoretical basis for such a treatment? In other words, why would someone reason that this technique would be any more effective than, say, shining light on the scalp, or the bottom of one's feet? (See *Light*, under **General Treatment Methods**.) And if it *does* work, what are the physiological mechanisms involved? How does it do what it does?

It's not everyday that we are asked to accept a miraculous-sounding solution to a long list of old problems where the solution is nearly as old as the problems themselves. To what shelf has this treatment of treatments been exiled? Was the technique misplaced and if so, why? Because if it *really is* effective, it's difficult to understand why so much time has passed without photoluminescence being in the mainstream of modern medicine. Many medical researchers who have studied photoluminescence believe the technique has been unfairly outdistanced by other less-deserving technologies, and should occupy its rightful place alongside the other tried-and-true beneficial therapies offered by 21st Century medicine.

Theoretical Backdrop: The Story Begins. In the late 1880s, Danish medical student Niels Ryberg Finsen (1860-1904) became interested in the effects of light upon the human body, and selected the ultraviolet portion of the spectrum for the experimental treatment of various ailments, mostly skin diseases. N.R. Finsen received his M.D. degree from the University of Copenhagen in 1890 at the age of 30, and in 1898 became a professor at that university. For the better part of his short 44 year life, Finsen studied the effects of UV, carbon arc and other wavelengths of light on the biological processes of organisms. He demonstrated an effective treatment for skin tuberculosis through the use of green light. He also made important discoveries in the area of skin pigmentation and the skin's susceptibility to light of different wavelengths.[1]

One of Finsen's most brilliant discoveries was the following: *hemoglobin, an iron-containing pigment of red blood cells, has the unique property of absorbing all wavelengths of ultraviolet light.*[2] What this means is that light is taken into the hemoglobin cells and involved in a chemical process (according to the Grotthus-Draper Law, the first law of photochemistry). The light is actually assimilated/metabolized by the body. However, the many specific ways the body uses the light remain unclear.

[Ultraviolet light is separated into several groupings of wavelengths, as follows: *Long Wave UV*, UV-A: 400-315 (nanometers) nm, black light; *Near UV*, UV-B:315-280 nm, sunburn radiation; *Middle UV*, UV-C: 280-100 nm, absorbed by air; *Short Wave UV*, far UV]

Dr. N.R. Finsen, known as the father of modern phototherapy, was the first Danish physician to receive the Nobel Prize in Medicine/Physiology (1903) "...in recognition of his contribution to the treatment of diseases with concentrated light radiation, whereby he has opened a new avenue for medical science."[3] The Finsen Institute in Copenhagen survives to this day, focusing on the study of cancer. (Phototherapy is the treatment of organisms with photons, i.e., light rays; a photon is a quantum, or particle, of light.)

One last note on N.R. Finsen. In 1893 Dr. Finsen found that "...*lengthy exposure of smallpox sufferers to the red light formed by exclusion of the violet end of the spectrum prevents the suppuration [formation] of the pustules, or formation of characteristic pockmarks.*"[4] This is an astounding fact, given the media publicity about bioterror events currently saturating our lives. Also note that the source of the information is unquestionably documented. The above quotation is taken from *The Encyclopedia Britannica.*

The person to stand on Finsen's shoulders and carry the research to the next level was the Russian scientist Dr. Alexander Gurwitsch (1874-1954). In the world of clever experiments, during the mid-1920s Alexander Gurwitsch performed one of the best. Gurwitsch mounted two onions perpendicularly in close proximity, the root tip of the first onion coming very close to but not touching the side of the root of the second. After a short time had elapsed, the side of the second onion's root at the point of near-contact was evaluated microscopically. It was discovered that at precisely the point of near-contact on the root of the second onion, a significant increase in cell mitosis (division, growth) had occurred in comparison to the opposite side of the second onion's root. Something was happening in that small, empty space between the two onions' roots that contributed to the unusual cell growth.

Gurwitsch placed a thin sheet of window glass between the two roots (and at other times some opaque materials) and the unusual effect disappeared. He then replaced these materials with a thin quartz sheet—and *voila*, the effect reappeared. "What's the difference," you might ask, "between ordinary glass and the quartz sheet Gurwitsch used that could have accounted for this on-and-off effect he observed?" It is a photodynamic property of quartz to allow the passage of certain wavelengths of ultraviolet (UV) light, whereas ordinary glass and opaque objects do not. Gurwitsch hypothesized that plant cells communicate with each other via certain wavelengths of light. He referred to this newly-discovered light source as "mitogenic radiation."[5]

Subsequently, he and his colleagues were able to demonstrate that mitogenic rays were indeed very weak photonic radiation emanating from cellular structures. They also developed a method of *indirectly* measuring the intensity and spectral distribution of the "rays." They showed that *the light given off by cells is in the ultraviolet portion of the electromagnetic spectrum*, and that each bodily organ produces light of a specific, discrete wavelength—all within the ultraviolet portion of the spectrum.[6]

The German researcher Dr. Fritz-Albert Popp began his research in the early 1970s and is still active today. Dr. Popp, presently of the International Institute of Biophysics in Neuss, Germany, has shown that all biological systems emit photons (light particles) ranging in the rate of output from only several to many thousands per second per square centimeter (sec/cm^2).[7] [In 2000, Drs. Masaki Kobayashi and Humio Inaba of the Tohoku Uni-

versity in Japan, demonstrated that living cells emit photons at the rate of 1-10,000/sec/cm^2][8] He and his colleagues have found that every change in the biological or physiological state of living systems is reflected by a corresponding change in photon emission.

Photoluminescence Emerges During Early 20th Century. "Photoluminescence" is a fairly recent term. Throughout its relatively short history the technique also has been referred to as Photochemotherapy, Photobiological therapy, Photodynamic therapy, Photo-oxidation, Photopheresis, Ultraviolet Blood Irradiation, each attempting to describe some treatment characteristic.

In the beginning, the technique itself simply may have represented the desire to apply a technology that was at least somewhat understood. It has been known for over 100 years that ultraviolet light (in the UV-C range of 254 nm) is a powerful disinfectant. The Japanese physician Dr. H. Noguchi demonstrated as early as 1906 that UV light inactivates the poisonous venom of both the cobra and rattlesnake.[9] UV light has been used for many years to purify water of a variety of pathogens including bacteria, viruses and protozoa. In fact, most anything can be sterilized effectively using UV radiation—simple ultraviolet light—including objects (e.g., surgical instruments), room air, and human skin.

It was perhaps a logical next step for researchers to investigate the disinfectant effects of UV irradiation in organisms having microbial infections of the blood. Referred to as hemo-irradiation, various experimental methods were employed in an attempt to destroy toxins within the blood using this technique. At first, mercury-vapor lamps were used to irradiate blood in petri dishes. Another method used the quartz-rod of a lamp as an applicator to stir a beaker of blood. Yet another method used a UV-irradiating quartz rod placed directly into an artery.[10]

In 1923, U.S. researchers tested UV blood irradiation—photoluminescence—on 40 dogs suffering from septicemia (infection of the blood by pathogenic microorganisms). Initially, the entire blood supply was irradiated, only to find that all the dogs died—presumably from shock. Thereafter, it was found that only a small portion of the total blood supply need be irradiated.[11]

After some experience was gained in the proper technique of administration, the researchers observed that the effects of the treatment were so unexpectedly beneficial they theorized additional physiological processes must be taking place. One of the early pioneers, Dr. Virgil Hancock, set forth several of the beneficial effects:[12]

1) An inactivation of toxins and viruses[13]
2) Destruction and inhibition of bacterial growth[14]
3) Increase in blood oxygen-combining power[15]
4) Activation of steroids[16]
5) Increased cell permeability[17]
6) Absorption of ultraviolet rays by the blood, and emanation of secondary irradiations[18]

A type of "induced secondary irradiation" occurs when blood is irradiated with ultraviolet light. This is a most unusual phenomenon, and is believed to be one of the principal mechanisms responsible for the dramatic effects produced. As Finsen demonstrated, hemoglobin—the iron-containing pigment of red blood cells that transports oxygen from the lungs to the tissues of the body—absorbs irradiated light energy over a broad range of UV wavelengths. These irradiated cells seem to "share the light" with some of their cellular brethren, so that other cells increase in photonic energy and "luminesce" in turn. This can be demonstrated by placing recently-irradiated blood in a thin-walled quartz vial (which passes UV-C wavelengths) and placing it in close proximity to UV-sensitive photographic film. The film quickly fogs over, indicating the presence of photonic UV energy within the blood.

Another pioneer in the field was Dr. E.W. Rebbeck, who personally administered over 3,000 UV blood irradiations. Rebbeck noticed that a dramatic increase in red blood cells often occurs following treatment—often as high as 1.2 million cells overnight, and tending to be accompanied by an increase in the white cell count. Dr. Rebbeck added to the list of beneficial results obtained and mechanisms of action defined:

❏ Activation of cortisone-like molecules, called sterols, into vitamin D.[19]

❏ Bacteria are killed directly by ultraviolet light and indirectly by increasing local and systemic resistance, an effect not entirely understood.[20] One of the main mechanisms of action may involve the formation of an autogenous (self-generated) vac-

cine that results from the destruction of bacteria within the irradiated blood sample.

❏ Restoration of normal chemical balances.

❏ In appropriate doses, it tends to correct cellular imbalances in the body.

❏ Disease-altered fat elements in the blood are restored to normal size and movement.

❏ UV radiation has cumulative effects. Each treatment builds on and enhances previous treatments.

❏ There are differences in sensitivity to UV radiation regarding systemic and skin effects.

❏ Sensitivity to light may be increased by certain drugs, such as sulfanilamide; foods such as buckwheat; and substances such as hematoporphyrin. In fact, a host of photosensitizing agents are known that can be administered as an adjunct to increase the effectiveness of treatment, often dramatically. Other photosensitizing agents include some amino acids, acridine dyes, adriamycin, chlorophyll, coal tar derivatives, hypericin, methylene blue, pentothiazine, porphyrins, quinine and tetracyclines.

❏ UV overdose produces depression, decreased resistance to bacterial infection, reduced bacteria-killing potency of the blood, and reduced hemoglobin. These levels are never approached in proper clinical practice.

❏ The action of UV may be immediate, delayed, markedly delayed or protracted.

The first article to detail the therapeutic efficacy of photoluminescence appeared in 1934. It was authored by Virgil Hancock and his colleague Emmett Knott, who was himself a great pioneer in the field. In 1944, Hancock and Knott made a presentation in Seattle, Washington at a meeting of the King County Medical Society. They offered the following explanations for the therapeutic benefits of the technique:[21]

1) Coagulation of bacteria caused by the creation of an "autogenous (self-generating) vaccine"
2) Immune enhancement: increased germicidal properties of the blood; increased antibodies
3) Luminescence: Induced secondary radiation produced by irradiated cells
4) Increased content of vitamin D and cholesterol in the blood plasma
5) Increased oxygen absorption by the blood

Over a span of several years Hancock and Knott reported many dramatic case histories. They treated a variety of ailments with remarkable success. By 1942, they had treated over 6,500 patients with photoluminescence, nearly all successfully, with no harmful side-effects. Not only was their work reported in scientific journals, but the most prestigious journals of their time. Dr. Rebbeck wrote in the early 1940s that Hancock and Knott "had in the irradiation of blood with ultraviolet spectral energy, a therapy of more pronounced value than any other method known to date."[22]

The therapeutic technique they used was simple and straightforward. A maximum of 1.5 milliliters of blood per pound of body weight was withdrawn (not more than 300 cc) into an air-tight circuit, with an anticoagulant added to prevent clotting. The blood circulated past an irradiation source, and was then re-injected into the patient through the same puncture site. The average time of exposure of the blood was only 10 seconds.

Types of Illnesses Treated. One of the most unusual phenomena associated with photoluminescence is the fact that the amount of pathogens killed during the direct radiation portion of treatment does not begin to account for the wide range of positive physiological effects. According to the Hancock and Knott method, only about 1/25th of the total blood volume (about 4%) is irradiated.

What happens to the remainder of the pathogens (~95%) which are never directly irradiated by the UV light? If direct radiation were the mechanism of microbial elimination, one would assume those pathogens not in the direct path of the UV photonic energy would live long, and prosper. On the contrary—and this is a fascinating aspect of UV blood irradiation—they do not! It's actually the re-injected blood which, through the various mechanisms discussed above (although still not totally understood), bolsters the immune system making it more effective against foreign invaders.

Further demonstrative of this unusual phenomenon are some of the experiments conducted by the early UV pioneers. In one such experiment, pathogens (bacteria) were mixed with blood and then irradiated for the length of time established by the Hancock and Knott protocol—about 10 seconds. The irradiation had virtually no effect on the microbes.[23]

Apparently such results encouraged skepticism about UV irradiation among many within the medical community. The early UV researchers probably entertained comments from their colleagues such as, "If your UV light won't kill bacteria in a petri dish, how do you expect it to produce any positive effects within the human body, eh?"

Pioneer researcher Dr. Henry Barrett sought to explain to his skeptical colleagues some of the understandings he had acquired during his personal use of the technique. Said Dr. Barrett:

> To those bacteriologists and others whose experience with ultraviolet energy has been largely confined to experiments consisting in the exposure of petri dish cultures to various sources of ultraviolet radiation, it is only fair to point out something that has apparently escaped many such an investigator, namely, the vast difference between inert gelatin and living, reacting animal tissue.[24]

With a degree of humility, as well as clarity, Barrett added:

> When we consider first of all the complexity of even the most simple photo-chemical processes and then reflect on the very complicated character of blood, consisting as it does of serum, red and white cells, platelets, chylomicrons [also called *somatids* by some modern researchers], antigens and antibodies, hormones, endocrine substances, enzymes, iron, phosphorous, calcium, and various pathogenic substances at times, bacterial and other toxins, and so forth, it seems somewhat foolhardy to undertake to say just what happens under the influence of ultraviolet radiation.[25]

One thing we do know is that the technique is effective against a broad range of maladies. The specifics of the mechanisms of action will unfold as new research brings deeper insights. It is known that the technique is 1) safe, 2) effective in treating a broad range of common ailments including serious diseases, 3) free of side effects, and 4) inexpensive compared to other treatments.

In 1939, Dr. George Miley studied the effects of UV irradiation on 97 patients suffering from various diseases. Miley observed the following:[26]

1) A 58% increase in venous oxygen within 10 minutes of treatment.

2) A 9% decrease in venous oxygen one-half hour following treatment. (This is theorized to be caused

by a "cleansing reaction" (the Herxheimer effect). 3) A 50% increase in venous oxygen one hour to one month following treatment.

During the late 1940s to the mid-1960s, American surgeon Robert Olney, M.D., studied photoluminescence, which he called Ultraviolet Blood Irradiation (UBI). Olney was a highly-respected surgeon whose studies were published in well-respected journals such as the *American Journal of Surgery* and the *Journal of the International College of Surgeons*.

Dr. Olney was a student of the works of Dr. Otto Warberg (1883-1970) of the Kaiser-Wilhelm-Institut für Biologie in Germany (currently the Max-Planck-Institut). Dr. Warberg was awarded the Nobel Prize in Physiology/Medicine in 1931 "for his discovery of the nature and mode of action of the respiratory enzyme."[27] Olney knew Warberg had found that a "blocking or impairment" of oxidation enzymes within cells produces an anaerobic (without oxygen) respiratory cycle involving fermentation of sugars within the cells—not the normal cycle of respiratory oxygenation. Warberg believed this lack of proper oxygenation within the cells is the primary cause of cancer. A corollary to this is that if the dangerous fermentative cycle can once again be replaced by the normal oxidative respiratory cycle, pathogenic organisms can revert to being non-pathogenic.

With this as his theoretical basis, Olney set out to investigate the effects of UBI on cancer patients. He reasoned that if cancer is the result of poor blood oxygenation, and that if UBI significantly increases oxygen blood levels, then he may have found an effective treatment for the dreaded disease. Through several studies, Olney (re-) established that blood oxygen levels are consistently low in most if not all pathological conditions, i.e., persons who are ill or immune-compromised, ranging from cancer patients to heavy cigarette smokers.

In the mid-1960s, Olney published a monograph reporting five case histories of cancer patients whom he treated using the identical technique as Knott, but Olney irradiated 500 ml of blood, and he used wavelengths in the ultraviolet-A range. That's "black light" folks! One case study follows:[28]

> D.P., a 30-year-old white male, was admitted to the hospital with a diagnosis of generalized malignant melanoma (a virulent form of skin cancer). Eleven years previously, a malignant melanoma had been removed from his right upper arm. When admitted to the hospital by Dr. Olney he had a tumor mass under the skin at the upper left chest just below the clavicle. Excision and biopsy revealed that the malignant melanoma had returned. He quickly developed metastases all over his body and his abdomen became very large from tumor growth. He had difficulty in breathing, had a constant cough and was obviously in serious condition. He was blue in the face and cancer could be felt throughout his abdomen.

> The patient was given ultraviolet blood irradiation therapy immediately and approximately every three days for about one week and then weekly. Within three weeks, the large tumor mass in his right armpit disappeared as well as a tumor on the right chest wall; the abdomen became definitely smaller and the tumor masses much less palpable. At the end of six weeks of treatment, the patient had no difficulty in breathing; his right leg, which had been extremely swollen, was normal and free of pain; and the abdomen had returned to normal size with no fluid or tumor masses palpable.

Following the case history, Dr. Olney commented about this patient:

> This case illustrates the very early, effective results of treatment with the whole program that we are now using for the treatment of all malignancy. This treatment is based upon the evidence that cancer is due to hypoxemia [low blood oxygen] and blocking of oxidation with the development of fermentation of sugars which causes the cancer's growth. It has been shown that all cancers have one common factor and that is fermentation of sugar in the enzymes and cells replacing normal oxidation. Reversal of this process back to normal oxidation is all-important.

A partial list of the types of illnesses photoluminescence treated effectively includes:[29]

+ AIDS/HIV
+ Any pathogenic substances in the blood, e.g., bacteria, viruses, fungi and parasites.
+ Appendicitis
+ Arthritis
+ Asthma
+ Autonomic nervous system balancing
+ Boils

◆ Cancer
◆ Generalized peritonitis
◆ Pneumonia
◆ Polio
◆ Septicemia
◆ Toxin neutralization (biowarfare agents—botulism, diphtheria, poisonous venoms, and tetanus)
◆ Tuberculosis
◆ Wound infections

Contemporary Researchers. Dr. William C. Douglass. In 1989 the well-known American physician Dr. William C. Douglass established a clinic in Uganda, Africa—a country hard-hit by HIV/AIDS. His choice of treatment was a combination of photoluminescence and intravenous hydrogen peroxide therapy, which he calls Photo-Oxidative therapy, or Photox. Douglass has written that,

> Word of the remarkable improvements seen in terminally ill patients with "slim" (African terminology for AIDS) has traveled across the country and the clinic is inundated with patients...We have proven in Africa, beyond a doubt, that photo-oxidation is the best treatment currently available for the treatment of AIDS...only lack of money prevents us from demonstrating that photo-oxidation is the best treatment currently available for AIDS and all infectious diseases.[30]

Dr. Douglass has administered hundreds of photoluminescence treatments in his medical practice, treating a wide variety of ailments. His treatment protocol is similar to the Knott technique, with one difference being that in one variation of his protocol he irradiates a smaller volume of blood—in the range of 10 cc. You can read Dr. Douglass' complete protocol—including the one in which he irradiates larger volumes of blood—in the recent edition of his book *Into the Light: The Exciting Story of the Life-Saving Breakthrough Therapy of the Age*, available either as an e-book or in hard copy. In the e-book version (but not the hard copy) there is a schematic diagram of an Ultraviolet Blood Irradiation apparatus which is very similar to the Knott apparatus, which irradiates larger volumes of blood. To purchase a state-of-the-art ultraviolet blood irradiation device, visit www.ozonegenerator.com. Click on "UV Instruments."

The e-book is the latest version of his book, and Dr. Douglass includes in it both a diagram of a simple blood irradiation device as well as a detailed description of his current clinical protocol. This information is included because he wants people to understand that in a time of dire emergency—such as a bioterror attack—all public medical facilities would likely be tremendously overburdened to the point of inaccessibility to the average citizen. In other words, if there really ever were such a catastrophic event as a biological attack or even a large-scale biological accident, chances are that you and your family would have to fend for yourselves.

While you wouldn't be able to self-administer a CAT Scan or personally initiate a course of chemotherapy (not that you'd want to—but even if you did, the necessary equipment and practical expertise is beyond the means of the average person), it is entirely within the means of most people to self-administer (or with the help of one other person) a course of treatment using ultraviolet light to irradiate the blood. Although Dr. Douglass cautions that self- (home-) administration should be attempted only in the case of an emergency, the technique does offer a possible means of protecting oneself and one's family *if all else fails*. The Boy Scout's motto is particularly relevant here: Be Prepared!

Dr. Douglass suggests that with little difficulty a handyman-type person would be able to construct the device he pictures. Although the device is fairly simple, if a true emergency were to manifest, a simpler apparatus and protocol could be useful. Dr. Douglass does describe a very simple protocol and apparatus in one variation of the technique, as follows:

> A 23- or 21-gauge butterfly needle is placed in an arm vein or the external jugular vein. Ten cc's of whole blood is withdrawn into a pure quartz syringe (Careful—they are very expensive and quite fragile.) [Quartz in this case is pure fused silica, necessary to pass UV at 254 nm. If using UV-A (black light), a regular glass syringe is adequate, as glass will pass this wavelength.] and put into the Photolume II instrument through a circular opening in the front of the machine. The syringe rotates slowly and is thus exposed to continuous ultraviolet light...The exposure time is three minutes. The syringe containing radiated blood is then withdrawn from the Photolume and reinjected intravenously. The original IV is kept open during the extracorporeal [out of the body] ultravio-

let irradiation by a heparin lock or by a slow hydrogen peroxide (0.015 solution) drip.[31]

Dr. Richard Edelson. The benefits of photoluminescence haven't escaped one contemporary researcher, Dr. Richard Edelson of the Department of Dermatology, Yale University. Edelson, who has labeled his technique "Extracorporeal Photopheresis (ECP)," is effectively treating a rare form of malignant cancer called cutaneous T-cell lymphoma (CTCL), the only disease for which UV blood treatment is officially sanctioned by the FDA. The typical survival rate of persons with CTCL is less than five years. Edelson's group obtained remissions of over 10 years using UV-A wavelengths.[32]

Edelson adds a photosensitizing agent to the blood which he believes increases the effectiveness of the procedure. Because the photosensitizing agent affects only cells having a nucleus, which red blood cells and platelets do not, Edelson's method separates white (nucleated) blood cells from the red cells and plasma (non-nucleated)—allowing the treatment to focus on the white cells.

Photoluminescence also appears promising in other areas, according to contemporary investigators. Using ECP, Costanzo-Nordin, *et al* reported that eight out of nine cardiac transplant rejections were reversed after one or two UV treatments. Edelson's technique also is effective both as a preventive adjunct to post-transplant immunosuppression and in the reversal of severe transplant rejection which is untreatable by all standard pharmacotherapy. Recalcitrant rejection in cardiac, pulmonary, renal (kidney), and hepatic (liver) transplant recipients has been reversed.[33]

Recent, small pilot studies have suggested the efficacy of UV irradiation in the treatment of atopic dermatitis, epidermolysis bullosa acquisita, inflammatory bowel disease, pemphigus vulgaris, rheumatoid arthritis, and systemic lupus erythematosus. Other indications are that the technique may be effective against AIDS-related complex, chronic hepatitis C, and multiple sclerosis.[34]

Although Edelson's technique is achieving impressive results, it is questionable whether the cost/benefit ratio warrants the use of such an expensive technique that virtually prices itself out of the range of any means of payment other than medical insurance. Further, even with all of the fancy, modern medical equipment in use today, contemporary practitioners seem not to have made significant improvements beyond the methods that were developed and utilized equally successfully more than 60 years ago which used techniques that are both extremely simple, very inexpensive and effective.

German Researchers. German physicians and medical researchers have recently reported significant improvement in vascular conditions when using ultraviolet blood irradiation, including peripheral arterial disease and Raynaud's disease (a vascular disease characterized by recurrent spasms of the capillaries). One study demonstrated a 124% increase in painless walking for patients with Stage IIb occlusive disease (Fontaine), as compared to 48% improvement with Pentoxifylline [a pharmaceutical drug designed to treat intermittent claudication (cramping pain in the legs when walking usually due to inadequate blood circulation—see *Cardiovascular Disease*) by reducing blood viscosity, thereby increasing microcirculatory blood flow].[35] UV blood irradiation improves claudication walking distances by 90% after a series of 10 treatments.[36] The authors also reported an 8% drop in plasma viscosity within the treated group, compared to no change in the Pentoxifylline group.

Frick reported an increase in prostacyclin (inhibits aggregation of platelets and dilates blood vessels) and a reduction in arteriosclerotic plaque. UV treatments were expanded to include circulatory diseases such as post-apoplexy (stroke), diabetes, venous ulcers and migraines. The researchers believe the biochemical effects are generated by the activation of molecular oxygen to singlet oxygen by UV energy. This active species of oxygen initiates a cascade of molecular reactions, resulting in the observed effects. Ultimately, this controlled oxidation process leads to a rise in the principle antioxidant enzyme systems of the body—*catalase, superoxide dismutase*, and *glutathione peroxidase*.[37] Contraindications included porphyria (an hereditary abnormality), photosensitivity, hemophilia, hyperthyroidism, and fever of unknown origin (but not pregnancy). The device utilized in this research was the Oxysan EN 400, manufactured by the Eumatron Company.

The following list summarizes the German findings concerning mechanisms of action and effects of Ultraviolet Blood Irradiation.[38] As we can see, each group of researchers from the early U.S.

pioneers to the present, put forth their own list of mechanisms which they believed are responsible for the beneficial effects of photoluminescence:

Biophysical and Chemical Effects
• Improvement of the electrophoretic movability of the red blood cells
• Elevation of the electrical charge on the red blood cells
• Lowering of the surface tension of the blood
• Origin of free radicals
• Elevation of the chemical illuminescence of blood

Hematologic Changes
• Increase in erythrocytes
• Increase in hemoglobin
• Increase in basophilic granulocytes
• Increase in lymphophocytes
• Decrease of thrombocytes

Hemostatic Changes
• Lowering of platelet aggregation
• Lowering of fibrin
• Normalization of fibrinolysis
• Tends to normalize fibrin-split products

Blood Parameter Changes
• Lowering of full-blood viscosity
• Lowering of plasma viscosity
• Reduction of elevated red blood cell aggregation

Metabolic Changes – Oxygen Utilization
• Increase in arterial pO_2
• Increase in venous pO_2
• Increase in arterial venous oxygen difference (increased oxygen release)
• Increase in peroxide count
• Increase in acid-buffering capacity and rise in blood pH
• Reduction in blood pyruvate content
• Reduction in blood lactate content
• Improvement in glucose tolerance
• Reduction in cholesterol count, transaminases, and creatine levels

Thermodynamic Changes
• Elevation of post stenotic arterial pressure
• Increase in volume of circulation

Improvement in Immune Defenses
• Increase in phagocytosis capability
• Increase in bacteriocidal capacity of blood
• Modulation of the immune status

Russian Researchers. Russian medical practitioners have been on the UBI bandwagon for some 30 years. Following the advent of costly antibiotic drugs, the Soviets were pressed to uncover alternative means of treating infection. Based on the early work of American engineer Emmett Knott and a sizable group of his medical colleagues, the Soviet physicians were able to bypass much time-consuming animal experimentation and move directly to human subjects.[39] They quickly discovered that UV blood irradiation is an effective technique in the treatment of far more than infectious diseases, and that the technique can be used on a multiplicity of additional ailments.

Physicians of the former USSR have administered over 500,000 treatments to over 100,000 patients as an adjunct to surgical operations. At the City Center for the Fotomodification of Blood in St. Petersburg, UV light therapy has cut the number of surgical complications by 50% and significantly reduced the necessity of antibiotics in severe trauma cases.[40] Cases have ranged from crushed kidneys to severe bleeding in the chest and abdominal cavities. Often the patient's own blood is collected from the wound site, irradiated, and then "auto-transfused" back to the patient.

The Soviets are using UV blood irradiation on severe burn victims with great success. Dr. V.M. Novopoltzeva of the Mordovsky University in Saransk, Russia, has treated many third degree burn cases with an apparatus similar to the Photolume III, an instrument being used in clinics around the world. Dr. Novopoltzeva and colleagues made the following observations:[41]

❍ The patients' general state improves almost immediately after UV blood re-infusion.
❍ Patients' appetites improve markedly.
❍ Severe pain subsides, and patients are often able to discontinue narcotic injections.
❍ Increase in the protein content of the blood usually following the first irradiation.
❍ Improved sleep due to the above changes.

A Ukranian study reports on the use of UBI in cases of ear, nose and throat disease (ENT). Dr. Filatov and colleagues at the Kharkov Medical Institute treated 173 patients with ENT diseases including chronic sinusitis, chronic middle ear infection, nasal furuncles (nose sores), and rhinogenic sepsis (often deadly blood poisoning due to a nasal infection). In most all cases the results were "extremely good." The study also notes that in cases of eardrum surgery, the UV patients' healing time was half that of the non-treated group.[42]

Bacterial endocardiasis, an infection of the heart valves, responds well to UBI. Ukrainian physician Dr. Krishtof has treated over 250 such cases with great success. Following treatment, 43 of the patients no longer needed surgical repair. Those who received UBI following surgery faired significantly better that their non-treated counterparts, including greatly-reduced recovery times.[43]

Physicians at the Sklifosovsky Institute for Urgent Medicine have effectively used UBI in the treatment of chemical toxicity. One hundred twenty eight patients were treated for either organophosphate or psychotropic drug toxicity, with the following results: 1) a 100% decrease in coma recovery time, 2) 50% fewer complications such as pneumonia, and 3) a 40% mortality reduction.[44]

The Krasnoyarsk Cancer Center has used UBI to treat post-operative cases of cancer of the rectum and colon. Of the 22 cases treated, the indications were as follows: 1) significant pain reduction often resulting in narcotics not being required on the first or second day following surgery, 2) no cases of adynamic ileus (paralysis of the intestines often following abdominal surgery), and 3) reduction in post-operative infections from 30% to 10%.[45]

Dr. Igor Dutkevich from Hospital 15 in St. Petersburg has treated patients with cancer of the bladder, kidney, lung and stomach. The results included 1) shortened hospital stays due to decreased recovery times, 2) a significant decrease in the frequency of post-operative complications (from 20% to 11%), and 3) a marked decrease in mortality (from 5.8% to 3%).[46]

Thirty-four patients were treated for hypertension (high blood pressure) at the Azerbaijan Republican Hospital in Baku. The criteria for selection were at least one of the following: 1) extremely high blood pressure, 2) treatment by anti-hypertensive drugs was ineffective, 3) patient could not tolerate anti-hypertensive drugs. Patients began an intensive course of photoluminescent therapy. A significant number of patients responded positively, averaging a 30% decrease in systolic and diastolic pressures. There was an accompanying reduction

of symptoms including chest pain, headaches, and dizziness. Improvements lasted at least 10 months with no evidence of vascular disease progression.[47]

A group of St. Petersburg physicians treated 145 patients who previously had a heart attack, and who currently had severe blockage of the arteries to the heart. All patients had not responded well to drug treatment. Following UBI treatment, 94% of the patients reported a "significant improvement," with accompanying reduction of pain (angina).[48]

At the Lenin Hospital, Dr. Lev Kukui and colleagues over a span of 15 years have treated over 250 patients having serious coronary heart disease. Ninety-five percent of those treated with UBI showed "at least a partial amelioration" of symptoms, and only 9% were unable to return to work. The dosage of nitroglycerine needed to prevent chest pain was reduced from 10 to an average of three tablets per day. Using red laser light (~690 nm) to irradiate the blood, Kukui's group was able to prevent heart attacks in 90% of patients having severe angina pain, while only 30% of the control group did not have a heart attack. Heart arrhythmia was successfully treated in 81% of the treatment group, compared to only 33% in the non-treated group.[49]

Dr. Levin and associates treated several cases of blockage of the leg arteries, a common problem of diabetics and heavy smokers. Eight of the 11 cases treated experienced significant pain relief accompanied by a reduction in pain medication; improved sleep and appetite; and improved healing of leg ulcerations.[50]

Some researchers believe that sensitive light-measuring devices will one day enable the early diagnosis of disease by the monitoring of light frequency emissions from cells. Diseased or compromised cells emit abnormal wavelengths of light which would be detected by these sensitive instruments. Also, *unhealthy cells give off more light* than their healthy counterparts. The blood of patients with cancer and diabetes, for example, emanate more light than the blood of healthy patients.

Smokers' cells, it has been found, emit twice as much light as their non-smoking counterparts. Their urine also gives off more light. Interestingly, within 24-hours of cessation of smoking, photon emission levels return to normal, apparently even if a person has been smoking for some time.[51] It is believed that the increased light production is caused by the increased production of free radicals within unhealthy cells. [High dose (5mg/day) folic acid taken over a one month period confers significant cardiovascular protection (increased arterial elasticity and lower blood pressure) to cigarette smokers].

Masaki Kobayashi of Tohoku University hopes that a new generation of photodetecting equipment such as *avalanche photodiodes* will boost the chances of detecting signals from individual photons from around 20% to 80% or greater. Equipment such as this could provide the breakthrough in sensitivity needed to develop a scanner capable of diagnosing disease via cellular photonic output.

Other researchers are developing new photoluminescent treatment techniques employing a broader range of the electromagnetic spectrum. Dr. Douglass, for example, is developing an apparatus that radiates all wavelengths of light ranging from 250 nm (germicidal UV) to 700 nm (red; just this side of infrared.) The theoretical understanding is that the body will then select the portion of the spectrum the irradiated blood sample needs for healing. He also is a proponent of adding photosensitizing agents to the blood to increase the effectiveness of the procedure.

Because Dr. Douglass is one of the principal living proponents of ultraviolet blood irradiation, it's only appropriate to conclude with his words:

> ...I hope many of you will join me in seeking to effect the widespread implementation of this miraculous technology, and to explore its possibilities further...Realizing those possibilities will mean the difference between health and sickness—and often, life and death—to millions of people. But it will mean the difference on an even larger scale. In the face of the AIDS epidemic, the very survival of our way of life is at stake. The key to the future health of our culture lies with widespread implementation of photoluminescence.[52]

Why isn't photoluminescence offered as a mainstream treatment in today's world? If effective, non-invasive therapies such as Photoluminescence are real, it's only fair they be made available to the needy public. It's unfortunate, however, that all too often—regardless of the reasons—much medical knowledge and understanding never reaches the surface of public awareness. To seasoned medical investigators this trend is as predictable as

snow is cold. Could Photoluminescence simply not have been allowed to prosper in the presence of an industry whose major entities dominate the playing field? Regardless of your personal conclusion, individuals can at least take advantage of what's now available, while hoping the future brings more forthrightness on the part of the medical establishment.

Contact Information. A state-of-the-art UBI apparatus is available at www.ozonegenerator.com. Click on "UV Instruments." If you are a medical professional wanting to be trained in the techniques of Ultraviolet Blood Irradiation, or if you would like to locate a UBI practitioner in your location, contact the International Oxidative Medical Association (IOMA; 800-235-4788) and/or the International Bio-Oxidative Medicine Foundation (IBOMF; 541-955-3372). These organizations conduct workshops and supply UBI equipment. A list for your area is available from IOMA or IBOMF.

PROLOTHERAPY

Flexible joints are comprised of cartilage-covered bone held in place by ligaments, strong bands of tissue that attach the articular extremities of bones to each other. Normal, healthy ligaments are taut, and hold the joints firmly in place. When ligaments become damaged, they become lax and allow too much movement within the joint—resulting in nerve fiber activation which causes pain and inflammation within the joint. Similarly, tendons are tough fibrous cords that connect muscle to bone, and can also cause inflammation when injured.

Prolotherapy is minimally-invasive, non-surgical ligament and tendon reconstruction. The goal of Prolotherapy, also called *sclerotherapy* and *reconstructive therapy*, is to re-tighten the ligaments and tendons of joints and other painful areas by shorting the collagen fibers within the connective tissues. By so doing, the structure causing the pain regains its normally-taut configuration, thereby eliminating the pain. Thus, Prolotherapy eliminates the root cause of pain.

This is accomplished by means of injections of a slightly irritating solution—usually glucose, dextrose, or saline (this varies slightly depending on the practitioner)—into the pain-causing areas where the ligaments and tendons attach to the bone. The injections are given by means of a slender, hair-like needle similar to those used in acupuncture. In effect, the injections simulate a new injury and trick the body into beginning new healing.

During the initial phase following the injection(s), the irritant causes inflammation and an immune reaction occurs. White blood cells (macrophages) and prostaglandins flock to the area and begin the work of helping to remove debris and foreign matter from the damaged area. Within a day or two, new collagen begins to proliferate and the ligaments and tendons begin to strengthen. Over a period of several weeks, this rebuilding (regeneration) process continues until the previously-weakened and relaxed connective tissues are returned to their normal, taut configuration—once again holding the joint(s) firmly in place in a manner similar to the pre-injury state. Research has shown that Prolotherapy increases ligament mass, thickness and cross-sectional area as well as strength.[1] It is this "proliferation" of new collagen within the ligaments and tendons from which the treatment derives its name "prolo."

One to several treatments are necessary to restore normal, pain-free functioning. The average number of treatments is about five, but ten or more may be required per each area treated, depending upon the severity of the problem. Each successive treatment results in the development of more tissue, causing the joint to become stronger and stronger. For many patients, even those who unsuccessfully have tried other treatment techniques such as drugs, chiropractic, physical therapy and even surgery, prolotherapy can provide near-miraculous results.

One of the most ardent supporters of Prolotherapy is Dr. C. Everett Koop, former Surgeon General of the United States. Dr. Koop describes his personal experience which saved his career as a practicing surgeon:

> When I was 40 years old, I was diagnosed in two separate neurological clinics as having intractable (incurable) pain...It was by chance that I learned Gustav A. Hemwall, M.D., a practitioner in the suburbs of Chicago, was an expert in Prolotherapy...To make a long story short, my intractable pain was not intractable and I was remarkably improved to the point to where my pain ceased to be a problem.[2]

Dr. Hemwall collected data on thousands of patients he treated over the years, and reported that 75.5% of the patients report complete recovery (cure), while an additional 24.3% reported general improvement. Only 0.2 % of the patients reported no improvement. Some quick addition shows that over 99% of Dr. Hemwall's patients significantly benefitted from Prolotherapy. Other studies have shown similar results.[3]

The Father of Prolotherapy, Dr. George Hackett, conducted research studies demonstrating the effectiveness of the technique. Published in 1958 in the third edition of his book *Ligament and Tendon Relaxation Treated by Prolotherapy*, Dr. Hackett evaluated Prolotherapy's effectiveness on 656 patients over a period of 19 years. The average duration of pain prior to treatment was 4.5 years, but ranged from three months to 65 years. Dr. Hackett reported that 12 years following the completion of the treatments, 82% of the patients considered themselves cured.[4]

Prolotherapy is an effective treatment for arthritis, back pain, carpal tunnel syndrome, chronic foot pain, fibromyalgia, frozen shoulder, herniated discs, loose joints, migraine headaches, neck pain, rotator cuff injuries, RSD pain, sciatica, sports injuries, tendinitis, tennis elbow, TMJ, and more.

Dr. Koop was so impressed with the results of Prolotherapy that he considered practicing the technique in his years following retirement from the University of Pennsylvania. That vision ended when President Reagan called on him to become Surgeon General. As to why not many physicians are aware of Prolotherapy, Koop states,

> In my opinion it is because medical folks are skeptical and Prolotherapy, unless you have tried it and proven its worth, seems to be too easy a solution to a series of complicated problems that afflict the human body and have been notoriously difficult to treat by any other method.[5]

To this we would add that medical techniques which don't handsomely profit either the pharmaceutical industry or the surgical community generally receive very little play. Because the technique is relatively unknown to the medical establishment, it is not usually covered by medical insurance.

To learn more about Prolotherapy, visit www.prolotherapy.org. To locate a prolotherapy practitioner in your location, call the American Association of Orthopedic Medicine (AAOM) at

(800)992-2063, or the American College of Osteopathic Pain Management and Sclerotherapy (ACOPMS) at (302)376-8080; or visit www.get prolo.com.

A modification of Prolotherapy has been developed by Nevada physician Dr. Frank Shallenberger. Known as Prolozone,® the technique uses a small amount of an oxygen and ozone gas mixture in place of the glucose, dextrose, or other solutions used in Prolotherapy. Because areas of injury, hence pain, are oxygen deprived, the administration of additional oxygen together with a small amount of the very reactive ozone gas causes an immediate boost in cellular energy production, tissue regeneration and repair, and a reduction in inflammation. According to Shallenberger and others who have used both techniques, Prolozone accomplishes in one session what normally takes several Prolotherapy sessions. Also, it requires less needle insertions per session—hence less pain—as the gas diffuses into an expanded area compared to the fluid solutions used in Prolotherapy. To learn more, visit www.antiagingmedicine.com/procedures.htm.

RESVERATROL

For the better part of the past 300 years, scientists have strived to "reverse engineer" the cell in an attempt to discover the genetic mysteries locked within its walls. The modern conception of genetics originated with the 19th Century Austrian monk Gregor Mendel, whose work confirmed that traits are inherited from one generation to the next in discrete informational units which interact in well-defined ways. In 1909, Danish botanist Wilhelm Johannsen used the term *gene* to describe these fundamental units of heredity, a term derived from the Greek words *genesis* (birth) or *genos* (origin). Simply stated, according to this current view of genetics, the various physical and behavioral characteristics of an organism—its *phenotypes*—are a function of variations in *genotype*, the organisms' specific set of genes, each set of which denotes a specific trait.

Each human inherits 23 sets of chromosomes from their parents, each chromosome being comprised of a single macro (large) molecule of DNA (deoxyribonucleic acid). DNA is a long polymer made up of more simple units called *nucleotides.*

DNA is a nucleic acid which contains the genetic instructions that guide living organisms to develop and function properly. The principal role of cellular DNA is the long-term storage of the information relating to reproduction of the organism, e.g., how to construct proteins, hormones, enzymes, RNA, other cell components, etc. The thousands of genes—arranged on strands of DNA—are the specific segments that carry this genetic information and, like a conductor, orchestrate all of the necessary components into the meaningful whole of life itself.

As a human fetus develops in the mothers' womb, thousands of genes direct the incredible growth process that is evolving. Following birth, many of these genes are naturally turned down/deactivated, while others activate and begin to direct a new set of growth and development tasks. Between the second and third decade of human life, many previously-activated genes begin to deactivate. As we age, there is a gradual loss of genetic power as more and more genes progressively deactivate in accordance with genetically-controlled mechanisms that govern their activity.

In addition to the natural biological mechanisms that deactivate genes, environmental factors also play a role. Lifestyle choices such as improper nutrition, excessive alcohol consumption, smoking, and lack of physical activity are factors that contribute to the aging process in several ways, but also by deactivating genes.

It is known that the reproductive capability and growth of organisms—genetics—can be altered by various other means. For example, researchers have known since the 1930s that the maximum lifespan of many species can be extended by reducing food consumption by 30-40% of normal intake, while at the same time providing sufficient nutrition. This area of research was originally proposed by the renowned gerontologist Dr. Roy Walford of U.C.L.A., and has come to be known as calorie restriction (CR), calorie restriction with optimal nutrition (CRON), or calorie restriction with adequate nutrition (CRAN). Researchers recently have discovered a genetic link to this phenomenon.

The positive health effects, and particularly CR's ability to extend maximum lifespan, have now been demonstrated in all species tested including fish, fruit flies, hamsters, mice, spiders, worms, and even yeast cells. There is ongoing research with rhesus and squirrel monkeys and, although it is too soon to draw a definitive conclusion, current observations suggest the response of primates to CR is almost identical to that of the other species tested. The noted effects include lower body temperatures; lower levels of glucose and insulin within the bloodstream; less chronic disease; and more youthful levels of various hormones including *dehydroepiandrosterone* (DHEA)—a chemical which has gained considerable attention in recent years as a possible longevity promoter.

Similar attempts in humans by life-extension enthusiasts using a self-administered CR protocol are ongoing. Because humans have a considerably longer lifespan in comparison to most other animals—and the relatively short duration of the ongoing human experiments—no final conclusions have been drawn regarding the human response to calorie restriction, although it is assumed the results will be similar to those already demonstrated in the many other animal species tested.

The life-extension effect of calorie restriction is dramatic, prolonging the life of laboratory animals by up to 60%, and yeast cells by up to 70%.[1] This would be equivalent to increasing the human lifespan to 140-160 years. There are several mechanisms apparently responsible for this effect. In both rodents and primates, the reduction of glucose and insulin levels and increased cellular sensitivity to insulin are among the most consistent responses noted, occurring within weeks of being initiated. The alteration of glucose and insulin levels as a result of CR implicate cellular metabolism as being intimately involved in the life-extension process. Although there are likely several mechanisms in play, the reduction of glucose and insulin levels may signal cells to adopt a "self-protective" mode, sensing that food supplies are scarce. Cellular maintenance and repair—i.e., preservation—may become the predominant metabolic focus, thereby enhancing cellular function, hence longevity.

Scientists recently identified a class of "longevity genes" called *sirtuins* (sir-TOO-inz)—derived from the term "silent information regulator proteins." They appear to be universal regulators of aging in all living organisms, i.e., they are the central regulators of the aging process. It is the activation or "switching on" of these genes by environmental cues including reduced glucose and insulin levels following calorie restriction that induce cellular changes such as adopting the protective mode of self preservation (as an adaptation technique), which includes the slowing of metabolism and enhancement of cellular respiration.[2]

Unfortunately, the degree of calorie restriction in humans necessary to accomplish a potential increase in lifespan and healthspan (the number of years we live a healthy life) would require a daily dietary intake of only about 1,750 calories. This austere, impractical regimen would be acceptable only to the most stalwart of individuals. For most Westerners, it would be tantamount to asking teenagers not to daydream about sex. For most of us, as they say, "It ain't gonna happen."

Spurred on by the great potential benefits of calorie restriction (and the reactivation of certain genes linked to the process) without the necessity of enduring a continuous state of semi-starvation, scientists have been searching for ways of mimicking the effects of CR without its attendant drawbacks. Of the various substances investigated as possible calorie restriction mimetics, one stands out as a leader—*resveratrol*, a substance first identified as recently as the early 1980s, and one that is destined to gain recognition as one of the most important health-giving substances ever identified.

A naturally-occurring compound, resveratrol is found in various food-stuffs and plants including berries, grapes, peanuts, pine trees, some herbs, and most notably in the root of the plant *Polygonum cuspidatum*. It occurs in a *cis* and *trans* molecular form, the trans form being biologically active. Chemically, resveratrol is classified a *polyphenol*, a broad group of plant-derived compounds further subdivided into other categories including the familiar group *flavonoids*, as well as *tannins, lignins,* and *phenylpropanoids*.

One common source of resveratrol is wine, a drink that has recently gained notoriety for promoting various important health benefits. In a study of 25,000 people, Danish researchers recently determined that wine drinkers reduce their overall risk of dying from any cause (all-cause mortality) by roughly 40%.[3] Consequently, some believe resveratrol may be at least partially responsible for this beneficial health effect. Because resveratrol forms in wine grapes in response to and as a defense against fungal infection, it is substantially present only in organic grapes—and predominately in red rather than white wines. Wine grapes grown by typical Western farming methods are treated so heavily with fungicides that resveratrol is produced only in very small quantities, e.g., less than one milligram per glass of red wine.

To qualify as a true calorie restriction mimetic, a substance must reduce the incidence of chronic diseases as well as activate genetic "switch" mechanisms which induce longevity, both of which occur in response to the calorie restriction protocol. Resveratrol seems to have both of these abilities by working through similar physiological mechanisms as CR. It is a powerful antioxidant, inhibiting low-density lipoprotein (LDL) oxidation and scavenging hydroxyl radicals—a highly-reactive radical with a half-life of only 10^{-9} seconds, but capable of damaging amino acids, lipids, and nucleic acids. It also preserves glutathione, the master antioxidant.

Resveratrol also boosts energy in the mitochondria, the reduction of which is a principal cause of aging and age-related chronic disease. Perhaps most interestingly, it is a gene expression modifier, as is calorie restriction. As such, both resveratrol and calorie restriction exert small quantitative effects on the level of expression of various genes. That is, they modulate (activate or inhibit) genetic pathways involved in lifespan extension. Resveratrol's life-extending capability may result from its ability to modify the SIRT2 gene, one of the family of sirtuin longevity-related genes.[4]

In the summer of 2003, Harvard researchers published a landmark study that shocked the anti-aging world.[5] The Harvard team demonstrated resveratrol—even in small amounts—is able to extend the life of yeast cells by 60-80%, as measured by the number of surviving generations. These results are similar to those obtained by caloric restriction. The researchers concluded that resveratrol activates a longevity gene in yeast cells in a fashion similar to the activation by calorie restriction of similar genes in the many animal species discussed. In other words, resveratrol extends survival by regulating a longevity gene or genes present in all life forms investigated, from yeast cells to humans. By means of a sophisticated technique known as *molecular pathway analysis*, both resveratrol-treated as well

as calorie-restricted animals show a significant overlap of modulated gene expression. Genes affected by resveratrol control over 100 key molecular pathways, including metabolism, DNA repair, and normal cell death. Apparently, it is the chemical structure of resveratrol rather than its other attributes (antioxidant properties, etc.) that is responsible for its gene-regulating ability.

In cancer studies, both in the laboratory (*in vitro*) and in animals (*in vivo*), resveratrol has been shown to inhibit cellular events associated with all three mechanisms of cancer formation—tumor initiation, promotion, and progression.[6] In laboratory cell cultures, it shows anti-cancer effects on many types cancer cells including breast, cervix, colon, esophagus, leukemia, lung, melanoma, neuroblastoma, ovary, pancreas, prostate, stomach, and thyroid.[7] Additionally, resveratrol increases the effectiveness of chemotherapeutic cancer drugs by sensitizing the targeted cancer cells, while at the same time reducing the toxic effects so characteristic of this class of drugs.[8]

In 2004, a group of Taiwanese researchers showed that resveratrol-fed laboratory mice experienced delayed skin tumor-induced tumor formation, with fewer tumors per animal compared to the untreated control group.[9] Other researchers treated rats implanted with hepatoma cells, one of the most aggressive forms of cancer. Tumor growth and metastasis were reduced in two studies.[10] Resveratrol was further shown to enhance the efficacy and reduce the toxicity of the anti-cancer drug 5-FU.[11] Significant anti-tumor effects were shown in lab animals implanted with glioma, a type of brain tumor. Positive effects included slower tumor growth, higher survival rates, and longer survival times.[12] It has been noted that the powerful antioxidant effects of resveratrol may inhibit healthy tissues from chemotherapy-induced damage.

Resveratrol also prevents many of the harmful effects caused by overeating and obesity. To learn more about this unusual benefit, see Resveratrol under **Diabetes.**

Although resveratrol has shown benefits in very small doses, at least 100 mg daily are recommended for maximum health benefits. One product that's highly recommended is Mega Potency Natural Resveratrol by Now Foods, which provides 200 mg of *trans* resveratrol per capsule.

SEANOL®

The Seanol story begins in the late 1980s at the University of Iowa, where three Ph.D.s of Korean decent were working on developing drugs for cardiovascular and Alzheimer's diseases. By the beginning of the 1990s, they had begun to question the conventional method of drug development which focuses only on strong inhibition of specific biochemical processes, often leading to more harm than benefit. This is especially true of chronic degenerative diseases including Alzheimer's, arthritis, cardiovascular diseases, and cancer.

One of the researchers had an interest in the physiological actions of what's referred to as "second metabolites" of land and sea plants. After five years of research focused primarily on compounds extracted from algae (seaweeds), he announced his success in isolating several new antioxidant compounds from edible algae. The three researchers confirmed the extracts' great potential as a superior natural agent with absolute safety and long-term efficacy in age-related chronic degenerative diseases.

They subsequently raised a total of $35 million in Korean government and private funding from 1999 through 2004 to perform further R&D. During this period, the researchers performed countless *in vitro*, *in vivo* and seven clinical trials in an attempt to determine for which medical indications the polyphenols worked most effectively. They discovered that Seanol has many superior properties beneficial to human vascular problems (cardio-, cerebro-, and penile), obesity, arthritis, osteoporosis, allergies, dementia, and other health problems. Their work is covered by many patents.

Seanol is the trade name for a standardized complex of 13 active fractions of polyphenol/phlorotannins which originate as secondary metabolites extracted from several brown and red algae, most notably *Ecklonia cava* (kajime). Their molecular structure represents a unique category of polyphenols as distinguished from those extracted from land-based plants.

Seanol is considered a flavonoid, which is a type of polyphenolic compound well known for their antioxidant properties. The power of antioxidants is a function of their specific molecular structure, which is comprised of connected rings. Polyphenols use these rings to capture stray elec-

trons from free radicals. The more rings, the more effective it is as an antioxidant. Most flavonoids have three connected rings. Green tea catechins, one of the most powerful antioxidants known, have four. The ring structure and the effectiveness of these other antioxidants pale in comparison to Seanol polyphenols, which have eight interconnected rings. As such, the Seanol molecule is a remarkable free radical scavenger, surpassing by 10-100 times the antioxidant ability of most other polyphenols.

The *Eklonia cava* alga from which the Seanol compounds are extracted grows at a depth of about 100 feet. Virtually all land-sourced polyphenols are water soluble, having a short half-life within the body of only 30 minutes. They also are significantly less able to cross the blood-brain barrier, the body's biological firewall which prevents unwanted substances from passing into the brain. Seanol compounds are 40% fat soluble (hydrophobic), and have a far greater ability to reach the brain and protect it from damaging free radicals. They also have a half-life of up to 12 hours, which allows them more time to do their work. Because of its unique structure and composition, Seanol has a profound effect on a wide variety of health challenges.

Vascular disease and hypertension. One of the important suspected causes of vascular disease and hypertension is thickened blood. Within the blood there is a special protein called plasmin that dissolves unwanted clots. Unfortunately, many people have inhibitors of this protein (known as *antiplasmin*) due to genetic disposition, excess weight, toxins, diet, and other factors. Seanol compounds block antiplasmin to free up normal dissolution of clots. Its activity is 40-200 times greater than several synthetic fibrinolytic compounds.

One study on Seanol compounds found a small but significant rise in the prothrombin time (PT) and a fall in fibrinogen levels. The PT is a common measure of blood thickness. Fibrinogen is the precursor protein to thrombin, the clot. Generally, a lower fibrinogen level means less inflammation and tendency to abnormally clot. A Korean Medical University open-label, six-week study[1] on 11 coronary artery disease (CAD) patients and 28 normal subjects using a Seanol product confirmed a very large increase in brachial blood flows for the CAD patients compared to normal subjects, with "flow-mediated dilation" increasing for the 11 CAD patients by a substantial 36% over six weeks of daily use, and a "nitroglycerin mediated dilation" increasing by 22% over the six week period. Normal subjects showed no statistically significant variation. What these results imply is that Seanol has a very large impact on normalizing blood flows for CAD patients whose atherosclerosis has restricted the flow of blood in the cardiovascular system.

Individuals with hypertension are often prescribed an ACE (angiotensin-converting enzyme) inhibitor medication. ACE inhibitors block a kidney enzyme system resulting in the generation of hypertension. Seanol compounds can potently suppress ACE. In a rat study,[2] Seanol was compared to the drug enalapril (Vasotec®). Seanol showed a similar blood pressure lowering profile to the drug. But unlike the rats given the drug, Seanol rats did not show a rebound in blood pressure when the subjects stopped taking the product. Seanol has more than 15 times the power to inhibit ACE as most land-based polyphenol compounds.

Artery disease. A human study[3] showed Seanol appears to scrub plaque off the vascular endothelium—the inner lining of the arteries—and also can regenerate vascular endothelium. The chemical nitric oxide (NO) dilates blood vessels. After six weeks of treatment, flow-mediated dilation and NO-mediated dilation increased by 60% and 50% respectively. This means Seanol can rejuvenate damaged endothelium.

This effect was further confirmed in a study on erectile dysfunction (ED). In an eight week study[4] of 31 men experiencing ED for more than six months, Seanol was compared with the drug Viagra® in the following parameters: orgasmic function, intercourse satisfaction, overall satisfaction, and erectile dysfunction. Seanol scored 87%, 74%, and 62%, and 66% respectively. Viagra scored 27%, 44%, 39%, and 66% respectively. No side effects were reported with Seanol use. Viagra works by inhibiting an enzyme that destroys NO's penile arterial dilating effects. Seanol's more favorable effect supports its optimization of NO function.

Many researchers accept the notion that coronary disease is not due to cholesterol. Cholesterol in the arterial walls is a secondary factor in relation to how it is handled by the body. The body's oxidation of vulnerable LDL cholesterol creates rancid products that incite damage to the endothelial lin-

ing of the arteries. Seanol is more potent in inhibiting the oxidation of LDL than green tea catechins. The strong lipid and cholesterol scavenging potential to scrub the endothelial lining of plaque in the blood vessels provides an additional benefit—reduced vasculitis (vascular inflammation).

Neuropathy. Increasingly, the scientific literature supports the notion that many forms of nerve pain (neuropathy) are caused by nerve pressure exerted by swollen, inflamed blood vessels adjacent to nerve fibers. A recent 40-patient, placebo-controlled, randomized clinical trial[5] on neuropathy confirmed Seanol's ability to reduce nerve pain by a significant 40% in just four weeks of daily usage, with an 80% response rate.

Cognitive impairment. Eight million Americans are believed to have "mild" cognitive decline. Most drugs have a high toxicity profile. Seanol compounds were found to increase the key memory neurotransmitter acetylcholine in animals by 140% in brain regions responsible for learning and memory. This response occurred in mice after only seven days of administration. Seanol compounds can easily neutralize the neurotoxic free radical *peroxynitrite* and reduce the associated inflammation.[6]

The National Institute of Health's National Institute on Aging labs in Baltimore, MD have completed rat model memory studies[7] of Seanol in which the compound evidenced a marked ability to inhibit beta-amyloid deposition in rat brains. (Fibrination of beta-amyloid proteins in particular regions of the brain is suspected of being a primary cause of memory loss and Alzheimer's Disease.) Further, their water maze tests showed marked improvement in short-term memory for Seanol-dosed rats as compared to placebo-administered rats.

Another study[8] found the velocity of blood flow in the carotid arteries can be increased from an average of 36.68 cm/sec. to 40.09 cm/sec. An EEG study on brain waves of healthy middle-aged volunteers found that Seanol compounds increase alpha waves. That is a highly significant and desirable effect in today's world, as alpha waves are an indicator of relaxation. Yet another study found Seanol compounds prevent sleepiness in bus drivers and in high school students during daytime driving and other activities.

Allergic lung disease. In a mouse study,[9] allergic inflammation was significantly reduced by

Seanol. Specifically, the migration of allergic cells (eosinophils) to the lungs was reduced by 75%. Inflammatory white blood cells were reduced by 50%. Mucus plugs in airways were reduced by 50%. These findings suggest Seanol can free one's lungs of mucous and acute inflammation. The increase in the number of airway epithelial lining cells was 75%. Fibrosis in lung tissue and smooth muscle cell thickness was reduced by 20% and 32% respectively. These findings suggest Seanol compounds can prevent or reverse the chronic progression of asthma, and potentially Chronic Obstructive Pulmonary Disease (COPD).

Arthritis. Seanol significantly reduced pain in a group of knee arthritis patients compared with the placebo group. With increasing concern, many have read of the problems with the COX (cyclooxygenase) inhibitory NSAID drugs (e.g., Celebrex®). LOX (lipo-oxygenase) is another set of oxygenase enzymes. This enzyme system is related to the generation of allergies, atherosclerosis and some cancers. Seanol compared almost identically to Celebrex in the ability to reduce PGE2—a potent inflammatory chemical derived from omega 6 fatty acids—by slowing down the LOX system. Its compounds have more than double the ability of resveratrol to inhibit LOX.[10] This was validated in a study of rabbit cartilage cells incubated with human inflammatory chemicals. Cells fed Seanol had up to an 80% reduction in degeneration.

Fibromyalgia. Fibromyalgia is a multi-symptomatic disorder affecting up to 10 million people in the U.S. From 2-4% of the population suffers from this disease. Fatigue, depression, lack of sleep, and loss of functional capacity are hallmarks of the disorder. Seanol was administered in an 8 week double-blind placebo-controlled study[11] to 36 participants in Korea and Washington state. Six patients had to discontinue the product due to mild diarrhea likely induced by magnesium in the product, while 29 completed the study with highly significant findings. Mean time to fall asleep was reduced by 47 minutes. Total nighttime sleep increased by 1.6 hours. Soundness of sleep improved by 80%. Energy improved by 71%. The number of self-reported "good days" increased by 2.25 days per week. The number of lost work days per week fell by 31 hours/week. Pain dropped by 31%. Global assessment of the general condition improved by 39%.

Improvement was noted at both moderate and high dosage levels of Seanol administration.

The improvement in sleep for fibromyalgia patients and the previously reported increased alertness for high school students and bus driver imply conflicting results but, in fact, are not. Seanol is stimulating ideal function—increased alertness as needed, and increased ability to sleep as needed. The more than 50 million Americans with various sleep disorders might well benefit from Seanol without the fear of addictive tendencies.

Obesity and Diabetes. Approximately 20 million Americans suffer from adult diabetes. In diabetic persons, high blood sugar leads to vascular complications. This occurs through an enzyme called *aldose reductase.* This enzyme is present in the eyes, nerves and many other parts of the body. Aldose reductase converts some of the excess glucose into a sugar alcohol. Sorbitol can build up in these critical cells and cause damage to vital tissues. In fact, recent research found that animals deficient in aldose reductase were protected from retinal complications of diabetes. Seanol compounds are potent inhibitors of this enzyme.

With respect to obesity, the body uses a key enzyme called DGAT as the final step in the synthesis of triglycerides (TG). TG measurements are a part of one's cholesterol panels. TG are circulating fat bodies that ultimately come to reside in one's fat cells. They are almost always elevated in diabetes. Seanol compounds can inhibit this enzyme by more than 50%. In animal tests[12] conducted by the University of Washington, suppressing DGAT led to reduced body fat and increased physical activity. Most importantly, it encouraged leanness in the animals and resistance to a high fat diet.

In human obesity tests,[13] 141 young adults were given a beverage containing Seanol at a daily dose of 200 mg. In only two weeks, average weight dropped over 1.09 kg, muscle mass increased over 1.13 kg, and body fat dropped 1.86 kg (1kg = 2.2 lbs). Body fat in this group dropped a highly statistically significant 7.48%. Seanol blocks fat creation and stimulates its combustion via an increase in muscle mass. The latest scientific research shows that fat in one's diet directly impairs the ability of the pancreas to manufacture insulin. A University of Washington mouse study showed Seanol reversed fat deposition in liver and pancreas cells. It showed that Seanol markedly inhibits Nf-kB (nuclear factor kappa beta) inflammation in the pancreas.[14]

A recent Harvard (Joslin School of Diabetes) mouse study[15] directly implicates excessive fat deposition in the mouse pancreas as "switching on" the Nf-kB inflammation pathway, resulting in full-blown type 2 diabetes and insulin insensitivity in the mice. Seanol reduces pancreas fat accumulation (through down-regulation of DGAT) which helps restore insulin production and therefore should help reverse type 2 diabetes. Also, if one's insulin metabolism is impaired, lipid and cholesterol metabolism will also be impaired. With Seanol one would expect cholesterol to improve as well.

In another study,[16] 39 adults averaging 55.6 years of age were given 100 mg of Seanol for six weeks. Their average cholesterol dropped from 228 to 224. LDL dropped from 141 to 135. The hard-to-raise HDL did in fact rise from 46.5 to 50.7, which was highly significant. Triglycerides fell from 215 to195. And the atherogenic index (total cholesterol—HDL) dropped a very significant 12.5%. All of this was achieved with no lifestyle changes.

The following is a summary of Seanol's primary metabolic benefits:

❏ Uniquely strong antioxidant scavenging of lipids, iron and cholesterol as well as free radicals from the cardiovascular system, thereby lowering risk of stroke and cardiovascular events, lowering cholesterol, and reducing vasculitis-caused neuropathy.

❏ Strong anti-plasmin inhibition effect (i.e., homogenizes blood flow, thereby lowering blood pressure and increasing arterial blood flow).

❏ Strong elastase agonist effect, thereby increasing the flexibility of the vascular system and helping normalize blood flow and blood pressure.

❏ Significant anti-inflammatory effect, by inhibition of the Nf-kB inflammatory pathway, which also serves to normalize blood glucose levels and lead to statistically-significant re-establishment of insulin sensitivity in the pancreas.

❏ Down-regulation (by 60%) of the DGAT enzyme responsible for lipid (fat) metabolism, thereby assisting in fat/weight loss.

❏ Significant analgesic effect in inhibiting the expression of the COX enzymes for arthritis, as well as for neuropathic and FMS/CFS pain.

❏ Inhibition of beta-amyloid brain plaque formation in mammals, thereby improving memory.

To learn more about Seanol, visit www.jprenew.com. Seanol is available as FibroBoost™ and Fibronol,™ although FibroBoost contains higher levels of Seanol. For a description of these products, visit www.jprenew.com/products.html.

SODIUM CHLORITE

For the better part of the past 90 years, a product generically referred to as "stabilized oxygen" has been marketed as a dietary supplement in the U.S. and other countries. It has been suggested these products produce their effectiveness as the result of increased blood oxygenation. When red blood cells are exposed to low doses of substances within these formulations, additional oxygen is released to tissues throughout the body. Many-to-most of these products incorporate or have as their main ingredient the substance *sodium chlorite*, chemically identified as $NaClO_2$.

Sodium chlorite is one of many oxides of the chemical *chlorine*, some others being *hypochlorous acid* (HOCl), *sodium chlorate* ($NaClO_3$), and *sodium perchlorate* ($NaClO_4$). Sodium chlorite is referred to as an *oxidant*, i.e., a substance which takes up (strips) electrons from other atoms and molecules. This can be particularly useful in treating various ailments and diseases when the disease microorganisms are more susceptible to the oxidants than the healthy host cells. *Antioxidants*, on the other hand, are substances which donate electrons. By donating electrons to oxidant atoms and molecules, these substances are able to quench dangerous free radicals within healthy cells. Thus, it is seen that both oxidants and antioxidants have their unique roles in maintaining a healthy body.

Many oxidants are well known for their healing properties, two examples of which are *allicin* from garlic and the herb *artemisinin*. Hyperbaric oxygen, iodine, and ultraviolet light (photoluminescence) are also powerful oxidizers, as described separately in this section. A variety of oxidants have been found to be powerful immune stimulants when taken internally in appropriate dosages. Exposure of the blood to these substances triggers the white blood cells to release cell signaling *cytokines* which sound an alarm to the immune system to increase the attack on microbial invaders such as viruses and bacteria. Activated immune cells naturally produce powerful oxidizing chemicals such as *hydrogen peroxide* (H_2O_2), *peroxynitrate* (OONO-), and hypochlorus acid. These chemicals strip electrons from the atoms and molecules of dangerous pathogens such as viruses, bacteria, fungi, and parasites, thus destabilizing and degrading them so that they either stop their growth or die.

Because of their ability to degrade and kill pathogens, various strong oxidants are powerful disinfectants, i.e., they are effective in treating ailments caused by viruses, bacteria, and other infectious microbes. A specific oxidant is effective against a pathogen to the extent the pathogen is more susceptible to the oxidant than are the healthy host cells. Sodium chlorite is one such oxidant that can be taken internally at levels that destroy harmful pathogens yet does not substantially degrade healthy cells. Although more research is needed, sodium chlorite may find application in treating many and varied pathogens responsible for a range of disease states including AIDS; arthritis; cancer; chronic fatigue; colds and flu; fungal infestation; hepatitis; Lyme disease; malaria; and many additional pathogen-induced ailments.

An important discovery about sodium chlorite was made recently by Jim Humble, a modern-day gold prospecting geologist. While deep in the remote jungles of South America, Humble encountered colleagues suffering from malaria, a disease caused by a group of protozoan parasites of the genus *Plasmodium*. Humble found he could significantly help his infected colleagues by giving them the stabilized oxygen he carried with him to purify the unclean water found in the remote work sites and villages he visited. As he gave these colleagues increasingly higher doses, the faster and more completely they regained their health.

This observation inspired Humble to increase the concentration of the sodium chlorite within the solution he was administering to his malaria-infected colleagues as well as the infected native villagers. The beginning point of his stabilized oxygen solution was about a 5% concentration. Over time, he increased the concentration to 28%, a level he felt was optimal. Humble made an additional important finding. He discovered that if he "activated" the sodium chlorite solution prior to administering it, the results were much more effective.

Activation of the solution is accomplished by acidifying it by the addition of an acid such as acetic acid, citric acid, lactic acid, tartaric acid, or a variety of other edible acids. Citric acid is easily obtained from healthfood stores as a powder, and fresh lemon juice accomplishes the same goal. (Ascorbic acid cannot be used as an activator, as it is an *anti*oxidant.) Following acidification/activation, the solution is then diluted with water prior to administration.

By acidifying the sodium chlorite, a more potent oxidant is formed—*chlorine dioxide* (ClO_2). Chlorine dioxide has long been recognized as one of the most powerful disinfectants known to man. While sodium chlorite has long been used as an ingredient in mouthwashes to clear oral bacteria and the odor and infection to which they contribute, acidified sodium chlorite is used in industry to disinfect meat, produce, and water.

Acidified sodium chlorite is the principal means of disinfecting the municipal water supplies of Europe. In the U.S., less expensive and potentially more harmful *elemental chlorine* is used. By reacting with other molecules, elemental chlorine is capable of producing byproducts which are toxic to humans. These toxic byproducts gain entry into the body through chlorinated drinking water and through showering with chlorinated water. Even though sodium chlorite and chlorine dioxide have names that sound similar to chlorine, due to the differences in their chemical structures they do not provide such toxic byproducts. For example, another chemical with a similar-sounding name is *sodium chloride* (NaCl), ordinary table salt.

Acidified sodium chlorite, by forming the more potent chlorine dioxide, may prove to be an invaluable tool in the fight against many forms of infectious diseases. It's inexpensive, easy to administer, and is not subject to the microbial resistance that plagues the use of modern antibiotics.

In his 2006 book *Breakthrough: The Miracle Mineral Supplement of the 21st Century*, Humble defines specific protocols for taking acidified sodium chlorite for a variety of specific disease states. He relates the stories of how he traveled to Africa where he totally cured thousands of malaria-infected Africans—by using a single dose of activated (acidified) sodium chlorite. He also tells the "sodium chlorite story" and gives a wealth of information that potential users will find important as a practical guide. The book also explains how to "self-prepare" ingestible sodium chlorite for human use using technical grade sodium chlorite, which is available from various chemical supply houses worldwide. Both Humble's book and 28% sodium chlorite solution can be purchased inexpensively on the internet from a variety of sources, some of them "Jim Humble approved" suppliers. For more information, visit http://mmsadvancedstudies.com and www.jimhumble.biz.

Sodium chlorite and chlorine dioxide are powerful oxidants, and further research is required to determine the safety of their long-term use. Therefore, erring on the side of caution would dictate that activated 28% sodium chlorite should not be taken continually (as a "maintenance dose") after the treatment protocol has been effectively applied for several days, weeks, or months, as the treatment may require. When treating long-term ailments such as chronic infection, antioxidants such as vitamin C can be taken 10-12 hours following sodium chlorite use to help insure a healthy antioxidant /oxidant balance. Because sodium chlorite is active within the body for roughly 12 hours, taking antioxidants prior to this waiting period could counteract sodium chlorite's beneficial effects.

In agreement with this approach is Tom Hesselink, M.D., a general practice physician practicing in Illinois and a chapter contributor to Jim Humble's book. Dr. Hesselink is an expert in chlorine chemistry, and cautions against unnecessary, continual or "maintenance" use of the powerful oxidant. His website is a compendium of useful sodium chlorite information. Particularly useful is his page dealing with suggestions for research protocols and precautions in the administration of oxides of chlorine: http://bioredox.mysite.com/CLOXhtml/CLOXprot.htm. Notwithstanding these common-sense and understandable precautions, Dr. Hesselink is a staunch advocate of continued research with sodium chlorite and chlorine dioxide, believing that in their use "...we may be on the verge of discovering the most potent and broad spectrum antibiotic yet known."[1]

THYMIC PROTEIN A

The body's first line of defense against all forms of illness is the immune system—a grand display of both biological complexity and simplicity. The job of the immune system is that of a protector/guardian, continuously in search of foreign intruders that can cause harm. Infective microbes such as viruses, bacteria, fungi, parasites, yeast, and other toxic substances continually challenge our immune defenses. In order to maintain good health, these defenses must have the ability to protect the body from infection from these potentially dangerous invaders by ridding them from the body. To the extent that immune function declines this does not happen, and disease and ill health follow.

When the immune system is challenged by pathogens such as viruses and bacteria, a vast array of complex systems goes into action to help the body avoid illness. It's only when these systems are functioning optimally that good health is maintained. Any medicinal agent that significantly boosts the power of the immune system's defenses could be of great benefit in the treatment of any disease caused by these invading pathogens. Many suggest the list of ailments with probable infective involvement would include the familiar names Alzheimer's disease, Parkinson's disease, multiple sclerosis, fibromyalgia, chronic fatigue syndrome, colds, influenza, lupus, and many others. Thymic Protein A offers a new level of immune enhancement.

The central control organ of the immune system is the *thymus gland*, a ductless gland located just beneath the breastbone in humans. The thymus is about the same size as the heart of a newborn, and grows rapidly during childhood. It peaks in size/mass at puberty, and thereafter begins to atrophy. By age 40, only a small fraction of the thymus remains intact. As the gland itself atrophies, its function declines proportionally. Laboratory animals whose thymus glands are removed (thymectomy) experience allergies; auto-immune diseases; cancer; failure to grow; immune suppression; infection; and neuromuscular paralysis.[1]

Because of its shrunken size in adult humans, the function of the thymus has been difficult for researchers to understand. It was only in the 1960s that the thymus began to be understood as a critical component of immunity. Its function has been described as a "finishing school" for T-lymphocyte cells, another important immune component that is manufactured in the bone marrow. T-lymphocytes migrate from bone marrow to the thymus where they mature, multiply, and become programmed to perform various functions.

One aspect of T-cell programming includes being differentiated into T-4 (also called CD-4 and helper) cells which initiate and control many key functions of the immune system, such as the production of cytokines and lymphokines (including interleukin-2 and interferon), other white blood cells, red blood cells, natural killer (NK) CD56 cells, and more T-4 cells. T-8 killer cells—which attack and destroy pathogens such as cancer cells and viruses, as well as T-8 suppressor cells, which help terminate attacks of the T-8 killers—are also differentiated in the thymus.

Since the discovery of the importance of the thymus to proper immune function, many attempts have been made to produce thymus extracts to boost the immune capability. These preparations are generally whole animal thymus which is ground, dried, strained, and prepared as a liquid or in capsules. Such preparations have been only marginally successful because they contain only fragments of the total complex of molecules responsible for the many critical immune functions governed by the thymus.

In the early 1980s, after eight years of intensive research, immunologist Terry Beardsley, Ph. D., was able to isolate the thymus' master molecule that produces the mixture of regulatory proteins from the thymus. Rather than extracted fragments of molecules, Beardsley isolated a substance which he named Thymic Protein A (TPA), a complete protein comprising a 500 amino acid chain.

Both the isolation and manufacturing processes are protected by U.S. patent 5,616,554: "Immune-enhancing Agent for Therapeutic Use in Immuno-compromised Hosts." By supplementing with Thymic Protein A, one is provided with a continuous source of pure, native biomolecules identical to those produced by an optimally-functioning thymus gland, according to Beardsley.

It is known that the body continues to produce the vital T-4 cells after the thymus becomes atrophied by about age 40. However, Beardsley has shown that even though there may be T-4 cells in the bloodstream, they are nonfunctional without being programmed by the appropriate thymic protein, which occurs only through direct contact with TPA. Because T-4 cells are the regulators of cell-mediated immunity, *they are able to up-regulate* the immune system to guard against pathogenic infection, *as well as down-regulate* the immune response in cases of auto-immune overactivation, depending on the specific needs of the body. TPA does not increase the activity or size of the thymus, but rather replaces the critical master protein molecule produced by a healthy thymus gland.

Dr. Beardsley has demonstrated the efficacy of TPA with both animals and humans *in vivo*. Initially working with laboratory animals, mice receiving grafted cultures of human thymus experienced a significant increase in T-cell population and immune function in comparison to the control group.[2] In a non-blinded pilot study of seven patients with elevated Epstein-Barr virus (EBV) titers, a significant reduction in the viral load was noted, suggesting that TPA may play a role in the treatment of this common infection which many believe is associated with Chronic Fatigue and Immune Dysfunction Syndrome (CFIDS).[3] In a study of 23 patients with clinical symptoms of CFIDS (and abnormal CD-8 subpopulations), 16 of the patients experienced normalization of the immune function with a corresponding improvement in clinical symptoms. The study authors concluded that "reinstitution of immune regulation with thymic protein A may ameliorate symptoms associated with CFIDS."[4]

Thymic Protein A is not derived from live animals, but is grown in cell cultures in only one laboratory in the world. The growth process was initially seeded from a single U.S. calf raised specifically for this purpose. All other proteins and fragments are filtered out, leaving only highly-purified TPA. As such, its potential to contain infective contaminants (including prions; see **Mad Cow Disease**) is virtually nonexistent, which cannot easily be said about other thymic extracts. One packet of product contains 4 micrograms (12 trillion active molecules) of freeze-dried TPA in a base of maltodextrin. The product is taken sublingually for both prevention and treatment. No adverse side-effects have ever been reported.

Thymic Protein A is available as ProBoost,® at www.proboostmed.com. For other sources and to learn more, search online for "thymic protein a."

Appendix A: Internet Ordering

Listed below, in alphabetical order, are several companies that sell nutritional supplements at a considerable discount. We've found these companies to provide excellent prices and service:

CompassioNet (New Jersey, USA)
(Specializes in Lane Labs products)
www.compassionet.com
(800)510-2010

DR Vitamin Solutions (Pennsylvania, USA)
(Specializes in Life Extension Foundation products)
www.drvitaminsolutions.com
(610)703-3185

Himalaya USA (Texas, USA)
(Specializes in Ayurvedic herbs)
www.himalayausa.com
(800)869-4640; (713)863-1622

iHerb.com (California, USA)
(Broadest selection. Highest recommendation)
www.iherb.com
(866)328-1171; (626)939-7800

Rain Tree Nutrition, Inc. (Nevada, USA)
(Specializes in rainforest herbals)
www.rain-tree.com
(800)780-5902; (775)841-4142

The Vitamin Shoppe (New Jersey, USA)
(Broad selection)
www.vitaminshoppe.com
(866)293-3367

Total Health Discount Vitamins (New York, USA)
(Broad selection. Also sells Standard Process products.)
www.totalhealthvitamins.net
(800)283-2833
Standard Process products are also available at
www.naturamart.com; (800)383-6008

Vitacost (Florida, USA)
(Broad selection)
www.vitacost.com
(800)381-0759; (561)752-8888

Web Vitamins (Connecticut, USA)
(Broad selection)
www.webvitamins.com
(800)919-9122

THE BOOK THAT NEVER GROWS OLD

With your purchase of *The Encyclopedia of Medical Breakthroughs & Forbidden Treatments*, you receive unlimited access to the Member's Area of our website, year after year. This password-protected area contains links to information that has become available since the last printing of *The Encyclopedia*. In this way we're able to keep our readers up to date on recent medical breakthroughs and other important medical information. *The Encyclopedia*, therefore, exists as a complete work in two locations: 1) in the physical world as a soft cover book (or online as an ebook), and 2) online in the Member's Area of our website. Without consulting the information contained within both venues, you will not have accessed the complete work.

"If it's not in the book, on our website you should look."

Please Visit Our Website Regularly for Important Updates at
www.medical-breakthroughs.com. Enter Username and Password.

Important Member's Area access: When you purchased *The Encyclopedia*, you were asked to create your unique access to the Member's Area. In addition, following your purchase you were emailed information on how to access the Member's Area had you not done so during the purchasing process. If at any time you need to acquire or recover your Username or Password, please visit medical-breakthroughs.com/support to submit a "Support Ticket" requesting additional information/directions.

To locate a holistic/integrative medical practitioner in your area,
contact the American College for Advancement in Medicine
at (800)532-3688, (949)309-3520, www.acam.org,
or the International College of Integrative Medicine at
(866)464-5226, (419)358-0273, www.icimed.com.

To order additional copies of *The Encyclopedia*
of Medical Breakthroughs & Forbidden Treatments,
visit www.RealMedicalHelp.com

Throughout the book, various statements have been made regarding the less-than-admirable actions of the hugely powerful and profitable pharmaceutical companies. These recitations are not simply isolated events of no basic consequence to the average person using pharmaceutical drugs. The following examples are illustrative of an industry whose financial bottom line all too often supersedes its capacity to care about its "valued" customers.

OFF-LABEL USE OF PRESCRIPTION DRUGS

Prescription drugs are approved by the U.S. Food and Drug Administration (FDA) for certain specific, limited uses. Approved drugs may also be used by physicians for uses other than those for which the drug is specifically approved. This is a practice known as an "off-label" use of the drug.

Off-label usage of drugs is a legal practice. In fact, it is often considered good medical practice for physicians to prescribe drugs for off-label uses, as it sometimes leads to new, important medical discoveries. On the other hand, the practice can be abused for the sake of profit, raking in millions to billions of dollars for the drug manufacturer while jeopardizing the health of the drug users.

In July of 2003, *Dateline NBC* aired an exposé regarding what it stated "may be one of the biggest medical deceptions in history."[1] In 1997, David P. Franklin, Ph. D., blew the whistle on the pharmaceutical giant Warner-Lambert (W-L) for crossing the line on the issue of off-label uses of pharmaceuticals. Although it's legal for doctors to use drugs for purposes other than those for which they are formally approved, it's illegal for a drug company to promote such off-label uses.

Over a number of years, W-L actively encouraged its sales staff, including Dr. Franklin—a former Research Fellow at Harvard Medical School—to actively promote the prescription drug Neurontin,® a drug approved as an anticonvulsive agent, for many uses other than its approved use—including uses which W-R was fully aware may be jeopardizing the health and lives of these patients.

In a voice-mail message that was entered as evidence in Dr. Franklin's law suit against W-L, a W-L executive informed the sales staff that in or-

der to make the drug profitable, they would have to promote Neurontin for a number of off-label uses, including pain relief, bipolar disorder, and other psychiatric uses such as ADHD for children.

Company executives understood full well that Neurontin is not effective in treating the additional disorders, and that there were safety-related issues as well. However, W-L forged ahead in spite of this, and was determined to pitch the drug for many off-label uses. Dr. Franklin began tape recording phone calls and messages from company executives, and caught the following gem from a W-L senior executive: "I don't want to hear that safety crap either...it's a great drug." Sales flourished, and Neurontin became a best-seller, raking in over USD $2 billion per year.

Pfizer, the company that acquired W-L in 2000, estimates that off-label use accounted for over 75% of the drug's sales. (Doctors, in fact, have been paid handsomely for holding seminars for other doctors for the expressed purpose of promoting off-label uses of prescription drugs.)

This feat was not accomplished without the complicity of many physicians, who participated in what was called a "shadowing program." W-L paid 75-100 doctors $350 each day they allowed a W-L sales rep to sit in during patient exams, and then give recommendations on what medications to prescribe. It's not clear whether or not these patients understood the "sit-ins" were sales reps.[2]

Warner Lambert is also accused of paying a professional marketing firm USD $12,000 to write journal articles—for publication in respected medical journals—painting Neurontin in a positive light. Further accusations claim W-L payed various doctors $1,000 each for agreeing to let their names be used as one of the co-authors of the articles.[3] In fact, it is common knowledge within the industry that pharmaceutical companies reward doctors handsomely for promoting their drugs—to the tune of billions of dollars annually.

To read the entire transcript of the *Dateline NBC* broadcast, Google "dateline david franklin."

JOURNAL ARTICLES

Picking up on the journal article theme, in September of 2001, 13 of the world's most prestigious medical journals spoke out against the transnational pharmaceutical conglomerates, accusing them of "distorting the results of scientific research for the sake of profits."[1]

The *Lancet*, the *New England Journal of Medicine*, the *Journal of the American Medical Association*, and 10 other well-known journals accused the drug giants of using their vast sums of money and power to tie up academic researchers with legal contracts which would make them unable to publish free and fair results of clinical trials investigating the safety and effectiveness of new drugs.

Included in the contracts are provisions which prevent the university scientists from having access to the raw data produced by the drug trials. This data is the only definitive way of assessing whether or not the drug is both safe and effective. Further, the researchers may have no input in the overall design of the trial, and may have only limited participation in the interpretation of the trial results. Even if the scientists do have substantial input into the various parameters of the clinical trials, the drug companies have the option of burying the results if they are unfavorable.

According to an article published in *The Guardian*, one of Britain's most respected investigative newspapers, editors of these journals state,

> ...the studies produced for publication may be skewed in the interest of the pharmaceutical company, which hopes to make big profits from a new drug.

Richard Horton, editor of the *Lancet*, said,

> Where the company controls the trial, the data, and the writing of the study, the research will be presented to favor the product that company makes. I think it happens all the time.

Some of the journal editors will be requesting those who submit articles for publication to sign a declaration accepting responsibility for the trial. If a company has "sole control" of the data, some of the journals will not publish the study.

Attorneys sometimes use what are called "weasel words," meaning some loopholes are left unplugged through which their clients can swim at some later date. "Sole control" sounds like one such loophole. In fact, a year after the tongue-lashing editorials were published in the 13 above-men-

tioned journals, a *New England Journal of Medicine* study revealed that articles submitted to the journals continue to fall short of the guidelines which are intended to provide unbiased reporting.[2]

Marcia Angell, former editor of the *NEJM*, told the *Wall Street Journal*,

> The academic community is still trying to have it both ways: to maintain their very close and very lucrative contacts with private industry while trying to respond to public concern about conflicts of interest.[3]

THE REVOLVING DOOR

Sometimes it happens serendipitously that former top-level employees of large corporations accidentally find their way into top positions of the U.S. government dealing with the same or even dissimilar areas of "expertise," and vice versa. This happens all too frequently, and often to the detriment of the public. One such occurrence—which exemplifies the practice—is related to the product Bovine Growth Hormone (rBGH).

Bovine Growth Hormone is used to increase the milk production of cattle. Since 1985 the FDA has allowed the sale of milk containing BGH without disclosing the presence of the hormone. Not uncharacteristically, the FDA claims that milk produced from cattle injected with BGH is safe for human use, although no long-term studies have been done. Currently, approximately 70% of all cattle in the U.S. receive BGH injections.[1]

The U.S. has long experienced a milk surplus which is subsidized by the government. At times, millions of dollars have been spent to slaughter cows to reduce this surplus. Does it make sense that chemicals such as BGH are being used to increase milk production? It has been reported that four companies invested over $1 billion to develop BGH:[2] American Cyanamid, Eli Lilly, Monsanto and Upjohn. Perhaps these companies need a decade or two to recover their investments.

Scientists and consumer groups have pointed out possible dangerous effects of BGH. The presence of BGH in the cow's bloodstream stimulates the production of another hormone, Insulin-like Growth Factor 1, or IGF-1. IGF-1 in cattle is chemically identical to IGF-1 in humans.[3] This hormone causes cells to divide. The question of concern is whether its increased presence within humans will cause an increase in cell division leading to tumor growth. Although more research is needed, one recent study suggests the consumption of milk treated with BGH may increase the risk of cancer in humans.[4]

In 1994 attorney Michael Taylor—FDA Deputy Commissioner for Policy—wrote the FDA's product labeling guidelines for BGH. The guidelines published in February 1994 virtually prohibited dairy companies from making any distinctions between dairy products containing BGH and those that don't. This was done by the FDA in an effort to keep the BGH dairy products from being "stigmatized" in the marketplace.

In March 1994, attorney Taylor was publically exposed as a former lawyer for Monsanto for seven years, working in the area of BGH "acceptability." One of Taylor's tasks was to investigate and render an opinion as to whether Monsanto could sue individual states or companies who sought to disclose to the public their products were BGH free. Another former Monsanto employee, Margaret Miller, Deputy Director of the FDA's Office of New Animal Drugs, worked on Monsanto's BGH safety studies until 1989.

Both Michael Taylor and Margaret Miller were the subjects of an investigation conducted by the U.S. General Accounting Office (GAO) in 1994 for their roles in the FDA's approval of Posilac,® Monsanto's version of BGH. The GAO found "no conflicting financial interest with respect to the drug's approval."[5]

A further example of the revolving door is discussed in the **Mad Cow Disease** section. Specifically, former U.S. Department of Agriculture Secretary Ann Veneman's spokeswoman was a former Director of Public Relations for the National Cattleman's Beef Association, and her Chief of Staff was the former chief lobbyist of that same organization. Elizabeth Johnson, USDA's Senior Advisor on Food and Nutrition, was also employed by that same organization in the capacity of Associate Director of Food Policy. Dr. Charles Lambert, USDA's Deputy Undersecretary for Marketing and Regulatory Programs, was formerly Chief Economist for National Cattleman's. Other revolving people include James Moseley, former Deputy Secretary of Agriculture, who was formerly a managing partner of Infinity Pork, LLC; Dr. Eric

Hentges, Director of the USDA's Center for Nutrition Policy and Pormotion, who was formerly Vice President of the National Pork Board and Director of Human Nutrition Research of the National Livestock and Meat Board; Donna Reifschneider, USDA's Administrator for Grain Inspection, Packers and Stockyards, who was formerly President of the National Pork Producer's Council; Mary Kirtley Waters, USDA's Assistant Secretary for Congressional Relations, who was formerly Senior Director and legislative council for ConAgra Foods; and Scott Charbo, USDA's Chief Information Officer, who was formerly President of mPower3, a ConAgra subsidiary.[6]

BLOOD FOR MONEY

The New York Times[1] recently reported on a blood-curdling story that unfolded in the 1980s. Cutter Biologicals, subsidiary of the German firm Bayer, A.G., manufactures a product called Factor VIII, a blood-clotting agent used to prevent uncontrolled bleeding in hemophiliacs. Factor VIII contains human blood plasma. In the early 1980s, it was discovered that HIV/AIDS could be transferred through the use of this and similar products.

Cutter quickly developed a process that removed the contamination of blood plasma with the AIDS virus, thus eliminating the threat of human-to-human transmission. However, a large supply of Factor VIII was already manufactured and was "on the shelf," waiting to be marketed.

There was now only one humane course of action to be taken: destroy the contaminated, unsafe, potentially life-threatening product. They instead exported the potentially-contaminated Factor VIII for sale to the Asian and South American markets. Furthermore, Cutter continued to manufacture the unsafe version for an additional five months.

Because of poor record keeping practices in the early 1980s, it's unknown how many lives were lost as a result of this unethical, inhuman business practice. No doubt it was in the hundreds, possibly thousands. One Taiwanese physician reported that in a single hemophiliac clinic in his country, 44 patients developed AIDS, 23 of whom died.

The parent company, Bayer, issued a statement saying that Cutter had acted "responsibly, ethically, and humanely." Again, war is peace. But the relatives of the afflicted and diseased didn't react peacefully. They instead sued Bayer to the tune of millions. To date, Bayer and three other companies that knowingly sold the contaminated product have paid out settlements totaling over USD $600 million. Cutter had only made $4 million by marketing the contaminated product. In this select case, crime didn't pay. On the other hand, these companies know that "you win some, you lose some"—but always with a net gain.

Getting wind of the issue, the U.S. FDA entered the scene. Whoooooa! Look out! Big Pharma trembles. Yet the end result was that the FDA simply explained to the guilty companies that it was unacceptable to sell knowingly-contaminated product...anywhere, even outside of the U.S. The FDA asked that the problem be settled "quickly and quietly," with no reason to alert the public, the medical community or the U.S. Congress. And so it was, until over 20 years later when *The New York Times* reported the incident in May of 2003.

VIOXX

The above stories are not isolated incidents within a community of pharmaceutical companies that profess their beneficent intentions toward those who take their medications—their loyal customers. On the contrary. Scenes similar to these stories have played out year after year, decade after decade, bringing into focus the fact that when huge profits are at stake, it's the consumer that's all too often left holding the short end of the stick. In the present case, the short end means an increased risk of sickness or death to those who take these drugs.

One further example illustrative of this point is the story of Vioxx, the prescription arthritis medication marketed by the giant pharmaceutical firm Merck & Company. Vioxx came to market in 1999, and was removed by the FDA in 2004 after it was learned (by the public, not Merck—they already knew) that the drug greatly increased the incidence of heart attacks and strokes. In the five years Vioxx was marketed, it caused 140,000 heart attacks or strokes in the U.S.—not counting other countries where it was sold—resulting in the death of a third of these victims.

When the surviving Vioxx victims initiated law suites, Merck chose to go to court rather than set-

tle privately, resulting in the company's internal documentation being made public—some 20 million pages of emails, memos, and medical reports. This paper trail made clear that the highest levels of both the medical researchers and the management at Merck knew full well that Vioxx was a flawed and harmful drug—even as the company raked in tens of billions in profits while the drug maimed and killed over 40,000 innocent and unsuspecting consumers. Lack of space limits our presentation of further details. However, an indelible impression will be made on those readers who take ten minutes to read the rest of the bone-curdling story of how Merck made a killing on Vioxx at www.prospect-magazine.co.uk/article_details.php?id=10425.

THE COST OF DRUGS

The pharmaceutical industry is a thriving enterprise—one of the most lucrative on the planet. According to *Fortune*[1] magazine, the 10 most profitable pharmaceutical companies in the world, including their Global 500 rankings, are: 1) Merck (50), 2) Johnson & Johnson (101), 3) Pfizer (106), 4) GlaxoSmithKline (119), 5) Novartis (214), 6) Aventis (238), 7) Roche Group (245), 8) Bristol-Myers Squibb (252), 9) Astra-Zenica (253), and 10) Abbott Laboratories (263). [(The much-discussed Pharmacia ranks #11 (281)].

All of these companies lie within the world's 265 most profitable corporations. This is quite a feat, given that there are literally millions of corporations globally. The combined revenues of these corporations in 2003 was over USD $270 billion.[2]

Two of the most important factors governing the amount of revenue generated by a corporation are: 1) Number of sales, and 2) Cost per sale. In the United States, where the price of pharmaceuticals far exceeds that of most other countries—even for identical products—the cost of drugs has become a controversial issue. Most Americans wonder why their prescription drugs are so expensive, and why they are required to pay such high prices in comparison to other countries. While it's true that the pharmaceutical companies spend hundreds of millions of dollars on clinical trials to test the safety and efficacy of each drug, the cost of this research isn't spread evenly over the countries selling these identical products.

The following examples of pricing inequalities were compiled by the Life Extension Foundation for the year 2003. Prices are given in U.S. dollars.[3]

❏ Augmentin® (12 count; 500 mg) sells in the U.S. for $52.62 compared to $9.89 in Europe.

❏ Cipro® (20 count; 500 mg) sells in the U.S. for $114.84 compared to $21.00 in Europe.

❏ Coumadin® (25 count; 5 mg) sells in the U.S. for $42.62 compared to $4.71 in Europe.

❏ Glucophage® (50 count; 850 mg) sells in the U.S. for $74.32 compared to $4.40 in Europe.

❏ Paxil® (28 count; 30 mg) sells in the U.S. for $83.36 compared to $48.36 in Europe.

❏ Pravachol® (28 count; 10 mg) sells in the U.S. for $85.62 compared to $27.00 in Europe.

❏ Premarin® (28 count; 0.6 mg) sells in the U.S. for $28.32 compared to $4.38 in Europe.

❏ Prilosec® (20 count; 20 mg) sells in the U.S. for $86.32 compared to $10.24 in Europe.

❏ Prozac® (14 count; 20 mg) sells in the U.S. for $56.62 compared to $14.80 in Europe.

❏ Synthroid® (50 count; 100 mcg) sells in the U.S. for $23.32 compared to $3.14 in Europe.

❏ Zocor® (28 count; 20 mg) sells in the U.S. for $118.68 compared to $48.36 in Europe.

The actual cost to the pharmaceutical companies of the generic ingredients that comprise the drugs sheds further light on the government-approved price gouging. Prices given for the year 2003 in USD for 100 count tablets/capsules.[4]

❖ Celebrex® 100 mg retail: $130.27; Cost of generic ingredients: $0.60; Markup: 21,712%

❖ Claritin® 10 mg retail: $215.17; Cost of generic ingredients: $0.71; Markup: 30,306%

❖ Lipitor® 20 mg retail: $272.37; Cost of generic ingredients: $5.80; Markup: 4,696%

❖ Paxil® 20 mg retail: $220.27; Cost of generic ingredients: $7.60; Markup: 2,898%

❖ Prevacid® 30 mg retail: $344.77; Cost of generic ingredients: $1.01; Markup: 43,136%

❖ Prozac® 20 mg retail: $247.47; Cost of generic ingredients: $0.11; Markup: 224,973%

❖ Xanax® 1 mg retail: $136.79; Cost of generic ingredients: $0.024; Markup: 569,958%

❖ Zithromax® 600 mg retail: $1,482.19; Cost of generic ingredients: $18.78; Markup: 7,892%

A markup of several hundred percent would be reasonable. This would represent a typical profit for the manufacturing sector. Several thousand to several hundred thousand percent is a bit presumptuous, and helps explain why these companies are the most profitable in the world. U.S. lawmakers simply allow pharmaceutical companies to price-gouge so that the pharmaceutical industry can reap huge rewards on the backs of the largely undiscerning American populace. The financial interests of the pharmaceutical companies are protected through legislation. The government—ostensibly for the people and by the people—is more accurately described as "for the corporations courtesy of the government." As payback, Big Pharma contributes handsomely to the campaign coffers of supportive representatives and senators.

Over the years, Americans have purchased tens of millions of dollars of prescription drugs from foreign countries, including Canada, in an attempt to make the dollar stretch farther. Annually, Americans buy more than USD$1 billion of drugs from Canada.[5] This practice came to a grinding halt with the December 2003 passage of the new Medicare bill which criminalizes this practice. According to statements made by top level U.S. FDA officials, the reason for the prohibition is not an economic concern, but rather an issue of safety. Canadian pharmaceuticals, according to the FDA, are inferior to U.S. pharmaceuticals and, as such, jeopardize the safety of Americans. Once again, the FDA is Johnny-on-the-spot to protect the health and welfare of the American citizen. (It was disclosed in 2008 that many of the pharmaceuticals sold to U.S. citizens by the largest U.S. pharmaceutical firm are actually manufactured in . . . China).

One glaring contradiction which makes clear the real intentions of the FDA is a loop-hole in the law, a waiver if you will, which permits U.S. government agencies such as the Department of Defense and the Veteran's Administration to continue buying hundreds of millions of dollars of Canadian pharmaceuticals annually.[6] Does this indicate that the issue of safety is really only a decoy whose true intention is to distract from the real reason individual Americans are prevented from purchasing

Canadian drugs, or does the FDA care more about private U.S. citizens more than it does about those employed by government?

At one point the pending Medicare bill contained provisions allowing Americans to purchase Canadian (and other foreign) drugs. But after all was said and done, these provisions were struck from the proposed bill. Congressional voting for the bill took place in a most unusual manner. Sherrod Brown, at the time a democrat from Ohio and ranking member of the Committee on Energy and the Commerce Subcommittee on Health, was present for the vote in the U.S. House of Representatives. Congressman Brown described to the *St. Louis Post Dispatch* newspaper what transpired during the wee hours of the morning as the vote was being taken. Such actions by elected government officials bring into question the true nature of American "democracy." Congressman Brown's article of December 18, 2003 as it appeared in the *St. Louis Post Dispatch*, is quoted below.

Democracy Crumbles Under Cover Of Darkness: House Republicans Bend Rules, Press For Votes During Wee Hours To Escape The Light of Accountability.

Never before has the House of Representatives operated in such secrecy: At 2:54 a.m. on a Friday in March, the House cut veterans benefits by three votes. At 2:39 a.m. on a Friday in April, the House slashed education and health care by five votes. At 1:56 a.m. on a Friday in May, the House passed the Leave No Millionaire Behind tax-cut bill by a handful of votes. At 2:33 a.m. on a Friday in June, the House passed the Medicare privatization and prescription drug bill by one vote. At 12:57 a.m. on a Friday in July, the House eviscerated Head Start by one vote. And then...at 12:12 a.m. on a Friday in October, the House voted $87 billion for Iraq.

Always in the middle of the night. Always after the press had passed their deadlines. Always after the American people had turned off the news and gone to bed. What did the public see? At best, Americans read a small story with a brief explanation of the bill and the vote count in Saturday's papers. But what did the public miss? They didn't see the House votes, which normally take...20 minutes, dragging on for as long as an hour as members of the Republican leadership trolled for enough votes to cobble together a majority.

They didn't see GOP leaders stalking the floor for whoever was not in line. They didn't see Speaker Dennis Hastert and Majority Leader Tom DeLay coerce enough Republican members into switching their votes to produce the desired result. In other words, they didn't see the subversion of democracy.

And late last month, they did it again. The most sweeping changes to Medicare in its 38-year history were forced through the House at 5:55 on a Saturday morning. The debate started at midnight. The roll call began at 3:00 a.m. Most of us voted within the typical 20 minutes. Normally, the speaker would have gaveled the vote closed. But...the Republican-driven bill was losing. By 4 a.m., the bill had been defeated 216-218, with only one member, Democrat David Wu, not voting. Still, the speaker refused to gavel the vote closed.

Then the assault began. Hastert, DeLay, Republican Whip Roy Blount, Ways and Means Chairman Bill Thomas, Energy and Commerce Chairman Billy Tauzin - all searched the floor for stray Republicans to bully. I watched them surround Cincinnati's Steve Chabot, trying first a carrot, then a stick; but he remained defiant. Next, they aimed at retiring Michigan congressman Nick Smith, whose son is running to succeed him. They promised support if he changed his vote to yes and threatened his son's future if he refused...

Many of the two dozen Republicans who voted against the bill had fled the floor. One Republican hid in the Democratic cloakroom. By 4:30, the browbeating had moved into the Republican cloakroom, out of sight of C-SPAN cameras and the insomniac public. Republican leaders woke President George W. Bush, and a White House aide passed a cell phone from one recalcitrant member to another in the cloakroom.

At 5:55, two hours and 55 minutes after the roll call had begun—twice as long as any previous vote in the history of the U.S. House of Representatives—two obscure western Republicans emerged from the cloakroom. They walked, ashen and cowed, down the aisle to the front of the chamber, scrawled their names and district numbers on green cards to change their votes...The speaker gaveled the vote closed; Medicare privatization had passed. You can do a lot in the middle of the night, under the cover of darkness.[7]

To view a *60 Minutes* exposé of this event, see www.youtube.com/watch?v=m17VkNIbymA.

Appendix C: Products Manufactured from Bovine and Other Animal Sources [1]

PRODUCTS FROM ADRENALS

cortisone - for arthritis, skin allergies, anti-inflammatory

epinephrine - aids in raising blood pressure, heart disorders, and allergies

PRODUCTS FROM BLOOD

adhesives

blood albumin - RH factor or typing

blood sausage

bone marrow

bone meal

cake mixes

deep-fry batters

egg substitute

fabric printing and dyeing

Fraction I - hemophelia

Fraction V - kills viruses

gravy mixes

imitation seafood

iron - anemia

leather-treating agents

livestock feed

minerals

pasta

plasma protein

plaster retardant

plywood adhesive

proteins - glue for automobile bodies

protein extracts - diagnostic microbiology

protein source in feeds

sticking agent

textile sizing

thrombin - blood coagualant

whipped toppings and coffee whiteners

PRODUCTS FROM BONES

bone charcoal

bone china

bone handles

bone jewelry

bone marrow - blood disorders

bone meal - calcium and phosphorous source

buttons

collagen and bone - plastic surgery

dried bones

fertilizer

glass

high grade steel

mineral source in feed

mineral source in supplements

pencils

porcelain enamel

soft cartilage - plastic surgery

water filters

whitener in refined sugar

xiphisternal cartilage - plastic surgery

PRODUCTS FROM BONE, HORNS, AND HOOVES

adhesives

bandage strips

buttons

cellophane wrap and tape

chessmen

collagen cold cream

combs

crochet needles

dice

dog biscuits

emery boards and cloth

fertilizer

gelatine capsules

gelatine desserts

glycerine

horn handles

ice cream, malts and shakes

imitation ivory

inedible bone meal

laminated wood products

livestock feeds

marshmallows

neatsfoot oil

ornaments

photographic film

piano keys

plant food

plywood and paneling

potted meats

shampoo and conditioner

wallpaper and wallpaper paste

PRODUCTS FROM BRAINS
anti-aging cream
cholesterol

PRODUCTS FROM FATS AND FATTY ACIDS (edible and inedible)
animal foods
antifreeze
biodegradable detergents
biodiesel
cellophane
cement
ceramics
chalk
chemicals
chewing gum
cosmetics
crayons
creams and lotions (sheep)
deodorants
detergents
explosives
fertilizer
fiber softeners
floor wax
glycerin
glycerol
herbicides
horse and livestock feeds
industrial oils and lubricants
insecticides
insulation
lard
linoleum
livestock feed
lubricants
makeup
matches
medicines
mink oil
nitroglycerine
oil polishes
ointment bases
oelo margarine
oleo shortening
oleostearin
paints
paraffin
perfumes
pet foods

pharmaceuticals
plasticizers
plastics
printing rollers
protein hair conditioner
protein hair shampoo
putty
rennet for cheese (sheep)
rubber products
shaving cream
shoe cream
soaps
solvents
stearic acid (sheep)
tallow for tanning
textiles
tires
water proofing agents
weed killers

PRODUCTS FROM GALLSTONES
ornaments

PRODUCTS FROM HAIR
air filters
artist's paint brush
felt and rug padding
insulation material
non-wovens
plastering material
textiles
upholstering material

PRODUCTS FROM HIDES AND SKINS
bandages
belts
candies and confectionery
collagen-based adhesives (from trimmings)
drum head (sheep)
emery boards
flavorings
gelatin
gelatin desserts
glues - for papermaking, bookbinding, cabinetmaking
ice cream
leather sporting goods
leather wearing apparel
luggage
marshmallows
mayonnaise

pharmaceuticals
photographic materials
pigskin garments, gloves, and shoes
porcine - dressings for burn victims
sausage casings
sheetrock
shoes and boots
upholstery
wallets
wallpaper
yogurt

PRODUCTS FROM HOG HEARTS
heart valves for human transplant

PRODUCTS FROM INTESTINES
instrument strings
medical sutures - surgery
sausage casings
tennis racquet strings

PRODUCTS FROM LIVERS
heparin - anti-coagulant, prevents gangrene
intrinsic factor - pernicious anemia
liver extract - treatment of anemia
Vitamin B12 - prevention of B-complex
   deficiencies

PRODUCTS FROM LUNGS
heparin - anti-coagulant, prevents gangrene

PRODUCTS FROM MANURE
fertilizer - used in gardens, lawns and farm
   cropland
minor minerals
nitrogen
phosphorous
potash

PRODUCTS FROM MILK/DAIRY
adhesives
animal feed
butter
carriers for human medicine
casein (proteins)
cheese and cheese products
cosmetics
cream
fats (lipids)
food ethanol
glue
ice cream and ice cream mixes
lactose (carbohydrates)

milk powder
pharmaceuticals
sherbet
sizing
specialty plastics
veterinary medicines
whey (proteins)
yogurt

PRODUCTS FROM OVARIES
estrogen
progesterone

PRODUCTS FROM PANCREASES
chymotrypsin - contact surgery
diastase - aids in starch digestion
glucagon - treats hypoglycemia
insulin - diabetes mellitus
pancreatin - aids digestion
trypsin - for burns, wounds, and infection
   - promotes healing, aids in protein digestion
   and in cleaning wounds

PRODUCTS FROM PITUITARY GLANDS
ACTH - arthritis, allergies, rheumatic fever, skin
   and eye inflammations
pressor hormone - regulates blood pressure
prolactin - promotes lactation
vasopressin - controls intestinal and renal
   functions

PRODUCTS FROM SPINAL CORDS
cholesterol - hormone products

PRODUCT FROM STOMACHS
pepsin - aids in protein digestion
rennet - aids in milk digestion

PRODUCTS FROM THYROIDS
bovine thyroid (Thyrar®) - a thyroid replacement
thyroid extract - hypothrodism
thyroid hormones
TSH - thyroid diagnosis

PRODUCTS FROM WOOL
asphalt binder
carpet
clothing
cosmetics
fabrics
felt
insulation
lanolin
medical ointments

paint and plaster binder
pelt products
rouge base
rug pads
upholstery
woolen goods
worsted fabric/yarns

OTHER MEDICAL AND HEALTH CARE PRODUCTS

antibodies (immunoglobins)
beef insulin
bovine collagen - used as injections to fill in scars
bovine fibrinolysin (Elase®) ointment - for use on necrotic tissue
bovine superoxide dismutase cream (Orgotein®) - cosmetic skin cream to prevent tissue aging
bovine thrombin (Thrombinar®) - clotting agent for blood
culture medium - diagnosis
fetal bovine serum - tissue cultures, vaccine manufacturing
hyaluronidase - efficient drug use

nitroglycerine
pegademase - bovine derivative (Adagen®)
 - for patients who are immuno-compromised
 - helps prevent white blood cells from breaking down.
pill capsules - GELATIN
PTH - control tetany
whole serum - vaccine manufacturing

GENERAL FOOD PRODUCTS FROM CATTLE, SHEEP, AND HOG FLESH

a huge variety of fresh, frozen, and pre-cooked meats and prepared and processed meat products

OTHER PRODUCTS FROM CATTLE SOURCES

airplane lubricants and runway foam
car polishes and waxes
hydraulic brake fluid
stearic acid - helps rubber in tires hold shape
steel ball bearings containing bone charcoal
textiles for car upholstery
various machine oils and viscous fluids

THE BOOK THAT NEVER GROWS OLD

With your purchase of *The Encyclopedia of Medical Breakthroughs & Forbidden Treatments*, you receive unlimited access to the Member's Area of our website, year after year. This password-protected area contains links to information that has become available since the last printing of *The Encyclopedia*. In this way we're able to keep our readers up to date on recent medical breakthroughs and other important medical information. *The Encyclopedia*, therefore, exists as a complete work in two locations: 1) in the physical world as a soft cover book (or online as an ebook), and 2) online in the Member's Area of our website. Without consulting the information contained within both venues, you will not have accessed the complete work.

"If it's not in the book, on our website you should look."

Please Visit Our Website Regularly for Important Updates at **www.medical-breakthroughs.com. Enter Username and Password.**

Important Member's Area access: When you purchased *The Encyclopedia*, you were asked to create your unique access to the Member's Area. In addition, following your purchase you were emailed information on how to access the Member's Area had you not done so during the purchasing process. If at any time you need to acquire or recover your Username or Password, please visit medical-breakthroughs.com/support to submit a "Support Ticket" requesting additional information/directions.

ENDNOTES

PART I: The Background

Preface

1. www.ndchealth.com, April 1, 2003.
2. Lasser, K., et al. "Timing of new black box warnings and withdrawals for prescription medications." *Journal of the American Medical Association.* Vol. 287, No. 17, May 1, 2002. http://jama.ama-assn.org/cgi/content/abstract/287/17/2215
3. Ibid.
4. Starfield, B. "Is U.S. health really the best in the world?" *Journal of the American Medical Association*, 284: 483-5, 2000; also Lararou, J., et al. "Incidence of adverse drug reactions in hospitalized patients: a meta-analysis of prospective studies." *Journal of the American Medical Association*, 279(15):1200-1205, April 15, 1998.
5. http://eurobserver.com/9/26973.
6. http://zia.hss.cmu.edu/miller/eep/news//vitpfix.mon.txt
7. Ibid.
8. Conner, Steve. *Glaxo Chief: Our Drugs Do Not Work On Most Patients.* Common Dreams News Center, Dec. 8, 2003. www.commondreams.org/cgi-bin/print.cgi?file=/headlines03/1208-02.htm; also http://bbc.co.uk/1/hi/health/3299945.stm
9. Ibid.
10. "Death By Medicine," Null, G., et al. *Life Extension*, pp. 1-2, August 2006. www.lef.org/magazine/mag2006/aug2006_report_death_01.htm (Null cites additional specific references.)
11. Ibid.
12. Null, as in Note 10.
13. Ibid.; http://rationalrevolution.net/articles/casualties_of_war.htm
14. www.businessweek.com/bwdaily/dnflash/content/jun2009/db2009064_666715.htm
15.http://en.wikipedia.org/wiki/Health_care_in_the_United_States (2008 statistic)
16. [Healthcare spending is 16% (as per Note 15) of 2008 GDP ($14.4 trillion) = $2.30 trillion] http://en.wikipedia.org/wiki/Health_care_in_the_United_States (2008 statistic) (The United States Department of Defense expenditures for fiscal year 2009 = $651.2 billion) http://en.wikipedia.org/wiki/United_States_Department_of_Defense (2009 statistic)
17. Wilper, A.P., et al. "Health insurance and morality in U.S. adults." *American Journal of Public Health*, 2009.
18. Ibid.
19. www.oecd.org/dataoecd/46/2/38980580.pdf (2007statistic)
20. http://en.wikipedia.org/wiki/List_of_countries_by_life_expectancy#List_by_the_CIA_World_Factbook_.282009_estimates.29 (2009 statistic)
21. www.photius.com/rankings/world_health_performance_ranks.html;www.photius.com/rankings/health_ranks.html (2000 statistic; latest available from WHO and still the primary reference.)
22. (Deaths caused by conventional medicine annually in U.S. = 800,000) Null, as in Note 10; (Deaths caused by automobiles annually in U.S.: ~40,000) www.edgarsnyder.com/car-accident/resources/statistics.html (2008 statistic)
23. (Deaths caused by conventional medicine annually in U.S.: 800,000) Null, as in Note 10; (Deaths caused by firearms annually in U.S., including both homicides and suicides: ~27,000) http://en.wikipedia.org/wiki/Gun_violence_in_the_United_States (2005 statistic)
24. (Deaths caused by conventional medicine annually in U.S.: 800,000) Null, as in Note 10; (Deaths caused by heart disease and cancer annually in U.S.: 631,636 and 559,888, respectively) www.cdc.gov/nchs/FASTATS/deaths.htm (2006 statistic)

Introduction

1. www.guardian.co.uk/medicine/story/0,11381,1062021,00.html
2. Rey, Roselyne. *The History of Pain.* Translated by Louise Elliott Wallace, J. A. Cadden, S.W. Cadden. Harvard University Press, 1999.

The Body-Mind-Body Loop

1. *Pain*, 90(1-2):191-9, 2001.
2. www.newscientist.com/news/news.jsp?id=ns99993767
3. Ibid.
4. Yue, G. and Cole, K.J. "Strength increases from the motor program: comparison of training with maximal voluntary and imagined muscle contractions." *Journal of Neurophysiology*, 67:1114-1123, 1992.
5. *Lancet*, 355(9199):233-4, 2000.
6. *The Wall Street Journal*, October 18, 1999.

Differences in Pain Perception

1. *Proceedings of the National Academy of Sciences* (DOI:10.1073/pnas.0136822100,10.1073/pnas.012682399
2. http://www.sciencemag.org/cgi/content/abstract/314/5807/1930
3. Ibid

Pain Relief Throughout History

1. Gurkirpal, S. "Recent considerations in Non-Streroidal Anti-inflammatory drug gastropathy." *American Journal of Medicine.* p. 31S, July 27, 1998.

PART II: Specific Ailments

Acquired Immune Deficiency Syndrome

1."The Secret Origin of AIDS and HIV: How scientists produced the most horrifying plague of all time - and then covered it up." Alan Cantwell Jr., M.D. Lecture series, 2000; www.whale.to/v/cantwell3.html.
2. Nduati, R., et al. "Effect of breastfeeding on mortality among HIV-1 infected women: A randomized trial."

Lancet, 357, 1651-1655, 2001.

3. Same as Note 1, p. ix.

4. UNAIDS/WHO Epidemiological Fact Sheet on HIV/AIDS and sexually transmitted infections: Senegal. 2000 update (revised).

5. Cowgill, U.M. "The distribution of selenium and mortality owing to acquired immune deficiency syndrome in the continental United States." *Biological Trace Element Research*, (56)43-61, 1997.

6. Taylor, E.W. "Selenium and viral diseases: Facts and hypotheses." *Journal of Orthomolecular Medicine*, 12(4):227-239, 1997.

7. Mariorino, M., et al. "Probing the presumed catalytic triad of a selenium-containing peroxidase by mutational analysis." Z. Ernahrungswiss, 37(Supp. 1), 118-121, 1998.

8. Ibid.

Alzheimer's Disease

1. www.alzheimers.org

2. Ibid.

3. Letter to HCFA by the Society of Nuclear Medicine in support of Alzheimer's PET scans, April 30, 2001; www.interactive.snm.org

4. Luchsinger, J.A., et al. "Caloric intake and the risk of Alzheimer's disease." *Archives of Neurology*, (59)1528-1563, 2002.

5. Travis, J. "Microbe linked to Alzheimer's disease—Chlamydia pneumoniae." *Science News*, Nov. 21, 1998.

6. From a speech given by Dr. Fudenberg at the NVIC International Vaccine Conference , Arlington, VA, 1997; www.mercola.com/2002/aug/14/alzheimers_eating.htm

7. Leong, C.W., et al. "Retrograde degeneration of neurite membrane structural integrity of nerve growth cones following in vitro exposure to mercury." *NeuroReport*, 12(4):733-737, 2001.

8. Ibid.

9. Ibid.

10. Ibid.

11. Ibid.

12. www.mercola.com/1998/archive/aluminum_and_alzheimer_prevention.htm

13. Ibid.

14. Verner, J., et al. "Chronic administration of aluminum-fluoride and sodium-fluoride to rats in the drinking water: alterations in neural and cerebrovascular integrity." *Journal of Brain Research*, Vol. 784, 1998.

15. Ibid.

16. Mullins, E. *Murder by Injection*. The National Council for Medical Research: Staunton, VA, 1995, p. 59.

17. A'o, Lono Kahuna Kupua, *Don't Drink the Water*, Kali Press: Pagosa Springs, CO, 1998, p.9.

18. Newsweek, February 5, 1990. Source: A'o, Lono Kahuna Kupua, *Don't Drink the Water*, Kali Press: Pagosa Springs, CO, 1998, p.49.

19. Veld, B.A., et al. "Nonsteroidal Anti-inflammatory Drugs and the risk of Alzheimer's disease." *New England Journal of Medicine*, (345):1515-1521, 2001.

20. Lim, G.P. "The curry spice cucurmin reduces oxidative damage and amyloid pathology in Alzheimer transgenic mouse." *Journal of Neuroscience*, 21(21):8370-8377, Nov. 1, 2001.

21. American Academy of Neurology, 54th Annual Meeting, Denver, CO, April 13-20, 2002

22. www.mayoclinic.com

23. Wilkins, D.J., et al. "Biochemical and clinical consequences of inhibiting coenzyme Q10 biosynthesis by lipid-lowering HMG-CoA reductase inhibitors (statins): A critical overview." *Advances in Therapy*, 15(4):218-228, July/Aug. 1998.

24. Merello, M., et al. "Effect of memantine on Parkinson's disease: A double-blind crossover randomized study." *Clinical Neuropharm.* 22(5):273-276, 1999.

25. Holter, S.M., et al. "Evidence for alcohol anti-craving properties of Memantine." *European Journal of Pharmacology*, 314(3):R1-2, 1996.

26. Results presented at the 52nd Annual Meeting of the American Academy of Neurology, San Diego, CA, April 29-May 6, 2000.

27. Winblad, B., et al. "Memantine in severe dementia: The benefit and efficacy in severely demented patients treated with Memantine." *International Journal of Geriatric Psychiatry*, 14(2):135-146, Feb. 1999.

28. Reiseberg, B., et al. "Memantine in moderate to severe Alzheimer's disease." *New England Journal of Medicine*, 348(14:1333-1341, April 3, 2003.

29. Woodruff-Pak, D.S., et al. "Nicotinic modulation in an animal model of a form of associative learning impaired in Alzheimer's disease." *Behavioral Brain Research*, 113(1-2):11-19, 2000.

30. Sramek, J.J., et al. "Efficacy of galantamine in the treatment of Alzheimer's disease." *Clinical Geriatrics*, 9(11):55-63, 2000.

31. Aerssens, J., et al. "APOE Genotype: No influence on galantamine treatment efficacy nor on rate of decline in Alzheimer's disease." *Dementia and Cognitive Geriatric Disorders*, 12:69-77, 2001.

32. Sierpina, V.S., et al. "Ginkgo Biloba." *American Family Physician*, 68:923-926, Sept. 1, 2003.

33. Ibid.

34. Hager, K., et al. "Alpha lipoic acid as a new treatment for Alzheimer's type dementia." *Archives of Gerontology & Geriatrics*, 32:275-282, 2001.

35. Xu, S.S., et al. "Efficacy of oral huperzine-A on memory, cognition, and behavior in Alzheimer's disease." *Chung Kuo Yao Li Hsueh Pao*, 16(5):391-395, 1995.

36. Zhang, Z., et al. "Clinical efficacy and safety of huperzine Alpha in treatment of mild to moderate Alzheimer's disease, a placebo-controlled, double-blind, randomized trial." *Zhoughua Yi Xue Za Zhi*, 82(14):941-944, July 25, 2002.

37. Sano, M., et al. "A controlled trial of selegiline, alpha-tocopherol, or both as treatment for Alzheimer's disease." *New England Journal of Medicine*, 336:1216-1222, 1997.

38. www.mercola.com

39. Derbyshire, D. "The helmet that could turn back the symptoms of Alzheimer's." *Daily Mail* (Online), January 25, 2008; http://www.dailymail.co.uk/health/article-510172/The-helmet-turn-symptoms-Alzheimers.html

40. Ibid.

41. Tobinick, E., et al. "Rapid cognitive improvement in Alzheimer's disease following perispinal etanercept administration." *Journal of Neuroinflammation*, doi:10.1186/1742-2094-5-2, January 2008.

42. Griffin, S. "Perispinal etanercept: potential as an Alzheimer's therapeutic." *Journal of Neuroinflammation*, doi: 10.1186/1742-2094-5-3, January 2008.

43. Ibid.

44. Zandi, P.P., et al. "Reduced risk of Alzheimer's disease in users of antioxidant vitamin supplements." *Archives of Neurology*, 61:82-88, 2004.

45. Snowden, D., et al. "Brain infarction and the clinical expression of Alzheimer's disease. The Nun Study." *Journal of the American Medical Association*, 277(10):813-817, March 12, 1997.

Amyotrophic Lateral Sclerosis (ALS)

1. "Lithium in Amyotrophic Lateral Sclerosis and Alzheimer's Disease." *Proceedings of the National Academy of Sciences USA.* 105:2052-2057, 2008; www.neura.net/images/pdf/Neura_V8I3_Lithium.pdf

Appendicitis

1. www.medicinenet.com/Appendicitis/page1.htm

Arthritis

1. Alexander, D. *Arthritis and Common Sense.* Simon & Shuster: New York, NY, 1954, p. 21.

2. Ibid., p. 23.

3. Gurkirpal, S. "Recent considerations in Non-Streroidal Anti-inflammatory drug gastropathy." *American Journal of Medicine.* P. 31S, July 27, 1998; also Wolfe, M.M., et al. "Gastrointestinal toxicity of nonsteroidal anti-inflammatory drugs." *New England Journal of Medicine.* 340:1888-1898, 1999.

4. Package insert for Celebrex, 819 058 000 P04025, Aug. 2003.

5. www.bcmfindings.net/vol1/is6/03june_n1.htm

6. White, L.C. *Merchants of Death: The American Tobacco Industry.* William Morrow: NY, NY, pp. 32-34, 1998.

7. Budenholzer, B. "Are COX-2 inhibitors inferior to NSAIDs?" *British Journal of Medicine.* 324:1287-1288, 2002.

8. Page, J., et al. "Consumption of NSAIDs and the development of Congestive Heart Failure in elderly patients." *Archives of Internal Medicine.*" 160:777-784, 2000.

9. Li, De-Kun, et al. "Exposure to non-steroidal antiinflammatory drugs during pregnancy and risk of miscarriage: population based cohort study." *British Medical Journal.* 327(7411):368, August 16, 2003.

10. Penglis, P.S., et al. "Differential regulation of prostaglandin E2 and thromboxane A2 production in human monocytes: implications for the use of cyclooxygenase inhibitors." *Journal of Immunology*, 165)3):1605-1611, Aug. 1, 2000; and Saklatvala, J. "Tumor necrosis factor alpha stimulates resorption and inhibits synthesis of proteoglycan in cartilage." *Nature*, 322(6079):547-549, Aug. 7-13, 1986.

11. Ronningen, H., et al. "Indomethacin treatment in osteoporosis of the hip joint." *Acta Orthopdica Scandanavica*, 50:168-174, 1979; Newman, N.M., et al. "Acetabular bone destruction related to non-steroidal anti-inflammatory drugs." *Lancet, ii*:11-13, 1985; Solomon, L. "Drug-induced arthropathy and necrosis of the femoral head." *Journal of Bone and Joint Surgery*, 55B:246-251, 1973.

12. Becker, M.A., et al. "Febuxostat compared with allopurinal in patients with hyperuricemia and gout." *New England Journal of Medicine*, 23(353):2450-2461, December 2005

13. Deal, C.L., et al. "Nutriceuticals as therapeutic agents in osteoarthritis. The role of glucosamine, chrondroitin sulfate, and collagen hydrolsate." *Rheumatic Disease Clinics of North America.* 25(2): 379-95, May 1999; and Gaby, A.R. "Natural treatments for osteoarthritis." *Alternative Medical Review.* 4:330-441, 1999.

14. Lippiello, L., et al. "In vivo chondroprotection and metabolic synergy of glucosamine and chondroitin sulfate." *Clinical Orthopedics.* 381:229-240, 2000.

15. Abedowale, A.O., et al. "Analysis of glucosamine and chondroitin sulfate content in marketed products and the Caco-2 permeability of chondroitin sulfate raw materials." *Journal of the American Medical Association.* 3:37-44, 2000.

16. www.jacoblab.com/msm_protocols.htm

17. Diehl, H.W., et al. "Cetyl Myristoleate isolated from Swiss Albino Mice: An apparent protective agent against adjuvant arthritis in rats." *Journal of Pharmaceutical Sciences.* Vol. 83, No. 3, March 1994. P-1 Surveillance for Asthma—United States 1960-1995, *Morbidity and Mortality Weekly Report*, April 24, 1998, 47(SS-1).

18. Ibid.

19. Bagga, H., et al. "Longterm effects of intraarticular hyaluronan on synovial fluid in osteoarthritis of the knee." *Journal of Rheumatology*, 33(5):946-950, May 2006.

20. www.bioiberica.com.

21. Henrotin Y.E., et al. "Avocado/soybean unsaponifiables increase aggrecan synthesis and reduce catabolic and proinflammatory mediator production by human osteoarthritic chondrocytes." *Journal of Rheumatology*, 30:1825–1834, 2003.

22. Appelboom J., et al. "Symptoms modifying effect of avocado/soybean unsaponifiables (ASU) in knee osteoarthritis." *Scandanavian Journal of Rheumatology*, 30:242–247, 2001.

23. Delecluse, C., et al, "Strength increase after whole-body vibration compared with resistance training." *Medicine and Science in Sports & Exercise.* 0195-9131, pp. 1033-1041, 2003.

24. Bosco, C.M., et al. "Hormonal responses to whole-body vibration in men." *European Journal of Physiology*, 81:449-54, 2000.

25. Flieger, J., et al. "Mechanical stimulation in the form of vibration prevents postmenopausal bone loss in variectomized rats." *Calcified Tissue International*, 63: 510-15, 1998.

26. www.ncbi.nlm.nih.gov/entrez/query.fcgi?db=PubMed &cmd=Display&dopt=pubmed_ pubmed&from_uid= 8185689

27. http://news.bbc.co.uk/2/hi/health/3247035.stm

28. Minas, T. "Autologous cultured chondrocyte grafting in focal defects of the knee," *American Journal of Knee Surgery*, 10:4, 1999.

29. Blau, L.W., "Cherry diet control for gout and arthritis." *Texas Reports on Biology and Medicine*, 8(3):309-311, 1950.

Asthma

1. "Asthma: A Concern for Minority Populations," National Institute of Allergy and Infectious Diseases. Jan. 1997.

2. www.about-asthma.com

3. Ibid.

4. www.cushing-help.com/prednisone-danger.htm

5. Redman, C.M., et al. "Nonprescription bronchial dilator use in asthma." *Chest*, 114:657-658, 1998.

6. *Journal of Family Practice, 40:121-122, 1995.*

7. Bowler, S.D., et al. "Buteyko breathing techniques in asthma: a blinded, randomized controlled trial." *Medical Journal of Australia*, 169:575-578, 1998.

8. *Tufts University Diet & Nutrition Letter*, Feb. 1996.

9. Johnston, C.S., et al. "Antihistamine effects and complications of supplemental vitamin C." *Journal of the American Dietetic Association*, 92 (8):988-989, 1992.

Autism

1. Parker, S.K., et. al. "Thimerosal-containing vaccines and autistic spectrum disorder: a critical review of published original data." *Pediatrics*, Vol. 114 No. 3, pp. 793-804, September 2004.

2. www.whale.to/vaccine/olmsted1.html

3. www.news.com.au/heraldsun/story/0%2C21985% 2C22864043-2862%2C00.html; and www.telegraph.co .uk/news/uknews/1567698/Cervical-cancer-drug-Gardasil-linked-to-deaths.html

4. Yasko, A., et al. *The Puzzle of Autism: Putting It All Together*, 2006.

5. From a speech given by Dr. Fudenberg at the NVIC International Vaccine Conference , Arlington, VA, 1997; www.mercola.com/2002/aug/14/alzheimers_eating.htm.

6. McGrath, J.J., et al. "Vitamin D—implications for brain development." *Journal of Steroid Biochemistry and Molecular Biology*, 89-90(1-5):557-560, May 2004.

7. Kalueff, A.V., et al., " The vitamin D neuroendocrine system as a target for novel neurotropic drugs." *CNS & Neurological Disorders—Drug Targets*, 5(3):363-371, June 2006.

8. Chez, M.G., et al. "Double-blind, placebo-controlled study of L-carnosine supplementation in children with autistic spectrum disorder." *Journal of Child Neurology*, Vol. 17, No. 11, November 2002.

Back

1. www.back.com/article-infuse.html?infusebox=yep

2. Ibid.

3. Ibid.

4. "Acupuncture for chronic low back pain: a randomized placebo-controlled study with long-term follow-up." *Clinical Journal of Pain*. 17(4):296-305, 2001; and Cheung, J. "Effect of electro-accupuncture on chronic painful conditions in general medical practice—a 4 years' study." *American Journal of Chinese Medicine*. 13(1-4):33-8, 1985.

5. www.cchs.net/health/health-info/docs/0800/ 0802.asp?index=4162

6. Ibid.

7. "Reduction in postoperative mortality and morbidity with epidural or spinal anesthesia: results from overview of randomized trials." *British Medical Journal*, 321 (7275):1,493, 2000.

8. Ibid.

9. "The Mainstreaming of Alternative Medicine." *Consumer Reports*. May 2000.

Burns

1. Grover, S.K, and Prasad, C.S. "Use of Madhu in Ayurveda." *Journal of the National Indian Medical Association*, 10: 7-10, 1985.

2. http://www.medbc.com/annals/review/vol_9/num_1/ text/vol9n1p33.htm

3. Molan, P.C., "Potential of honey in the treatment of wounds and burns." *American Journal of Clinical Dermatology*." 2(1):13-9, 2001.

4. Subrahmanyam, M. "Topical application of honey in treatment of burns." *British Journal of Surgery*, 78(4):497-8, April 1991.

5. Subrahmanyam, M. "A prospective randomized clinical and histological study of superficial burn wound healing with honey and silver sulfadiazine." *Burns*. 24(2):157-61, Mar. 1998.

6. Kamenicek, V., et al. "Systemic enzyme therapy in the treatment and prevention of post-traumatic and post-operative swelling." *Acta Chir Traumatol Cech*, 68(1):45-9, 2001.

7. www.celltran.co.uk

8. http://medlib.med.utah.edu/kw/ibc/minor_burns/ frcontent.html

Cancer

1. Olsen, Ole and Gotzsche, Peter C. "Cochrane review on screening for breast cancer with mammography." *Lancet*, Vol. 358, October 20, 2001, pp. 1340-42 (research letter); Horton, Richard. "Screening mammography – an overview revisited." *Lancet*, Vol. 358, pp. 1284-85 (commentary), October 20, 2001.

2. Baines, C. "Mammography screening: Are women really giving informed consent?" *Journal of the National Cancer Institute*, 95(20): 1508-1511 ("Counterpoint" by A.O. Berg: pp. 1511-1512; "Countering the Counterpoint" by C. Baines: pp. 1512-1513), October 15, 2003.

3. Miglioretti D.L., et al. "Radiologist characteristics associated with interpretive performance of diagnostic mammography." *Journal of the National Cancer Institute*, 99:1854-1863, 2007.

4. "Predicting the cumulative risk of false-positive mammograms." *Journal of the National Cancer Institute*, 92(20): 1,657-1,666, 2000.

5. breastthermography.com/breast_cancer_facts.htm

6. Ibid.

7. Ibid.

8. Ibid.

9. Ibid.

10. www.iact-org.org/patients/breastthermography/what-is-breast-therm.html

11. Nyirjesy, I., et al. "Clinical observation, mammography, and thermography in the diagnosis of breast carcinoma." *Thermology*. 1:170-173, 1986.

12. iact-org.org/articles/articles-review-btherm.html

13. "Elevated levels of anti-malignin antibody are quantitatively related to longer survival in cancer patients." *Protides Biol. Fluids*, 31:739-747, 1984; and "Determination of anti-malignin antibody and malignin in 1,026 cancer patients and controls: relation of antibody to survival." *J. Medicine* 13:49-69, 1982.

14. "Increased accuracy of anti-malignin antibody determination in unstored sera permits screening." *Cancer Detection and Prevention* 11:No. 1/2, 85, 1987. Also, Note 4 above.

15. http://www.bcaction.org/Pages/SearchablePages/1996Newsletters/Newsletter 037E.html

16. Same as Note 5.

17. "Determination of anti-malignin in patients with suspicious mammograms." *Proceedings of the American Association of Cancer Research* (31: A 1550, 1990).

18. "Early detection and monitoring of cancer with the anti-malignan test." *Cancer Detection and Prevention*, 18(1):65-78, 1994.

19. Honn, K.V., et al. "Prostacyclin: a potent antimetastatic agent." *Science*. 212:1270-1272. 1981

20. Gorelik, E. "Augmentation of the antimetastatic effect of anticoagulant drugs by immunostimulation in mice." *Cancer Research*. 47:809-815. 1987.

21. Thornes, R.D. "Adjuvant therapy of cancer via the cellular immune mechanism of fibrin by induced fibrinolysis and oral anticoagulants." *Cancer*. 35:91-97. 1975.

22. Honn, as per Note 19.

23. Zelikoff, J.T., et al. "Studies on the anti-tumor promoting activity of naturally occurring substances. IV.Pd-II[(+0 anomalin, (+) praeruptorin B], a seselin-type coumarin, inhibits the promotion of skin tumor formation by 12-O-tetradecanoylphorbol-13-acetate in 7,12-dimethylbenz[a]anthracene-initiated mice." *Carcinogenesis*. 11:1557-1561, 1990.

24. Knudsen, K.A., et al. "Trigramin, an RGD-containing peptide from snake venom, inhibits cell-substratum adhesion of human melanoma cells." *Experimental Cell Research*, 179:42-49, 1988.

25. Tuszynski, G.P., et al. "Isolation and characterization of antistasin. An inhibitor of metastasis and coagulation." *Journal of Biological Chemistry*. 262:9718-9723, 1987.

26. George, J. and Shattil, S. "The clinical importance of acquired abnormalities of platelet function." *The New England Journal of Medicine*. 324:27. 1991.

27. Strum, S., et al. "Modified Citrus Pectin Slows PSA Doubling Time: A Pilot Clinical Trial." Presented at the International Conference on Diet and Prevention of Cancer May 28-June 2, 1999 Tampere, Finland.

28. Eliaz, I. "The Potential Role of Modified Citrus Pectin in the Prevention of Cancer Metastasis." *Clinical Practice of Alternative Medicine*. Vol. 2, No. 3, Fall 2001.

29. Briggs, S. "Modified Citrus Pectin May Halt Metastasis." *Nutrition Science News*. May, 1997. http://vitamintrader.com/articles1997_05_ ModCit.html

30. Strum, as in Note 27.

31. Eliaz, as in Note 28.

32. Strum, as in Note 27.

33. *Pharmacology and Applications of Chinese Materia Medica*, Vol. 2.

34. Eliaz, I. "The Role of Modified Citrus Pectin in the Prevention of Cancer Metastases." *Townsend Letter for Doctors and Patients*. July 1999, pp.64-66.

35. Platt, D., et al. "Modulation of the lung colonization of B16-F1 melanoma cells by citrus pectin." *Journal of the National Cancer Institute*. 84(6):438-432, Mar. 18,1992.

36. Pienta, K.J. et al. "Inhibition of spontaneous metastasis in a rat prostate cancer model by oral administration of modified citrus pectin." *Journal of the National Cancer Institute*. Mar. 1, 87(5): 348-353, 1995.

37. Naik, H. Pilat, M., et al. "Inhibition of in vitro tumor cell-endothelial adhesion by modified citrus pectin: A pH modified natural complex carbohydrate." *Proceedings of the Annual Meeting of the American Association of Cancer Research*. 36:A377, 1995.

38. Strum, S., et al. "Modified citrus pectin slows PSA doubling time: A pilot clinical trial." *International Conference on Diet and Prevention of Cancer*, Tampere, Finland, May 1999.

39. Weiss, T. "Modified citrus pectin induces cytotoxicity of prostate cancer cells in co-cultures with human endothelial monolayers." *Int'l. Conference on Diet and Prevention of Cancer*, Tampere, Finland, May 1999.

40. Hayashi, A. Et al. "Effects of daily oral administration of quercitin chalcone and modified citrus pectin." *Alternative Medical Review*. 5(6):546-552, Dec. 2000.

41. Hittelett, A., et al. "Upregulation of galectins-1 and -3 in human colon cancer and their role in regulating cell migration." *International Journal of Cancer*, 103(3): 370-379, Jan. 2003.

42. Lahm, H., et al. "Comprehensive galectin fingerprinting in a panel of 61 human tumor cell lines by RT-PCR and its implications for diagnostic and therapeutic procedures." *Journal of Cancer Research and Clinical Oncology*, 127(6):375-386, 2001.

43. Nangia-Makker, P., et al. "Inhibition of human cancer cell growth and metastasis in nude mice by oral intake of modified citrus pectin." *Journal of the National Cancer Institute*, 94(24):1859-1862, Dec. 18, 2002.

44. O'Driscoll, L., et al. "Galectin-3 expression alters adhesion, motility and invasion in a lung cell line in vivo." *Anticancer Research*, 22(6A):3117-3125, Nov-Dec 2002.

45. Hitelett, as in Note 41.

46. Guess, B. et al. "Using splines to detect changes in PSA doubling times." *The Prostate*. 54(2):88-94, 2003.

47. John, Constance, et al. "Truncated galectin-3 inhibits tumor growth and metastasis in orthotopic nude mouse model of human breast cancer." *Clinical Cancer Research*. Vol. 9, 2374-2383, June 2003.

48. Keller, E., D.V.M, Ph. D., *Journal of the National Cancer Institute*, 95(12),839-841, 878-889, June 18, 2003. http://jncicancerspectrum.oupjournals.org/jnci/

49. Rath, Matthias. *Cancer*. MR Publishing, Inc.: Santa Clara, CA, 2001, p.28.

50. Ibid.

51. Ibid.

52. Ibid., pp. 30-31.

53. Ibid, pp. 44-45.

54. Astedt, B., et al. "Treatment of advanced breast cancer with chemotherapeutics and inhibition of coagulation and fibrinolysis." *Acta Med. Scand.* 201: 491-493, 1997.

55. Astedt, B., et al. "Arrest of growth of ovarian tumor by tranexamic acid." *Journal of the American Medical Association*. 238: 154-155, 1977.

56. Some, H., et al. "Treatment of advanced ovarian cancer with fibrinolytic inhibitor (tranexamic acid)." *Acta Obstetrica et Gynecologica Scandinavica*. 59: 285-287.

57. Tonnesen, H., et al. "Effect of cimetidine on survival after gastric cancer." *Lancet*, 2(8618):990-992, October 1988.

58. Adams, W.J., et al. "Short-course cimetidine and survival with colorectal cancer." *Lancet*, 344(8939-8940):1768-1769, December 1994.

59. Matsumoto, S., et al. "Cimetidine increases survival of colorectal cancer patients with high levels of sialyl Lewis-X and sialyl Lewis-A epitope expression on tumor cells." *British Journal of Cancer*, 86(2):161-167, January 2002.

60. Moss, R.W., *The Cancer Industry*, New York, NY: Equinox Press, 1999; and Moss, R.W., *Questioning Chemotherapy*, New York, NY: Equinox Press, 1995.

61. Moss, *The Cancer Industry*, p. 43.

62. www.lef.org/protocols/prtcl-026.shtml

63. Ibid.; also Moss, *The Cancer Industry*, p. 64.

64. Morgan, G., et al. "The contribution of cytotoxic chemotherapy to 5-year survival in adult malignancies." *Clinical Oncology*, 16(8):549-560, December 2004.

65. Ibid.

66. Moss, same as Note 60; and Day, Lorraine, *Cancer Doesn't Scare Me Anymore* (Video); www.drday.com

67. Pierce, Tanya H., *Outsmart Your Cancer: Alternative Non-Toxic Treatments That Work*, Thoughtworks Publishing: Stateline, NV, 2004, p. 7.

68. Moss, same as Note 60.

69. Moss, *Questioning Chemotherapy*, p. 163.

70. Sheridan, James V., Personal Writings, as quoted in Pierce, *Outsmart Your Cancer*, Note 67.

71. Sheridan, J.V., et al., "How Does Entelev/Cancell Work: A Layman's Explanation." *Journal of the Bio-Electro-Magnetics Institute*, Vol. 3, No. 3, p. 37, April 1992.

72. Pierce, pp. 125-126.

73. Brewer, K.A., "The High pH Therapy for Cancer, Test on Mice and Humans," *Pharmacology Biochemistry and Behavior*, Vol. 221, Supplement 1, pp. 1-5, 1984; also www.mwt.net/~drbrewer/highpH.htm

74. Ibid.

75. Ibid.

76. Ibid; and Pierce, as in Note 67.

77. Ibid.

78. Warburg, Otto. "The Prime Cause and Prevention of Cancer" (Revised Lindau Lecture), www.whale.to/a/warburg.html

79. www.cancertutor.com/Cancer/Budwig.html

80. Budwig, J., *"Der Tod des Tumors, Band II"* (*"The Death of Tumors, Vol. II"*), Transcribed interview, broadcast Sept. 11, 1967 by Süddeutscher Rundfunk Stuttgart (Germany).

81. Roehm, D.C., "The Bio Electron, Re-Examining the Work of Johanna Budwig", *Townsend Letter for Doctors and Patients*, July 1990, p. 480.

82. Willner, R.E., *The Cancer Solution*, Peltec Publications: Boca Raton, FL, 1994.

83. www.alkalizeforhealth.net/Ltijuanacancerclinics.htm

84. www.medsafe.govt.nz/profs/Datasheet/f/Fentanyl citrateinjUSP.htm

85. "Randomised crossover trial of transdermal fentanyl and sustained release oral morphine for treating chronic non-cancer pain." *British Medical Journal*, 322:1-7, 2001.

86. www.medicalnewstoday.com/articles/163732.php.

87. www.medtronics.com/hic/cancer.html

88. www.norml.org.

Cardiovascular Disease

1. www.cdc.gov/nccdphp/bb_heartdisease/index.htm

2. "The Regeneration Game." *New Scientist*, Sept. 27-Oct. 3, p. 42, 2003.

3. www.americanheart.org/presenter.jhtml?identifier=4741

4. Ibid.

5. Ibid.

6. Jensen, Bernard. *Empty Harvest: Understanding the Link Between Our Food, Our Immunity, and Our Planet*. Avery Publishing Group Inc.: Garden City Park, NY, 1990, p. 126.

7. www.americanheart.org/presenter.jhtml?identifier=475

8. Bachmaier, K., et al. "Chlamydia infections and heart disease linked through antigenic mimicry." *Science*. 283:1335–1339, 1999. Also http://ourworld.compuserve.com/homepages/CarolASThompson/CMVHD.htm

9. *New England Journal of Medicine*, Vol. 340, 1999.

10. Cheng, J., et al. "Cytomegalovirus infection causes an increase of arterial blood pressure." *PLoS Pathogens*. Published online May 2009.

11. Ibid.

12. Rubio, A.R., et al. "Nitric oxide, an iceberg in cardiovascular physiology: far beyond vessel tone control." *Archives of Medical Research*, 35(1):1-11, Jan-Feb 2004.

13. http://www.cimit.org/vplaque.html

14. Stampfer, M.J., et al. "A prospective study of plasma homocyst(e)ine and risk of myocarial infarction in US physicians." *Journal of the American Medical Association*, 268(7):877-81, 1992.

15. McCully, Kilmer. *The Homocysteine Revolution: A Bold New Approach to the Prevention of Heart Disease*. McGraw Hill, 1999.

16. Libby, P. "Atherosclerosis: A New View." *Scientific American*, pp. 47-55. May, 2002.

17. Ibid.

18. Ibid.

19. Ibid.

20. Ibid.

21. www.americanheart.org/presenter.jhtml?identifier=4741

22. Robinson, K., et al. "Hyperhomocysteinemia and low pyridoxal phosphate. Common and independent reversible risk factors for coronary artery disease." *Circulation*. 92(10);2825-2830, Nov. 15, 1995.

23. Verhoef, P, Stampfer, M.J., et al. "Homocysteine metabolism and risk of myocardial infarction: relation with vitamins B6, B12, and folate." *American Journal of Epidemiology*. 143(9): 845-859, May 1, 1996.

24. Zeng, X., et al. "Homocysteine mediated expression and secretion of monocyte chemoattractant protein-1 and interleukin-8 in human monocytes." *Circulation Research*, 93(4): 311-320, Aug. 22, 2003.

25. Ridker, P.M. "Comparison of C-reactive protein and low-density lipoprotein cholesterol levels in the prediction of first cardiovascular events." *New England Journal of Medicine*. Vol. 347(20): 1557-1565, Nov. 14, 2002.

26. Vivekananthan, D., et al. *Journal of the American College of Cardiology*, (42): 831-841, Sept. 3, 2003.

27. www.clevelandclinic.org/heartcenter/pub/history/future/mri.asp; http://new.reillycom.com/diagnostic/article_print.php?ID=86.

28. King, S.B., et al. "A ramdomized trial comparing coronary angioplasty with coronary bypass surgery." *New England Journal of Medicine*, 331:1044-1045, 1994; and Yusif, S., et al. "Effect of coronary artery bypass surgery on survival: an overview of 10-year results from randomized trials by the coronary artery bypass surgery trialists collaboration." *Lancet*. 344:563-570, 1994.

29. Braunwald, E. "Coronary-artery surgery at the crossroads" (editorial). *New England Journal of Medicine*. 297(12): 661-663, 1977.

30. Selnes, O.A., et al. "Coronary artery bypass surgery and the brain." *New England Journal of Medicine*. 44(6): 451-452, Feb. 8, 2001.

31. Newman, F.M., et al. "Longitudinal assessment of neurocognitive function after coronary-artery bypass surgery." *New England Journal of Medicine*. 344(6): 395-402, Feb. 8, 2001.

32. Van Vlaanderen, E. "A new view on heart disease." *Cortland Forum*, pp. 150-156, Mar. 2000.

33. "CASS Principal Investigators and Their Associates: Myocardial infarction and mortality in the coronary artery surgery study (CASS) randomized trial." *New England Journal of Medicine*. 310:750-758, 1984; and Alderman, E.L., et al. "Ten-year follow-up of survival and myocardial infarction in the randomized coronary artery surgery study (CASS)." *Circulation*, 82:1629-1646, 1990.

34. Hueb, W. "Two-to eight-year survival rates in patients who refused coronary artery bypass grafting." *American Journal of Cardiology*. 63:155-159, 1989.

35. Coronary Artery Surgery Study; as in Note 33.

36. Ibid.

37. Ibid.

38. Faloon, W. Startling New Findings about Homocysteine. *Life Extension*, pp. 11-16, Nov. 2003.

39. Majeed, M., et al. *Turmerc and the Healing Curcuminoids*. Keats Publishing: New Caanan, CT, 1996.

40. de Lorgeril M., et al. "Mediterranean alpha-linolenic acid-rich diet in secondary prevention of coronary heart disease." *Lancet*. 143:1454–1459, 1994.

41. Leaf, Alexander. "Dietary prevention of Coronary Heart Disease." *Circulation*. 99:733-735, 1999.

42. Enig, Mary. "Trans fatty acids: An update." *Nutrition Quarterly*. 17(4): 79-95, 1993.

43. Abramson, J., et al. "Are lipid-lowering guidelines evidence-based?" *Lancet*, 369:168-169, 2007.

44. *Journal of the Association of Physicians of India*, 42(2):287-9, 1994.

45. *International Journal of Cardiology*, 49(3):191-9, 1995.

46. Ibid.

47. *Indian HJ of Physiological Pharmacology*, 42(1): 101-6, 1998.

48. *Journal of the Association of Physicians of India*, 49:231-5, 2001.

49. *International Journal of Cardiology*, 67(2):199-24, 1998.

50. *Indian Journal of Experimental Biology*, 35(5):478-82, 1997.

51. *Journal of Ethnopharmacology*, 62(2):173-82, 1998.

52. www.melhorn.de/Strophhormon2/

53. Ibid.

54. www.wrf.org/news/news0016.htm

55. Ibid.

56. Ibid.

57. Ibid.

58. *Cayenne* (Newsletter), Volume 1, Number 12, Date unknown; http://www.healthfree.com/dr_jon_christopher_cayenne.html#1

59. Jones, K., et al. "Peripheral nociception associated with surgical incision elicits remote nonischemic cardioprotection via neurogenic activation of protein kinase C signaling." *Circulation*, 120:S1-S9, 2009; www.sciencedaily.com/releases/2009/09/090914173010.htm

60. www.healthyhotline.com/natto.html

61. Ibid.

62. Sumi, H. Healthy Microbe "Bacillus natto." Japan Biological Sciences Laboratory Co. Ltd.

63. Fujita, M., et al. *Biology Pharmacy Bulletin*, 18(10):1387-91, 1995.

64. www.healthyhotline.com/natto.html

65. Sumi, H., et al. "Enhancement of the fibrinolytic activity in plasma by oral administration of nattokinase." *Acta Haematol.* 84(3):139-143, 1990.

66. Maruyama, M., and Sumi, H. "Effect of natto diet on blood pressure." *JTTAS*, 1995.

67. Suzuki, Y., et al. "Dietary supplementation with fermented soybeans suppresses intimal thickening." *Nutrition*, 19(3):261-264, 2003.

68. www.allergyresearchgroup.com/news/letters/ARGFocusAug02.pdf

69. *Journal of Vascular Investigation*, 4:129-136, 1998.

70. www.drlam.com/A3R_brief_in_doc_format/chelation.cfm#top

71. Cranton, Elmer, M..D., *Bypassing Bypass: The New Technique of Chelation Therapy*. 2nd Edition, Hampton Roads Publishing Co. 1997.

72. Klimoz, A.N., et al "Essential phospholipids vs. nicotinic acid in the treatment of patients with Type IIIb hyperlipoproteinemia and ischemic heat disease." *Cardiovascular Drugs & Therapy.* 9:779-784, 1995.

73. Rath, M., et al. "Nutritional supplement program halts progression of early coronary atherosclerosis documented by ultrafast computed tomography." *Journal of Applied Nutrition*, 48:68-78, 1996.

74. Aviram, M., et al. "Pomegranate juice consumption for 3 years by patients with carotid artery stenosis reduces common carotid intima-media thickness, blood pressure and LDL oxidation." *Clinical Nutrition*, 23(3):423-433, June 2004.

75. Cloarec, M., et al. "GliDODin, a vegetal sod with gliadin, as preventative agent vs. atherosclerosis, as confirmed with carotid ultrasound-B imaging." *Allergy & Immunology*, 39(2):45-50, February 2007.

76. Hermann, F., et al. "Dark chocolate improves endothelial and platelet function." *Heart*, 92(1):119-120, January 2006.

77. *Chinese Traditional and Herbal Drugs*, pp. 251, 268.

78. Bliznakov, E., et al. *The Miracle Nutrient Coenzyme Q10*. Bantam Books: New York, NY, 1986.

79. Ibid.

80. Ibid.

81. Ibid.

82. www.eecp.com

83. Ibid.

84. Vaccarino V., et al. "Pulse pressure and risk for myocardial infarction and heart failure in the elderly." *Journal of the American College of Cardiology*, 36: 130-8, 2000.

85. Franklin, S.S., et al. "Does the relation of blood pressure to coronary heart disease risk change with aging? The Framingham Heart Study." *Circulation*, 103(9):1245-1249, March 2001.

86. Beltrami, A.P., et al. "Evidence that human cardiac myocytes divide after myocardial infarction." *New England Journal of Medicine*, No. 23, Vol. 344:1750-1757, June 7, 2001.

87. www.nhlbi.nih.gov/new/press/01-06-06.htm

88. Ibid.

89. Ibid.

90. Ibid.

91. Orlic, D., et al. "Bone marrow cells regenerate infarcted myocardium." *Nature*, 410:701-705, 2001.

92. Ibid.

93. Wyatt, D.A., et al. "Purine-enhanced asanguineous cardioplegia retards adenosine triphosphate degradation during ischemia and improves post ischemic ventricular function." *Journal of Thoracic and Cardiovascular Surgery*, 97(5):771-778, May 1989.

94. Hegewald, M.G., et al. "Ribose infusion accelerates thallium redistribution with early imaging compared with late 24-hour imaging without ribose." *Journal of the American College of Cardiology*, 18(7):1671-1681, December 1991.

95. www.bioenergy.com/Ribose_Heart_Health.html

96. "Hard Work Pays Off: Stroke Expert Says Intense Therapy Can Help Stroke Patients Regain Function in Their Arms." Commentary by Dr. Edward Taub. Special to ABCNEWS.com; http://abcnews.go.com/sections/living/DailyNews/stroke_constraint_therapy_TAUB020222.html; also Liepert, J., et al. "Treatment-induced cortical reorganization after stroke in humans." *Stroke.* 31:1212-1216, 2000.

97. Ibid.

98. Nudo, R.J., et al. "Use-dependent alterations of movement representations in primary motor cortex of adult squirrel monkeys." *Journal of Neuroscience.* 16:785-807, 1996.

99. Ellis-Behnke, R., et al. "Nano neuro knitting: Peptide nanofiber scaffold for brain repair and axon regeneration with functional return of vision." *Proceedings of the National Academy of Sciences*, Vol. 103, No. 13, 5054-5059, March 28, 2006.

100. "Nanotech helps blind hamsters see." BBC News, March 14, 2006; http://news.bbc.co.uk/2/hi/science/nature/4801728.stm.

101. Ellis-Behnke, R., et al. "Nano hemostat solution: Immediate hemostasis at the nanoscale." *Nanomedicine: Nanotechnology, Biology, and Medicine*, 2(2006), 207-215,

August, 2006; http://www.hku.hk/fmri/index/journals/So_Nanomedicine_2006.pdf

102. Sarkamo T., et al. "Music listening enhances cognitive recovery and mood after middle cerebral artery stroke." *Brain*, 131:866-876, 2008.

103. www.newscientist.com/article.ns?id=dn3619; *Science News*, Vol. 172, No. 2, July 14, 2007; *Stroke*, doi: 10.1161/01.STR.0000068170.80517.B3.

104. Ibid.

105. Feldman, H.A., et al. "Impotence and its medical and psychosocial correlates: results of the Massachusetts Male Aging Study." *Journal of Urology*, 151(1):54-61, January 1994.

106. Montorsi, P., et al. "Association between erectile dysfunction and coronary artery disease. Role of coronary clinical presentation and extent of coronary vessel involvement: the COBRA trial." *European Heart Journal*, 27(2):2632-2639, November 2006.

107. Stanislovov, R. "Treatment of erectile dysfunction with pycnogenol and L-argenine.: *Sex Marital Therapy*, 29(3):207-213, May-June 2003.

108. De Andrade, E., et al. "Study of the efficacy of Korean red ginseng in the treatment of erectile dysfunction." *Asian Journal of Andrology*, 9(2):241-244, 2007.

109. Jain, P., et al. "Testosterone supplementation for erectile dysfunction: results of a meta-analysis." *Journal of Urology*, 164(2):371-375, August 2000.

110. Feldman, as in Note 105.

111. Reiter, W.J., et al. "Dehydroepiandrosterone in the treatment of erectile dysfunction: a prospective, double-blind, randomized, placebo-controlled study." *Urology*, 53(3):590-594, March 1999.

112. Cavallini, G., et al. "Carnitine versus androgen administration in the treatment of sexual dysfunction, depressed mood, and fatigue associated with male aging." *Urology*, 63(4):641-646, April 2004.

113. Ang, H.H., et. al. "Evaluation of the potency activity of aphrodisiac in *Eurycoma longifolia Jack*." *Phytotherapy Research*, 15: 435-436, 2001; and Ang, H.H., et al. "Sexual pleasure enhancement of *Eurycoma longifolia* Jack—A comparison study." The Proceedings of the Seminar on Medicinal and Aromatic Plants, pp: 96, 2002.

Cataracts

1. www.nei.nih.gov/health/cataract_facts.htm

2. www.bionational.com/cataract.html

3. Zhoo, C., et al. "Prevention of acetaminophen-induced cataract by a combination of diallyl disulfide and N-acetylcysteine." *Journal of Ocular Pharmacology and Therapy*. 14(4):345-355, Aug. 1998.

4. www.allaboutvision.com

5. Babizhayev, M.A., et al. "Efficacy of N-Acetylcarnosine in the treatment of cataracts." *Drugs R&D*, 3(2):87-103, 2002; Babizhayev, M.A., et al. "N-Acetylcarnosine, a natural histidine-containing di-peptide, as a potent ophthalmic drug treatment for human cataracts." *Peptides* (USA), 22(6):979-994, 2001.

6. Ibid.

7. www.visionworks.com

Chronic Fatigue and Fibromyalgia

1. *Merriam Webster's Medical Dictionary*, Merriam Webster, Inc.: Springfield, Ma, 1995, p. 117.

2. Ibid., p. 236.

3. Berg, et al. *Blood Coagulation and Fibrinolysis*, 10:435-438, 1999.

4. Ibid.

5. Ibid.

6. Ibid.

7. Ibid.

8. www.hemex.com/cfs/lab_guide.html; http://www.springboard4health.com/notebook/health_hypercoagulation_ill.html

9. http://news.bbc.co.uk/1/hi/health/1014089.stm

10. *Journal of Pharmacology Science*, 51: 592-593, 1962.

11. *American Journal of Medical Science*, 243: 758-769, 1962.

12. Ibid; and *Clinical Medicine*, pp. 85-90, Jan. 1964.

13. Breggin, Peter, M.D., et al. *Talking Back to Prozac: What Doctors Aren't Telling You about Today's Most Controversial Drug*. St. Martin's Press, 1995.

14. Puttini, P.S., et al. "Primary fibromyalgia syndrome and 5-hydroxy-l-tryptophan." *Journal of Internal Medicine Research*, 20:182-9, 1992.

15. Jacobsen, S., et al. "Oral S-adenosylmethionine in primary fibromyalgia. Double-blind clinical evaluation." *Scandinavian Journal of Rheumatology*, 20: 294-302, 1991.

16. Bennett, R.M., et al. "A randomized, double-blind placebo-controlled study of growth hormone in the treatment of fibromyalgia." *American Journal of Medicine*. 104(3): 227-31, Mar 1998. St. Amand, R.P., *What Your Doctor May Not Tell You About Fibromyalgia*, New York: Warner, 1999.

17. St. Amand, R.P., *What Your Doctor May Not Tell You About Fibromialgia*. Warner Books, 2003.

18. Teitelbaum, J.E., et al. "The use of D-ribose in chronic fatigue syndrome and fibromyalgia: A pilot study." *Journal of Alternative and Complementary Medicine*, Vol. 12, No. 9, pp. 857-862, 2006.

Cirrhosis of the Liver

1. Lieber, C.S. "Relationships between nutrition, alcohol use, and liver disease." *Alcohol Research & Health*. 27:220-231, 2003.

2. Turecky, L., et al. "Plasma lipid parameters in patients with alcoholic fatty livers after treatment with essential phospholipids." *Bratisl Lek Listy*, 104:227-231, 2003.

Colds and Flu

1. "Avian Flu Hysteria Is for the Birds Says Hudson Expert." November 17, 2005. Press Release: U.S. Newswire. releases.usnewswire.com/printing.asp?id=56915.

2. "An Epidemic of Overreaction." Siegel, Mark, M.D. Los Angeles Times (online), Oct. 11, 2005.

3. "Experts Dismiss Scare Over Bird Flu." Chun, Diane,

Gainesville Sun (online), Nov. 1, 2005; www.gainesville.com/apps/pbcs.dll/article?AID=/20051101/LOCAL/51101021/1078/news

4. Madjid, M. "Influenza as a bioweapon." *Journal of the Royal Society of Medicine*, 97(7):345-6, July 2003.

5. "Vaccine Revenues Expected to Reach $10 billion by 2006." Yahoo News, Jan. 7, 2003.

6. Jefferson, T., et al. "Efficacy and effectiveness of influenza vaccines in elderly people: a systematic review." *Lancet*, 366(9492):1165-1174, October 2005.

7. Yahoo News, January 7, 2003, as in Note 5.

8. FluMist package insert.

9. Ibid.

10. www.healthfreedomusa.org/index.php?page_id=279.

11. Bright, R.A., et al. "Incidence of adamantine resistance among influenza A (H3N2) viruses isolated worldwide from 1994-2005: a cause for concern." *Lancet*, 366(9492):1175-1181, October 2005.

12. Ibid.

13. www.fda.gov/cder/consumerinfo/druginfo/tamiflu.htm

14. Ibid.

15. www.tamiflu.com/sideeffects.aspx

16. www.fda.gov/cder/news/relenza/default/htm

17. *Infectious Diseases*, Prague, Abstract #1271392, April 26-30, 1994.

18. Ferley, J.P., et al. "A controlled evaluation of a homeopathic preparation in the treatment of influenza-like syndromes." *British Journal of Clinical Pharmacology*, 27(3): 329-335, 1989.

19. Papp, R., et al. "Oscillococcinum in patients with influenza-like syndromes." *British Homeopathic Journal*, 87:69-76, 1989.

20. www.babyboomers-seniors.com/dec01/immune.html

21. Cannell, J.J., et al. "Epidemic influenza and Vitamin D." *Epidemiology and Infection*, 134:1129-1140, 2006.

22. Ibid.

23. Ibid; www.lef.org/magazine/mag2007/sep2007_report_vitamind_01.htm; www.vitamindcouncil.org.

24. Cannell, J.J., as in Note 23.

25. Ibid.

26. Chan, M.C.W., et. al. "Proinflammatory cytokine responses induced by influenza A (H5N1) viruses in primary human alveolar and bronchial epithelial cells." *Respiratory Research* (online), 6:135, November 11, 2005.

27. www.allisure.com/AllisureSMPC.pdf.

28. Vetvicka, Vaclav, et. al. "An evaluation of the immunological activities of commercially available B1,3-glucans." *Journal of the American Nutraceutical Association*. Vol. 10, No. 1, 2007.

Diabetes

1. Rosen, O.M. "After Insulin Binds." *Science*. 273:1452-1457, 1987.

2. www.diabetes.org

3. Ibid.

4. Reuters Health. "a third of Americans Have Pre-diabetes Syndrome." Aug. 27, 2002.

5. Ibid.

6. Ibid.

7. Borch-Johnson, K., et al., "Relation between breastfeeding and incidence of insulin-dependent diabetes mellitus." *Lancet*, 2:1083-86, 1984; and Gerstein, H.C. "Cow's milk exposure and type I diabetes mellitus. A critical overview of the clinical literature." *Diabetes Care*, 17(1):13-19, 1994.

8. Classen, J.B., et al. "Association between Type I diabetes and Hib vaccine." *British Journal of Medicine*. 319: 1133, 1999.

9. Menkes, J.H., et al. "Workshop on complications of pertussis and pertussis vaccination." *Neuropediatrics*, 21(4): 171-176, 1990; and Murphy, T.V., et al. "Intussusception among infants given an oral rotavirus vaccine." *New England Journal of Medicine*. 344(8):564-572, 2001.

10. Wautier, J.L. "Advanced glycation end products, their receptors and diabetic angiography." *Diabetes Metabolism*, 27(5): 536-42, 2001.

11. Stadtman, E.R. "Protein oxidation and aging." *Science*. 257(5074):1220-1224, August 28, 1992; Stadtman, E.R., et al. "Protein oxidation." *Annals of the New York Academy of Science*, 899:191-208, 2000; and Berlett, B.S., et al. "Protein oxidation in aging, disease, and oxidative stress." *Journal of Biological Chemistry*, 272(33):20313-20316, August 15, 1997.

12. www.diabetes.org

13. Bjornholt, J.V., et al. "Fasting blood glucose: an underestimated risk factor for cardiovascular death." *Diabetes Care*, 22(1):45-49, 1999.

14. www.quickmedical.com

15. Malhotra, A.K. "Effect of Diabecon in diabetic patients with microalbuminuria." *The Indian Practitioner*, 52(9):595-597, 1999; also Whitaker, Julian. *Dr. Whitaker's Guide to Natural Healing*. Prima Publishing: Rocklin, CA, p. 225.

16. www.rezulin-lawsuit-news.com

17. http://insider.ucsf.edu/2003/aug/index.shtml

18. Winkler, G., et al. "Effectiveness of different benfotiamine dosage regimens in the treatment of painful diabetic neuropathy." Arzneimittelforschung, 49(3): 220-224, March 1999; and Stracke, H., et al. "A benfotiamine-vitamin B combination in treatment of diabetic polyneuropathy." *Experimental Clinical Endocrinology & Diabetes*, 104(4): 311-6, 1996.

19. Brownlee, M. "Benfotiamine blocks three major pathways of hyperglycemic damage and prevents experimental diabetic retinopathy." *Natural Medicine*, 9(3): 294-99, 2003.

20. Brownson C, et al. "Carnosine reacts with a glycated protein." *Free Radicals in Biology & Medicine*, 15;28(10):1564-70, May 2000; and Hipkiss AR, et al. "A possible new role for the anti-ageing peptide carnosine." *Cellular and Molecular Life Sciences*, 57(5):747-53, May 2000.

21. Hipkiss, A.R., et al. "Pluripotent effects of carnosine,

a naturally-occurring dipeptide." *Annals of the New York Academy of Sciences*, 854:37-53, November 20, 1998.

22. Nguyen, Q.D., et al. "Supplemental oxygen improves diabetic macular edema: a pilot study." *Investigative Ophthalmology & Visual Science*, (45)2:617-24, Feb. 2004.

23. Knowler, W.C., et al. "Reduction in the incidence of type 2 diabetes with lifestyle intervention or metformin." *New England Journal of Medicine*, 346:393-403, 2002; and www.diabetes.org.

24. Jensen, Bernard. *Empty Harvest: Understanding the Link Between Our Food, Our Immunity and Our Planet.* Avery Publishing Group Inc., 1990, p. 45.

25. Wiley, H.W. *The History of a Crime Against the Food Law: The Amazing Story of the National Food and Drug Law Intended to Protect the Health of the People, Perverted to Protect Adulteration of Foods and Drugs,*1929.

26. Toeller, M., et al. "Protein intake and urinary albumin excretion rates in the EURODIAB IDDM complications study." *Diabetologia.* 40-10:219-1226, Oct. 1997.

27. Berry, E.M. "Dietary fatty acids in the management of diabetes millitus." *American Journal of Clinical Nutrition.* 66 Supplement 4:S991-997, Oct. 1997.

28. Anderson, R., et al. "Elevated intake of supplemental chromium improves glucose and insulin variables in individuals with Type II diabetes." *Diabetes.* 46:1786-1791, 1997.

29. Cheng, N., et al. "Follow-up survey of people in China with Type II diabetes mellitus consuming supplemental chromium." *Journal of Trace Elements in Experimental Medicine.* 12:55-60, 1999.

30. Anderson, R. "Chromium, glucose intolerance and diabetes." *Journal of the American College of Nutrition."* 17(6):548-555, 1998.

31. Bailey, C.J., et al. "Cerasee, a traditional treatment for diabetes. Studies in normal and streptozotocin diabetic mice." *Diabetes Research*, 2:81-84, 1985.

32. Rao, B.K. "Antidiabetic and hypolipidemic effects of Momordica cymbalari Hook. Fruit powder in alloxan-diabetic rats." *Journal of Ethnopharmacology*, 67:103-109, 1999.

33. Safdar, M., et al. "Effects of various doses of cinnamon on blood glucose in diabetic individuals." *Pakistan Journal of Nutrition*, 3(5):268-272, 2004; and Khan, A., et al. "Cinnamon improves glucose and lipids of people with type 2 diabetes." *Diabetes Care*, 26(12):3215-8, Dec 2003.

34. Shanmugasundaram, E.R.B., et al. "Possible regeneration of the islets of langerhans in streptozotocin-diabetic rats given *gymnema sylvestre* leaf extracts." *Journal of Ethnopharmacology*, 30(3):265-279, 1990; and Shanmugasundaram, E.R.B., et al. "Use of *Gymnema sylvestre* leaf extract in the control of blood glucose in insulin-dependent diabetes mellitus." *Journal of Ethnopharmacology*, 30(3):281-294, 1990.

35. Baskaran, K., et al. "Antidiabetic effect of a leaf extract from Gynema sylvestre in non-insulin-dependent diabetes mellitus patients." *Journal of Ethnopharmacology*, 30:295-

305, 1990.

36. Amiel, S.A. "Intensified insulin therapy." *Diabetes Metabolism Review.* 9:3-24, 1993.

37. Lazarow, A. , et al "Protection against diabetes with nicotinamide." *J Lab Clin Med* 36:249–258, 1950

38. Andersen, H.U., et al. "Nicotinamide prevents interleukin-1 effects on accumulated insulin release and nitric oxide production in rat islets of Langerhans." *Diabetes.* 43:770–777, 1994.

39. Pocoit, F., et al. "Nicotinamide—Biological actions and therapeutic potential in diabetes prevention." *Diabetologia*, 36:574-576, 1993; and Cleary, J.P. "Vitamin B3 in the treatment of diabetes mellitus: Case reports and review of the literature." *Journal of Nutritional Medicine.* 1:217-225, 1990; *Lancet*, 1(8533):619-620, 1987.

40. Bingley, P.J., et al. "Nicotinamide and insulin secretion in normal subjects." *Diabetologia* 36:675–677, 1993.

41. Belury, M.A., et al. "The conjugated linoleic acid (CLA) isomer, t10c12-CLA, is inversely associated with changes in body weight and serum leptin in subjects with Type 2 diabetes mellitus." *Journal of Nutrition*, 133: 257S-260S, 2003.

42. Collene A.L., et al. "The effects of a nutritional supplement containing *Salacia oblonga* extract and insulinogenic amino acids on postprandial glycemia, insulinemia, and breath hydrogen responses in healthy adults." *Nutrition*, 21: 848-54, 2005.

43. Baur J.A., et al. "Resveratrol improves health and survival of mice on a high-calorie diet." *Nature.* 16;444(7117):337-42, November 2006.

44. Ibid.

45. Dind, E., et al. "Sex differences of exogenous sex hormones and risk of type II diabetes." *Journal of the American Medical Association*, 295(11):1288-1299, March 15, 2006.

46. Kapoor, D., et al. "Testosterone therapy improves insulin resistance, glycemic control, visceral adiposity and hycholesterolaemia in hypogonadal men with type 2 diabetes." *European Journal of Endocrinology*, 154(6):899-906, June 2006.

47. Razavi, R., et al. "TRPV1+ sensory neurons control beta cell stress and islet inflammation in auto-immune diabetes." *Cell*, 127: 1123-1135, 2006.

48. www.naturalnews.com/021345/html

49. www.celltran.co.uk

50. Dawson, J.B. "Massage for Leg Ulcers." *American Family Physicain*, 57(11):2628-2629, 1998.

Emphysema

1. Hind, M., and Maden, M., "Retinoic acid induces alveolar regeneration in the adult mouse lung." *European Respiratory Journal*, Vol. 23, Issue 1, pp. 20-27, 2004.

2. Lamson, D.W., et al. "The use of nebulized glutathione in the treatment of emphysema: a case report." *Alternative Medicine Review*, Vol. 5 No. 5, pp. 429-431. 2000.

3. Ibid, p. 430.

Gallbladder

1. Breneman, J.C. "Allergy elimination diet as the most effective gallbladder diet." *Ann All.* 26:83-87, 1968.
2. Ibid.
3. Nassauto, G., et al. "Effect of silibinin on biliary lipid composition: Experimental and clinical study." *Journal of Hepatology.* 12:290-295, 1991.

Glaucoma

1. www.nei.nih.gov/health/glaucoma/glaucoma_facts.htm
2. Vision Disorders. *Townsend Letter for Doctors and Patients*, #231, Oct. 2002, p. 54. Excerpted from Goldberg, B. *Alternative Medicine: The Definitive Guide*, 2nd Edition, 2002.
3. Ibid, p. 56.
4. Collin, J. Letter from the Publisher, *Townsend Letter for Doctors and Patients*, #231, Oct. 2002, p. 16.
5. www.nei.nih.gov/health/glaucoma/glaucoma_facts.htm
6. Vision Disorders, as in Note 2, p. 56.
7. Eye M.D.S. Discuss New Possibilities for the Prevention and Treatment of Blindness. *Townsend Letter for Doctors and Patients*, #231, p. 20, Oct. 2002.
8. Vino, M., et al. "Oral treatment of glaucoma with vitamin C." *Eye, Ear, Nose, Throat Monthly*, 46:1502-1508, 1967.
9. Vision Disorders, as in Note 2, p. 55.
10. Ibid.
11. Ibid, p. 20.

Gulf War Syndrome

1. Morahan, L. Vets Group Wants Rumsfeld Out Over Alleged Shipment to Iraq. CBSNews.com, Oct. 8, 2002, www.cnsnews.com/ViewPentagon.asp?Page=%5CPentagon%5Carchive%5C200210%5CPEN0021008a.html
2. *Blood Coagulation & Fibrinolysis*, 11:673-678, 2000.
3. Nicolson, G.L. and Nicolson, N.L., "Summary of Persian Gulf War Illness Pilot Study On Mycoplasmal Infections In Veterans and Family Members," 1997.

Hair Loss

1. Physician's Desk Reference (PDR), Thompson Healthcare, 2004.
2. Tobin, D.J., et al. "Antibodies to hair follicles in alopecia areata." *Journal of Investigative Dermatology.* 102(5):721-724, May 1994.
3. Ibid.
4. www.curetage.com
5. www.medicinenet.com/minoxidil/article.htm
6. www.nlm.nih.gov/medlineplus/druginfo/uspdi/202649.html#SXX16
7. Walker, M. *Bald No More*, Kensington Books: New York, NY, 1998, pp. 155-165.
8. Ibid, p. 163.
9. Ibid, pp. 112-113

10. Maddin, W.S., et al. "The biological effects of a pulsed electrostatic field with specific reference to hair." *International Journal of Dermatology*, Vol. 29, No. 6, July-August, 1990.
11. Ito, M., et al. "Wnt-dependent de novo hair follicle regeneration in adult mouse skin after wounding." *Nature*, 447: 316-321, 2007.

Hepatitis

1. www.pegasys.com
2. Ibid.
3. http://hepatitis-central.com
4. Ibid.
5. www.pegasys.com
6. www.nlm.nih.gov/medlineplus/druginfo/uspdi/202509.html#Brands; www.pegasys.com
7. Cathcart, R.F. "The method of determining proper doses of vitamin C for the treatment of disease by titrating to bowel tolerance." *Journal of Orthomolecular Psychiatry.* 10:125-132, 1981.
8. Ibid.
9. Ibid.
10. Murata, A. "Viricidal activity of vitamin C: Vitamin C for prevention and treatment of viral diseases." First Intersectional Congress International Association Microbiology Society. Vol. 3, Hasagawa, T. U Press: Tokyo, pp. 432-442, 1975.
11. Burgsteiner, C. "Cure for hepatitis? 'Physician, heal thyself,' and he did." *Journal of the Medical Association of Georgia.* 80:21-22, 1991.
12. Pizzorno, J., and Murray, M. *A Textbook of Natural Medicine*, Vol II. John Bastyr College Publications: Seattle, WA, 1988.
13. Ibid.
14. Murray, M. *The Healing Power of Herbs.* 2nd Edition, Prima Publishing, 1995.
15. Mascarella, S., et al. "Therapeutic and antolipoperoxidant effects of silybin-phosphatidylcholine complex in chronic liver disease: Preliminary results." *Current Therapeutic Research*, 53(1):98-102, 1993.
16. Cabot, S., *The Liver Cleansing Diet*, 1998.
17. Monograph: Glutathione, Reduced (GSH), *Alternative Medicine Review*, Vol. 6, No. 6, p. 603, 2001.

Herpes

1. www.valtrex.com/about-herpes/genital-herpes.htm
2. Reyes, M., et al. "Acyclovir-resistant genital herpes among persons attending sexually transmitted disease and human immunodeficiency virus clinics." *Archives of Internal Medicine*, 163(1):76-80, Jan. 2003.
3. U.S. Patent 501, 732. www.uspto.gov
4. U.S. Patent 592,735. www.uspto.gov
5. U.S. Patent 824,320. www.uspto.gov
6. U.S. Patent 1, 044,201. www.uspto.gov
7. U.S. Patent 3,368,155. www.uspto.gov
8. U.S. Patent 3,467,076. www.uspto.gov
9. U.S. Patent 4,323,056. www.uspto.gov

10. U.S. Patent 4,665,898. www.uspto.gov
11. U.S. Patent 4,616,640. www.uspto.gov
12. U.S. Patent 4,932,421. www.uspto.gov
13. U.S. Patent 5,188,738. www.uspto.gov
14. *Science News*, Vol. 139, March 30, 1991.
15. McAuliffe, Sharon. "Electrocuting the AIDS Virus: A Safer-Yet Blood Supply." *Longevity*, Dec. 1992.
16. Douglass, W.C., *Hydrogen Peroxide—Medical Miracle*. Second Opinion Publishing, 1996.
17. Walker, Morton. *DMSO: Nature's Healer*. Avery Publishing Group: Garden City Park, NY, p. 59.
18. Ibid., p. 215.
19. Rath, Matthias. *Cancer*. MR Publishing, Inc.: Santa Clara, CA, 2001, p. 14-15.
20. Ibid.
21. Weissman, G. And Claiborne, R. *Cell Membranes: Biochemistry, Cell Biology and Pathology*. Harper Publishing Company, 1979.
22. Ibid.
23. Rath, p. 38-62.
24. Kagan, C. "Lysine therapy for herpes simplex." *Lancet*. 1(37): 1974.
25. Yacenda, J. *The Herpes Diet*. Pamphlet. Felmore, Ltd., Tunbridge Wells.
26. Rath, p. 62.
27. Rath, Matthias. *The Heart*. MR Publishing, Inc.: Santa Clara, CA, 2001, p. 153.
28. Rath, *Cancer*, p. 62.
29. Ibid., p. 63.
30. Ibid., p. 68.
31. Ibid., pp. 40-41.
32. Ibid., p. 62.
33. Ibid., p. 38.
34. Ibid.
35. www.coldsore-inhibitor.com
36. Ibid.
37. Ibid.
38. http://iptq.com/mh02.htm

Hot Flashes

1. Trace Minerals in the Environment, The National Institute of Environmental Health Sciences, Department of Health, Education and Welfare, Volume 5: Indium, pp. 9, 537.
2. U.S. Patent 6,007,847 to George A.H. Bonadio, 1997.
3. www.vital-nutrients.com/indium.htm
4. Ibid.
5. Schroeder, H., et al. "Interactions of Trace Metals in Mouse and Rat Tissues; Zinc, Chromium, Copper and Manganese With 13 Other Elements." *Journal of Nutrition*; and Schroeder, et al. *Journal of Nutrition*, Vol. 101: 1431-1438, 1971.
6. Barnes, B.O. *Hypothyroidism: The Unsuspected Illness*. Lawrence Galton, 1976.
7. Kunin, R.A. "Clinical uses of iodide and iodine." *Nutritional Healing*, July 1998.
8. "Isoflavones from Red Clover (Promensil) Significantly Reduce Menopausal Hot Flush Symptoms compared with Placebo," *Maturitas*, 42:187-193, 2002.
9. Ingels, Darin, N.D. "Red Clover Extract Reduces Hot Flashes in Menopausal Women," *Healthnotes Newswire*, Oct. 10, 2002.
10. "Phytoestrogen Supplements for the Treatment of Hot Flashes: The Isoflavone Clover Extract (ICE) Study." *Journal of the American Medical Association*, Vol. 290, pp. 207-214, July 9, 2003.
11. www.newmediaexplorer.org/sepp/2003/07/25/prescribing_a_placebo.htm
12. Ibid.
13. Ibid.

Indigestion

1. Cowan, Tom, M.D., *Wise Traditions in Food, Farming and the Healing Arts* (the quarterly magazine of the Weston A. Price Foundation), Winter 2002.
2. Ibid.
3. Hayakawa, A., Inoue, M., et al, "Clinical Evaluation of Z-103 on gastric ulcer." *Japanese Pharmacology Therapy*, 20(1):1-18, Jan. 1992.
4. Odashima, M., et al. "Induction of a 72-kDa heat-shock protein in cultured rat gastric mucosal cells and rat gastric mucosa by zinc L-carnosine." *Digestive Disorders Science*, 47(12):2799-2804, Dec. 2002.
5. Pereira, R.D. "Regression of gastroesophageal reflux symptoms using dietary supplementation with melatonin, vitamins and amino acids: comparison with omeprazol." *Journal of Pineal Research*, 41(3):195-200, October 2006.
6. Willette, R.C., et al. "Purified d-limonene: an effective agent for the relief of occasional symptoms of heartburn." Unpublished study; as reported in *Life Extension*, "Natural relief from heartburn," September 2006.
7. Ibid.
8. Ibid.

Irritable Bowel Syndrome

1. Irfan, S., et al. "Efficacy of New Diarex in Diarrhea," *The Indian Practitioner*. 54(7):497-499, July 2001.
2. Lakshmi, P., et al. "Clinical Evaluation of New Diarex in acute and chronic diarrhea." *The Antiseptic*, 98(10):371-372, Oct. 2001.
3. Tiwari, S., et al. "Clinical Study on the Trial Drug New Diarex in Cases of Irritable Bowel Syndrome," *Indian Journal of Clinical Practice*, 12(7):53-56, Dec. 2001.
4. Nichols, T.W., et al. "Improvement in mucosal integrity and function in IBD patients and reduction of GI symptoms in HIV patients with dietary peptides from hydrolyzed white fish." *Regulatory Peptides*. 108(1):31, 2002.
5. Walker, A.F. "Artichoke leaf extract reduces symptoms of irritable bowel syndrome in a post-marketing surveillance study." *Phytotherapy Research*, 15(1):58-61, 2001.
6. www.alcat.com/index.html
7. Thompson, W.G. "Probiotics for irritable bowel

syndrome: a light in the darkness." *European Journal of Gastroenterology & Hepatology*, 13(10):1143-1147, 2001.

Kidney Stones

1. Freitas, A. M., et al. "The effect of *Phyllanthus niruri* on urinary inhibitors of calcium oxalate crystallization and other factors associated with renal stone formation." *BJU International*. 89(9): 829–34, 2002; and Calixto, J. B. "Antispasmodic effects of an alkaloid extracted from *Phyllanthus sellowianus*: a comparative study with papaverine." *Braz. J. Med. Biol. Res.* 17(3–4): 313–21, 1984.

Leg Cramps

1. www.drmirkin.com/archives/6752.html
2. Ibid.
3. Man-Son-Hing, M. "Quinine for nocturnal leg cramps: a meta-analysis including unpublished data." *Journal of General Internal Medicine*. 13(9):600-6, Sept. 1998; and Man-Son-Hing, M., "Meta-analysis of efficacy of quinine for treatment of nocturnal leg cramps in elderly people." *British Medical Journal*, 310:6971:13-17, Jan. 1995.
4. Cathcart, R.F. "Vitamin E and Leg Cramps." *Journal of the American Medical Association*, Vol. 219, No. 2, Jan. 10, 1972.

Lyme Disease

1. www.cdc.gov/ncidod/dvbid/lyme/
2. Burgdorfer, W. "How the discovery of *Borrelia burgdorferi* came about." *Clinical Dermatology*, 11(3):335-338, July-Sept. 1993.
3. www.cdc.gov/ncidod/dvbid/lyme/
4. Ibid.
5. Ibid.
6. Medical Diagnostic Laboratories, www.mdlab.com.
7. www.cdc.gov/ncidod/dvbid/lyme/qa.htm
8. Dattwyler, R.J., et al. "Ceftriaxone compared with doxycycline for the treatment of acute disseminated Lyme disease." *New England of Medicine*, 337(5): 289-294, July 31, 1997.
9. www.cdc.gov/ncidod/dvbid/lyme/
10. Mattman, L. *Cell Wall Deficient Forms: Stealth Pathogens*, 3rd Edition, Lewis Publishers, Inc., 2000.
11. Ibid.; and www.bowen.org.
12. Mattman, as in Note 10.
13. Cowden, W.L., et al. Pilot Study of Samento (Pentacyclic Alkaloid-Chemotype of Uncaria tomentosa) for the Treatment of Lyme Disease. Presented at the International Symposium for Natural Treatment of Intracellular Micro Organisms, Munich, Germany, March 29, 2003.
14. Ibid.
15. Central Florida Research, Inc.; http://central floridaresearch.com.
16. www.wildernetwork.org/complexities_of_Lyme.html
17. Cowden, as in Note 13.

Macular Degeneration

1. "Vision Disorders." *Townsend Letter for Doctors &*

Patients. #231, Oct. 2002, p. 55.
2. Thomson, L.R., et al. "Long term dietary supplementation with zeaxanthin reduces photoreceptor death in light-damaged Japanese quail." *Experimental Eye Research*, Vol. 75, Issue 5, pp. 529-542(14), November 2002.
3. www.eri.harvard.edu
4. Ibid.
5. Macular Degeneration Foundation. www.eyesight.org
6. Macular Degeneration: A Leading Cause of Vision Loss. Investigating the Effects of Abnormal Blood Flow, Press Release, University of Pennsylvania Medical Center, May 1998.
7. "Initial results of microcurrent stimulation in the treatment of Age Related Macular Degeneration." Kondrot, E. *Townsend Letter for Doctors & Patients*. #231, Oct. 2002, pp. 65-67.
8. Ibid., p. 95.
9. "A randomized, placebo-controlled, clinical trial of high-dose supplementation with vitamins C and E, beta carotene, and zinc for Age-Related Macular Degeneration and vision loss: AREDS Report No. 8." Age-Related Eye Disease Study Research Group. *Archives of Ophthalmology*, 119:1417-1436, Oct. 2001.
10. Thomson, L.R., as in Note 2.
11. Bone, R.A., et al. "Lutein and zeaxanthin dietary supplements raise macular pigments of these carotenoids in humans." *Journal of Nutrition*, 133(4):992-998, April 2003.

Mad Cow Disease

1. Hadlow, William, DVM. "An Overview of Scrapie in the United States," *Journal of the American Medical Association*. Vol. 196, No. 10, May 15, p. 1676, 1990.
2. Hulse, V., *Mad Cows and Milk Gate*. Marble Mountain Publishing: Phoenix, OR, p. 36, 1996.
3. Fox, N. *Spoiled: The Dangerous Truth About a Food Chain Gone Haywire*, BasicBooks: New York, NY, p. 294, 1997.
4. Mathews, D. "Bovine Spongiform Encephalopathy." *Journal of the Royal Society of Health*. Feb. 1991, pp. 3-5.
5. Brown, P., et al. "Resistance of scrapie infectivity to steam auto-claving after formaldehyde fixation and limited survival after ashing at 360 degrees C: Practical and theoretical implications." *Journal of Infectious Diseases*, 1990, pp. 161, 467-472.
6. Hulse, p. 18.
7. Fox, p. 303. [Fox's source: Zane, Peder, J. "It Ain't for Meat; It's for Lotion," *The New York Times*. May 5, 1996.]
8. Carrel, Chris. "Mad Cows Ate My Brain." *Seattle Weekly*. March 12, 1998, p. 27.
9. Rampton, Sheldon and Stauber, John. *Mad Cow U.S.A.* Common Courage Press: Monroe, ME, 1997.
10. Blakeslee, Sandra. "Disease Fear Prompts New Look at Rendering." *The New York Times*, March 11, 1997.
11. Fox, p. 304.

12. Hulse, p. 21.

13. Deley, Suzanne. "Mad Cow Disease Panicing Europe as Incidents Rise." *The New York Times*, Dec. 1, 2000, p. A1.

14. Hulse, p. 28.

15. Ibid., p. 30.

16. "BSE Experts Give Up Beef," *Agscene*. No. 102, Spring, 1991.

17. Hulse, p. 30.

18. Ibid., p. 134.

19. Hueston, William, et al. "Bovine Spongiform Encepholopathy," *Animal Health Insight*, pp. 1-7, 1992.

20. Fox, p. 295.

21. Hulse, p. 16.

22. Ibid., p. 60.

23. Carrel, p. 27.

24. Hulse, p. 105.

25. Fox, p. 307.

26. *Food Chemical News*, June 3, 1996.

27. Fox, p. 312. [Fox's source: McNair, Joel. "Experts Argue Over BSE Measures," *Agri-views*, Sept. 16, 1993.]

28. Ibid., p. 311.

29. Ibid., p. 312.

30. Marsh, R.F., et al. "Epidemiology and experimental studies on a new incident of transmissible mink encephalopathy," *Journal of General Virology*, pp. 72, 589-594, 1991.

31. Meilke, James. "Millions at Risk from CJD," *The Guardian*, Sat. Jan. 8, 2000.

32. Hulse, p. 26.

33. Ibid., p. 19.

34. http://organicconsumers.org/madcow/Greger122403.cfm

35. Hulse, p. 28.

36. *The Observer*. Oct. 22, 2000; www.newsunlimited.co.uk; [Cited in *Nexus*. "Vaccines Contaminated with Mad Cow Disease?" Jan.-Feb. 2001, p. 9]; www.nexusmagazine.com

37. "Mad Cow Disease and Makeup, New Fears." CBC, Toronto, Tues., Jan. 23, 2001.

38. Mullins, E. *Murder by Injection*, National Council for Medical Research: Staunton, VA, p. 140-142, 1995.

39. *Lancet*. July 7, 1990.

40. Boller, Francis, et al. "Diagnosis of Dementia: Clinicalpathologic Correlations." *Neurology*. 39(1):769, Jan. 1989.

41. Hulse, p. 114; Manuelidis, E. and L. Manuelidis. "Suggested links between different types of dementias: Creutzfeldt-Jakob disease, Alzheimer disease, and retroviral CNS infections." *Alzheimer Disease and Associated Disorders*, pp. 100-109, 1989.

42. Ibid., p. 60; Rampton, Sheldon and Stauber, John. *Mad Cow U.S.A.* Common Courage Press: Monroe, ME, p. 150, 1997; Original source: USDA/APHIS, "Bovine Spongiform Encephalopathy: Rendering Policy," pp. 6-10, 1991.

43. Rampton, pp. 215-218.

44. FDA Center for Veterinary Medicine News Release, January 10, 2001; General Accounting Office, GAO Report to Congressional Requesters. *Mad Cow Disease: Improvements in the Animal Feed Ban and Other Regulatory Areas Would Strengthen U.S. Prevention Efforts*. GAO-02-183, January 2002.

45. Carrel, pp. 30-32; Rampton, Sheldon and Stauber, John. *Mad Cow U.S.A.* Common Courage Press: Monroe, ME, 1997

46. Rampton, p. 217.

47. Stauber, J. (Co-author of *Mad Cow USA*), "It's The Cow Feed, Stupid." www.Common Dreams.org, Jan. 3, 2004.

48. Ibid.

49. Carrel, pp. 30-32.

50. Ridgeway, J. "Slaughterhouse Politics: Ranchers fought rules that might have prevented mad cow." *The Village Voice*, Dec. 31, 2003-Jan. 6, 2004.

51. Ibid.

52. Schlosser, E. (Author of *Fast Food Nation*), "The Cow Jumped Over The USDA." *The New York Times* Op-Ed, Jan. 2, 2004.

53. Ibid.

54. Ibid.

55. Ibid.

56. Ibid.

57. Ibid.

58. Ibid.

59. Prusiner, S., et al. *Proceedings of the National Academy of Sciences*, 99:3812-3817, March 2002.

60. Ibid.

61. Joint WHO/FAO/OIE Technical Consultation on BSE. OIE Headquarters, Paris, France, June 11-14, 2001.

62. European Commission Press Release, ip/00/432. Brussels, Belgium, May 3, 2000.

63. Testimony of Peter Lurie, M.D., M.P.H., Deputy Director of Public Citizen's Health Resource Group, before the Consumer Affairs Foreign Commerce and Tourism Subcommittee. Senate Commerce, Science and Transportation Committee, April 4, 2001, Wash., D.C.

64. Testimony of Caroline Smith DeWaal, Director of Food Safety before the Senate Committee on Commerce, Science and Transportation Hearing on *"Mad Cow Disease: Are Our Precautions Adequate?"* April 4, 2001, Washington, D.C.

65. National Cattleman's Beef Association. Presence of Central Nervous System (CNS) Tissue in Advanced Meat Recovery (AMR) Products, April, 2001.

66. Ibid.

67. USDA. Analysis of 2002 FSIS Bovine AMR. Products Survey Results. Feb. 2003. www.fsis.usda.gov/OA/topics/AMRAnalysis.pdf

68. Sparks Companies. Advanced Meat Recovery Systems—An Economic Analyses of Proposed USDA Regulations, July 1999.

69. Center for the Science in the Public Interest. *Nutrition Health Letter*, June 2001.

70. *Village Voice*, same as Note 50.

71. Ibid.

72. St. Clair, J. *Been Brown So Long It Looked Like Green To Me.*" Common Courage Press, 2003.

73. Ibid.

74. Daly, D.J., et al. "Use of a marker organism to model the spread of central nervous system tissue in cattle and the abattoir environment during commercial stunning and carcass dressing." *Applied and Environmental Microbiology.* 68(2):791-798, Feb. 2002.

75. St. Clair, as per Note 72.

76. Sherman, Mark. U.K. *Lab Confirms Mad Cow Case U.S.,* Yahoo! News, Dec. 25, 2003; *The New York Times,* Dec.25, 2003.

77. Ibid.

78. Mitchell, Steve. *"More Deadly Lies—Did USDA Even Test 20,000 Cattle?" USDA Refuses to Release Mad Cow Test,* United Press International, Dec. 24, 2003.

79. Ibid.

80. Ibid.

81. FDA. "Substances Prohibited from Use in Animal Food or Feed; Animal Proteins Prohibited in Ruminant Feed." Proposed Rule, 21 CFR Part 589, Docket No. 96N-0135, Jan. 3, 1997.

82. Ibid.

83. "BSE may cause more CJD cases than thought." *New Scientist.* Nov. 28, 2002, www. newscientist.com/news/ news.jsp?id=ns99993122.

84. "Sheep consumption: a possible source of spongiform encephalopathy in humans." *Neuroepidemiology,* (4):240-249, 1985.

85. Dawson, M., et al. "Primary parenteral transmission of bovine spongiform encephalopathy to the pig." *Veterinary Record,* 127:338, 1990.

86. *National Hog Farmer,* Feb. 15, 2002.

87. Davanipour, Z., et al. "A case-control study of Creutzfeldt-Jalob disease. Dietary risk factors." *American Journal of Epidemiology,* Vol. 122, No. 3, pp. 443-451, 1985.

88. *Dateline NBC,* March 14, 1997.

89. Creutzfeldt-Jakob disease surveillance in the U.K.: Sixth Annual Report 1997. Edinburgh, Scotland: National CJD Surveillance Unit, 1998.

90. Davanipour, as in Note 87.

91. Same as Note 89.

92. Boller, F., et al. "Creutzfeldt-Jakob disease: A case control study." *American Journal of Epidemiology,* (98):381-384, 1973.

93. *Food Chemical News* pp. 57-59, July 5, 1993.

94. Fischer, M.B. "Binding of disease-associated prion protein to plasminogen." *Nature.* 408:479-483, 2000.

95. http://news.bbc.co.uk/1/hi/health/424000.stm

96. www.gradipore.com

97. Peretz, D., et al. "Antibodies inhibit prion propagation and clear cell cultures of prion infectivity." *Nature.* 412:739-743, 2001.

98. Mallucci, G. "Depleting neuronal PrP in prion infection prevents disease and reverses spongiosis." *Science,* 301:871-874, 2003.

99. Foot, Richard, *Montreal Gazette CanWest News Service,* Sept. 27, 2003.

100. Glatzel, M., et al. "Extraneural pathologic prion protein in sporadic Creutzfeldt-Jakob disease." *New England Journal of Medicine,* 349(19):1812-1820, Nov. 6, 2003.

101. Vince, Gaia. "Volcanic pool enzyme kills prions." *New Scientist.* July 29, 2003. www. newscientist.com/ news/print.jsp?id=ns99993999.

Migraines

1. www.migraines.org.

2. *Townsend Letter for Doctors and Patients,* 202:104-6, 2000.

3. *Der Freie Artz,* 3:44-9, 1996.

4. Same as Note 2.

5. www.onlineallergycenter.com/headaches22/

6. Blum, J.M., et al. "Herbal homeopathic support for the treatment of migraine-type headache symptoms." *Executive Summary.* NatureWell, Inc., LaJolla, CA, Aug. 29, 2001.

7. Gobel, H., et al. "Effects of peppermint and eucalyptus oil on neurophysiological and experimental algesimetric headache parameters." *Cephalgia,* 14(3):228-234, 1994.

8. Plastic Surgery Effective in Eliminating/Decreasing Migraine Headaches. American Society of Plastic Surgeons, Press Release, July 13, 2002.

9. Schoenen, J., et al. "High-dose riboflavin as a prophylactic treatment of migraine: Results of an open pilot study." *Cephalgia,* 14:328-329, l994.

Multiple Sclerosis

1. www.mult-sclerosis.org

2. Ibid.

3. www.ecureme.com/emyhealth/data/Multiple_Sclerosis.asp

4. Riise, T., et al. "Smoking is a risk factor for multiple sclerosis." *Neurology,* 61:1122-1124, 2003.

5. Sandyk, R. "Successful treatments of multiple sclerosis with magnetic fields." *International Journal of Neuroscience.* pp. 237-250, Oct. 1992.

Osteoporosis

1. Kanis, J.A., et al. "The diagnosis of osteoporosis." *Journal of Bone Mineral Research.* 9:1137-1141, 1994.

2. *Hospital Diagnosis and Therapy Audit.* MediMedia USA: Yardley, PA, 1995-2003.

3. http://osteoed.org/faq/male/male_prevalence.html

4. Cluett, J. Hip Fracture: Information about a broken hip. http://orthopedics.about.com/cs/hipsurgery/a/brokenhip.htm

5. Same as Note 3.

6. Same as Note 4.

7. Ibid.

8. Davis, J.W., et al. "Ethnic, anthropometric, and lifestyle associations with regional variations in peak bone

mass." *Calcified Tissue International.* 65(2):100-105, Aug., 1999; also Hu, J.F., et al. "Dietary calcium and bone density among middle-aged and elderly women in China." *American Journal of Clinical Nutrition.* 58(2):219-227, Aug., 1993.

9. Lips, P. "Epidemiology and predictors of fractures associated with osteoporosis." *American Journal of Medicine.* 103(2A):3S-8S; discussion 8S-11S; and Xiaoge, D., et al. "Bone mineral density differences at the femoral neck and Ward's triangle: a comparison study on the reference data between Chinese and Caucasian women." *Calcified Tissue International.* 67(3):195-198, 2000; and Memon, A., et al. "Incidence of hip fracture in Kuwait." *International Journal of Epidemiology.* 5:860-865, 1998.

10. Fujita, T., et al. "Comparison of osteoporosis and calcium intake between Japan and the United States." *Proceedings of Social and Experimental Biology and Medicine,* 200(2):149-152, 1992; and Lau, E.M., et al. "Admission rates for hip fracture in Australia in the last decade." *Medical Journal of Australia,* 158(9):604-606, 1993; and Paspati, I., et al. "Hip fracture epidemiology in Greece during 1977-1992." *Calcified Tissue International,* 62(6):542-547, 1998.

11. Xu, L., et al. "Very low rates of hip fracture in Beijing, People's Republic of China." The Beijing Osteoporosis Project. *American Journal of Epidemiology,* 144(9):901-907, 1996.

12. Fescanich, D., et al. "Milk, dietary calcium, and bone fractures in women: a 12-year prospective study." *American Journal of Public Health.* 87:992-997, 1997.

13. Cumming, R.G., et al. "Case-control study of risk factors for hip fractures in the elderly." *American Journal of Epidemiology.* 139:493-503, 1994.

14. Brown, S.E. *Better Bones, Better Body,* Keats Publishing: New Caanan, CT, 2000.

15. Lorenc, R.S., et al. "Evaluation of bone mass in children in a national sample of the population." *Pol Tyg Lek,* 48 Supplement 3:16-19, Nov. 1992; Ling, X, et al. "Vertebral fractures in Beijing, China: the Beijing osteoporosis project." *Journal of Bone Mineral Research,* 15(10):2019-2025, Oct. 2000; Wang, Q, et al. Bone mineral density in immigrants from southern China to Denmark: a cross-sectional study." *European Journal of Endocrinology,* 134(2):163-167, 1996; Hagaiwara, S., et al. "Quantification of bone mineral content using dual-photon absorptiometry in a normal Japanese population." *Journal of Bone Mineral Research,* 4(2)217-222, April 1989; Dibba, B., et al. "Effect of calcium supplementation on bone mineral accretion in Gambian children accustomed to a low-calcium diet." *American Journal of Clinical Nutrition,* 71(2):544-549, 2000.

16. Jilka, R.L., et al. "Osteoblast programmed cell death (apoptosis): modulation by growth factors and cytokines." *Journal of Bone Mineral Research,* 13(5):793-802, 1998.

17. *Hospital Diagnosis and Therapy Audit,* MediMedia, USA: Yardley, PA, 1995-2003.

18. McClung, M., et al, "Alendronate prevents postmenopausal bone loss in women without osteoporosis." *Annals of Internal Medicine,* 128(4):253-261, Feb. 15, 1998; Hosking, D., et al. "Prevention of bone loss with Alendronate in postmenopausal women under 60 years of age." *New England Journal of Medicine.* 338:485-492, Feb. 19, 1998.

19. "Aldronic acid in primary prevention." *Prescrire Int,* 9(47): 70-72, June 2000.

20. Funayama, H., et al. "Elevation of histidine decarboxylase activity in the mandible of mice." *Archives of Oral Biology,* 45(9):787-795, Sept. 2000.

21. Blank, M.A., et al. "Gastric damage in the rat with nitrogen-containing biophosphates depends on the pH." *Alimentary Pharmacology & Therapeutics.,* Sept. 14, 2000; Lanza, F.L. "Placebo-controlled, randomized, evaluator-blind endoscopy study of risedronate vs aspirin in healthy postmenopausal women." *Alimentary Pharmacology & Therapeutics,* 14(12):1163-1170, Dec. 2000.

22. Larsen, K.O., et al. "Esophageal lesions associated with diphosphonates." *Tidsskr Nor Laegeforen,* Aug 2000; Lucinai, J., et al. "Esophagitis associated with use of aldronate in 5 postmenopausic patients." *Acta Gastroenterol Latinam,* May 2001.

23. Halabe, A., et al. "Liver damage due to alendronate." *New England Journal of Medicine,* 343:365-366, Aug. 3, 2000.

24. "Raloxifene and prevention of vertebral fracture: mainly when estrogen is contraindicated." *Prescrire Int,* 9(50):190-191, Dec. 2000.

25. "Raloxifene: new preparation. Not better than estrogen." *Prescrire Int,* 8(44):165-167, Dec. 1999.

26. Pritchard, K.I., et al. "Raloxifene: handle with care." *Canadian Medical Association Journal,* 165(2):151-153, July 2001.

27. Needle, S.J.M., et al. "Raloxifene affects brain activation patterns in post-menopausal women during visual encoding." *Journal of Clinical Endocrinology and Metabolism,* 86(3):1422, March 2001.

28. Liggett, N.W., et al. "The incidence, epidemiology and aeteology of osteoporosis." *Hospital Pharmacist,* Vol. 7, No. 3, pp. 62-86, March 2000 Special Features.

29. Dawson-Hughes, B., et al. "A controlled trial of the effect of calcium supplementation on bone density in post-menopausal women." *New England Journal of Medicine,* 323:878-883, 1990; Reid, I.R., et al. "Effect of calcium supplementation on bone loss in post-menopausal women." *New England Journal of Medicine,* 328:460-464, 1993.

30. Liggett, N.W., et al. "The incidence, epidemiology and aeteology of osteoporosis." *Hospital Pharmacist,* Vol. 7, No. 3, pp. 62-86, March 2000 Special Features.

31. www.ibiblio.org/pub/academic/medicine/alternative-healthcare/faqs/FAQ:-Vitamin-Supplementation

32. Plotnikoff, G. "Lack of vitamin D linked to pain." *Mayo Clinic Proceedings.* Vol. 78, pp. 1463-1470, December 2003.

33. Vitamin K and Osteoporosis. Presented at The Second

Thorne Holst Symposium in Nutrition, Nov. 14-15, 2002, Grand Hotel, Oslo, Norway.

34. http://news.bbc.co.uk/1/hi/health/912855.stm

35. *Journal of Natural Health.* Vol. 9, No. 1, 2003.

36. Meunier, P.J., et al. "The effects of strontium ranelate on the risks of vertebral fracture in women with postmenopausal osteoporosis." *New England Journal of Medicine*, 350:459-468, Jan. 29, 2004.

37. Elias, A.N., et al. "Immobilization osteoporosis in paraplegia." *Journal of the American Paraplegia Society*, 15(3):163-170, July, 1992.

38. Chow, R., et al. "Effect of two randomized exercise programmes on bone mass of healthy post-menopausal women." *British Medical Journal.* 295:1441-1444, 1987.

39. Smith, R. "Exercise and osteoporosis." *British Medical Journal.* 290:1163-1164, 1985.

40. Feskanich, D., et al. "Walking and leisure-time activity and risk of hip fracture in postmenopausal women." *Journal of the American Medical Association.* 288:2300-2306, Nov. 13, 2002.

41. Arjmandi, B.H.., et al. "Flaxseed supplementation positively influences bone metabolism in postmenopausal women." *Journal of the American Nutraceutical Association*, Vol. 1, No. 2:27-32, 1998.

42. Svanberg, M., et al. "Dietary xylitol prevents ovariectomy-induced changes of bone inorganic fraction in rats." *Bone Mineralization*, 26:81-88, 1994.

43. Mattila, P., et al. "Increased bone volume and bone mineral content in Xylitol-fed aged rats." *Gerontology*, 47:300-305, 2001.

44. Horowitz, M. "Cytokines and estrogen in bone: anti-osteoporotic effects." *Science*, 260:626-628, 1993; Ralston, S.H. "Analysis of gene expression in human bone biopsies by polymerase chain reaction: Evidence for enhanced cytokine expression in postmenopausal osteoporosis." *Journal of Bone Mineral Research*, 9:883-890, 1994.

45. Sellman, S. *Hormone Heresy: What Women Must Know About Their Hormones*, 2000.

46. Weiderpass, E., et al. "Low-potency oestrogen and risk of endometrial cancer: a case-control study." *Lancet*, 353:1824-1828, May 29, 1999.

47. Ross, R., et al. "Effect of Hormone Replacement Therapy on breast cancer risk: estrogen versus estrogen plus progestin." *Journal of the National Cancer Institute*, 92:328-332, Feb. 16, 2000.

48. Hulley, S., et al. "Randomized trial of estrogen plus progestin for secondary prevention of coronary heart disease in postmenopausal women." *Journal of the American Medical Association*, 280(7):605-613, August 19, 1998.

49. Ibid.

50. Schumaker, S., et al. "Estrogen plus progestin and the incidence of dementia and mild cognitive impairment in postmenopausal women." *Journal of the American Medical Association*, 289:2651-2662, 2003.

51. Prior, J.C. "Progesterone and the prevention of osteoporosis." *The Canadian Journal of Ob/Gyn & Women's Health Care*, 3.4:178-184, 1991.

52. Lee, J.R. "Osteoporosis reversal: The role of progesterone." *International Clinical Nutrition Review*, 10.3:384-391, 1990; Lee, J.R. "Is natural progesterone the missing link in osteoporosis prevention and treatment?" *Medical Hypotheses*, 35:316-318, 1991.

53. Snyder, P.J., et al. "Effects of testosterone treatment on bone mineral density in men over 65 years old." *Journal of Clinical Endocrinology and Metabolism*, 84:1966-1972, 1999.

54. www.medicinenet.com/calcitonin/article.htm

55. Ibid.

56. Frassetto, L.A., et al. "Worldwide incidence of hip fracture in elderly women: relation to consumption of animal and vegetable foods." *Journal of Gerontology Series A: Biological Science and Medical Science*, 55(10):M585-592, 2000; Munger, R.G., et al. "Prospective study of dietary protein intake and risk of hip fracture in postmenopausal women." *American Journal of Clinical Nutrition*, 69(1):147-152, Jan. 1999.

57. Fox, D. "Hard Cheese." *New Scientist*, Dec. 15, 2001.

58. Frassetto, as in Note 56.

59. Sellmeyer, S., et al. "A high ratio of dietary animal to vegetable protein increases the rate of bone loss and the risk of fracture in postmenopausal women." *American Journal of Clinical Nutrition*, 73(1):118-122, Jan. 2001; Sellmeyer, S., et al. "Dietary ratio of animal to vegetable protein and rate of bone loss and risk of fracture in postmenopausal women." *American Journal of Clinical Nutrition*, 74(3):411-412, Sept. 2001.

60. Remer, T., et al. "Potential renal acid load of foods and its influence on urine pH." *Journal of the American Dietetic Association.* 95:791-797, 1995; www.vegan society.com/downloads/dietandbone.pdf

61. Ibid; http://home.bluegrass.net/~jclark/alkaline_foods.htm

62. Winter, R. *A Consumer's Dictionary of Food Additives.* 4th edition, Random House, Inc.: New York, NY, 1994.

63. Washington Post, Feb. 27, 2001, p. HE10.

64. Wyshak, G. "Teenaged girls, carbonated beverage consumption, and bone fractures." *Archives in Pediatric Adolescent Medicine*, 154:610-613, 2000.

65. Eaton, B. and Shostak, M. *The Paleolithic Prescription*, 1988.

66. Fox, as in Note 57.

67. Liggett, as in Note 30.

Parkinson's Disease

1. www.ninds.nih.gov

2. Ibid.

3. www.ivanhoe.com/channels/p_channelstory.cfm?storyid=8175

4. Tanner, C.M. Drug-induced movement disorders in Extrapyramidal Disorders. In *Handbook of Clinical Neurology*, Vol. 5. Edited by Vinken, P.J., et al. Elsevier: Amsterdam, Holland, pp. 185-204, 1986.

5. Hammerstad, J., et al. "Parkinson's disease: surgical

options." *Current Neurology & Neuroscience Reports*, 1(4):313-319, July 2001.

6. Sechi, G., et al. "Reduced intravenous glutathione in the treatment of early Parkinson's disease." *Progress in Neuropsychopharmacology & Biological Psychiatry*. 20(7):1159-1170, Oct. 1996.

7. www.wjla.com/news/stories/0504/147299.html

8. Shults, C.W., et al. "Effects of coenzyme Q10 in early Parkinson's disease: evidence of slowing of the functional decline." *Archives of Neurol.*, 59(10):1541-1550, 2002.

9. Rosenberg, R.N. "Mitochondrial therapy for Parkinson's disease." *Archives of Neurology*, 59:1523, 2002.

10. HP-200 in Parkinson's Disease Study Group. "An alternative treatment for Parkinson's disease: Results of a multi-center clinical trial." *Journal of Alternative & Complementary Medicine*, 1(3):249-255, 1995.

11. Ibid.

12. www.ivanhoe.com/channels/p_channelstory.cfm? storyid=8175

13. Bjorklund, L.M. "Embrionic stem cells develop into functional dopaminergic neurons after transplantation in a Parkinson's rat model." *Proceedings of the National Academy of Sciences*, 99(4):1755-1757, Feb. 2002.

14. www.bbc.co.uk, April 9, 2002.

15. Birkmayer JGD, et al. "Nicotinamide adenine dinucleotide (NADH)—a new therapeutic approach to Parkinson's disease: Comparison of oral and parenteral application." *Acta Neurol Scand* 87: Suppl.146:32-35, 1993.

16. Address to the American Academy of Neurology, April 16, 2002.

17. de Rijk, M.C., et al. "Dietary antioxidants and Parkinson's disease: The Rotterdam Study." *Archives of Neurology*, 54(6), June 1997.

18. www.reutershealth.com, Nov. 26, 2001.

19. Chen, H., et al. "Nonsteroidal Anti-inflammatory Drugs and the risk of Parkinson's disease." *Archives of Neurology*, 60(8):1059-1064, 2003.

20. Majeed, M., et al. *Turmeric and the Healing Curcuminoids*. Keats Publishing: New Caanan, CT, 1996.

Poison Ingestion

1. Spiller, H.A., et al. "Evaluation of administration of activated charcoal in the home." *Pediatrics*. 108:e100-e100, Dec. 2001.

Prostate

1. http://health.yahoo.com/health/dc/000381/0.html

2. www.bhj.org/journal/1999_4103_july99/SP_395.htm

3. Ibid.

4. www.ebglaw.com/files/8995_article_564.pdf

5. www.laserscope.com

6. Ibid.

7. Holmberg, L., et al. "A randomized trial comparing radical prostatectomy with watchful waiting in early prostate cancer." *New England Journal of Medicine*. 347(11):781-9, 2002.

8. Steineck, G., et al. "Quality of life after radical prostatectomy or watchful waiting." *New England Journal of Medicine*. 347(11):790-6, 2002.

9. www.drmirkin.com

10. Stamey, T.A., et al. "Preoperative prostate specific antigen levels between 2 and 22 ng./ml. correlate poorly with post-radical prostatectomy cancer morphology." *Journal of Urology*, 167(1): 103-11, 2002.

11. Ibid.

12. www.peenuts.com/learning_center.html

13. Ibid.

14. www.drmirkin.com

15. Same as Note 12.

16. Ibid.

17. Ibid

18. Ibid.

19. Ibid.

20. Rhodes, L., et al. "Comparison of finasteride (Proscar), a 5-reductase inhibitor, and various commercial plant extracts in vitro and in vivo 5-reductase inhibition." *The Prostate*. 22:43-51, 1993.

21. Champault, G., et al. "A double-blind trial of an extract of the plant Serenoa repens in benign prostatic hyperplasia." *British Journal of Clinical Pharmacology*, 18:461-462, 1984.

22. Carraro, J.C., et al. "Comparison of phytotherapy (permixon) with finasteride in the treatment of benign prostatic hyperplasia: a randomized international study of 1,098 patients." *The Prostate*. 29:231-240, 1996.

23. Barlet, A., et al. "Efficacy of Pygeum Africanum extract in the medical therapy of urination disorders due to benign prostatic hyperplasia: evaluation of objective and subjective parameters. A placebo-controlled double-blind multicenter study." *Wiener Klinische Wochenschrift*. 102:667-673, 1990.

24. Hirano, T., et al. "Effects of stinging nettle roots and their steroidal components on the Na+, K+ ATPase of the benign prostatic hyperplasia." *Planta Medica*. 60: 30-33, 1994.

25. Berges, R.R., et al. "Randomized, placebo-controlled clinical trial of beta-sitosterol in patients with benign prostatic hyperplasia." *Lancet*. 345:1529-1532, 1995; and Klippel, K.F., et al. "A multi-center, placebo-controlled, double-blind clinical trial of beta-sitosterol (Phytosterol) for the treatment of benign prostatic hyperplasia." *British Journal of Urology*. 80:427-432, 1997.

26. www.bcn4life.com

27. "Crinum latifolium, a promising and highly effective treatment for BPH, health and life." *Journal of Health Ministry of Vietnam*, N 207, December 20, 2002.

28. Doan Thu Nhu. "Crinum latifolium in treatment of benign hypertrophy of prostate and cancers." *Journal of Health and Life of Vietnamese Health Ministry*, N 148, December 10, 2002.

29. "Crinum latifolium extract has a very good therapeutic effect on benign hyperthrophy of prostate (BHP)." Vietnamese Central State News Agency September 22, 2005; www.vietnamnet.vn.

30. Holden, F.C. "The Elliot Treatment: A new method of applying vaginal heat." *American Journal of Obstetrics and Gynoclolgy*, 22: 87-96, 1931; Lewis, L.G. "Treatment of prostatitis by local heat: The Elliot Treatment Regulator." *Journal of Urology* 25: 681-686, 1936.
31. www.laserscope.com/surgical/consumers/procedure.html
32. Ibid.
33. Kaltas, H. "Too Hot for Cancer." *Alternative Medicine*, Sept. 2002.
34. Ibid.

Psoriasis

1. Muller, K. et al. *Planta Medica*, 61(1): 74-75, 1995.
2. Misik, V., et al. "Lipoxygenase inhibition and antioxidant properties of protoberbine and aporphine alkaloids isolated from Mahomia aquifolium." *Planta Medica*, 61(4): 372-373, 1995.
3. Gieler, U., et al. *Journal of Dermatological Treatment.* 6(1): 31-34, 1995.
4. Kilham, C. "Oil of Tamanu (*Calophyllum inophyllum*): An Overview." *Total Health*, March, 25(1), 2003.
5. www.new-chapter.com
6. Itoigawa, M., et al. "Cancer chemoprotective agents, 4-phenylcoumarins from calophyllum inophyllum." *Cancer Letters*, 169(1): 15-19, Aug. 10, 2001.
7. Spino, C., et al. "Anti-HIV coumarins from caolphyllum seed oil." *Bioorganic Medicine Chemical Letters*, 8(24): 3475-3478, Dec. 15, 1998.

Scoliosis

1. www.scoliosis.org

Sleep Apnea

1. www.ninds.nih.gov/health_and_medical/disorders/sleep_apnea.htm
2. Ibid.
3. www.sleeping-tips.com/american-sleep-disorder-association.htm

Spinal Cord Injuries

1. Goldsmith, H., et al. "Spinal cord vascularization by intact omentum." *American Journal of Surgery*, 129:262-265, 1975; Goldsmith, H. "Omental transposition to brain of stroke patients." *Stroke.* July-Aug., 10(4): 471-472, 1979; Goldsmith, H., et al., "Vasoactive neuro-chemicals identified in omentum." *British Journal of Neurosurgery.* 1:359-364, 1987.
2. Ibid.
3. www.lightparty.com/Health/Spinal.html
4.Byrnes, K.R., et al. "Low Power Laser Irradiation Promotes Axonal Growth In An Animal Model Of Acute Spinal Cord Injury." *Society for Neuroscience Abstract* 26(1):304; 2000; Byrnes, K.R., et al. "Cellular invasion following spinal cord lesion and low power laser irradiation." *Lasers Surgery in Medicine*, S14: 11; 2002.
5. Walker, Morton, D.P.M. *DMSO: Nature's Healer.* Avery Publishing Group Inc: Garder City Park, New York. p. 50, 1993.
6. Ibid., pp. 143-147.
7. Ibid., p. 153.
8. Ibid., p. 154.
9. www.lightparty.com/Health/Spinal.html
10. Walker, p. 153.
11. www.lightparty.com/Health/Spinal.html
12. Ibid.
13. Walker, p. 55.
14. Ibid.
15. Wilson, Clare. "Old drug offers hope of new growth in spinal cord." *New Scientist* magazine, December 13-19, 2003.
16. Bittner, G.D., et al. *Journal of Neuroscience*, 19(7)2442-2554, April 1, 1999.
17. Shi, R., et al. "Acute repair of crushed guinea pig spinal cord by polyethylene glycol." *Journal of Neurophysiology*, Volume 81, No. 5, pp. 2406-2414, 1999; Borgens, R.B. and Shi, R. "Immediate recovery from spinal cord injury through molecular repair of nerve membranes with polyethylene glycol." *FASEB Journal*, January 2000.
18. Laverty, P.H., et al. "A Preliminary Study of Intravenous Surfactants in Paraplegic Dogs Polymer Therapy in Canine Clinical SCI." *Journal of Neurotrauma*, December 2004.
19. Ibid.

Stress

1.www.stressdirections.com/corporate/stress_organizations/stress_statistics.html
2. www.guardian.co.uk/france/story/0,11882,1080507,00.html
3. Ibid.
4. www.cmcsb.com/tranquil.htm
5. www.drugawareness.org; and Breggin, Peter, M.D., et al. *Talking Back to Prozac: What Doctors Aren't Telling You about Today's Most Controversial Drug.* St. Martin's Press, 1995.
6. Sahley, B.J., *GABA: The Anxiety Amino Acid.* Pain and Stress Publications: San Antonio, TX, 1998. p. 11.
7. Ibid.
8. Ibid., pp. 14, 34.
9. Ibid., p. 22.
10. Juneja, L., et al. "L-theanine: a unique amino acid of green tea and its relaxation effect in humans." *Trends in Food Science & Technology.* 10: 199-204, 1999; and Yofogoshi, H, et al. "Effect on theanine r-glutamylethylamide, on brain monoamines and striatal dopamine release in conscious rats." *Neurochemical Research.* 23: 667-73. 1998.
11. Ibid.
12. Juneja, as in Note 10.
13. *Biosciences, Biotechnology, Biochemistry.* 62(4): 816-17, 1998.
14. *Neurochemistry Resources.* 23(5): 667073, 1998.
15. Ibid.
16. *Pharmacopsychiat*, 30: 1-5, 1997.

17. www.supplementquality.com/news/kava_toxicologist.html

18. www.irisherbal.com/nwsltrarchive.html

19. Darbinyan, V., et al. "Rhodiola rosea in stress-induced fatigue: a double-blind cross-over study of a standardized extract SHR-5 with a repeated low-dose regimen on the mental performance of healthy physicians during night duty." *Phytomedicine.* 7(5): 365-71, Oct. 2000.

20. Spasov, A., et al. "A double-blind, placebo-controlled pilot study of the stimulating and adaptogenic effect of Rhodiola rosea SHR-5 extract on the fatigue of students caused by stress during an examination period with repeated low-dose regimen." *Phytomedicine*, 7(2): 85-9, April 2000.

21. www.anti-aging-guide.com/RhodiolaRosea.html

22. Linh, P., et al. "Quantitative determination of salidroside and thyrosol from the underground part of Rhodiola rosea by high performance liquid chromatography." *Archives of Pharmaceutical Research.* 23(4):349-52, Aug. 2000.

23. McAuliffe, S. "The Black Box-Secret....Treatment of Rock Superstars." *Omni Magazine.* Vol. 5, No. 4, 1983.

24. Madden, R. and Kirsch, D. "Low-intensity electrostimulation improves human learning." *American Journal of Electromedicine.* 4(2):41-45, 1987; and Gibson, T., et al. "Cranial application of low level transcranial electrotherapy vs. relaxation instruction in anxious patients." *American Journal of Electromedicine.* 4(1):18-21, 1987. Also doctoral dissertation, California School of Professional Psychology, 1983.

25. Smith, R.B. *Neural Stimulation,* 1985.

26. Smith, R.B. "Is microcurrent stimulation effective in pain management? An additional perspective." *American Journal of Pain Management,* 11(2):62-66, 2001.

27. Ibid.

28. Ibid.

29. Shapiro, F. *EMDR: The Breakthrough Therapy for Overcoming Anxiety, Stress, and Trauma.* BasicBooks: New York, NY, 1997; Shapiro, F. *Eye-Movement Desensitization and Reprocessing: Basic Principles, Protocols, and Procedures.* 2nd Ed., Guilford Press: New York, NY, 2001; www.emdr.com; www.induced-adc.com.

30. Addolorato, G. et al. "Effectiveness and safety of baclofen for maintenance of alcohol abstinence in alcohol-dependent patients with liver cirrhosis: randomised, double-blind controlled study." *Lancet,* 370(9603):1915-1922, Dec. 8, 2007.

31. "Ten years of therapy in one night." *The Guardian,* Saturday, September 20, 2003, http://books.guardian.co.uk/print/0,3858,4756137-99946,00.html

32. www.ibogaine.org/history.html

33. *The Guardian,* as in Note 31.

34. Linde, et al. "St John's wort for depression: An overview and meta-analysis of randomized clinical trials." *British Medical Journal.* 313(7052): 253, 1996.

35. Erasmus, Udo. *Fats that Heal, Fats that Kill.* Alive Books, 2000.

36. Ibid.

37. Kiefer, D. "Omega-3 fatty acids." *Life Extension,* p. 34, Dec. 2003.

38. Ibid.

39. http://www.medpagetoday.com/Psychiatry/Depression/tb/3877

40. Zarate, C.A. "A randomized trial of an *N*-methyl-D-aspartate antagonist in treatment-resistant major depression." *Archives of General Psychiatry.* 63:856-864, 2006.

41. www.usatoday.com/news/health/2003-09-02-pet-benefits_x.htm

42. "Machines roll in to care for elderly." *New Scientist.* May 15-21, 2004.

Stuttering

1. www.kidsource.com/ASHA/Stuttering.html

2. http://serendip.brynmawr.edu/bb/neuro/neuro01/web2/Walker.html

3. Ibid.

4. www.speecheasy.com

Teeth and Gums

1. http://newsfromrussia.com/science/2004/05/04/53752.html

2. Judd, Gerald. *Good Teeth, Birth to Death: The Prescription for Perfect Teeth.* Gerald Judd, 1997.

3. Cortellini, P., et al. "A minimally invasive surgical technique with an enamel matrix derivative in the regenerative treatment of intra-bony defects: a novel approach to limit morbidity." *Journal of Clinical Periodontology,* 34:87-93, 2007.

4. Zafiropoulous, G.G., et al. "Treatment of intrabony defects using guided tissue regeneration and autologous spongiosa alone or combined with hydroxyapitite/beta-tricalcium phosphate bone substitute or bovine-derived xenograft." *Journal of Periodontology,* 78:2216-25, 2007.

Tuberculosis

1. Mitnick, Carole D., et al. "Extensively drug-resistant tuberculosis: A comprehensive treatment." *New England Journal of Medicine,* 359(6):563-574, August 7, 2008.

Varicose Veins

1. www.quantumhealth.com/news/vein_go_away.html

2. Annoni, F., et al. "Venotonic activity of escin on the human saphenous vein." *Arzneim-Forsch,* 29;672-5, 1979.

3. Diehm, C., et al. "Comparison of leg compression stockings and oral horse chestnut-seed extract therapy in patients with venous insufficiency." *Lancet.* 347: 292-294, 1996.

4. Ellingwood, Finley. *The American Materia Medica, Therapeutics and Pharmacognosy,* 1919.

Vision Disorders

1. www.myclearvision.com/210.asp?nav=200

2. Ibid.

3. Ibid.

4. Ibid.

5. Vision Disorders. *Alternative Medicine: The Definitive Guide*, 2nd Edition, 2002; www.alternativemedicine.com

6. Ibid.

7. Ibid.

8. Ibid.

9. Ibid.

10. Ibid.

11. Ibid.

12. Ibid.

13. Ibid.

14. Lavine, J., *The Eye Care Sourcebook*, Contemporary Books, 2001.

15. www.refractec.com

Warts

1. Facade, D.R., et al. "The efficacy of duct tape vs cryotherapy in the treatment of verruca vulgaris (the common wart)." *Archives of Adolescent Pediatric Medicine*, 156:971-974, 2002.

PART III: Pain Relievers

DMSO

1. Walker, Morton. *DMSO: Nature's Healer*. Avery Publishing Group, Inc.: Garden City Park, New York, 1993, p. 35.

2. Ibid.

3. Ibid., p. 51.

4. Edelson, E. "DMSO." *Daily News*, June 9, 1980, p. 35.

5. Ibid., p. 64.

Electricity

1. www.bodyclock.co.uk/questions.html#TENS

2. Ibid; and www.paintechnology.com/046.htm

Farabloc

1. Clement, D.B., et al. "Alleviation of pain with the use of Farabloc, an electromagnetic shield: A review." *BC Medical Journal*, 43(10), pp. 573-577, December 2001.

2. Ibid, p. 574.

3. Zhang, J., et al. "The efficacy of Farabloc, an electromagnetic shield, in attenuating delayed-onset muscle soreness." *Clinical Journal of Sports Medicine*, 10(1):15-21, Jan 2000.

Light

1. www.painxequine.com/polychromatic.htm

2. www.promolife.com/products/lightp.htm

3. www.painxequine.com/Questions.htm; and www.painxequine.com/wound_healing_3.htm

4. Beckerman, H., et al. "The efficacy of laser therapy for musculoskeletal skin disorders: A criteria-based meta-analysis of randomized clinical trials." *Physical Therapy*, 72(7):483-91, July 1992.

5. *NASA News*, Marshall Space Flight Center News Release 00-36, Dec. 18, 2000.

6. Ibid.

7. Ibid.

8. Clark, Sir Arthur. "Beyond Gravity." *National Geographic*, p.2-29, Jan. 7, 2001; and *NASA News*, Marshall Space Flight Center News Release 00-36, Dec. 18, 2000.

Magnets

1. www.lashotochiropractic.com/magneticdevices/

2. Ibid.

3. www.magneticosleep.com

4. Nakagawa, K. "Magnetic field deficiency syndrome and magnetic treatment." *Japanese Medical Journal*, No. 2745, Dec. 4, 1975; Cox, A. "Magnetic field reversals." *Scientific American*, pp. 44-54, 1967; Gubbins, D., et al. "The secular variation of the Earth's magnetic field." *Nature*, Vol. 317, Oct. 31, 1985.

5. www.magneticosleep.com

6. Ibid.

7. Ibid.

8. Ibid.

9. Alfano, A., et al. "Static magnetic fields for treatment of fibromyalgia: A double-blind, randomized controlled trial." *Journal of Alternative and Complementary Medicine*, 7(1):53-64, 2001.

Pain Neutralization Technique

1. www.kaufmantechnique.com/index.html

Penetran + Plus

1. Hadley, M.T., et al. "A topically applied quanterrnary ammonium compound exhibits analgesic effects for orthopedic pain." *Alternative Medicine Review*, 3(5): 361-6, 1998.

Sphenopalatine Ganglion Block

1. Chan-laio, Mingi, Dept. Of Anesthesia, Jen-Ai Hospital, Taichung, Taiwan, R.O.C. "Sphenopalatine block: A simple but underutilized therapy for pain control." www.pain-management.org.tw/s-pain05.htm

2. Ibid.

Urine

1. Rey, Roselyne. *The History of Pain*. Translated by Louise Elliott Wallace, J. A. Cadden, S.W. Cadden. Harvard University Press, 1999.

PART IV: General Treatment Methods

Acupuncture

1. http://users.med.auth.gr/~karanik/english/main.htm

Bowen Therapy

1. www.mercola.com/nst/explain.htm

Del Immune V

1. www.delimmune.com; Personal conversations with John Sichel; Martinjuk, N.B., et al. "Blasten—the preparation with immunomodulating properties."

Presented at the conference: Actual Problems of New Drug Development, St. Petersburg, Russia, November 21-23, 1996; Vospjakov, V.G., et al. "Effect of Blastolen on hemopoietic cells." *HIV/AIDS and Related Problems*, Vol. 5, Issue 1, 2001; and Vospjakov, V.G., et al. Blasten—new immunomodulator of natural origin." *HIV/AIDS and Related Problems*, Volume. 5, Issue 1, 2001.

Hyperbaric Oxygenation Therapy
1. www.hhi-kc./whatis.htm.; www.drcranton.com/hbo.htm
2. Ibid.
3. Ibid.
4. Thom, S., et al. "Stem cell mobilization by hyperbaric oxygen." *American Journal of Physiology-Heart and Circulatory Physiology.* 290:H1378-H1386, 2006.

Insulin Potentiation Therapy
1. http://www.nobel.se/medicine/laureates/1923/
2. Rosen. *Science.* 273:1452-1457, 1987.
3. Hauser, Ross, M.D., and Hauser, Marion, M.S., R.D. *Treating Cancer with Insulin Potentiation Therapy.* Beulah Land Publishing: Oak Park, IL, 2002, p. 112.
4. www.iptcancer.com/cancer_pain_treatments.htm
5. Ibid.
6. Hauser, p. 342.
7. Gregory, W. "Chemotherapy of advanced breast cancer: outcome and prognostic factors." *British Journal of Cancer*, 1993, 68:988-995.
8. Hoffman, E. *Cancer and the Search for Selective Biochemical Inhibitors.* CRC Press, 2000. Crewdson, J. "Cancer-drug treatment: less might prove more." *Chicago Tribune*, April 2, 2000.
9. Ibid.
10. Evenson, B. "Discovery could win war on cancer." *National Post*, April 1, 2000.
11. Hauser, p. 80; Papa, V. "Elevated insulin receptor content in human breast cancer." *Journal of Clinical Investigation*, 1990, 86:1503-1510.
12. Aslabaster, O. "Metabolic modification by insulin enhances methotrexate cytotoxicity in MCF-7 human breast cancer cells." *European Journal of Oncology*, 1981, 13:1223-1228.
13. Cullin, J. "Insulin-like growth receptor expression and function in human breast cancer." *Cancer Research*, 50:48-53, 1990; and Hauser, p. 81.
14. Spring-Mills, E. "Immunoreactive hormones in human breast tissues." *Surgery*, Dec. 1983:946-950.
15. Hauser, pp. 91, 112.
16. Ibid., p. 258.
17. www.contemporarymedicine.net
18. Hauser, pp. 90-91, 112-113.
19. Hauser, pp. 91-92.
20. Adapted from Hauser, pp. 91-92; and McKimmell, R.G., et al. *The Biological Basis of Cancer.* Cambridge University Press, 1999.
21. Hauser, p. 138; and www.iptq.com

22. *Cellular Cancer Therapy*, Drs. Peréz García I & II.
23. Ibid.
24. Hauser, p. 137; *Catalogue of Services*. Immunosciences Lab, Beverly Hills, pp. 9-10, 2001.
25. Ibid., p. 138.
26. Ibid., p. 139.
27. Ibid., p. 138; Paquette, Jean-Claude, M.D. *Medicine of Hope*, 1999.
28. Hauser, p. 142. Hausers' source: *Catalogue of Services*. Immunosciences Lab, Inc., Beverly Hills, CA, 2001.
29. Ibid., p. 143.
30. Ibid., p. 144.
31. Ibid., 145.
32. http://www.nobel.se/chemistry/laureates/1993/
33. Ford, D. "The microbial causes of rheumatoid arthritis." *Journal of Rheumatology*, 18:1441-1442, 1991; Rook, G. "A reappraisal of the evidence that rheumatoid arthritis and several other idiopathic diseases are slow bacterial infections." *Annals of Rheumatic Diseases.* 52:S30-S38, 1993.
34. Brightman, M. "Morphology of blood-brain interfaces." *Experimental Eye Research*, 25:1-6, 1971.
35. Hauser, p. 85.
36. Partridge, W. "Receptor-mediated peptide transport through the blood-brain barrier." *Endocrinology Review.* 1986, 7:314-330; and Van Houten, M., et al. "Insulin binds to brain blood vessels in vivo." *Nature*, 282:623-628, 1979.
37. Frank, H. "Enhanced insulin binding to blood-brain barrier in vivo and to brain microvessels in vitro in newborn rabbits." *Diabetes*, 34:728-733, 1985.
38. Hauser, p. 148.
39. Ibid., pp. 63-65.
40. www.iptq.com/mexcert.htm
41. Hauser, p. 13.

Iodine
1. Szent-Györgyi, A., *Bioenergetics*. Academic Press, New York, p. 112, 1957.
2. Wright, J.V. "One mineral can help a myriad of conditions from atherosclerosis to 'COPD' to zits." www.tahoma-clinic.com/iodide.shtml
3. Abraham, G.E., et al. "Optimum levels of iodine for greatest mental and physical health." *The Original Internist*, 9:5-20, 2002.
4. Abraham, G.E., et al. "Measurement of urinary iodide levels by ion-selective electrode: Improved sensitivity and specificity by chromatography on anion-exchange resin." *The Original Internist*, 11(4):19-32, 2004.
5. Abraham, G.E., et al. "Orthoiodosupplementation: Iodine sufficiency of the whole human body." *The Original Internist*, 9:30-41, 2002.
6. Abraham, G.E. "The safe and effective implementation of orthoiodosupplementation in medical practice." *The Original Internist*, 11:17-36, 2004.
7. Abraham, G.E. "The concept of orthoiodosupplementation and its clinical implications." *The Original Internist*,

11(2):29-38, 2004.

8. Abraham, G.E. "The historical background of the iodine project." *The Original Internist*, 12(2):57-66, 2005.

9. Brownstein, D. "Clinical experience with inorganic, non-radioactive iodine/iodide." *The Original Internist*, 12(3):105-108, 2005.

10. Flechas, J.D. "Orthoiodosupplementation in a primary care practice." *The Original Internist*, 12(2):89-96, 2005.

11. Kelly, F.C. "Iodine in Medicine and Pharmacy Since its Discovery – 1811-1961." *Proceedings of the Royal Society of Medicine*, 54:831-836, 1961.

12. Wolff, J. "Iodide goiter and the pharmacologic effects of excess iodide." *American Journal of Medicine*, 47:101-124, 1969.

13. Ghent, W.R., et al. "Iodine replacement in fibrocystic disease of the breast." *Canadian Journal of Surgery*, 36:453-460, 1993.

Neural Therapy

1. Faber, W.J., et al. *Pain Pain Go Away*, Ishi Press International: Menlo Park, CA, 2000; and www.milwaukeepainclinic.com/NeuralTherapy.asp

2. Ibid.

3. Ibid.

4. Ibid.

Nutrition: Toxicities & Deficiencies

The Other Face of Progress

1. Beasley, J.D., et al. *The Kellogg Report*, Institute of Health Policy and Practice, The Bard College Center, 4:171, 1989.

2. Timbrel, J.A. *Principles of Biochemical Toxicology*, 2nd ed., Washington, D.C.: Taylor and Francis, 1992.

3. U.S. Environmental Protection Agency, 1991. Toxics in the Community: National and Local Perspectives; The 1989 Toxics Release Inventory National Report, Office of Toxic Substances, Washington, D.C.; www.lib.umich.edu/govdocs/stenv.html

4. Selikoff, Irving. "Second Sunday." NBC Television, March 9, 1969.

5. Mandal, Veronique. Housework Makes Women Sick: From Detergents to Cosmetics, Home Is Where the Cancer Is. *Windsor Star*, Sept. 20, 2003.

6. Ibid.

7. Ibid.

8. Litovitz, T.L., et al. 1996 Annual Report of the American Association of Poison Control Centers Toxic Exposure Surveillance System, 15:447-500, 1997.

9. Mandal, as in Note 5.

10. Lowe, C. *Toxic Food*. Avon Books, 1990, p. 8.

11. Rosenstock, L., et al. "Chronic central nervous system effects of acute organophosphate pesticide intoxication." *Lancet*, 338:223-227, 1991.

12. Ibid.; *Pesticides: A Toxic Time Bomb in Our Midst*, Marvin J. Levine, Praeger Publications, 2007.

13. EPA Study. "Unfinished Business: A Comparative Assessment of Environmental Problems." Feb. 1987.

14. Wilson, D. "Fear in the Fields." *The Seattle Times*.

July 3, 1997, pp. 1-2.

15. www.ndchealth.com, April 1, 2003.

16. Starfield, B. "Is U.S. health really the best in the world?" *Journal of the American Medical Association*, 284:483-5, 2000; also Lararou, J., et al. "Incidence of adverse drug reactions in hospitalized patients: a meta-analysis of prospective studies." *Journal of the American Medical Association*, 279(15):1200-1205, April 15, 1998.

17. Ibid.

18. www.ewg.org/reports/bodyburden2/execsumm.php

19. Ibid.

20. www.ewg.org/reports/bodyburden2/part3.php, p. 1.

21. Ames, B., et al. "Ranking Possible Carcinogenic Hazards," *Science* 236 (1987), p. 275.

22. Hlleman, B. "Multiple Chemical Sensitivity." *Chemical & Engineering News*. July 22, 1991, pp. 26-42.

23. Steventon, G.B., et al. "Xenobiotic metabolism in Parkinson's disease." *Neurology*. 39:883-887, 1998; and Steventon, G.B., et al. "Xenobiotic metabolism in Alzheimer's disease." *Neurology*. 40:1095-1098, 1990.

24. Quig, D. "Cysteine Metabolism and Metal Toxicity." *Alternative Medicine Review*. Vol. 3, No. 4, 1998, pp. 262-263.

25. Technical Bulletin. Detoxification: Clinical Perspective. HealthComm International, Inc., 2000. www.healthcomm.com.

26. Ibid.

27. www.atdonline.org/atd/Detoxification.pdf. (Ask the Doctor Online)

28. www.botanical.com/botanical/mgmh/b/burdoc87.html

29. www.healthyhealing.com/aisle170p.html

30. www.healthyhealing.com/aisle175p.html

31. McKinnon, R.A., et al. "Localization of cytochromes P450 in human tissue: Implications for chemical toxicity." *Pathology*, 28:148-155, 1996.

32. www.atdonline.org

33. Ibid.

34. Ibid.

35. Ibid.

36. Technical Bulletin. Detoxification:Biochemistry. HealthComm International, Inc., 2000. www.healthcomm.com.

37. Timbrel, as in Note 2.

38. Percival, M. "Nutrition support for detoxification." *Applied Nutrition Science Reports*. Nov. 1999.

39. Boyd, E.M., et al. "Lindane toxicity and protein-deficient diet." *Archives of Environmental Health*. 17:156-163, 1968; and Boyd, E.M., et al. "Toxicity of captan and protein-deficient diet." *Journal of Clinical Pharmacology*. 8:225-234, 1968.

40. Anderson, K.E., et al. "Dietary regulation of cytochrome P450," *Annual Review of Nutrition*, 11:141-167, 1991.

41. Ibid.

42. Ibid.

43. Percival, as in Note 38, p. 4.

44. Ibid.

45. Ibid., p. 5.

46. Technical Bulletin. Detoxification:Biochemistry, as in Note 36.

47. Ibid.

48. Kidd, P. "Glutathione: Systemic protectant against oxidative and free radical damage." *Alternative Medicine Review*, 2(3):156, 1997.

49. Cook, G.C., et al. "Results of a controlled clinical trial of glutathione in cases of hepatic cirrhosis." *Gut*, 6:472-476, 1965.

50. Kidd, p. 159.

51. Bremmer, H.J., et al. *Disturbances of Amino Acid Metabolism: Clinical Chemistry and Diagnosis.* Baltimore-Munich: Urban and Schwartzberg. pp. 80-82, 1981.

52. Kidd.

53. Ibid; also "Glutathione, reduced (GSH)," *Alternative Medicine Review*, 6(6):601, 2001.

54. Kidd, p. 158.

55. Ibid.

56. Ibid., p. 159.

57. Droge, W., et al. "Functions of glutathione and glutathione disulfide in immunology and immuno-pathology." *FASEB Journal*. 8: 1131-1138, 1994.

58. Fidelus, R.K., et al. "Glutathione and lymphocyte activation: A function of aging and auto-immune disease." *Immunology*, 61:503-508, 1987.

59. Lomaestro, B.M., et al. "Glutathione in health and disease: pharmacotherapeutic issues." *Annals of Pharmacotherapy*. 29:1263-1273, 1995.

60. Ibid.

61. Meister, A. "Minireview: Glutathione-ascorbic acid antioxidant system in animals." *Journal of Biological Chemistry*, 269(13):9397-9400, April 1, 1994.

62. Tarp, U. "Selenium and the selenium-dependent glutathione peroxidase in rheumatoid arthritis." *Danish Medical Bulletin*, 41(3):264-274, June 1994.

63. Bounous, G., et al. "Dietary whey protein inhibits the development of dimethylhydrazine-induced malignancy." *Clinical Investigation in Medicine*. 11:213-217, 1988.

64. Newberne, P.M., et al. "Acute and chronic effects of aflatoxins B1 on the liver of domestic and laboratory animals: A review." *Cancer Research*, 29:236-250, 1969; and Djuric, J., et al. "In vivo and in vitro formation of glutathione conjugates from the K-region epoxides of 1-nitropyrene." *Carcinogenesis*. 8:1781-1786, 1987.

65. Weber, C.F. "Final common pathways in neuro-degenerative diseases: regulatory role of glutathione cycle." *Neurosciences Biobehavioral Review*. 23:1079-1086, 1999; and Prasad, A., et al. "Glutathione reduces endothelial dysfunction and improves nitric oxide bioavailability." *Journal of the American College of Cardiology*, 34:507-514, 1999.

66. Stamler, J.S., et al. "Biological chemistry of thiols in the vasculature and in vascular-related disease." *Nutrition Reviews*. 54:1-30, 1996.

67. Miura, K. "Cystine uptake and glutathione level in endothelial cells exposed to oxidative stress." *American Journal of Physiology*, 262:C50-58, 1992.

68. Amano, J., et al. "Salutary effect of reduced glutathione on renal function in coronary artery bypass operation." *Journal of the American College of Surgery*, 179:714-720, 1994.

69. Kidd, P.M., et al. "Cell membranes, endithelia, and atherosclerosis: the importance of dietary fatty acid balance." *Alternative Medical Review*, 1(3):148-167, 1996.

70. Technical Bulletin. Detoxification: Clinical Perspective, as in Note 25.

71. Gull, M., et al. "Cellular and clinical implications of glutathione." *Indian Journal of Experimental Biology*, 38:625-634, 2000.

72. Ibid.

73. Sen, C.K. "Glutathione homeostasis in response to exercise training and nutritional supplements." *Molecular Cell Biochemistry*, 196:31-42, 1999.

74. Ibid.

75. Ibid.

76. Ibid.

77. Lands, L.C., et al. "Effect of a cysteine donor on muscular performance." *Journal of Applied Physiology*, 87(4): 1381-1385, 1999.

78. Anderson, M.E. "Glutathione and glutathione delivery compounds." *Advancements in Pharmacology*, 38:65-78, 1997.

79. Pace, G.W., et al. "The role of oxidative stress in HIV disease." *Free Radicals in Biology and Medicine*. 19:523-528, 1995.

80. Anderson, as in Note 78.

81. Loguercio, C. "Alteration of erythrocyte glutathione, cysteine, and glutathione synthetase in alcoholic and non-alcoholic cirrhosis." *Scandanavian Journal of Clinical Laboratory Investigations*, 52:207-213, 1992.

82. Shigesawa, T., et al. "Significance of plasma glutathione determination patients with alcoholic and non-alcoholic liver disease." *Journal of Gastroenterology and Hepatology*, 7:7-11, 1992; and Seifert, C.F., et al. "Correlation of acetaminophen and ethanol use, plasma glutathione concentrations and diet with hepatotoxicity." *Pharmacotherapy*, 14:376-377, 1994.

83. Monograph: Glutathione, Reduced (GSH), *Alternative Medicine Review*, Vol. 6, No. 6, 2001, p. 603.

84. Suter, P.M., et al. "N-acetylcysteine enhances recovery from acute lung injury in man." *Chest*, 105:190-194, 1994.

85. Lamson, D.W., et al. "The use of nebulized glutathione in the treatment of emphysema: a case report." *Alternative Medicine Review*, Vol. 5, No. 5, 2000.

86. Beal, M.F. "Aging, energy and oxidative stress in neurodegenerative diseases." *Annals of Neurology*, 38:357-366, 1995.

87. Jenner, P. "Oxidative damage in neurodegenerative disease." *Lancet*, 344:796-798, 1994.

88. Sano, M., et al. "A controlled trial of selegiline, alpha-tocopherol, or both as treatment for Alzheimer's disease.

The Alzheimer's Disease Cooperative Study." New England Journal of Medicine, 336:1216-1222, 1997.

89. Witschi, A., et al. "The systemic availability of oral glutathione." *European Journal of Clinical Pharmacology,* 43:667-669, 1992.

90. Aw, T., et al. "Oral glutathione increases tissue glutathione in vivo." *Chemical-Biological Interactions,* 80:89-97, 1991.

91. Iantomasi, T., et al. "Glutathione metabolism in Chron's disease." *Biochemical Medical Metabolism in Biology,* 53:87-91, 1994.

92. Perlmutter, D. BrainRecovery. com. The Perlmutter Health Center, 2000.

93. Buhl, R., et al. "Oxidant-protease interaction in the lung. Prospects for antioxidant therapy." *Chest,* 110:267S-272S, 1996.

94. Lomaestro, as in Note 59.

95. Buhl, as in Note 93.

96. Kidd, as in Note 48.

97. Traber, J., et al. "In vivo modulation of total and mitochondrial glutathione in rat liver." *Biochemical Pharmacology,* 43:961-964, 1992.

98. Spied, C.D., et al. "Influence of N-acetylcysteine on direct indicators of tissue oxygenation in septic shock patients: results from a prospective, randomized, double-blind study." *Critical Care Medicine,* 22:1738-1746, 1994.

99. Van Zandwijk, N. "N-acetylcysteine (NAC) and glutathione (GSH): antioxidant and chemoprotective properties, with special referance to lung cancer." *Journal of Cell Biochemistry* Supplement, 22:24-32, 1995.

100. Kidd, as in Note 48.

101. "New study shows supplement raises glutathione levels and balances immune system." Chronic Fatiguesupport.com, Nov. 7, 2000.

102. Lomaestro, as in Note 59.

103. Ibid.

104. Almasio, P. et al. "Role of S-adenosyl methionine in the treatment of intrahepatic cholestasis." *Drugs,* 40(Supplement 3):111-123, 1990.

105. Monograph: Glutathione, Reduced (GSH), as in Note 83.

106. Flickstein, A. "Health Mate infrared saunas." *Townsend Letter for Doctor's and Patients.* #202, pp. 66-70, 2000.

107. www.sunlightsaunas.com/detox.htm

108. Ibid.

109. Ibid.

110. Ibid.

111. Gard, Z., et al. "Literature review and comparison studies of sauna/hyperthermia in detoxification." *Townsend Letter for Doctor's and Patients.* June 1992; Fletcher, D.J. "Warming Up To Far-InfraRed," *Alternative Medicine,* Issue 39, January 2001.

112. Ibid.

Superfoods

113. www.neutraceuticalsworld.com/Nov021.htm

114. Belay, A. "The potential application of Spirulina (Arthrospira) as a nutritional and therapeutic supplement in health management." *Journal of the American Nutraceutical Association,* Vol.5, No. 2, pp. 28-48, Spring 2002.

115. Kamen, B. "What has been the world's largest wasted food resource has shown significant therapeutic value in treating cardiovascular conditions, arthritis, diabetes and many other illnesses." *Alternative Medicine.* July 2001.

Enzymes

116. Howell, E, et al. *Enzyme Nutrition: The Food Enzyme Concept,* 1986.

117. Ibid.

118. Ibid.

119. Ibid.

120. Dr. med. Nat. Wrba. *Enzymes—A drug of the future: Strengthening the immunological system with enzyme therapy.* Ecomed Verlagsgesellschaft, AG & CO. KG, 1998.

121. Howell, as in Note 116.

122. www.isga-sprouts.org/nutritio.htm

123. www.neutraceuticalsworld.com/Sept021.htm

124. Stalknecht, G.F., et al. Alternative wheat cereals as food grains: Einkorn emmer, spelt, kamut, and triticale. In J. Janick (ed.), *Progress in New Crops,* ASHS Press: Alexandria, VA, pp-156-170, 1996.

125. Chavan, J.K., et al. "Nutritional improvement of cereals by fermentation." *CRC Critical Review in Food Science and Technology.* 28(5): 401-437, 1989.

126. Howell, as in Note 116.

Minerals

127. Passwater, R., et al. *Trace Elements, Hair Analysis and Nutrition.* Keats Publishing, Inc.: New Canaan, CT, 1983.

128. Mindell, E. *What You Should Know About Trace Minerals.* Keats Publishing, Inc.: New Canaan, CT, 1997; Berger, P. *The Healing Power of Minerals, Special Nutrients, and Trace Elements.* Prima Publishing: Rocklin, CA, 1997.

129. Mindell, as in Note 128.

130. de Langre, J. *Seasalt's Hidden Powers.* Happiness Press: Magalia, CA, 1994.

Essential Fatty Acids

131. Erasmus, Udo. *Fats that Heal, Fats that Kill.* Alive Books, 2000; Murray, M., et al. *Understanding Fats and Oils: Your Guide to Healing with Essential Fatty Acids,* 1996.

132. Ibid.

133. Ibid.

134. Mantzioris, E., et al. "Biochemical effects of a diet containing foods enriched with n-3 fatty acids." *American Journal of Clinical Nutrition.* 72: 42-48, 2000.

135. Das, U. "Essential fatty acids and osteoporosis." *Nutrition,* 16:386-390, 2000.

136. McCarty, M. "Magnesium taurate and fish oil for

prevention of migraine." *Medical Hypothesis*, 47(6):461-466, Dec. 1996.

137. Belluzzi, A., et al. "Effect of an enteric-coated fish-oil preparation on relapses in Chron's disease." *New England Journal of Medicine*. 334:1557-1560, 1996.

138. Same as Note 131.

Phytonutrients

139. Goldberg, I. *Functional Foods, Designer Foods, Pharmafoods, Nutraceuticals*. Chapman & Hall: NY, NY, 1994.

140. Balentine, D., et al. "Role of medicinal plants, herbs, and spices in protecting human health." *Nutritional Review*, 57(9):S41-S45, 1999.

141. Rita, R. "Pilot study: Food nutritional supplement increases antioxidant levels in the blood." *Journal of the American Nutraceutical Association*, Vol. 4, No. 2, pp. 44-48.

142. Mehta, J., "Intake of antioxidants among American Cardiologists." *American Journal of Cardiology*, Vol. 79, Issue 11, pp. 1558-1560, June 1, 1997.

143. Joshipura, K., et al. "The effect of fruit and vegetable intake on risk of coronary heart disease." *Annals of Internal Medicine*, 134(12):1106-1114, June 19, 2001.

144. Jacobs, R., Jr., et al. "It's more than an apple a day: an appropriately-processed, plant-centered dietary pattern may be good for your health." *American Journal of Clinical Nutrition*, 72(4):899-900, Oct. 1, 2000.

145. Arab, L., et al. "Lycopene and cardiovascular disease." *American Journal of Clinical Nutrition*, 79(1): 47-53, January 2004.

146. McKeown, K., et al. "Whole grain intake and risk of ischemic stroke in women." *Nutrition Review*, 59(5):149-158, May 2001.

147. Ibid.

148. www.vegsource.com/esselstyn/reversal01.htm

149. Birt, D., et al. "Dietary agents in cancer prevention: flavonoids and isoflavonoids." *Pharmacology & Therapeutics*. 90:157-177, 2001.

150. Michaud, D., et al. "Fruit and vegetable intake and incidence of bladder cancer in a male prospective cohort study." *Journal of the National Cancer Institute*. 91(7):605-613, 1999.

151. Ley, Beth. *Phytonutrients: Medicinal Nutrients Found in Food*. BL Publications, 1998; Mozian, Laurie Deutsch, *Foods that Fight Disease: A Simple Guide to Using & Understanding Phytonutrients to Protect & Enhance Your Health*. Avery Publishing Group, 2001; Bland, J., et al. *The 20-Day Rejuvenation Diet Program With The Revolutionary Phytonutrient Diet*. McGraw Hill/ Contemporary Books, 2000; and Beling, S. *PowerFoods: Good Food, Good Health with Phyto- chemicals, Nature's Own Energy Boosters*. Harper Collins, 1998.

152. Liebman, B. "Lessons from China." *CSPI Nutrition Action Health Letter*, p. 6, December 1990.

153. Brody, J. "The nutrient that reddens tomatoes appears to have health benefits." *The NY Times*, March 12, 1997.

Probiotics

154. Gupta, P., et al. "Is lactobacillus GG helpful in children with Crohn's disease? Results of a preliminary, open-label study." *Journal of Pediatric Gastroenterology and Nutrition*, 31(4):453-457, Oct. 2000.

155. Trenev, Natasha. *Probiotics: Nature's Internal Healers*. Avery Penguin Putnam, 1998; Brudnak, M.A. *The Probiotic Solution: Nature's Best-Kept Secret for Radiant Health*. Dragon Door Publications, 2003; Lipski, E. et al. *Digestive Wellness*. McGraw Hill/Contemporary Books, 1999.

156. Ibid.

157. Ibid.

Fiber

158. Kaman, B., *New Facts About Fiber*, Nutrition Encounter, 1992.

159. Ibid.

160. www.neutraceuticalsworld.com/Sept021.htm

161. Kamen, as in Note 158.

162. Ibid.

163. Walker, A. "What causes appendicitis?" *Journal of Clinical Gastroenterology*, 12(2):127-129, 1990.

164. Smith, B., et al. "Lactulose in the treatment of symptomatic diverticular disease: a comparative study with high-fibre diet." *British Journal of Clinical Practice*. 44(8):314, Aug. 1990.

165. Simin, L. "Whole-grain consumption and risk of coronary heart disease: Results from the Nurses' Health Study." *Am. J of Clinical Nutrition*." 70:412-419, 1999.

166. Kamen, as in Note 158.

Exercise

167. Booth, F., et al. "Waging war on modern chronic diseases: primary prevention through exercise biology." *Journal of Applied Physiology*. Vol. 88, Issue 2, pp. 774-787, Feb. 2000.

168. Ibid.

169. Colditz, G., et al. Harvard Center for Cancer Prevention Report. Dec. 11, 1997; www.hsph.harvard. edu/facres/cldz.html

170. McGinnis, J. "Actual causes of death in the United States." *Journal of the American Medical Association*, 270:2207-2212, 1993.

171. Paffenbarger, R., et al. "The association of changes in physical-activity level and other lifestyle characteristics with mortality among men." *New England Journal of Medicine*. 328:538-545, 1993.

172. Hu, F., et al. "Physical activity and risk of stroke in women." *Journal of the American Medical Association*. 283(22):2961-2967, June 14, 2000.

173. Taylor-Tolbert, et al. "Ambulatory blood pressure after acute exercise in older men with essential hypertension." *American Journal of Hypertension*. 13(1):44-51, 2000.

174. Diabetes Prevention Program Research Group. "Reduction in the incidence of Type 2 diabetes with lifestyle intervention or metformin." *New England Journal*

of Medicine. 346(6):393-403, 2002.

175. Manson, J. Et al. "A prospective study of exercise and incidence of diabetes among US male physicians." *JAMA.* 268:63-67, 1992.

176. Blumenthal, J., et al. "Effects of exercise training on older patients with major depression." *Archives of Internal Medicine.* 159(19):2349-2356, Oct. 1999.

177. Colditz, as in Note 169.

178. Leitzmann, M., et al. "The relation of physical activity to risk for symptomatic gallstone disease in men."*Annals of Internal Medicine*, 128:417-425, 1998.

179. McGuire, D., et al. "A 30-year follow-up of the Dallas Bed Rest and Training Study: I & II." *Circulation.* 104:1350-1366, Sept. 2001.

180. Kramer, K. Beckman Institute for Advanced Science and Tech.; www.beckman.uiuc.edu/faculty/kramer.html.

181. Gutman, J. Glutathione (GSH): Your Body's Most Powerful Healing Agent. Gutman & Schettinin, Inc.: Montreal (Quebec) Canada, 2000.

182. Egger, G., et al. "Estimating historical changes in physical activity levels." *Medical Journal of Australia*, 175:635-636, 2001.

Olive Leaf Extract

1. Walker, M. *Olive Leaf Extract.* Kensington Publishing Group: New York, NY. 1997, pp. 34-37, 41.

2. Ibid., p. 45.

3. Ibid., p. 54.

4. Ibid., pp. 65-68. Dr. Walker lists 25 sources of documentation, pp. 213-214.

Photoluminescence

1. Douglass, W.C., *Into the Light*, Second Opinion Publishing, Inc., 1997, p. 274.

2. www.nobel.se/medicine/laureates/1903/finsen-bio.html; Douglass, W.C., M.D. *Into the Light*, Second Opinion Press, 1997, p.33.

3. www.nobel.se/medicine/laureates/1903/

4. www.britannica.com/nobel/micro/209_43.html

5. Gurwitsch, A., 'Die Natur des Specifischen Erregurs der Zeliteilung', Roux, Archiv: 100; 11, 1923; Gurwitsch, A., "Invisible Irradiations of Organisms," *Protoplasma*--Monographin, Burlin, Borntraeger, Vol. 9, 1936; www.21stcenturysciencetech.com/articles/summ01/Biophysics /Biophysics.html

6. www.21stcenturysciencetech.com/articles/summ01/Biophysics/Biophysics.html; Douglass, W.C., *Into the Light*, Second Opinion Publishing, Inc., 1997, p. 33.

7. Popp, F.A., "Experimental investigations on ultraweak photon emission from biological systems." In: Schram, Eric P., Stanley, P.(eds.): *Proceedings International symposium on analytical applications of bioluminescence and chemiluminescence*, Brüssel, 1978, pp. 601-617.

8. Kobayashi, M and Inaba, H., "Photon statistics and correlation analysis of ultraweak light originating from living organisms." *Applied Optics*, 2000, Vol. 39, p. 183; Kobayashi, M and Inaba, H. et al, "In vivo imaging of spontaneous ultraweak photon emission from a rat's brain," *Neuroscience Research*, 1999, Vol. 34, p. 103.

9. Noguchi, H. "The Photodynamic Action of Eosin and Erythrosin Upon Snake Venom," *Journal of Experimental Medicine*, 6:252-267, 1906.

10. Douglass, p. 253.

11. Ibid., p. 13.

12. Hancock, Virgil, M.D. "Treatment of Blood Stream Infection with Hemo-Irradiation," *American Journal of Surgery*, 58:336, 1942.

13. Macht, "Contributions to Photopharmacology or the Application of Plant Physiology to Medical Problems," *Science*, 71:303- 304, March 21, 1930.

14. Zinsser, et al. *Textbook of Bacteriology*, New York, NY: Appleton Century Company, Inc.,1939.

15. Miley, George, M.D. "The Ultraviolet Irradiation of Auto-Transfused Human Blood, Studies of the Absorption Value." *American Journal of Medical Science*, Vol. 14, 1938-1939.

16. Duggar, *Biological Effects of Radiation*, New York: McGraw-Hill Book Company, pp. 323-335.

17. Ibid.

18. Luckiesh, M. And Pacini, A.J. *Light and Health*, Baltimore: The Williams and Wilkins Company, 1926, pp. 61-91.

19. Duggar, as in Note 16.

20. Ellis and Wells, *The Chemical Action of Ultraviolet Rays*, New York, NY: The Chemical Catalogue Company, 1925.

21. Hancock, V.K., M.D. and Knott, E.K. "Irradiated Blood Transfusion in Treatment of Infections," *Northwest Medicine*, 33:200, 1934.

22. Rebbeck, E.W. "Ultraviolet Irradiation of Auto-Transfused Blood in the Treatment of Acute Peritonitis, General," The *Hahnemannian* [Hospital and Medical School] *Monthly*, April, 1941.

23. Guttmacher and Mayer, *American Review of Tuberculosis*, 10:170, October, 1924.

24. Barrett, H.A. "Five Years' Experience with Hemo-irradiations." *American Journal of Surgery*, 61: 42-53, 1943.

25. Ibid.

26. Miley, G. "The Ultraviolet Irradiation of Auto-transfused Human Blood: Studies in Oxygen Absorption Values." *American Journal of Medical Science*, Vol. 14, 1938-1939.

27. www.nobel.se/medicine/laureates/1931/

28. Douglass, p. 141.

29. Ibid., pp. 44-48, 70-91, 95-106, 117-150, 169-178, 297-314.

30. Ibid., pp. 313-314.

31. Ibid., p. 256.

32. Edelson R., et al. "Treatment of cutaneous T-cell lymphoma by extracorporeal photochemotherapy. Preliminary results." *New England Journal of Medicine*, 1987 Feb. 5; 316(6):297-303.

33. Costanzo-Nordin, M.R., et al. "Successful treatment

of heart transplant rejection with photopheresis." *Transplantation*, 1992 Apr; 53(4): 80815; Costanzo-Nordin, M.R., et al. "Photopheresis versus corticosteroids in the therapy of heart transplant rejection. Preliminary clinical report." *Circulation*, 1992 Nov; 86(5 Suppl): II242-50.

34. www.emedicine.com/derm/topic566.htm

35. Pohlmann, et al. "Wirksamkeit Von Pentoxifyllin und der Hamatogenen Oxydationstherapie," *Natur-und GanzheitsMedizin*, 1992; 5:80-4. Source of Notes 35-37: Rowen, R.J. "Ultraviolet Blood Irradiation: The Cure that Time Forgot," *International Journal of Biosocial Medical Research*, Vol. 14(2). 115-132, 1996.

36. Paulitschke, Turowski, and Lerche, Ergebnisse der Berliner HOT/UVB - Bergleichsstudie bei Patienten mit peripheren arterielien Durchblutungsstorungen, *Z. gesamte Inn. Med.*, No. 47, 1992, pp. 148-153.

37. Frick, G., "A Linke: Die Ultraviolet bestrahlung des Blutes, ihre Entwicklung und derzeitiger Stand.," *Zschr-arztl.*, Forth. 80, 1986.

38. Rowen, R.J. "Ultraviolet Blood Irradiation: The Cure that Time Forgot," *International Journal of Biosocial Medical Research*, Vol. 14(2). 115-132, 1996.

39. Douglass, p. 234.

40. Ibid., p. 235.

41. Ibid., p. 236.

42. Ibid., p. 238.

43. Ibid., p. 239.

44. Ibid., p. 240.

45. Ibid.

46. Ibid., p. 241.

47. Ibid., p. 242.

48. Ibid.

49. Ibid., p. 243.

50. Ibid.

51. Rahm, Otto. "The Physio-chemical Basis of Biological Irradiations," *Cold Spring Harbor Symposia and Quantitative Biology*," Vol. 2, pp. 226-232.

52. Douglass, p. 252, 1934.

Prolotherapy

1. Hauser, R.A., et al. *Prolo Your Pain Away: Curing Chronic Pain With Prolotherapy*. Beulah Land Press: Oak Park, Il, 2000, p.43.

2. Ibid., pp. 15-16

3. Ibid., p. 42.

4. Hackett, G.S. *Ligament and Tendon Relaxation Treated by Prolotherapy*, 1958.

5. Hauser, p. 15.

Resveratrol

1. Ingram, D.K., et al. "Development of calorie restriction mimetics as a prolongevity strategy." *Annals of the New York Academy of Sciences*, 1019:412-423, June 2004.

2. Ferguson, L.R. "Role of plant polyphenols in genomic stability." *Mutation Research*, 475:89-111, 2001.

3. Grónback, M., et al. "Type of alcohol consumed and mortality from all causes, coronary heart disease, and cancer." *Annals of Internal Medicine*. 133(6):411-419, 2000.

4. Kaeberline, M., et al. "Substrate-specific activation of sirtuins by resveratrol." *Journal of Biological Chemistry*, 280(17):17038-17045, April 29, 2005; and Guarente, L., et al. "Calorie restriction—the SIR2 connection." *Cell*, 120(4):473-482, Feb. 25, 2005.

5. Howitz, K.T., et al. "Small molecule activators of sirtuins extend *Saccharomyces cerevisiae* lifespan." *Nature*, 425(6954):191-196, August 24, 2003.

6. Jang, M., et al. "Cancer chemopreventive activity of resveratrol, a natural product derived from grapes." *Science*, 275:2118-2120, 1997.

7. Aggarwal, B.B., et al. "Role of resveratrol in prevention and therapy of cancer: preclinical and clinical studies." *Anticancer Research*, 24(5A):2783-2840, Sept. 2004.

8. Cal, C., et al. "Resveratrol and cancer: chemoprevention, apoptosis, and chemo-immunosensitizing activities." *Current Medical Chemistry—Anti-Cancer Agents*, 3(2):77-93, 2003.

9. Fu, Z.D., et al. "Chemopreventive effect of resveratrol to cancer." 23(8):869-873, *Ai Zheng*, 2004.

10. Miura, D., et al. "Hypolipidemic action of dietary resveratrol, a phytoalexin in grapes and red wine, in hepatoma-bearing rats." *Life Sciences*, 73(11):1393-1400, 2003.

11. Wu, S.L., et al. "Effect of resveratrol and in combination with 5-FU on murine liver cancer." *World Journal of Gastroenterology*, 10(20):3048-3052, 2004.

12. Tseng, S.H., et al. "Resveratrol suppresses the angionenesis and tumor growth of gliomas in rats." *Clinical Cancer Research*, 10(6):2190-2202, 2004.

Seanol

1. Fukayama, Y., et al. "Structure of an anti-plasmin inhibitor, eckol, isolated from the brown algae ecklonia kurome okamura and inhibitory activities of its derivatives on plasmin inhibitors." *Chemistry and Pharmacology Bulletin*, 37:349-353, 1989.

2. Hyun, A.J., et al. "Angiotensin-converting enzyme 1 inhibitory activity of phlorotannins from *Eklonia stolonifera*." Fisheries Science, 72(6): 1292-1299.

3. Fukayama, Y., et al., as in Note 1.

4. Becker, A.J., et al. "Plasma levels of angiotensin ll during different penile conditions in the cavernous and systemic blood of healthy men and patients with erectile dysfunction." *Urology*, 58(5):805-810, November 2001.

5. Shibata, T., et al. "Inhibitory effects of brown algal phlorotannins on secretory phospolipase a2s, lypoxigenases, and cycloxygenases." *J Applied Psychology*, 15: 61-66, 2003.

6. Lee, B. Unpublished research, Hanbat National University, Korea. National Institute of Aging, National Institutes of Health, 2004.

7. Ibid.

8. "Effect of Mo'Baron hemopoiesis, endothelial function,

endochrinological profile, and daily activities in adults." Jang, Y., Cardiology Division, College of Medicine, Yonsei University, Seoul Korea, November 2001.

9. "Effect of KLS (renamed Seanol-AL) on allergen-induced murine asthma model." Chi, E. Chairman, Dept. of Histopathology, University of Washington, 2005.

10. Shin, H.C., et al. "An antioxidative and antiinflammatory agent for potential treatment of osteoarthritis from *Ecklonia cava.*" *Archives of Pharmacology Research*, 29(2)165-171, February 2006.

11. Same as Note 5.

12. "The beneficial effects of feeding Seanol-based Drink "X2" in a fat mouse model study." Chi, E. Dept. Of Pathology, University of Washington, November 2006.

13. Seanol—Obesity/DGAT Research Notes, Shin, H.C. LiveChem Inc., Seoul, Korea, 2005.

14. Same as Note 12.

15. Ibid.

16. Same as Note 8.

Sodium Chlorite

1. *Breakthrough: The Miracle Mineral Supplement of the 21ˢᵗ Century.* 2ed. J. Humble. 2006. An Overview: p. 25.

Thymic Protein A

1. "Thymic Protein A: Its development may signal a new tool for rejuvenating immune function." *Life Extension Foundation* magazine, July 1997.

2. Hays, E.F. and Beardsley, T.R. "Immunologic effects of human thymus stromal grafts and cell lines." *Clinical Immunology and Immunopathology*, 33(3):381-390, 1984.

3. Riordan, N.E., et al. "Pilot study of the effects of thymus protein on elevated Epstein-Barr virus titers." Project RECNAC, Bio-Communications Research Institute. *Townsend Letter for Doctors & Patients*, February/ March, 1998.

4. Rosenbaum, M.E., et al. "Improved immune activation markers in chronic fatigue and immune dysfunction syndrome (CFIDS) patients treated with Thymic Protein A." *Journal of Nutritional & Environmental Medicine*, (11):241-247, 2001.

APPENDIX B

Off Label Use of Drugs

1. "Drug Giant Accused of False Claims." *Dateline NBC*, July 11, 2003; msnbc.com.

2. "Suit Says Company Promoted Drug in Exam Rooms." *The New York Times*, May 5, 2002; nytimes.com.

3. "Drug Giant Accused of False Claims." *Dateline NBC*, July 11, 2003; msnbc.com.

Journal Articles

1. www.guardian.co.uk/medicalscience/story/0,1129, 549562,00.html

2. "A national survey of provisions in clinical trial agreements between medical schools and industry sponsors." *New England Journal of Medicine*, 347(17): 1,335-1,341, 2002.

3. "Study Lashes Medical Schools for Drug-Research Conflict." *Wall Street Journal*, October 24, 2002.

Revolving Door

1. Hulse, V. *Mad Cows and Milkgate*. Marble Mountain Publishing: Phoenix, AZ, 1996, p. 232.

2. Ibid., p. 231.

3. Ibid., p. 238.

4. Ibid.

5. Quotation from the 1994 GAO report, as reported by www.edmonds-institute.org/door.html

6. http://ga3.org/bushgreenwatch/join.html?rk= G1qRleK16GRC

Blood for Money

1. Bogdanich, W., et al. "2 Paths of Bayer Drug in 80s: Riskier Type Went Overseas." *The New York Times*, May 22, 2003; www.nytimes.com.

The Cost of Drugs

1. www.fortune.com/fortune/global500/industrysnap shot/0,15133,37,00.html

2. Ibid.

3. Faloon, W. "Jerry Falwell Attacks Life Extension Foundation," *Life Extension*, October, 2003.

4. Ibid.

5. Thompson, J. CBC News Online, November 17, 2003, www.cbc.ca

6. Bowers, C. *Inside Story*. CBS News, December 9, 2003.

7. www.pwww.org/articleprint/4572

APPENDIX C

1. Adapted from www.rense.com/general6/cow.htm

Index